Integrating AI, Extended Reality, and Wearable Sensors in Mental Healthcare

Richard Lamb
University of Georgia, USA

IGI Global
Scientific Publishing
Publishing Tomorrow's Research Today

Vice President of Editorial	Melissa Wagner
Director of Acquisitions	Mikaela Felty
Director of Book Development	Jocelynn Hessler
Production Manager	Mike Brehm
Cover Design	Jose Rosado

Published in the United States of America by
IGI Global Scientific Publishing
701 East Chocolate Avenue
Hershey, PA, 17033, USA
Tel: 717-533-8845 | Fax: 717-533-7115
Website: https://www.igi-global.com E-mail: cust@igi-global.com

Library of Congress Cataloging-in-Publication Data

Names: Lamb, Richard, 1976- editor
Title: Integrating AI, extended reality, and wearable sensors in mental healthcare / edited by Richard Lamb.
Description: Hershey, PA : IGI Global Scientific Publishing, [2026] | Includes bibliographical references and index. | Summary: "This book explores how artificial intelligence, extended reality, and wearable sensors are transforming mental healthcare. By integrating ethical design, clinical validation, and multimodal technologies, it presents a comprehensive framework for personalized, accessible, and adaptive care across all stages of life-from pediatrics to geriatrics"-- Provided by publisher.
Identifiers: LCCN 2026002220 (print) | LCCN 2026002221 (ebook) | ISBN 9798337349978 h/c | ISBN 9798337349985 s/c | ISBN 9798337349992 ebook
Subjects: LCSH: Mental health services--Technological innovations | Artificial intelligence--Medical applications | Mixed reality--Industrial applications | Wearable technology--Industrial applications
Classification: LCC RC480.5 .I58 2026 (print) | LCC RC480.5 (ebook)
LC record available at https://lccn.loc.gov/2026002220
LC ebook record available at https://lccn.loc.gov/2026002221

British Cataloguing in Publication Data
A Cataloguing in Publication record for this book is available from the British Library.

Table of Contents

Foreword

It is both a distinct honor and a genuine pleasure to offer this forward for the remarkable work of Dr. Richard Lamb, a volume that, for the better part of my years observing the evolution of mental health care, I have come to recognize as both a milestone and a guiding beacon for the field. In a time when technology increasingly permeates every facet of our daily lives, this text stands as a careful, thoughtful, and necessary examination of the ways in which emerging tools, artificial intelligence, extended reality, and related digital innovations, may enhance the care we provide to those we serve. This is not a work written merely to catalog new innovations or to impress; rather, it is a work grounded in purpose, guided by the principles of ethical responsibility, clinical prudence, and human dignity.

I write this forward not merely as a professional endorsement, but as someone whose clinical identity has been shaped through years of direct service in rural and underserved communities. In these settings, the realities of mental health care are shaped as much by geography, infrastructure, and scarcity as by clinical theory or evidence-based practice. Distance itself becomes a barrier to care; transportation is often unreliable or unavailable; and access to broadband, so frequently assumed in discussions of digital health, is inconsistent at best. Stigma, too, persists quietly, reinforced by cultural norms that discourage vulnerability and by the lack of anonymity in small communities where everyone knows one another. These are not abstract challenges or policy talking points. They are lived experiences that shape whether individuals seek care at all, how long they wait before doing so, and the degree of trust they are willing or able to bring into the therapeutic relationship.

In such environments, one learns quickly that effective mental health care extends far beyond diagnosis and treatment planning. It is rooted in presence, patience, and the slow cultivation of trust over time. Progress is often incremental and nonlinear, requiring clinicians to balance evidence-based interventions with cultural humility, flexibility, and an appreciation for the social contexts that shape both suffering and resilience. Care is rarely confined to the therapy room; it unfolds across families, workplaces, schools, and faith communities, and it is shaped by economic pressures and generational narratives that cannot be captured in a chart note. It is from this vantage point, grounded in relational work and lived complexity, that I approached Dr. Lamb's work, and it is from this same vantage point that I found his scholarship not only rigorous, but deeply attuned to the human realities of care.

The humanistic quality of this work is one of its most compelling and enduring strengths. It reflects a philosophy of care that does not seek to force change upon individuals, but rather to accompany them as they navigate their own processes of understanding, adaptation, and growth. This orientation aligns closely with the foundational insights of Carl Rogers, whose person-centered approach emphasized empathy, authenticity, and respect for the individual's lived experience. Rogers famously wrote, *"To be what one is, is to enter fully into being a process,"* a statement that captures the essence of human growth as something unfolding, relational, and deeply contextual. Dr. Lamb's work mirrors this humanistic ethos by meeting people where they are, honoring their histories, capacities, and constraints, while creating conditions in which growth, agency, and healing can emerge organically rather than being imposed.

One of the central strengths of this volume is its unwavering recognition that the ethical, legal, and social dimensions of digital mental health care are not secondary considerations to be addressed after innovation has occurred, but foundational principles that must guide development from the outset. As technologies grow increasingly capable of observing, predicting, and influencing human behavior, the responsibilities borne by clinicians, researchers, and developers expand accordingly. Dr. Lamb insists, rightly, that innovation without ethical grounding risks eroding the very values mental health care seeks to uphold. Transparency, accountability, privacy protection, and procedural justice are presented not as optional features or regulatory hurdles, but as essential conditions for trust, legitimacy, and long-term sustainability.

Throughout my own career, I have been reminded repeatedly that tools, no matter how sophisticated, are only as effective as the integrity and intention with which they are deployed. In communities where mistrust of institutions may be longstanding or well earned, even the most elegant technologies can fail if they are perceived as intrusive, opaque, or misaligned with local values and needs. Dr. Lamb's insistence on embedding ethical safeguards at every stage of design and implementation reflects a deep understanding of this reality. His work consistently reframes digital mental health tools not as replacements for human care, but as extensions of it, capable of amplifying reach, sensitivity, and insight while preserving the primacy of the therapeutic relationship.

The book's treatment of artificial intelligence is particularly noteworthy for its careful balance of promise and restraint. Dr. Lamb presents AI not as a panacea, but as a set of tools with specific affordances and clearly articulated limitations. He explores how machine learning systems can support early detection and screening by identifying subtle linguistic, behavioral, and contextual patterns associated with emerging mental health concerns. Smartphone-based monitoring, passive data collection, and natural language processing offer new avenues for identifying risk earlier than traditional methods often allow, potentially reducing delays in care and enabling more timely intervention. There is something quietly remarkable in the idea that everyday digital behaviors, how long we pause before responding to a message, how our typing cadence shifts, or how patterns of engagement change over time, may offer meaningful signals about emotional and cognitive states.

Dr. Lamb approaches these possibilities with both scientific rigor and ethical caution, emphasizing that such data must always be interpreted within context and governed by clear consent, transparency, and robust privacy protections. Used responsibly, these tools offer clinicians additional sources of information, signals rather than conclusions, that can inform compassionate inquiry and proactive support. In the domain of treatment personalization, the text situates AI within the broader movement toward precision mental health care. By integrating clinical history, behavioral data, and biological markers, adaptive models may help predict which interventions are most likely to benefit a given individual at a particular moment in time. This approach offers a thoughtful alternative to trial-and-error treatment selection, potentially reducing patient burden and improving outcomes, while never displacing the clinician's role as interpreter, collaborator, and ethical decision-maker.

Extended reality (XR), encompassing virtual, augmented, and mixed realities, represents another area in which the book makes a substantive contribution. Dr. Lamb presents XR not as a technological novelty, but as a clinically grounded modality with specific, evidence-informed applications. Virtual reality–based exposure therapy, skills rehearsal, and psychoeducation are discussed with careful attention to both empirical support and practical considerations. The importance of screening for contraindications, monitoring tolerance, and pacing interventions is emphasized, underscoring that immersion must always be guided by patient safety, readiness, and informed choice. One can readily imagine a patient gradually engaging with a feared stimulus within a controlled environment, a clinician nearby, attentive to subtle cues and ready to adjust the process as needed, an image that captures the essence of responsible innovation.

Beneath these discussions lies a strong theoretical foundation grounded in cognitive science, systems theory, and the biopsychosocial model. Dr. Lamb demonstrates how neuroadaptive systems can be informed by learning mechanisms, cognitive architectures, and multimodal measurement strategies that integrate behavioral observation, physiological signals, and contextual data. Mental health is framed not as a static condition, but as a dynamic, evolving process shaped by development, culture, environment, and lived experience. Adaptive systems, he argues, must be designed with this complexity in mind, respecting developmental constraints and cultural variability if they are to be both effective and just.

Equally compelling is the book's systemic perspective on implementation. Technology adoption is not treated as a singular event, but as an ongoing process requiring alignment with organizational workflows, infrastructure capacity, reimbursement structures, and community resources. Dr. Lamb emphasizes iterative pilot studies, interdisciplinary collaboration, and continuous evaluation, not only of technical performance, but of relational outcomes such as trust, perceived dignity, engagement, and continuity of care. These insights resonate strongly with my own experience, where even the most promising innovations can falter if they are introduced without regard for the rhythms, constraints, and values of the systems into which they are placed.

Equity and inclusion are woven throughout the text with clarity and intention. Dr. Lamb confronts directly the risk that neuroadaptive technologies, if implemented without care, may inadvertently exacerbate existing disparities. He offers concrete strategies to mitigate these risks, including co-design with underserved populations, early integration of equity goals into development processes, and the establishment of measurable benchmarks for access and impact. Having witnessed how well-intentioned interventions can reinforce inequities when context is overlooked, I find this commitment both necessary and deeply affirming.

The volume further advances a participatory vision for the future of mental health care, one that centers the voices of those with lived experience. Community advisory panels and stakeholder consultations are presented not as symbolic gestures, but as essential mechanisms for surfacing values, fears, and priorities that shape acceptable and effective interventions. These insights are translated into governance principles, design constraints, and implementation strategies that honor autonomy and dignity. This approach reflects a belief I have long held: that the most durable and ethical solutions emerge not from top-down mandates, but from genuine collaboration with the communities we seek to serve.

Ethical considerations surrounding predictive and anticipatory neuroadaptive systems are explored with particular depth. When technologies are capable of inferring vulnerability or risk before an individual is consciously aware of it, questions of autonomy, consent, and surveillance become unavoidable. Dr. Lamb offers a thoughtful roadmap for navigating these tensions, advocating for layered and revocable consent, meaningful human oversight, and mechanisms that keep control firmly in the hands of patients. In rural practice, where trust is both precious and fragile, such frameworks are not theoretical ideals but practical necessities.

Throughout the book, a consistent guiding principle emerges with quiet clarity: technology must remain in service to people, never the reverse. Whether discussing artificial intelligence, extended reality, or broader neuroadaptive systems, Dr. Lamb continually returns to the lived experience of patients, their histories, fears, hopes, and aspirations. This human-centered orientation resonates profoundly with my own work and reflects a lineage of humanistic thought that sees the whole person, embedded in relationship and community, striving toward meaning, belonging, and contribution.

In conclusion, this volume articulates a vision of mental health care that is ethical, inclusive, relational, and forward-looking. Neuroadaptive systems are positioned not as replacements for clinicians or communities, but as partners that can extend capacity while honoring human judgment and connection. Evaluation frameworks attend not only to efficiency and accuracy, but to dignity, trust, and social impact. Readers are invited to imagine a future in which innovation and justice are inseparable, and in which intelligence is guided by wisdom.

I can state without hesitation that this work represents a landmark contribution to the literature on digital mental health. Dr. Lamb brings together analytical rigor, clinical insight, and ethical foresight in a manner that is both rare and deeply compelling. As someone who has spent much of my career working alongside underserved populations, I am particularly struck by the care with which equity, participation, and contextual sensitivity are treated throughout the text.

It is with the deepest enthusiasm, therefore, that I endorse this book. Dr. Richard Lamb has provided the field with a work that is at once innovative, discerning, and profoundly humane. For clinicians, researchers, policymakers, and technologists alike, this volume offers not only guidance, but a call to responsibility. It charts a path toward digital mental health systems that are ethical, equitable, and effective, systems that extend our capacity to listen, to understand, and to care for one another. It is a future worth pursuing, and most certainly worth building.

Jason O. Perry
Department of Interdisciplinary Professions, East Carolina University, USA

Preface

OVERVIEW OF THE SUBJECT MATTER

The field of mental health care is undergoing a profound transformation driven by the convergence of advanced digital technologies—artificial intelligence (AI), extended reality (XR), and wearable sensors. This book explores the integration of these technologies into mental health practice, research, and education, presenting a comprehensive framework for digital therapeutics that are adaptive, personalized, and ethically grounded.

Digital mental health care is no longer a futuristic concept but a present reality reshaping how mental health is understood, assessed, and treated. The integration of AI enables predictive analytics and decision support, XR offers immersive therapeutic environments, and wearable sensors provide continuous, real-time physiological and behavioral monitoring. Together, these modalities form neuroadaptive systems that dynamically sense, interpret, and respond to users' cognitive and emotional states, enabling closed-loop interventions that are timely, precise, and scalable. This transformation addresses longstanding challenges in mental health care, including access barriers, workforce shortages, stigma, and fragmented service delivery. For example, AI-driven algorithms can detect early signs of depression or anxiety through natural language processing of speech and text, while XR-based exposure therapy can help individuals confront phobias or traumatic memories in controlled, immersive environments. Wearable devices, such as EEG headbands or heart rate monitors, allow clinicians to track stress responses and cognitive load in real time, enabling interventions that are both proactive and personalized.

Beyond clinical applications, these technologies have profound implications for education and workforce development. Training programs for mental health professionals increasingly incorporate XR simulations to teach crisis intervention skills, while AI-powered platforms provide adaptive learning experiences tailored to individual competencies. This integration ensures that future clinicians are equipped to navigate a technology-enhanced care environment.

However, the promise of digital mental health is accompanied by significant ethical, legal, and social considerations. Issues such as data privacy, algorithmic bias, and equitable access demand rigorous attention. For instance, AI models trained on biased datasets risk perpetuating disparities in diagnosis and treatment, while XR interventions must account for cultural sensitivity and inclusivity. Moreover, the reliance on continuous data collection raises questions about consent, autonomy, and the boundaries of surveillance in therapeutic contexts. The book situates these innovations within a biopsychosocial and systems theory framework, emphasizing the importance of interdisciplinary collaboration, rigorous validation, and inclusive design. It advocates for a balanced approach that harnesses technological potential while safeguarding human dignity and therapeutic integrity. By weaving together theory, empirical evidence, and practical guidance, this volume provides a roadmap for integrating digital technologies into mental health care responsibly and effectively.

WHERE THE TOPIC FITS IN THE WORLD TODAY

Mental health disorders remain a leading cause of disability worldwide, with unmet needs exacerbated by global crises such as the COVID-19 pandemic, geopolitical instability, and economic uncertainty. According to the World Health Organization, depression and anxiety alone cost the global economy over $1 trillion annually in lost productivity. These staggering figures underscore the urgency of scalable, innovative solutions that transcend traditional models of care. Digital therapeutics offer unprecedented opportunities to expand access, personalize care, and enhance outcomes across diverse populations and settings—from pediatric to geriatric care, from schools to workplaces, and even in remote or underserved regions.

The rapid adoption of telehealth and mobile health applications during the pandemic has laid the groundwork for more sophisticated digital ecosystems that integrate AI, XR, and wearable biosensors. These technologies extend care beyond traditional clinical environments into homes, schools, and communities, supporting continuous monitoring and just-in-time adaptive interventions. For example, AI-driven chatbots can provide immediate cognitive-behavioral support, XR environments can deliver immersive exposure therapy for PTSD, and wearable sensors can detect physiological markers of stress or cognitive overload in real time. Together, these innovations enable proactive, data-informed care rather than reactive, episodic interventions. However, this digital shift occurs amidst significant challenges. The digital divide threatens to widen disparities, leaving rural and low-income populations behind. Regulatory frameworks lag behind technological innovation, creating uncertainty around reimbursement, liability, and standards of care. Ethical dilemmas around consent, data governance, and algorithmic fairness demand urgent attention, particularly as AI systems increasingly influence clinical decision-making. Furthermore, cultural and linguistic diversity introduces complexities in designing inclusive and accessible digital tools.

This book addresses these complexities by offering a roadmap for responsible innovation that balances technological potential with human-centered values. It advocates for equity-driven design, rigorous validation, and transparent governance, ensuring that digital mental health solutions enhance, not compromise, the therapeutic relationship. By situating these technologies within global health priorities and ethical imperatives, the book positions digital mental health as a transformative force capable of reshaping care delivery for generations to come.

TARGET AUDIENCE

This volume is intended for a broad interdisciplinary audience engaged in the evolving landscape of digital mental health care, including:

- **Clinicians and Mental Health Professionals:** Psychiatrists, psychologists, counselors, social workers, and allied health providers seeking to integrate digital therapeutics into practice safely and effectively.
- **Researchers and Academics:** Scholars in psychology, neuroscience, computer science, biomedical engineering, and health informatics interested in the theoretical foundations, empirical evidence, and methodological innovations in digital mental health.
- **Technology Developers and Engineers:** Professionals designing AI algorithms, wearable devices, XR environments, and integrated platforms who require clinical insights and ethical frameworks to guide development.
- **Policy Makers and Health Administrators:** Leaders responsible for regulatory oversight, reimbursement policies, and health system integration who must navigate the complexities of digital mental health implementation.
- **Educators and Trainers:** Faculty and program developers preparing the next generation of clinicians and technologists with competencies in digital health.
- **Caregivers and Advocates:** Individuals supporting patients and communities who seek to understand the implications and opportunities of digital mental health tools.

IMPORTANCE OF EACH CHAPTER

Chapter 1: The Digital Shift in Mental Health Care

This foundational chapter introduces the systemic transformation underway in mental health care, driven by AI, XR, and wearable sensors. It situates digital therapeutics within global health priorities, outlines technological capabilities, and highlights ethical and operational challenges. The chapter sets the stage for the detailed explorations that follow, emphasizing how these innovations are reshaping care delivery models, reducing barriers to access, and enabling proactive interventions. Real-world examples of telehealth adoption and emerging digital ecosystems illustrate the urgency and potential of this shift.

Chapter 2: Theoretical Foundations of Neuroadaptive Systems

Explores cognitive science, systems theory, and the biopsychosocial model as the conceptual backbone for neuroadaptive technologies. It emphasizes the integration of multimodal measurement and adaptive algorithms, providing a scientific framework for understanding and designing responsive mental health interventions. This chapter also addresses how dynamic feedback loops between physiological, behavioral, and cognitive data inform personalized care strategies.

Chapter 3: Ethics, Equity, and Privacy in Digital Mental Health

Addresses the critical ethical dimensions of digital mental health, including data governance, algorithmic bias, and equitable access. It proposes operational principles—transparency, accountability, and justice—and discusses the moral imperatives that must guide technology development and deployment. Practical case studies highlight the consequences of neglecting these principles and offer strategies for inclusive design and regulatory compliance.

Chapter 4: Artificial Intelligence in Mental Health Practice

Focuses on AI applications such as predictive analytics, natural language processing, and decision support systems. It discusses clinical integration, bias mitigation, and the balance between automation and human oversight, illustrating AI's potential and limitations in mental health care. Examples include AI-driven triage tools and conversational agents for crisis intervention.

Chapter 5: Extended Reality for Immersive Therapy

Examines XR modalities (VR, AR, MR) as transformative tools for exposure therapy, skills training, and embodiment interventions. The chapter covers clinical protocols, safety considerations, ethical governance, and implementation strategies to harness XR's therapeutic potential responsibly. It also explores gamification and immersive learning environments for pediatric and trauma-focused care.

Chapter 6: Wearable Sensors and Psychophysiological Monitoring

Details the use of wearable biosensors (EEG, HRV, GSR, fNIRS) for continuous monitoring of physiological correlates of mental health. It discusses data quality, integration with AI, clinical applications, and ethical considerations, emphasizing the role of wearables in precision and adaptive care. Examples include stress detection in workplace settings and early identification of cognitive decline.

Chapter 7: Multimodal Integration: Building Closed-Loop Systems

Explores the convergence of AI, XR, and wearable sensors into integrated neuroadaptive ecosystems. It highlights technical requirements for interoperability, timestamp synchronization, and clinician oversight, alongside ethical safeguards and implementation science frameworks. This chapter envisions future systems capable of real-time intervention based on multimodal data streams.

Chapter 8: Pediatric and Adolescent Mental Health

Focuses on developmental considerations in digital mental health, highlighting age-appropriate interventions, consent complexities, and the use of gamified XR and AI-driven screening tools. It emphasizes family-centered care and long-term outcome monitoring, addressing unique challenges such as digital literacy and safeguarding.

Chapter 9: Adult Mental Health and Workplace Stress

Addresses the impact of modern work environments on mental health, exploring digital therapeutics for burnout prevention, resilience training, and cognitive behavioral therapy in workplace settings. It discusses organizational culture, ethical data use, and integration strategies, offering models for scalable employee wellness programs.

Chapter 10: Geriatric Mental Health and Cognitive Decline

Examines the unique challenges of mental health care for older adults, including neurodegenerative disorders and social determinants. It explores digital tools for early detection, continuous monitoring, cognitive training, and caregiver support, emphasizing dignity and accessibility in design.

Chapter 11: Clinical Trials and Evidence-Based Validation

Provides a roadmap for rigorous evaluation of digital mental health interventions, covering trial design adaptations, regulatory considerations, and the importance of inclusive, pragmatic research to ensure safety, efficacy, and equity. It also addresses emerging standards for digital health validation.

Chapter 12: Training Clinicians for Tech-Enhanced Practice

Outlines essential competencies, certification pathways, and educational frameworks for preparing clinicians to integrate digital tools into practice. It addresses barriers to adoption and strategies for ongoing professional development, including simulation-based training and XR-enhanced learning.

Chapter 13: Designing for Engagement and Accessibility

Explores user experience and interface design principles that promote usability, emotional attunement, and sustained engagement. It emphasizes inclusive design, cultural sensitivity, ethical UX, and the mitigation of cognitive load and digital fatigue, ensuring tools remain effective and humane.

Chapter 14: Scaling Digital Mental Health Solutions

Discusses implementation science frameworks, stakeholder engagement, policy alignment, and sustainability planning necessary for scaling digital mental health interventions equitably and effectively across diverse settings. It includes strategies for integrating solutions into public health systems and global markets.

Chapter 15: The Future of Neuroadaptive Mental Health Care

Synthesizes technological, clinical, and ethical trajectories shaping the next decade. It anticipates advances in multimodal systems, federated learning, and immersive environments, while addressing emerging risks and advocating for participatory governance and global standards. This chapter concludes with a vision for a mental health ecosystem that harmonizes innovation with compassion.

CONCLUSION: IMPACT ON THE FIELD AND CONTRIBUTION TO THE SUBJECT MATTER

This book offers a comprehensive, interdisciplinary roadmap for the digital transformation of mental health care. By integrating foundational theory, cutting-edge technology, ethical imperatives, and practical implementation strategies, it advances the field toward a future where mental health support is personalized, adaptive, accessible, and equitable.

The convergence of AI, XR, and wearable sensors into neuroadaptive systems represents a paradigm shift from reactive, episodic care to continuous, context-aware intervention. This shift holds promise for improving outcomes across the lifespan, from early childhood to older adulthood, and across diverse clinical and community settings. For example, AI-driven predictive analytics can identify early warning signs of relapse in individuals with mood disorders, while XR-based exposure therapy can provide immersive, controlled environments for trauma recovery. Wearable sensors, capable of monitoring heart rate variability, galvanic skin response, and neural activity, enable clinicians to track stress and cognitive load in real time, creating opportunities for timely, data-informed interventions.

Importantly, the book emphasizes that technological innovation must be matched by rigorous validation, ethical governance, and human-centered design. Without these safeguards, the promise of digital mental health could be undermined by unintended consequences such as algorithmic bias, inequitable access, and erosion of trust in care systems. The chapters collectively advocate for transparency in algorithm development, participatory design involving patients and clinicians, and robust regulatory frameworks that prioritize safety and equity. These principles are not optional—they are foundational to ensuring that digital mental health tools serve as bridges to healing rather than barriers to care.

By providing detailed guidance on clinical integration, training, engagement, and scaling, this volume equips clinicians, researchers, developers, and policymakers with the knowledge and tools necessary to navigate the complexities of digital mental health. It addresses practical questions such as: How can clinicians incorporate AI-driven decision support without compromising the therapeutic alliance? What competencies must future mental health professionals develop to work effectively in tech-enhanced environments? How can organizations implement XR-based interventions while safeguarding patient privacy and minimizing digital fatigue? These discussions move beyond theoretical speculation to actionable strategies grounded in evidence and best practices.

The book also underscores the importance of inclusivity and cultural sensitivity in digital mental health design. Technologies must be adaptable to diverse linguistic, cultural, and socioeconomic contexts to avoid reinforcing existing disparities. For instance, AI models trained on homogeneous datasets risk misdiagnosing or overlooking symptoms in underrepresented populations. Similarly, XR environments must reflect cultural norms and values to ensure relevance and engagement. By foregrounding these considerations, the book positions equity as a central pillar of innovation rather than an afterthought.

Looking ahead, the integration of neuroadaptive systems into mental health care signals a future where interventions are not only personalized but anticipatory—where technology predicts and mitigates crises before they escalate. Advances in federated learning will enable secure, decentralized data sharing across institutions, enhancing predictive accuracy while preserving privacy. Emerging modalities such as haptic feedback and brain-computer interfaces may further enrich therapeutic experiences, offering new pathways for cognitive and emotional regulation. Yet, as these frontiers expand, so too does the responsibility to ensure ethical stewardship, interdisciplinary collaboration, and global standards that safeguard human dignity.

Ultimately, this work contributes to shaping a future of mental health care that is not only more effective and scalable but also more compassionate, just, and attuned to the lived realities of those it serves. It invites readers to envision a mental health ecosystem where technology amplifies, not replaces, the human touch, where data informs care without dictating it, and where innovation is guided by empathy as much as by efficiency. In doing so, the book lays the groundwork for a new era of mental health practice; one that harmonizes scientific rigor, technological sophistication, and unwavering commitment to the well-being of individuals and communities worldwide.

Richard Lamb
University of Georgia, USA

Acknowledgement

I would like to express my deepest gratitude to my family and friends for their unwavering support and encouragement. I also extend my thanks to the Neurocognition Science Laboratory at the University of Georgia for fostering an environment of innovation and collaboration. Finally, I am grateful for the opportunity to pursue research that advances mental health and neurodevelopmental care, particularly for veterans and children a mission that remains central to my work.

Section 1
Foundational Frameworks

Chapter 1
The Role of Digital Technologies in Mental Health Care

ABSTRACT

This chapter introduces the convergence of artificial intelligence (AI), extended reality (XR), and wearable biosensors as a paradigm shift in mental health care. Moving beyond episodic, clinic bound models, it frames digital mental health as a transition toward continuous, adaptive, and precision oriented systems of care. The chapter establishes foundational concepts including dynamic consent, data stewardship, algorithmic bias, and human centered design, setting expectations that technology must augment rather than replace clinical judgment. By outlining both the promise and the risks of digital transformation, this chapter provides a conceptual and ethical anchor for the volume.

THE ROLE OF DIGITAL TECHNOLOGIES

In recent years, the convergence of digital technologies has created new opportunities to address persistent challenges in mental health care. This convergence implies not only the availability of multiple tools, but also the need for interoperability and coordinated design across platforms. Integration points and data governance rules must be clearly specified by design teams, and vendors should provide documented APIs and data schemas to support safe and effective integration (Rajpal, 2025). Early pilot implementations should include feasibility assessments, privacy safeguards, and equity checks to ensure responsible deployment. The integration of artificial intelligence (AI), extended reality (XR), and wearable biosensors represents a paradigm shift—one that moves beyond incremental innovation to fundamentally reshape how

DOI: 10.4018/979-8-3373-4997-8.ch001

mental health is conceptualized, monitored, and treated (Singh & Chandra, 2025). These technologies offer the potential to enhance diagnostic precision, personalize interventions, and extend the reach of services beyond traditional clinical environments (Johnson et al., 2021). To ensure safety and efficacy, clinical validation and user-centered testing must precede any deployment of digital therapeutics (Glass et al., 2022).

Context of Global Urgency

This digital transformation is unfolding against a backdrop of significant global need. Mental health disorders rank among the leading causes of disability worldwide, affecting individuals across all age groups. The COVID-19 pandemic further exacerbated these challenges, exposing vulnerabilities in existing care infrastructures and accelerating the adoption of digital modalities. Teletherapy, once considered a niche service, became essential during periods of lockdown and social isolation (Mulukuntla, 2025). Before adopting new platforms, it is critical to quantify the local burden of mental health disorders to ensure alignment with public health priorities. Moreover, systems must protect continuous data streams with end-to-end encryption to safeguard patient privacy and maintain trust in digital care environments (Kumar, 2025).

Wearable Sensors and Real-Time Monitoring in Digital Mental Health Care

Wearable sensors are rapidly transforming the landscape of digital mental health care by enabling continuous, real-time monitoring of physiological signals that reflect emotional, cognitive, and behavioral states (Elfouly & Alouani, 2025). These technologies—ranging from wrist-worn devices to EEG headbands, functional near infrared spectroscopy (fNIRS), and smart textiles—offer clinicians and researchers a dynamic window into the psychophysiological processes underlying mental health conditions (Huang et al., 2024). When thoughtfully integrated into therapeutic systems, wearable sensors support adaptive, personalized interventions that respond to the user's moment-to-moment needs, thereby enhancing both clinical precision and user engagement (Huang et al., 2024).

Among the most commonly used physiological signals in mental health applications are heart rate variability (HRV) electrodermal activity (EDA) and electroencephalography (Berardi et al., 2024; Hickey et al., 2021). HRV reflects autonomic nervous system balance and is a sensitive marker of stress, emotional regulation, and resilience (Crameri et al., 2021). EDA measures changes in skin conductance associated with sympathetic arousal, providing insight into emotional intensity and reactivity. EEG and fNIRS captures electrical activity and hemodynamic changes in the brain, offering temporally precise data on attention, cognitive workload, and affective processing (Sharma & Meena, 2024). These signals, when interpreted within a structured clinical framework, can inform diagnosis, monitor treatment progress, and guide moment-to-moment therapeutic adjustments (Sharma & Meena, 2024).

To ensure the accuracy and reliability of these data streams, baseline calibration and ongoing validation must be conducted for each user (Clemens-Meyer et al., 2021). Physiological signals are highly individualized, influenced by factors such as age, medication, fitness level, and comorbid conditions. Without proper calibration, sensor data may yield misleading interpretations, potentially compromising clinical decision-making (Tsai et al., 2025). For example, a low HRV reading may indicate stress in one individual but fall within normal limits for another (Immanuel et al., 2023). Establishing a personalized baseline—ideally through resting-state measurements and repeated sampling across contexts—is essential before integrating sensor data into therapeutic workflows (Mackey et al., 2025). Validation should be repeated periodically to account for changes in physiology over time, especially in longitudinal care settings.

When integrated with digital therapeutic platforms—such as mobile apps, virtual reality (Robinson et al., 2024) environments, or conversational agents—wearable sensors enable closed-loop interventions (Ghanim et al., 2023). These systems adapt dynamically to the user's physiological and emotional state, creating a feedback loop that enhances therapeutic responsiveness. For instance, a VR-based mindfulness application may adjust its visual and auditory environment in response to elevated EDA, signaling heightened arousal. Similarly, an AI-driven chatbot may modify its tone, pacing, or content based on real-time HRV data, offering more calming or directive responses depending on the user's stress level (Mitsea et al., 2024). These adaptive capabilities allow interventions to be delivered at the right moment, in the right format, and with the appropriate intensity—an approach that aligns with principles of precision medicine and person-centered care.

Figure 1. A conceptual model of a closed-loop neuroadaptive system showing the flow from user sensing to AI interpretation to adaptive intervention

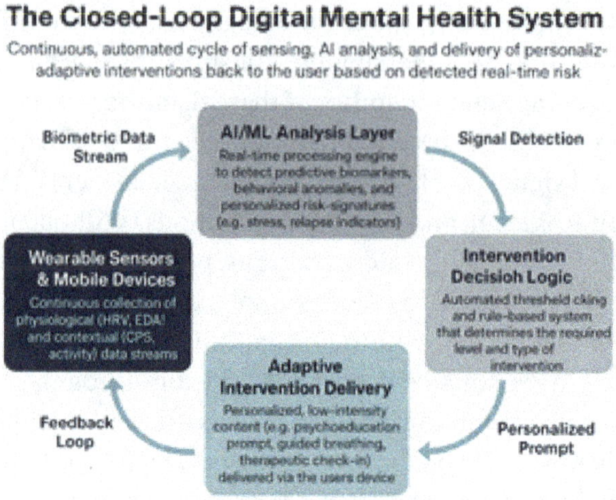

Beyond moment-to-moment adaptation, wearable sensors generate longitudinal datasets that reveal patterns in emotional regulation, sleep quality, activity levels, and stress reactivity (Shah et al., 2021). These data can inform treatment planning, monitor progress, and detect early signs of relapse or deterioration (Moriarty et al., 2022). For example, a sustained decline in HRV over several days may indicate emerging depressive symptoms, prompting a clinician to initiate a check-in or adjust the treatment plan (Pruden, 2025). In research contexts, these datasets support the development of predictive models that link physiological markers to clinical outcomes, enabling earlier and more targeted interventions (Lazarou & Exarchos, 2024).

However, the integration of wearable sensors into mental health care raises important ethical, legal, and technical considerations, particularly around data governance (Ghadi et al., 2025). Biometric datasets are inherently sensitive, containing information that can reveal not only mental health status but also patterns of behavior, location, and social interaction (Jiao, 2024). To protect user privacy, these datasets must be governed by clearly defined retention limits and access controls. Data should be encrypted both in transit and at rest, and access should be restricted to authorized personnel based on role-specific permissions (Chennupati, 2025). Institutions must establish transparent policies regarding data storage duration, secondary uses, and user rights to access, correct, or delete their data (Ikwuanusi et al., 2023). These policies should be reviewed regularly and updated in response to evolving legal standards and technological capabilities.

(Godfrey et al., 2021). Users should be made aware of what data is being collected, how it will be used, who will have access, and what safeguards are in place to protect their privacy (Layode et al., 2024). Consent should be dynamic, allowing users to modify their preferences over time as their understanding evolves or as the system changes. For vulnerable populations—such as children, individuals with cognitive impairments, or those in crisis—additional safeguards may be necessary to ensure that consent is truly informed and voluntary. Consent materials should be written in plain language, include visual aids where appropriate, and be accessible across literacy levels and languages.

From a technical standpoint, wearable sensors must meet rigorous standards for accuracy, reliability, and interoperability (Canali et al., 2022). Devices should be validated against gold-standard clinical instruments, and their performance should be tested across diverse populations and settings (Ferrar et al., 2021). Interoperability is particularly important in integrated care environments, where sensor data must be seamlessly shared across platforms, electronic health records (EHRs), and clinical dashboards (Hughes & Kalra, 2023). Vendors should provide documented APIs, data schemas, and integration protocols to facilitate safe and effective data exchange (Pal et al., 2020). Systems should also include timestamp synchronization across data streams to support multimodal analysis and reduce interpretive ambiguity (Basystiuk et al., 2024).

Usability is another critical factor in the success of wearable sensor interventions (Smuck et al., 2021). Devices must be comfortable, unobtrusive, and easy to use, especially for individuals with sensory sensitivities, motor impairments, or limited digital literacy. Battery life, data transmission reliability, and user interface design all influence adherence and data quality (Baumann et al., 2024). Usability testing with representative users should be conducted during the design and pilot phases to identify and address barriers to engagement. Feedback from users should inform iterative improvements to hardware, software, and support materials. Accessibility features—such as adjustable font sizes, voice prompts, and multilingual interfaces—should be standard, not optional.

In clinical practice, wearable sensors can be used to support a range of therapeutic modalities (Ferrara, 2024). In exposure therapy, for example, physiological data can help clinicians monitor the client's arousal level and adjust the intensity or duration of the exposure accordingly (Back et al., 2022). In biofeedback interventions, users learn to regulate their physiological responses through real-time feedback, enhancing self-awareness and emotional control. In telehealth settings, wearable sensors can provide clinicians with objective data to complement self-report and behavioral observations, improving the accuracy of remote assessments and interventions (Hilty et al., 2021). These applications are particularly valuable in high-volume or resource-constrained settings, where real-time data can help prioritize care and allocate resources more effectively (Almadani et al., 2025).

The use of wearable sensors also opens new possibilities for population-level mental health monitoring (Akinode et al., 2025). Aggregated, anonymized data can reveal trends in stress, sleep, and activity across communities, informing public health strategies and resource allocation (Wang et al., 2022). For example, during a natural disaster or public health crisis, wearable data could help identify populations at elevated risk for mental health deterioration, enabling targeted outreach and support (Volckens et al., 2023). However, such applications must be carefully governed to prevent misuse, discrimination, or erosion of trust. Data-sharing agreements should include equity safeguards, and public reporting should be transparent and accessible (Holly et al., 2023).

To realize the full potential of wearable sensors in mental health care, interdisciplinary collaboration is essential (Hassan Almansour et al., 2024). Clinicians, engineers, data scientists, ethicists, and users must work together to design systems that are clinically meaningful, technically robust, and ethically sound (Goktas & Grzybowski, 2025). Training programs should equip mental health professionals with the skills to interpret physiological data, integrate it into treatment planning, and communicate its significance to clients (Wibberly, 2024). Likewise, developers must understand the clinical context in which their tools will be used, ensuring that design decisions support therapeutic goals and respect user autonomy (Bayor et al., 2025).

ETHICAL, LEGAL, AND SOCIAL CONSIDERATIONS IN DIGITAL MENTAL HEALTH CARE

The digital transformation of mental health care introduces a complex array of ethical, legal, and social considerations that must be addressed with deliberate care. As artificial intelligence (AI), extended reality (XR), and wearable sensors become increasingly embedded in clinical practice, the potential for innovation is matched by the risk of exacerbating existing disparities, violating privacy, and outpacing regulatory safeguards (Akhtar & Rawol, 2025). Each deployment of digital mental health technologies should undergo a multidisciplinary ethics review to evaluate risks, ensure equitable access, and align with the core values of person-centered care.

Data privacy remains one of the most pressing ethical concerns (Renuka et al., 2025). Digital mental health tools often collect sensitive biometric, behavioral, and contextual data—ranging from heart rate variability and electrodermal activity to speech patterns and geolocation (Tizzard, 2025; Saksena et al., 2021). Systems must implement end-to-end encryption, role-based access controls, and transparent data retention policies (Mohammad, 2021). Users should be empowered to understand what data is being collected, how it will be used, and who will have access (Kang & Exworthy, 2022). Consent must be explicit, revisable, and context-sensitive, especially for vulnerable populations such as children, individuals with cognitive impairments, or those in crisis. In addition, biometric monitoring must be accompanied by clear consent protocols that specify both primary and secondary data uses (Zenker et al., 2022).

Algorithmic bias presents another critical challenge. AI models trained on non-representative datasets may produce inaccurate or inequitable outcomes, particularly for marginalized populations (Panarese et al., 2025). For example, a chatbot trained primarily on English-speaking, urban populations may misinterpret distress signals from rural, non-English-speaking users. Facial recognition tools may misclassify expressions in neurodivergent individuals or people of color. To mitigate these risks, developers must conduct fairness audits, validate models across diverse demographic subgroups, and publish performance metrics disaggregated by race, gender, age, and other relevant factors. Clinical deployment should include human oversight for all safety-critical decisions, ensuring that AI augments rather than replaces clinician judgment (Morey et al., 2025). Model outputs should include interpretable explanations or confidence metrics to support clinician interpretation and accountability (Allgaier et al., 2023).

Equitable access to digital mental health care is also constrained by the persistent digital divide. Factors such as income, geography, and digital literacy influence whether individuals can benefit from digital therapeutics. In rural areas, broadband access may be limited; in low-income communities, smartphones or wearable devices may be unaffordable; and among older adults or those with disabilities, digital interfaces may be inaccessible (Correa et al., 2021). To address these disparities, digital mental health initiatives must include accessibility testing across relevant user groups, offer low-bandwidth alternatives, and provide multilingual, culturally adapted interfaces. XR sessions used clinically should be paired with clinician monitoring to ensure safety and therapeutic alignment, particularly when immersive environments may provoke strong emotional responses (Morgan et al., 2025).

The rapid pace of technological development often outstrips the creation of regulatory frameworks and evidence-based guidelines, creating uncertainty for clinicians, patients, and policymakers (Anklam et al., 2022). Regulatory mapping and compliance verification must be completed prior to jurisdictional deployment. Institutions should establish clear protocols for data governance, clinical oversight, and ethical review (Bibi, 2024). In the absence of formal regulation, professional organizations and academic institutions must take the lead in developing interim standards and best practices. Deployment plans should also include contingency protocols for data loss, service degradation, and adverse events to ensure continuity of care and system resilience (Boda & Allam, 2022).

Despite these challenges, the integration of digital technologies into mental health care offers a compelling vision for the future. To ensure responsible innovation, each deployment should be guided by a success criterion that includes measurable outcomes for access, effectiveness, and equity. Pilot systems must include diverse participant samples to ensure generalizability and fairness. Results should be transparently reported before scaling, allowing for evidence-based refinement and public accountability (Adepoju & Adepoju, 2025). Digital mental health invites clinicians to re-examine therapeutic relationships, clinical workflows, and the very nature of mental health practice (Verma et al., 2023). It challenges traditional models of episodic, in-person care and opens the door to continuous, adaptive, and personalized interventions. However, this transformation must remain grounded in ethical practice, scientific rigor, and person-centered care. Technologies should be designed not only for efficiency but for empathy, equity, and empowerment.

To support responsible deployment, institutions should adopt a planning rule: map local service gaps before deploying digital interventions. This ensures that technology is used to address real needs rather than to replicate existing inequities. For example, in communities with long waitlists for therapy, telehealth platforms may improve access; in populations with high stigma, anonymous digital screening tools may lower barriers to care. However, without careful mapping, digital tools may simply reinforce the status quo or divert resources from more pressing needs. Digital initiatives should also be aligned with public health priorities to ensure strategic relevance and sustainability.

The convergence of AI, XR, and wearable sensors represents a paradigm shift—not merely an incremental improvement (Lamb et al., 2025). These technologies offer the potential to enhance diagnostic accuracy, personalize treatment, and extend the reach of mental health services beyond traditional clinical settings (Omiyefa, 2025). Expected outcomes should be clearly defined: improved access, greater personalization, and earlier detection of distress. Implementation plans must include contingency protocols and performance metrics to evaluate personalization features and system responsiveness.

AI, in particular, has emerged as a powerful tool in this context. Machine learning algorithms can analyze vast datasets to identify patterns that may elude human clinicians—such as subtle changes in speech, facial expressions, or behavioral patterns that signal the onset of depression or anxiety (Chen et al., 2022). Natural language processing (Li et al., 2025) enables the development of conversational agents that can provide psychoeducation, monitor mood, and deliver elements of cognitive behavioral therapy (CBT). These tools are not intended to replace human therapists but to augment their capabilities and extend their reach. All safety-critical decisions must be subject to human oversight, and clinicians should retain final authority over diagnosis and treatment.

XR technologies—including virtual reality (Fischer et al., 2025) and augmented reality (AR)—offer immersive environments that can be tailored to individual therapeutic needs (Radanliev, 2025). Virtual Reality (VR) exposure therapy allows individuals to confront and process traumatic memories in a controlled and safe setting, while Augmented Reality (AR) applications can enhance mindfulness practices or support social skills training by overlaying digital cues onto real-world interactions. These experiences are not only engaging but can be precisely calibrated to match the user's emotional and cognitive state. Clinical use of XR must include accessibility testing, clinician supervision, and safety protocols for motion sickness, dissociation, and emotional overload (Kourtesis, 2024).

Wearable sensors add another layer of insight by enabling continuous, real-time monitoring of physiological signals (Ma et al., 2025). Devices that track HRV, EDA, or EEG can provide valuable data on stress levels, emotional arousal, and cognitive workload (Boffet et al., 2025). When integrated into digital therapeutic systems, these sensors allow for the creation of closed-loop interventions—systems that adapt in real time based on the user's current state. For instance, a VR meditation app might adjust its environment based on the user's heart rate, or an AI-driven chatbot might modify its tone and content in response to detected stress signals (Jain & Jain, 2025). To support accurate analysis, sensor and app data must be synchronized with timestamp alignment, and biometric monitoring must be governed by explicit consent and clearly defined data use policies (Ross et al., 2022).

In conclusion, the ethical, legal, and social dimensions of digital mental health care are not peripheral—they are foundational. As the field evolves, it must do so with a commitment to transparency, accountability, and justice. Technologies must protect privacy, promote equity, and preserve the therapeutic relationship. By embedding ethical safeguards into every stage of development and implementation, we can ensure that digital mental health care serves not only as a tool for innovation but as a bridge to more inclusive, effective, and compassionate care.

To ensure ethical use of emerging technologies in mental health care, systems must synchronize timestamps across sensor and app data to support accurate multimodal analysis (Chaabene et al., 2025). Users must also provide explicit consent for biometric monitoring and any secondary uses of their data, with clear documentation of data governance policies (Leivaditis & Sepetis, 2025). The promise of these technologies lies not only in their individual capabilities but in their potential for integration. Multimodal systems that combine artificial intelligence (AI), extended reality (XR), and wearable sensors can deliver highly personalized and responsive care (Kostadimas et al., 2025). These neuroadaptive systems represent a new frontier in mental health, where interventions are dynamic, context-aware, and tailored to the unique needs of each individual (Islam & Bae, 2024). To support this vision, institutions must develop an enterprise-level integration roadmap that specifies technical standards, governance structures, and clinician training requirements. This roadmap should include interoperability protocols, data security measures, and contingency plans for system failure or degradation (Adegoke et al., 2025). Performance metrics must be established to evaluate the effectiveness of personalization features, including symptom reduction, functional improvement, and user satisfaction. These metrics should be reviewed regularly and used to guide iterative refinement of digital tools and platforms. The ethical, legal, and social dimensions of digital mental health care are not peripheral—they are foundational. As the field evolves, it must do so with a commitment to transparency, accountability, and justice. Technologies must be designed and deployed in ways that protect privacy, promote equity, and preserve the therapeutic relationship. Ethical safeguards must be embedded into every stage of development and implementation, from initial design to post-deployment monitoring. This includes requiring early stakeholder engagement and independent ethics review to ensure that diverse perspectives inform system design and deployment.

Issues of data privacy, algorithmic bias, and equitable access must be addressed proactively to ensure that technological innovation does not exacerbate existing disparities. The digital divide—driven by factors such as income, geography, and digital literacy—poses a significant barrier to the widespread adoption of digital therapeutics. Moreover, the rapid pace of technological development often outpaces the creation of regulatory frameworks and evidence-based guidelines, creating uncertainty for clinicians, patients, and policymakers alike (Ong et al., 2025). To address these gaps, cross-sector advisory panels should be convened to guide implementation, bringing together experts in clinical care, ethics, law, technology, and public health. Despite these challenges, the integration of digital technologies into mental health care offers a compelling vision for the future. To realize this vision responsibly, pilot programs must be designed with equity in mind and include robust evaluation frameworks. Diverse participant samples should be prioritized to ensure generalizability, and pilot results should be transparently reported to inform wider adoption. This approach supports evidence-based refinement and fosters public trust in digital mental health innovations. Digital transformation invites a reimagining of therapeutic relationships, clinical workflows, and the very nature of mental health itself (Hiland, 2021). It challenges traditional models of episodic, in-person care and opens the door to continuous, adaptive, and personalized interventions. As we explore the possibilities and limitations of these tools, it is essential to ground our efforts in ethical practice, scientific rigor, and human-centered design. Technologies must be developed not only for efficiency but also for empathy, equity, and empowerment.

This chapter introduces the foundational concepts that will be explored in greater depth throughout the book. It provides a historical overview of mental health care, outlines the current challenges facing the field, and highlights the transformative potential of digital therapeutics (Hiland, 2021). By examining the intersection of

AI, XR, and wearable technologies, we aim to illuminate a path forward—one that embraces innovation while remaining anchored in the core values of empathy, equity, and evidence-based care (Reddy, 2025).

Understanding the digital transformation of mental health care requires more than a technical perspective; it demands an appreciation of the field's complex historical evolution and the lessons embedded within it (Bond et al., 2023). Historical analysis is not merely descriptive—it serves as a strategic tool for informing present implementation choices and mitigating risks. By examining past failures and successes, we can extract principles that map directly to operational safeguards and evaluation criteria for contemporary systems. Over centuries, mental health care has undergone a series of paradigm shifts, each shaped by prevailing scientific, societal, and technological influences. These shifts have not only reflected changing attitudes toward mental illness but have also determined the structure and delivery of care. Linking these historical trajectories to modern governance design ensures that innovation does not repeat the mistakes of earlier reforms (Cristofaro & Giardino, 2025). For example, the consequences of deinstitutionalization—where systemic changes outpaced community resource development—underscore the need for coordinated planning and transition metrics in today's digital initiatives. In this sense, history becomes a blueprint for ethical deployment, reminding us that technological progress must be accompanied by infrastructure, policy, and equity safeguards (Chithra & Bhambri, 2024).

HISTORICAL CONTEXT

The earliest approaches to mental illness were deeply rooted in cultural and spiritual frameworks. In antiquity, mental disorders were commonly attributed to supernatural forces or moral transgressions, shaping both social responses and care settings (Subu et al., 2022). Treatments were often spiritual or punitive, including rituals, exorcisms, or confinement, reflecting a worldview where illness was seen as a breach of divine or moral order. The Hippocratic tradition in ancient Greece marked an early move toward medicalization, positing that mental disorders resulted from imbalances in bodily humors. While this framework introduced a naturalistic perspective, it remained limited by the scientific understanding of its era. Comparing these early models to modern biopsychosocial frameworks offers clinicians a critical lens for understanding how explanatory paradigms influence treatment design and stigma reduction today. The Middle Ages witnessed a regression in humane treatment, with mental illness frequently interpreted as demonic possession or divine punishment (El Khoury-Malhame et al., 2025). Social labeling reinforced exclusionary legal and custodial practices, leading to widespread ostracism and confinement under harsh conditions. It was not until the Enlightenment that more compassionate approaches began to emerge (Gilbert & Van Gordon, 2023). Reformers such as Philippe Pinel in France and William Tuke in England championed "moral treatment," emphasizing structured environments, compassion, and respect for individual dignity. These principles laid the groundwork for institutional care and remain relevant to modern person-centered care and therapeutic milieu design. However, the moral treatment movement also illustrates a recurring theme in mental health history: the tension between idealistic reform and practical implementation. While its principles were progressive, resource limitations and inconsistent application often undermined its effectiveness—a cautionary lesson for today's digital interventions, which must balance aspirational goals with operational feasibility.

The 19th and early 20th centuries saw the proliferation of asylums, intended as therapeutic refuges for those with mental illness. Initially envisioned as structured environments promoting recovery, many institutions became overcrowded and underfunded, devolving into custodial facilities where care was minimal. This failure highlights the importance of evaluating institutional capacity before concluding therapeutic value—a principle equally applicable to digital systems, which require robust infrastructure and governance to avoid becoming symbolic rather than functional solutions. During this period, psychiatry began to establish itself as a medical specialty, with competing theoretical models—including psychoanalysis and biological psychiatry—shaping clinical practice (Gilbert & Van Gordon, 2023; Abdul Rahman et al., 2023). A major turning point occurred in the mid-20th century with the advent of psychopharmacology. The introduction of antipsychotic and antidepressant medications revolutionized treatment and catalyzed the deinstitutionalization movement. Large psychiatric hospitals were closed in favor of community-based care, guided by principles of autonomy and social integration. However, insufficient investment in community resources left many individuals without adequate support, resulting in cycles of hospitalization, homelessness, and involvement with the criminal justice system. These failures underscore the need for coordinated community service planning, transition metrics, and funding commitments when implementing systemic reforms—a lesson that should inform digital transformation strategies today (Mahon, 2023). Modalities such as cognitive behavioral therapy (Brasier et al., 2025) and dialectical behavior therapy (Singh & Chandra, 2025) gained prominence, providing structured, effective interventions for a broad range of mental health conditions. These therapies emphasized the interplay of cognition, behavior, and emotion, and established a foundation for the digital adaptation of psychological interventions. Randomized trials and manualized treatments introduced reproducibility safeguards, and fidelity monitoring remains essential when adapting these interventions to digital formats. As we move toward AI-driven and XR-enabled therapeutic ecosystems, these historical lessons remind us that innovation must be coupled with rigorous evaluation, ethical oversight, and equitable access—principles that are as relevant today as they were in the era of institutional reform.

Figure 2. Example of integrated digital mental health ecosystem

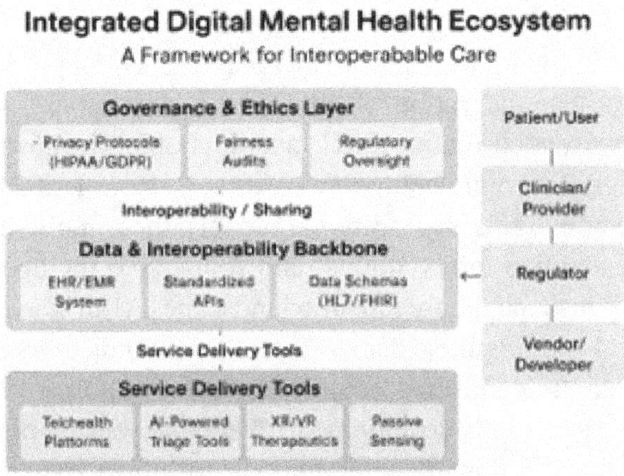

THE DIGITAL ERA: FROM COMPUTER-ASSISTED THERAPY TO MOBILE HEALTH

The late 20th and early 21st centuries marked the entry of digital technology into mental health care, introducing tools that extended therapeutic reach beyond traditional clinical settings. Early computer-assisted therapy programs were largely static, replicating established therapeutic models without significant interactivity or adaptability. These systems provided structured exercises and psychoeducational content but lacked the dynamic responsiveness that characterizes modern digital interventions. As internet access expanded, online forums, self-help platforms, and teletherapy services proliferated, creating new pathways for individuals to seek support. Pragmatic trials during this period demonstrated improved access for underserved populations, though engagement often remained inconsistent without human facilitation—a finding that continues to inform hybrid care models today. The widespread adoption of smartphones in the 2010s ushered in a new wave of mobile health (Weiner et al., 2025) applications, enabling users to track symptoms, practice mindfulness, and access therapeutic content on demand. These tools significantly increased accessibility, particularly for individuals facing geographic, financial, or social barriers to in-person care. However, rapid expansion also raised concerns regarding quality assurance, data privacy, and regulatory oversight (Kargarandehkordi et al., 2025). To address these challenges, operational standards must require apps to disclose evidence levels, data practices, and clinical validation status upfront, ensuring transparency and informed decision-making for both clinicians and users.

The Current Digital Transformation

In recent years, the integration of advanced technologies—such as artificial intelligence (AI), extended reality (XR), and wearable biosensors—has ushered in a new era of digital mental health care (Akhtar & Rawol, 2024). Unlike earlier efforts that focused on digitizing traditional models, these innovations enable real-time monitoring, adaptive interventions, and immersive therapeutic experiences that fundamentally reshape the therapeutic landscape. AI-driven tools can analyze complex behavioral and linguistic data to detect subtle indicators of distress, while XR technologies create controlled environments for exposure therapy, mindfulness training, and social skills development. Wearable sensors provide continuous physiological feedback, allowing interventions to adjust dynamically based on heart rate variability, electrodermal activity, or other markers of emotional arousal (Saganowski et al., 2022). This convergence of modalities supports closed-loop systems that personalize care in ways previously unattainable. However, integration demands more than technical capability; it requires cross-disciplinary governance, interoperability standards, and rigorous validation protocols. Before scaling, pilot programs must demonstrate safety, efficacy, and equitable performance across diverse populations. Validation checklists should include usability testing, bias audits, and contingency planning for data loss or service degradation. These measures ensure that technological innovation enhances care without compromising ethical principles or widening disparities.

Lessons From History and Future Directions

This historical overview underscores the dynamic and evolving nature of mental health care, revealing a consistent pattern: progress often introduces new challenges shaped by the interplay of scientific advancement and societal values (Henderson & Bekhuis, 2023; Souther & Boughton, 2025). Each era—from the moral treatment movement to the rise of psychopharmacology—offers lessons that remain relevant today (Pinel, 1793; Wykes et al., 2019). The failures of overcrowded asylums caution against scaling without infrastructure; the shortcomings of deinstitutionalization highlight the necessity of coordinated community supports; and the success of evidence-based psychotherapies demonstrates the value of reproducibility and fidelity monitoring (Stirman, 2022; Marriott et al., 2025). These lessons must be translated into explicit governance, training, and evaluation protocols for digital systems (Martí-Noguera, 2025; World Economic Forum, 2022). Operational design principles should include capacity planning, equity audits, and transparent reporting of outcomes. Clinician training must emphasize digital literacy, ethical oversight, and the integration of multimodal data into treatment planning (American Psychiatric Association, 2023; Price & Van Heerden, 2025). Evaluation frameworks should prioritize not only clinical efficacy but also accessibility, cultural relevance, and user experience (Jones, 2024; Bunyi et al., 2021). By embedding these safeguards, the field can harness the transformative potential of technology while remaining anchored in the core values of empathy, equity, and evidence-based care (Bapat & Jog, 2025; Spahl & Rubeis, 2025). The directive is clear: publish pilot findings transparently, engage stakeholders early, and adopt adaptive governance models that evolve alongside technological innovation (Society for Digital Mental Health, 2025). In doing so, mental health care can move beyond digitization toward a truly responsive, inclusive, and ethically grounded system—one that honors its historical lessons while embracing the possibilities of the future (Martí-Noguera, 2025; World Economic Forum, 2022).

Current Challenges in Mental Health Care

Despite decades of progress in understanding and treating mental health conditions, the global mental health care system continues to face profound and multifaceted challenges. These challenges span operational, clinical, and technological domains, each exerting measurable influence on access, equity, and quality of care (Langat, 2025; Saxena, 2016; Price & Van Heerden, 2025). Stakeholders must therefore begin every intervention with a baseline assessment of system metrics—including provider-to-population ratios, wait times, and digital infrastructure—before introducing new solutions. Every proposed digital innovation should be explicitly linked to documented service gaps, ensuring that technology addresses real needs rather than amplifying existing inequities. This framing is essential as the field moves toward integrating digital therapeutics into routine practice.

One of the most persistent barriers is the widespread lack of access to mental health services. In low- and middle-income countries, resources are often scarce or entirely absent; even in high-income settings, access remains constrained by geography, cost, and systemic inefficiencies. Rural and remote communities frequently lack mental health professionals altogether, forcing individuals to travel long distances or endure extended wait times for care. Urban environments, while better resourced, are not immune—long waitlists and high out-of-pocket costs continue to impede timely access.

To address these gaps, regional provider-to-population ratios should be mapped prior to planning, and operational strategies should prioritize telehealth and task-sharing models where workforce shortages are most acute (County Health Rankings & Roadmaps, 2025; Sangraula et al., 2024). The shortage of trained professionals—including psychiatrists, psychologists, counselors, and social workers—further exacerbates this problem, particularly in subspecialties such as child and adolescent mental health, geriatric psychiatry, and culturally competent care. Scalable training and supervision models for non-specialist providers offer a pragmatic solution, but their effectiveness depends on robust quality assurance. Systems should therefore track referral completion rates and treatment fidelity to ensure responsiveness and safety.

Stigma remains a powerful deterrent to help-seeking, even amid growing public awareness. Mental illness is often associated with shame or perceived weakness, leading to internalized guilt and avoidance. Fear of discrimination in employment, education, or social relationships compounds these barriers. Needs assessments should therefore include stigma metrics, and interventions should deploy anonymous, culturally adapted digital screening tools to lower barriers to first contact. Cultural beliefs and norms also shape how mental health is understood and addressed. In some communities, symptoms are interpreted through spiritual or religious frameworks, prompting individuals to seek help from traditional healers rather than medical professionals. Language barriers, mistrust of health systems, and lack of culturally sensitive services further limit engagement. Every digital intervention protocol should embed cultural adaptation requirements and involve co-design with community stakeholders prior to rollout (Naderbagi et al., 2024; Brotherdale et al., 2024). These measures ensure that technology does not replicate the cultural blind spots of traditional systems.

FRAGMENTATION AND SYSTEMIC BARRIERS

Mental health care is often fragmented, with services dispersed across multiple providers and institutions. This fragmentation leads to poor coordination, duplication of services, and gaps in treatment—particularly for individuals with complex or co-occurring conditions such as substance use disorders. Transitions between levels of care (e.g., inpatient to outpatient) are frequently poorly managed, increasing the risk of relapse or disengagement. Systems should implement single-point referral directories to reduce navigation burden and monitor successful transition rates at discharge as a core quality metric. Digital tools such as electronic health records (Johnson et al., 2021) have the potential to improve coordination, but their implementation remains inconsistent. Many systems lack interoperability, making it difficult to share information across providers. Privacy regulations, while essential, can inadvertently create barriers to collaboration. Procurement policies should therefore require interoperability standards, and governance frameworks must establish data-sharing agreements with role-based access controls to balance confidentiality with continuity of care (Megahed Ibrahim et al., 2024; Ostrowski & Goldberg, 2022). Chronic underfunding remains a major impediment to effective mental health care. In many countries, mental health receives a disproportionately small share of health budgets, often concentrated in inpatient settings rather than community-based or preventive services. Insurance coverage is frequently inadequate, resulting in high out-of-pocket costs, limited provider networks, and restrictions on session limits—barriers that disproportionately affect low-income populations. Systems should quantify current mental health spending as a percentage of total health budgets, advocate for parity laws, and explore bundled payment models for integrated care.

Policy frameworks often lag behind evolving population needs. Outdated legislation and fragmented strategies hinder integration of mental health into broader health and social systems. Stakeholders should map outdated laws, prioritize reforms based on public health impact, and establish measurable policy milestones tied to funding commitments. Sustained investment and political will are essential to modernize legislation and align policy with technological innovation, including AI, XR, and wearable sensors (Tabassum et al., 2025; Xing et al., 2025). These challenges are not isolated—they interact in ways that compound inequities. Workforce shortages amplify access barriers; stigma and cultural misalignment reduce engagement; fragmentation undermines continuity; and underfunding constrains innovation. Digital technologies offer promising solutions, but their success depends on strategic alignment with documented gaps, rigorous evaluation, and governance frameworks that prioritize equity and ethical integrity. As mental health systems evolve, operational readiness, cultural responsiveness, and policy reform must advance in tandem with technological innovation.

DIGITAL DIVIDE AND TECHNOLOGICAL BARRIERS

While digital technologies offer promising avenues for expanding access and improving care, they also introduce new challenges. Before implementing digital interventions, assess community-level broadband availability and device ownership to ensure feasibility. The digital divide—the gap between those with and without access to technology—remains a significant barrier, particularly for individuals in rural areas, older adults, and those with lower socioeconomic status. Lack of access to smartphones, reliable internet, or digital literacy skills can limit the reach and effectiveness of digital mental health interventions. Deploy low-bandwidth solutions and telephone-based protocols where connectivity is limited. Many digital tools are not designed with inclusivity in mind. Ensure applications include multilingual options and low-literacy modes to maximize inclusivity. Language, literacy, and cultural relevance are often overlooked in the development of mental health apps and platforms, which may fail to engage or meet the needs of diverse populations. Accessibility features for individuals with disabilities are also frequently lacking. Incorporate accessibility features such as screen-reader compatibility and adjustable font sizes during development.

Quality, Regulation, and Data Security The rapid proliferation of digital mental health tools has significantly outpaced the development of regulatory frameworks and evidence-based standards (Scholle, 2024; Bezyl, 2024). Thousands of mental health apps are available to consumers, yet only a small fraction have undergone rigorous evaluation for safety, efficacy, or data security (Agarwal et al., 2025; Watson, 2025). This lack of oversight creates substantial risks for users and complicates clinical decision-making, as providers struggle to identify trustworthy interventions amid a crowded and uneven marketplace (Mescher et al., 2025; APA, 2025). To address this gap, app listings should disclose evidence levels and evaluation status upfront, enabling clinicians and users to make informed choices (Agarwal et al., 2025). Procurement policies should prioritize tools supported by peer-reviewed evidence and transparent privacy practices, ensuring that adoption aligns with clinical integrity and ethical standards (APA, 2025).

Data privacy and security represent critical pillars of responsible digital mental health care (Surani et al., 2023; APA, 2024). These tools frequently collect highly sensitive information—ranging from mood logs and behavioral patterns to biometric signals such as heart rate variability and electrodermal activity (GDPR Advisor, 2025; Watson, 2025). Protecting this data is not optional; it is foundational to maintaining trust and safeguarding user rights (Stanford Law School, 2025). Systems must therefore implement a security baseline that mandates encryption in transit and at rest for all clinical data, coupled with robust key management protocols (HIPAA vs GDPR, 2025). Beyond technical safeguards, governance frameworks should require periodic third-party security audits to verify compliance and detect vulnerabilities before they result in harm (APA, 2025). Quality assurance and data protection are inseparable from the ethical deployment of digital mental health tools. Evidence disclosure, rigorous evaluation, and enforceable security standards must become non-negotiable requirements—not aspirational goals—if digital therapeutics are to fulfill their promise without compromising safety or equity (Watson, 2025).

Provider Well-Being and Systemic Sustainability The mental health workforce is experiencing unprecedented strain, a challenge that threatens both the sustainability of care systems and the quality of patient outcomes. Clinicians across disciplines face mounting caseloads, administrative burdens, and the emotional toll of treating individuals in crisis. These pressures contribute to burnout, turnover, and diminished clinical performance—trends that have accelerated in the wake of global crises such as the COVID-19 pandemic (CDC, 2023; Crocker et al., 2023). To address these risks proactively, organizations should monitor clinician workload and burnout indicators monthly, using standardized measures to inform staffing decisions and resource allocation. Digital tools offer promising avenues for alleviating some of these burdens. Automation of routine documentation, integration of decision-support systems, and flexible telehealth arrangements can reduce administrative load and improve work-life balance. However, these technologies must be implemented thoughtfully. Poorly designed systems can inadvertently increase cognitive load, disrupt workflows, or create new layers of complexity. To prevent such outcomes, deployment should follow a pilot-first approach, incorporating clinician co-design and iterative feedback cycles to ensure usability and alignment with real-world clinical needs (National Academy of Medicine, 2020).

Supporting provider well-being is not only a moral imperative but a clinical necessity (Lyndon, 2015; Aiken et al., 2023). Burnout impairs judgment, reduces empathy, and elevates the risk of errors—effects that reverberate across patient safety and organizational performance (Dima, 2025; Simbo AI, 2025). Institutions should provide confidential mental health services and peer supervision for staff, creating safe spaces for reflection and emotional processing. Workforce sustainability metrics, including retention rates and satisfaction scores, should be integrated into technology ROI assessments, ensuring that innovation enhances rather than erodes clinician well-being. Systemic sustainability also demands a shift in evaluation priorities. Health systems should pair integrated service metrics with clinical outcomes, recognizing that efficiency, coordination, and workforce stability are as critical as symptom reduction (Aiken et al., 2023). Planning for digital transformation must include cross-sector stakeholder convenings before major rollouts, fostering alignment among clinicians, administrators, technologists, and policymakers. This collaborative approach ensures that digital solutions address real-world constraints rather than introducing new layers of complexity.

Access and Workforce Gaps: A Persistent Barrier Despite decades of progress, access to mental health care remains one of the most pressing global challenges. In many low- and middle-income countries, resources are scarce or nonexistent; even in high-income settings, access is often constrained by geography, cost, and systemic inefficiencies. Rural and remote communities frequently lack mental health professionals, forcing individuals to travel long distances or endure extended wait times for care. Urban areas, while better resourced, are not immune—long waitlists and high out-of-pocket costs continue to impede timely access. To address these gaps, systems should collect baseline data on wait times and travel distances before implementing interventions (NASHP, 2025). Operational strategies should prioritize telehealth and task-sharing models where workforce shortages are most acute (BHM

Healthcare Solutions, 2025). Expanding brief telephone interventions can serve as a temporary mitigation strategy to reduce waitlists and maintain continuity of care. Longer-term solutions require scaling supervised paraprofessional programs to extend reach, particularly in underserved regions. These models must include robust quality assurance, with systems tracking service quality across task-shared models to ensure safety and effectiveness.

Stigma remains a powerful deterrent to help-seeking, even amid growing public awareness campaigns. Mental illness is often associated with shame or perceived weakness, leading to internalized guilt and avoidance. Fear of discrimination in employment, education, or social relationships compounds these barriers. Needs assessments should therefore include stigma metrics, and interventions should deploy anonymous, culturally adapted digital screening tools to lower barriers to first contact (Naderbagi et al., 2024; Ellis et al., 2022). Cultural beliefs and norms also shape how mental health is understood and addressed. In some communities, symptoms are interpreted through spiritual or religious frameworks, prompting individuals to seek help from traditional healers rather than medical professionals. Language barriers, mistrust of health systems, and lack of culturally sensitive services further limit engagement. Programs should hire cultural liaisons for community engagement and adaptation, and every digital intervention protocol should embed cultural adaptation requirements (Nittas et al., 2023; Sit et al., 2020). Uptake and satisfaction should be evaluated across cultural groups, ensuring that interventions are inclusive and equitable.

FRAGMENTATION AND SYSTEMIC BARRIERS

Mental health care is often fragmented, with services dispersed across multiple providers and institutions. This fragmentation leads to poor coordination, duplication of services, and gaps in treatment—particularly for individuals with complex or co-occurring conditions such as substance use disorders. Transitions between levels of care (e.g., inpatient to outpatient) are frequently poorly managed, increasing the risk of relapse or disengagement. Systems should implement integrated care navigators to coordinate services for complex patients and simulate common transition scenarios to identify failure points before scaling new models. Digital tools such as electronic health records (Kim & Backonja, 2025) have the potential to improve coordination, but their implementation remains uneven. Many systems lack interoperability, making it difficult to share information across providers. Privacy regulations, while essential, can inadvertently create barriers to collaboration. Procurement policies should therefore require interoperability certification for new systems, and governance frameworks must establish data-sharing agreements with role-based access controls (CMS, 2024; World Economic Forum, 2022; ASPE, 2024). Quality measures should include tracking redundant assessments as an indicator of system inefficiency. These challenges—workforce strain, access inequities, stigma, cultural misalignment, fragmentation, and underfunding—are not isolated. They interact in ways that compound systemic vulnerabilities. Digital technologies offer promising solutions, but their success depends on strategic alignment with documented gaps, rigorous evaluation, and governance frameworks that prioritize equity and ethical integrity. As mental health systems evolve, operational readiness, cultural responsiveness, and policy reform must advance in tandem with technological innovation.

ECONOMIC AND POLICY CONSTRAINTS

Despite the promise of digital solutions, economic and policy barriers continue to constrain the mental health care system. Before procurement, organizations should quantify digital program costs and expected savings, ensuring that investments align with both fiscal responsibility and clinical impact (Berardi et al., 2024; Loud, 2025). Mental health services remain chronically underfunded relative to their burden of disease, with many countries allocating only a small fraction of total health budgets to mental health care. Funding is often concentrated in inpatient facilities, limiting the development of community-based, preventive, and early intervention programs that are critical for reducing long-term morbidity (Omiyefa, 2025; GAO, 2022). To avoid short-termism, procurement policies should require multi-year funding commitments for digital pilots, enabling sufficient time for evaluation and iterative refinement. Insurance coverage represents another significant barrier. While mental health parity laws have improved access in some regions, many individuals still face high out-of-pocket costs, restricted provider networks, and limitations on the number of covered sessions. These constraints disproportionately affect low-income populations and those without stable employment or insurance, exacerbating inequities in access to care (GAO, 2022; APA Services, 2025). To mitigate these disparities, payers should negotiate reimbursement for remote monitoring and brief digital contacts, recognizing their role in continuity of care and early intervention. Furthermore, pilot evidence should be aligned with advocacy for scalable reimbursement models, ensuring that successful innovations transition from experimental projects to sustainable components of routine care (SAMHSA CFRI, 2023; ASPE, 2023).

Policy frameworks often lag behind the rapidly evolving needs of the population. Many mental health laws remain outdated or inconsistently enforced, resulting in fragmented service delivery and inadequate protection for individuals with mental health conditions. A first step toward modernization is to inventory relevant laws and prioritize gaps for reform, focusing on those with the greatest public health impact

(WHO, 2025; NASHP, 2024). Implementation should include cross-agency strategic plans with measurable targets, integrating mental health into broader health and social systems to improve coordination and efficiency. Accountability mechanisms are essential: governments and institutions should publish annual progress reports tied to funding disbursements, creating transparency and reinforcing commitments to reform. In addition to modernization, duplication and fragmentation within existing policies must be addressed. Systems should reconcile overlapping regulations to reduce implementation friction, which often delays innovation and burdens providers with conflicting compliance requirements. Stakeholder engagement is critical to this process. Policymakers should convene service users, providers, and community representatives to co-create reform agendas, ensuring that legislative changes reflect lived experience and clinical realities (NAMI, 2024; Penn LDI, 2022). Without these commitments—sustained investment, political will, and inclusive governance—the potential benefits of emerging technologies such as AI, XR, and wearable sensors will remain unrealized, and disparities in access and quality of care will persist (WHO, 2025; APA Services, 2025).

TECHNOLOGICAL GAPS AND THE DIGITAL DIVIDE

Digital technologies hold significant promise for improving mental health care, yet they introduce new challenges—most notably, the persistent digital divide. This divide refers to the gap between individuals who have reliable access to digital tools and those who do not, and it remains a substantial barrier to equitable mental health care delivery. Populations most affected include those living in rural areas, older adults, individuals with lower socioeconomic status, and people with severe mental illness, who may lack access to smartphones, broadband internet, or the digital literacy skills necessary to use these technologies effectively. Before any rollout, systems should conduct local needs assessments to survey device ownership and connectivity, ensuring that interventions are grounded in the realities of community infrastructure.

The consequences of digital exclusion are far-reaching. Individuals without adequate digital access are often unable to benefit from telehealth, online therapy, or digital self-management tools, leading to delays in care, poorer health outcomes, and exacerbation of existing mental health disparities. For example, during the COVID-19 pandemic, the rapid shift to remote mental health services highlighted how digital exclusion can compound isolation, limit access to support, and increase the risk of untreated mental health conditions. To mitigate these risks, health systems should develop access plans that include device loan programs and community access points, ensuring that technology-enabled care does not become a privilege reserved for the digitally connected. Equity must be measurable: programs should report service reach by connectivity strata, making disparities visible and actionable.

Beyond infrastructure, inclusivity in design remains a critical challenge. Many digital mental health tools fail to account for language diversity, literacy levels, and cultural relevance, resulting in platforms that do not engage or meet the needs of diverse populations. Accessibility features for individuals with disabilities are also frequently lacking, further limiting usability. To address these gaps, procurement specifications should mandate multilingual interfaces and low-literacy modes, and developers should incorporate universal design principles from the outset. Compliance audits should certify accessibility standards pre-deployment, ensuring that inclusivity is not an afterthought but a core design requirement.

Bridging the digital divide requires a multifaceted approach that extends beyond device distribution. Infrastructure development is essential, but so too is the cultivation of digital literacy and the creation of culturally and linguistically appropriate tools. Programs should partner with telecom providers and community organizations to expand broadband access, while simultaneously funding community digital navigators who can provide sustained support for individuals unfamiliar with technology. These navigators can assist with device setup, troubleshoot connectivity issues, and guide users through digital mental health platforms, reducing attrition and improving engagement.

INTEGRATING MENTAL HEALTH CARE INTO DIGITAL EQUITY INITIATIVES

Integrating mental health care into broader digital equity initiatives is critical for preventing the deepening of health disparities in the digital age. Policy frameworks should align mental health technology adoption with national and regional strategies for digital inclusion, ensuring that investments in AI, XR, and wearable sensors do not bypass the populations most in need (Robinson et al., 2024; Kim & Backonja, 2025; Berardi et al., 2024). Monitoring systems should track engagement by socioeconomic indicators, enabling continuous evaluation of whether digital interventions are reaching underserved groups or reinforcing existing inequities (Jones, 2024; Jena, 2024). While digital innovations have the potential to transform mental health care, their benefits will only be fully realized if efforts are made to ensure equitable access and inclusive design for all individuals. This requires coordinated action across infrastructure, policy, design, and training domains, supported by measurable equity metrics and sustained community engagement.

QUALITY AND REGULATION OF DIGITAL INTERVENTIONS

The rapid expansion of the digital mental health market has significantly outpaced the establishment of regulatory frameworks and quality standards (Agarwal et al., 2025; Armontrout et al., 2018). Thousands of mental health apps and digital tools are available for download, yet only a small fraction have undergone rigorous evaluation for safety, efficacy, or data security (Shahsavar & Choudhury, 2025; Liu & Schueller, 2023). This lack of oversight poses substantial risks, as users may inadvertently rely on interventions that are ineffective, unproven, or potentially harmful (Glass et al., 2022). To address this gap, systems should require apps to display evidence levels and data policies prominently, enabling transparency and informed decision-making (Agarwal et al., 2025; Shahsavar & Choudhury, 2025). Health systems should also develop trusted formularies for clinician recommendation, ensuring that only validated tools are integrated into care pathways (Liu & Schueller, 2023; Gkintoni et al., 2025).

The Transparency Imperative

Transparency is the cornerstone of trust in digital mental health care. Consumers and clinicians alike need clear, accessible information about the evidence base supporting a given tool, its intended use, and its data governance practices (Camacho et al., 2022; Price & Van Heerden, 2025). App stores and health system procurement portals should mandate prominent disclosure of evidence levels, privacy policies, and evaluation status, using standardized labels that allow quick comparison across products (Camacho et al., 2022; Berardi et al., 2024). This approach mirrors nutrition labeling in food systems—providing essential information at a glance to guide informed choices. Without such transparency, users are left to navigate a marketplace dominated by marketing claims rather than scientific validation (Babu & Joseph, 2025).

Challenges for Clinicians and Health Systems

For clinicians, the proliferation of digital tools presents a dual challenge: identifying high-quality interventions and integrating them into clinical workflows (Berardi et al., 2024; Smith et al., 2023). The absence of standardized evaluation criteria and certification processes complicates these tasks. Many clinicians hesitate to recommend apps because they cannot verify safety or efficacy, while others rely on anecdotal evidence or patient preference, introducing variability and risk (Hall et al., 2024). Health systems should therefore develop curated formularies of approved digital tools, similar to medication formularies, based on rigorous review of clinical evidence, usability, and security (Liu & Schueller, 2023; Gkintoni et al., 2025). Procurement policies should include checklists requiring peer-reviewed evidence and independent security audits, ensuring that adoption aligns with ethical and clinical standards (Berardi et al., 2024; Hall et al., 2024). Regulatory bodies are beginning to address these gaps, but progress remains inconsistent across jurisdictions (Ball et al., 2025; Löchner et al., 2025). Harmonization efforts should involve clinicians, patients, and technology developers in regulatory design, ensuring that frameworks are both clinically relevant and practically implementable (Price & Van Heerden, 2025).

Data Privacy and Security: A Non-Negotiable Standard

Data privacy and security remain paramount concerns in digital mental health care (Iwaya et al., 2023; Inkster et al., 2023). These tools frequently collect sensitive personal information, including mood, behavioral patterns, geolocation, and biometric data (Alhammad et al., 2024; Khoo et al., 2024). Protecting this data requires robust safeguards: systems should implement minimum encryption standards for data in transit and at rest, coupled with audit logging to track access and modifications (Iwaya et al., 2023). Compliance should not rely on vendor self-attestation; instead, health systems must enforce third-party security certification for clinical deployments, creating an independent layer of accountability (Inkster et al., 2023). Transparent privacy policies, strong encryption, and adherence to legal and ethical standards are essential for maintaining trust and protecting individual rights (Khoo et al., 2024). Consent processes must also evolve to reflect the complexity of digital data flows. Users should be offered clear opt-in mechanisms for secondary data use, with granular controls that allow them to specify which data streams can be shared and for what purposes. Dynamic consent models—where users can revisit and revise their choices over time—should replace static, one-time agreements that fail to account for evolving technologies and user preferences (Lay et al., 2025).

Research Priorities and Evidence Generation

The evidence gap in digital mental health care is stark (Livieri et al., 2025; Baka et al., 2025). While thousands of apps claim therapeutic benefits, few have been subjected to randomized controlled trials or real-world effectiveness studies (Camacho et al., 2022; Hall et al., 2024). To close this gap, funding agencies and health systems should prioritize comparative effectiveness research on certified versus uncertified apps, generating data that informs both clinical practice and policy (Mulukuntla, 2025). Pragmatic trials embedded in routine care settings can provide insights into usability, engagement, and outcomes across diverse populations

(Baka et al., 2025). These studies should report not only symptom reduction but also functional improvements, equity impacts, and cost-effectiveness metrics (Livieri et al., 2025). Clinicians should be advised to consult institutional formularies before recommending apps, ensuring that patient care is grounded in validated tools rather than marketing claims (Liu & Schueller, 2023). Continuing education programs should include training on digital health literacy, regulatory standards, and ethical considerations, equipping clinicians to navigate this rapidly evolving landscape (Smith et al., 2023). While digital interventions offer significant promise—particularly through technologies such as AI, XR, and wearable sensors—their safe and effective implementation depends on the development of robust regulatory frameworks, standardized quality measures, and strong data protection protocols (Ball et al., 2025; Löchner et al., 2025). A practical roadmap should publish phased standards and timelines for compliance, guiding developers, clinicians, and policymakers toward a future where innovation is matched by accountability and equity (Price & Van Heerden, 2025). Key steps include:

Phase 1: Mandatory transparency labeling for all mental health apps, including evidence level and privacy practices (Kumar, 2025).
Phase 2: Certification programs for clinical-grade digital tools, incorporating usability, accessibility, and security audits (Cruz-Gonzalez et al., 2025).
Phase 3: Integration of certified tools into health system formularies, supported by reimbursement models and clinician training.
Phase 4: Continuous monitoring through post-market surveillance, bias audits, and dynamic consent evaluations.

By embedding these safeguards into the digital mental health ecosystem, stakeholders can ensure that technology serves as a bridge to better care—not a barrier that amplifies risk and inequity.

BURNOUT AND WORKFORCE WELL-BEING

The mental health workforce is under unprecedented strain, a reality that threatens both the sustainability of care systems and the quality of patient outcomes. Clinicians across disciplines are managing high caseloads, navigating increasing administrative demands, and bearing the emotional weight of treating individuals in crisis. These pressures contribute to elevated rates of burnout and workforce turnover, which undermine provider well-being and compromise care quality. To address these risks proactively, organizations should implement regular workload reviews and redistribute tasks as needed, ensuring that staffing models reflect real-time demand and prevent chronic overload. The COVID-19 pandemic magnified these vulnerabilities, exposing systemic gaps in support structures and underscoring the urgent need for resilience-building strategies. Digital tools—including AI-driven platforms, electronic health records (EHRs), and telehealth solutions—offer potential avenues to alleviate some of these burdens (Crocker et al., 2023; Simbo AI, 2025). However, their implementation must be deliberate and evidence-informed (National Academy of Medicine, 2020; Hall et al., 2024). Pilot automation features before wide rollout to prevent workflow disruption, as poorly designed systems can inadvertently increase administrative complexity or disrupt clinical workflows, exacerbating stress rather than relieving it (Elfouly & Alouani, 2025). Governance frameworks should include clinician-reported usability as a go/no-go metric, ensuring that technology adoption enhances rather than hinders care delivery. When thoughtfully deployed, automation of routine administrative tasks, enhanced clinical decision support, and flexible work arrangements can reduce workload and improve work-life balance (Huang et al., 2024). Yet these benefits hinge on co-design principles. Health systems should include clinicians in tool selection and workflow integration, recognizing that frontline providers are best positioned to identify practical barriers and usability concerns. Co-design fosters trust, improves adoption, and ensures that technology serves as an enabler rather than an additional source of strain.

WHY WELL-BEING MATTERS FOR CARE QUALITY

Prioritizing the well-being of mental health professionals is not only vital for sustaining the workforce but also for safeguarding care quality. Burnout has been linked to impaired clinical judgment, diminished empathy, and a higher risk of errors—effects that reverberate across patient safety and treatment outcomes (Dima, 2025; Aiken et al., 2023). Organizations should provide protected time for reflective practice and supervision, creating structured opportunities for clinicians to process complex cases, share strategies, and maintain emotional resilience. These practices are not optional; they are evidence-based interventions that reduce burnout and improve retention (Lyndon, 2015; Hall et al., 2024). To operationalize these priorities, health systems should track clinician well-being metrics longitudinally, using validated instruments to monitor trends and identify emerging risks. These data should inform resource allocation, guiding investments in staff support programs and workload redistribution (Simbo AI, 2025). Institutions should fund dedicated staff wellness programs, including confidential mental health services, peer support groups, and resilience training. These initiatives signal organizational commitment to clinician well-being and create a culture where seeking support is normalized rather than stigmatized. Systemic sustainability requires embedding workforce well-being into governance structures. Health systems should make staff well-being a board-level performance indicator, elevating it to the same level of importance as financial metrics and clinical outcomes (National Academy of Medicine, 2020). This shift reframes well-being from an individual responsibility to an organizational priority, aligning leadership accountability with frontline realities. Furthermore, digital transformation strategies must include post-deployment workforce impact assessments, evaluating whether new technologies reduce administrative burden or inadvertently increase stress. These assessments should be iterative, informing continuous improvement and preventing harm.

DIGITAL TRANSFORMATION AS A DOUBLE-EDGED SWORD

The Role of Technology in Modernizing Mental Health Care

The integration of technology into mental health care represents a critical evolution, driven by the increasing complexity and scale of mental health needs globally. Traditional systems are often unable to keep pace with rising demand, workforce shortages, and the need for personalized, accessible care. To ensure meaningful progress, organizations should align technology priorities with population health goals and clinician capacity, avoiding fragmented adoption that fails to address systemic gaps. In this context, digital technologies provide innovative pathways for diagnosis, treatment, monitoring, and ongoing support—positioning themselves as essential complements to the expertise of human clinicians rather than replacements. A guiding principle for implementation is clear: design technologies to augment clinical judgment and preserve the therapeutic alliance, ensuring that human connection remains central to care (Price & Van Heerden, 2025; Ball et al., 2025). Digital tools—including telehealth platforms, mobile applications, artificial intelligence (AI), extended reality (XR), and wearable sensors—are reshaping the mental health landscape (Tabassum et al., 2025; Xing et al., 2025). Before introducing new solutions, health systems should catalog existing tools and their intended user populations, creating a comprehensive inventory that prevents duplication and supports strategic integration. These technologies extend the reach of mental health services, facilitate timely interventions, and enable more individualized and data-driven approaches to care (Liu & Schueller, 2023). For example:

Telehealth and mobile applications increase accessibility, allowing individuals to receive support regardless of geographic barriers or mobility limitations.

AI-driven platforms enhance clinical decision-making, support early identification of risk, and personalize treatment recommendations (Ni & Jia, 2025; Auf et al., 2025; Cruz-Gonzalez et al., 2025).

Extended reality (Cushnan et al., 2024) creates immersive therapeutic environments for interventions such as exposure therapy and skills training (Lamb et al., 2025; Li et al., 2025).

Wearable sensors enable real-time monitoring of physiological and behavioral indicators, supporting proactive and adaptive care (Elfouly & Alouani, 2025; Shen et al., 2025; Brasier et al., 2025).

Interoperability and Evidence-Driven Adoption

To ensure interoperability and scalability, every category of tool should include clear integration plans, specifying data standards, security protocols, and compatibility with electronic health records (Adegoke et al., 2025; Sadeh et al., 2023). Without these safeguards, digital ecosystems risk becoming siloed, undermining continuity of care and increasing clinician burden (Ball et al., 2025). Together, these innovations form the foundation of a digitally enabled mental health ecosystem—one that offers new opportunities to improve outcomes, reduce disparities, and support both patients and providers in an increasingly complex care environment. However, technology adoption must be evidence-driven (Liu & Schueller, 2023). Health systems should prioritize research that evaluates effectiveness across real-world settings, moving beyond controlled trials to understand usability, engagement, and equity impacts in diverse populations (Baka et al., 2025; Livieri et al., 2025).

The integration of technology into mental health care is not merely a trend—it is a necessary evolution in response to global challenges. Yet, this evolution must be guided by principles that protect care quality and clinician well-being. Digital tools should augment rather than replace human expertise, extending reach and enhancing decision-making without eroding the relational core of therapy (Price & Van Heerden, 2025). Planning frameworks should include contingency funds for technology maintenance and upgrades, recognizing that sustainability depends on ongoing investment rather than one-time procurement. Adoption strategies should also require pilots with defined outcome targets and written workflows, ensuring that implementation is measured, iterative, and aligned with clinical priorities (Ball et al., 2025). Stakeholder engagement is critical to success. Health systems should involve patients in setting success criteria for pilots, ensuring that technology addresses real needs and reflects user preferences (Clemens-Meyer et al., 2021). Similarly, clinicians must play an active role in co-design, providing insights into workflow integration and usability. These collaborative processes reduce resistance, improve adoption, and foster trust in digital transformation initiatives (Tsai et al., 2025).

Domains of Impact

Telehealth and Mobile Applications Telehealth platforms have become indispensable, particularly in the wake of global disruptions such as the COVID-19 pandemic. They reduce geographic barriers, increase scheduling flexibility, and support continuity of care during crises (Smith et al., 2023; Hall et al., 2024). Mobile applications complement these services by offering self-guided interventions, symptom tracking, and psychoeducation. However, quality assurance remains essential. Systems should require transparent disclosure of evidence levels and privacy practices, enabling clinicians and patients to make informed choices (Camacho et al., 2022; Shahsavar & Choudhury, 2025).

Artificial Intelligence (Fanarioti & Karpouzis, 2025) AI-driven tools enhance precision and scalability in mental health care (Price & Van Heerden, 2025; Ball et al., 2025). Machine learning algorithms can detect subtle indicators of distress in speech, text, or behavioral patterns, enabling early intervention (Löchner et al., 2025). Decision-support systems synthesize patient data to recommend evidence-based treatment options, while conversational agents provide low-intensity support between sessions (Gkintoni et al., 2025). Yet, these benefits depend on rigorous validation and ethical safeguards. AI deployment must include bias audits, explainability features, and clinician oversight, ensuring that algorithms augment rather than override human judgment (Hall et al., 2024; Inkster et al., 2023).

Extended Reality (Ricciardi & Zomaya, 2025) XR technologies—including virtual reality (Immanuel et al., 2023) and augmented reality (AR)—create immersive environments for therapeutic interventions (Carl et al., 2019; Lindner et al., 2024). VR exposure therapy allows patients to confront fears in controlled settings, while AR overlays digital cues onto real-world contexts to support skill practice. These tools can enhance engagement and accelerate progress, but they require clinician training, safety protocols, and accessibility testing to prevent adverse effects such as cybersickness or emotional overload (Lindner et al., 2024).

Wearable Sensors Wearable devices enable continuous monitoring of physiological signals such as heart rate variability, electrodermal activity, and sleep patterns (Xing et al., 2025; Alhammad et al., 2024). These data streams support adaptive interventions, alert clinicians to emerging risks, and empower patients through biofeedback (Mackey et al., 2025). However, integration demands robust data governance, including encryption, consent frameworks, and interoperability standards (Iwaya et al., 2023; Lay et al., 2025). Without these safeguards, wearable technologies risk becoming intrusive or inequitable (Robinson et al., 2024).

Building a Sustainable Digital Ecosystem

The promise of technology lies not in isolated tools but in integrated systems that deliver seamless, person-centered care. Achieving this vision requires strategic alignment with population health goals and clinician capacity, ensuring that technology priorities address real needs rather than creating redundant solutions. Interoperability must be a core design principle, enabling secure data exchange across platforms to reduce fragmentation and support continuity of care (Adegoke et al., 2025; Sadeh et al., 2023). Governance structures should embed usability testing, workforce impact assessments, and ethical oversight into every stage of implementation, while evaluation frameworks must extend beyond efficacy to examine engagement, cultural relevance, and cost-effectiveness in real-world contexts (Ball et al., 2025). Sustainability depends on forward-looking funding models that account for maintenance, upgrades, and training, preventing obsolescence and ensuring long-term viability (Price & Van Heerden, 2025). By integrating these elements—strategic alignment, interoperability, governance, evaluation, and sustainability—health systems can create a digital ecosystem that strengthens care delivery, supports clinicians, and advances equity. Technology is reshaping mental health care, offering unprecedented opportunities to expand access, personalize interventions, and enhance clinical decision-making (Löchner et al., 2025; Smith et al., 2023). Yet, these benefits will only be realized if innovation is guided by principles of equity, usability, and human-centered design. Digital tools should serve as enablers—not replacements—of therapeutic relationships, augmenting clinician expertise while preserving empathy and trust. By embedding governance, interoperability, and stakeholder engagement into every stage of implementation, health systems can create a future where technology strengthens—not strains—the fabric of mental health care.

Telehealth and Mobile Mental Health Applications

Telehealth has emerged as one of the most visible and widely adopted modalities in digital mental health care, offering a lifeline for individuals who might otherwise face insurmountable barriers to accessing services (Hall et al., 2024; Smith et al., 2023). This approach encompasses a spectrum of remote delivery methods, including video conferencing, telephone consultations, and secure messaging platforms. Teletherapy, in particular, has seen substantial growth, enabling individuals to connect with licensed mental health professionals from the privacy and comfort of their own homes. The advantages of telehealth are significant: it reduces geographic and transportation barriers, increases scheduling flexibility, and is especially beneficial for individuals with mobility limitations, social anxiety, or caregiving responsibilities. To optimize access, providers should schedule flexible hours to accommodate diverse patient schedules, ensuring that telehealth does not replicate the rigidity of traditional in-person care. The COVID-19 pandemic underscored the value of telehealth, as it ensured continuity of mental health services during periods of widespread disruption to in-person care. However, equity considerations remain paramount; systems should provide private access points for clients lacking confidential home spaces, such as designated rooms in community centers or clinics, to prevent privacy concerns from becoming a barrier to engagement. Mobile mental health applications (mHealth apps) further broaden access to support and intervention, leveraging the ubiquity and portability of smartphones to deliver care anytime and anywhere. These apps offer a diverse array of features, including mood and symptom tracking, guided meditation, cognitive behavioral therapy (Ghanim et al., 2023) exercises, journaling, and crisis support resources. Some applications are designed for self-guided use, while others integrate seamlessly into clinician-directed care plans, creating hybrid models that combine digital convenience with professional oversight. To ensure quality and transparency, developers should include clear evidence statements and privacy disclosures within the app, enabling users and clinicians to make informed choices (Camacho et al., 2022; Shahsavar & Choudhury, 2025). Clinicians, in turn, should monitor app usage trends during follow-up sessions, using engagement data to inform treatment planning and identify barriers to adherence (Mitsea et al., 2024). Despite these benefits, the rapid proliferation of mental health apps presents notable challenges. Many available tools lack rigorous clinical validation, and the quality and accuracy of content can vary widely (Hall et al., 2024; Babu & Joseph, 2025). This variability makes it difficult for users to identify trustworthy and effective resources, and clinicians may hesitate to recommend apps in the absence of clear evidence for efficacy and safety (Shah et al., 2021). To mitigate these risks, health systems should mandate pilot testing with target user groups before wide release, ensuring that apps meet usability and cultural relevance standards (Moriarty et al., 2022). Procurement policies should prefer tools supported by clinical trial evidence and robust data governance practices, reinforcing accountability and safeguarding user trust (Pruden, 2025). As the field continues to evolve, there is an urgent need for standardized evaluation frameworks, regulatory oversight, and seamless integration of digital tools with broader health care systems to ensure both quality and safety for users (Löchner et al., 2025). The ongoing maturation of telehealth and mobile applications represents a critical step toward a more accessible, responsive, and patient-centered mental health care ecosystem. These technologies have demonstrated their potential to expand reach, reduce disparities, and enhance continuity of care, but their success depends on thoughtful implementation and continuous evaluation. Health systems should track access improvements and user satisfaction over time, using these metrics to guide iterative refinements and ensure that digital solutions deliver on their promise of equity and effectiveness.

The Promise of AI in Mental Health Care

AI-driven tools offer several compelling advantages (Dehbozorgi et al., 2025; Cruz-Gonzalez et al., 2025). Machine learning algorithms can analyze vast and complex datasets—such as electronic health records, speech samples, and behavioral patterns—to identify subtle markers of mental health conditions that might elude human observation (Baydili et al., 2025; Ni & Jia, 2025). For example, changes in language use, tone of voice, or facial expression may signal the onset of depression or anxiety long before these symptoms become clinically apparent (Malgaroli et al., 2023; Spytska, 2025). By detecting these early indicators, AI systems can support timely intervention, reducing the risk of symptom escalation and improving long-term outcomes (Humayun et al., 2025). Natural language processing (Lazarou & Exarchos, 2024) enables conversational agents and chatbots to engage users in dialogue, provide psychoeducation, and deliver structured therapeutic exercises based on evidence-based modalities such as cognitive behavioral therapy (Humayun et al., 2025; Balcombe, 2023; Vaidyam et al., 2019). These tools can operate asynchronously, offering immediate support to individuals who may be reluctant to seek in-person care due to stigma, cost, or logistical barriers. Importantly, AI-driven conversational agents can serve as a bridge to more intensive care, guiding users toward professional help when risk thresholds are crossed (Spytska, 2025). AI also enhances clinical decision-making through predictive analytics and decision-support systems (Auf et al., 2025). By synthesizing patient data—including demographic variables, symptom profiles, and treatment histories—AI can generate personalized recommendations for pharmacological and psychotherapeutic interventions (Okposio et al., 2025). In high-volume settings such as emergency departments or primary care clinics, these tools can help prioritize cases, allocate resources efficiently, and reduce clinician cognitive load. Despite its transformative potential, AI must be implemented thoughtfully to avoid unintended consequences (Tavory, 2024; Saeidnia et al., 2024). Health systems should adopt a pilot-first approach, testing AI tools in controlled environments before scaling to routine practice. Pilots should include defined outcome targets, usability assessments, and workflow integration plans, ensuring that technology aligns with clinical priorities and does not disrupt established processes (Ball et al., 2025). Clinician involvement is critical; systems should include clinicians in tool selection and co-design, leveraging their expertise to identify practical barriers and optimize user experience (Ghadi et al., 2025). Governance frameworks should embed clinician-reported usability as a go/no-go metric, preventing the adoption of tools that increase administrative burden or compromise care quality. Furthermore, AI deployment must include bias audits and explainability features, enabling clinicians to understand how algorithms generate recommendations and to contest outputs when necessary (Funda, 2025; Freyer et al., 2024). Transparency is essential for maintaining trust—not only among clinicians but also among patients, who must be informed about the role of AI in their care.

Ethical and Practical Considerations

The integration of AI into mental health care raises complex ethical questions related to privacy, autonomy, and equity (Saeidnia et al., 2024). AI systems often rely on sensitive data streams, including speech patterns, facial expressions, and biometric signals (Baydili et al., 2025). Protecting this data requires robust safeguards, including encryption in transit and at rest, audit logging, and role-based access controls (Jiao, 2024). Consent processes must evolve to reflect the complexity of AI-driven care, offering clear opt-in mechanisms for secondary data use and dynamic consent models that allow users to revise their preferences over time (Chennupati, 2025). Algorithmic bias represents another critical challenge. AI models trained on non-representative datasets may produce inaccurate or inequitable outcomes, particularly for marginalized populations (Humayun et al., 2025; Lacmanovic & Skare, 2025). For example, a chatbot trained primarily on English-speaking, urban populations may misinterpret distress signals from rural or non-English-speaking users. Facial recognition tools may misclassify expressions in neurodivergent individuals or people of color. To mitigate these risks, developers must conduct fairness audits, validate models across diverse demographic subgroups, and publish performance metrics disaggregated by race, gender, age, and other relevant factors (Funda, 2025). Clinical deployment should include human oversight for all safety-critical decisions, ensuring that AI augments rather than replaces clinician judgment (Tavory, 2024).

Applications Across the Care Continuum

AI is being applied across multiple domains of mental health care, from early detection and screening to treatment personalization and relapse prevention (Dehbozorgi et al., 2025; Cruz-Gonzalez et al., 2025). In early detection, machine learning algorithms analyze linguistic and behavioral data to identify patterns associated with emerging mental health conditions (Malgaroli et al., 2023; Ni & Jia, 2025). For example, smartphone-based monitoring systems can track changes in typing speed, scrolling behavior, and app usage patterns—digital biomarkers that correlate with mood and cognitive function (Ikwuanusi et al., 2023). These insights enable proactive outreach, reducing reliance on self-report and minimizing delays in care. In treatment personalization, AI models synthesize multimodal data to predict which interventions are most likely to be effective for a given individual (Baydili et al., 2025). By integrating clinical, behavioral, and biological signals, these models support stratified care pathways, matching patients with the right level and type of support at the right time (Sun et al., 2025). This approach aligns with the broader movement toward precision medicine, offering a data-driven alternative to trial-and-error treatment selection (Baydili et al., 2025). AI also supports continuous monitoring and adaptive intervention through just-in-time adaptive interventions (Godfrey et al., 2021; van Genugten et al., 2025). These systems leverage real-time data from wearable sensors and mobile apps to deliver context-sensitive prompts, such as relaxation exercises during periods of heightened physiological arousal (Layode et al., 2024). By coupling sensing with intervention, JITAIs create closed-loop systems that respond dynamically to user needs, enhancing engagement and improving outcomes. While AI offers powerful capabilities, there is a risk of over-reliance on technology at the expense of human connection (Canali et al., 2022). Mental health care is deeply relational, and therapeutic alliances play a critical role in treatment outcomes. Replacing or minimizing human interaction may undermine the emotional support and empathy that are central to healing. To mitigate this risk, digital tools should be positioned as complements—not substitutes—for human care (Vaidyam et al., 2019). Hybrid models that combine AI-driven support with clinician oversight offer a balanced approach, preserving the relational core of therapy while leveraging the efficiencies of technology (Spytska, 2025). Safeguards should include minimum human contact thresholds, ensuring that patients receive regular opportunities for face-to-face or synchronous interaction. Systems should also incorporate patient preference checks, allowing individuals to choose their preferred modality and adjust settings over time. These measures reinforce autonomy and prevent the erosion of trust in care relationships.

Toward a Responsible AI Ecosystem

Building a responsible AI ecosystem in mental health care requires coordinated action across technical, clinical, and policy domains (Saeidnia et al., 2024). Key priorities include: Transparency: Require apps and platforms to display evidence levels, privacy policies, and algorithmic limitations prominently (Camacho et al., 2022; Freyer et al., 2024). Accountability: Establish governance structures that include clinicians, ethicists, and patient representatives, ensuring that diverse perspectives inform system design. Equity: Conduct bias audits and validate models across demographic subgroups, publishing disaggregated performance metrics to promote fairness (Funda, 2025; Lacmanovic & Skare, 2025). Security: Implement encryption, audit logging, and third-party compliance certification for all clinical deployments (Iwaya et al., 2023; Inkster et al., 2023). Evaluation: Fund comparative effectiveness studies of certified versus uncertified tools, generating evidence to guide procurement and policy decisions (Humayun et al., 2025; Auf et al., 2025). Sustainability: Include contingency funds for maintenance, upgrades, and retraining, recognizing that AI systems require ongoing investment to remain safe and effective (Price & Van Heerden, 2025). Artificial Intelligence holds immense promise for modernizing mental health care, offering tools that can enhance precision, scalability, and personalization. Yet, this promise will only be realized if innovation is matched by accountability, equity, and human-centered design (Smith et al., 2023; Tavory, 2024). AI should serve as a partner—not a replacement—in therapeutic relationships, augmenting clinician expertise while preserving empathy and trust (Spytska, 2025). By embedding ethical safeguards, usability standards, and continuous evaluation into every stage of development and deployment, health systems can harness the transformative potential of AI without compromising the values that define mental health care (Löchner et al., 2025). The future of AI in this domain is not about replacing clinicians—it is about empowering them to deliver care that is more responsive, inclusive, and effective than ever (Vaidyam et al., 2019).

Extended Reality (Ferrar et al., 2021) for Immersive Therapy

Extended reality (XR), which encompasses virtual reality (VR), augmented reality (AR), and mixed reality (MR), offers immersive environments that are transforming therapeutic experiences (Carl et al., 2019; Lindner et al., 2024). These technologies enable users to engage with simulated scenarios that are interactive, controlled, and customizable—making them particularly valuable for exposure therapy, skills training, and psychoeducation. Before initiating XR-based interventions, clinicians should perform safety screening and contraindication checks, ensuring that patients are suitable for immersive experiences and mitigating risks such as motion sickness or dissociation (Hughes & Kalra, 2023). VR has been extensively studied in the treatment of anxiety disorders, post-traumatic stress disorder Post-Traumatic Stress Disorder (PTSD) and phobias. In VR exposure therapy, individuals confront feared stimuli in a safe and controlled virtual environment, allowing for gradual desensitization and tailored pacing based on patient tolerance (Carl et al., 2019). For example, a veteran with PTSD might revisit a combat scenario in VR, guided by a therapist who adjusts intensity and pacing to maintain therapeutic safety. To ensure fidelity and effectiveness, health systems should require competency-based XR training for therapists using exposure protocols, equipping clinicians with the skills to manage immersive environments and respond to adverse reactions (Lindner et al., 2024). Augmented reality (Basystiuk et al., 2024) overlays digital content onto the real world, enhancing therapeutic exercises and mindfulness practices (Lindner et al., 2024). For instance, AR can visualize breathing patterns during relaxation training or provide real-time feedback during social skills practice. These applications are particularly engaging for younger users and can be integrated into daily life in meaningful ways. Developers and clinicians should ensure AR content is legible and non-distracting, maintaining clarity while avoiding sensory overload. Beyond individual therapy, XR holds promise for group interventions, psychoeducation, and clinician training (Carl et al., 2019). Virtual environments can simulate social interactions, model coping strategies, or provide immersive learning experiences for trainees (Lindner et al., 2024). As XR hardware becomes more affordable and accessible, its integration into mainstream mental health care is likely to accelerate (Löchner et al., 2025). However, adoption must be accompanied by rigorous evaluation. Programs should measure the transfer of skills from XR to real-world contexts, confirming that immersive experiences translate into functional improvements outside the virtual setting (Carl et al., 2019). Despite its potential, XR requires careful attention to usability, accessibility, and clinical appropriateness (Lindner et al., 2024). Motion sickness, sensory overload, and technological barriers can limit effectiveness for some users. Moreover, therapeutic content must be grounded in evidence-based principles and delivered within a supportive framework (Löchner et al., 2025). Clinicians should document potential side effects and alternatives during informed consent, ensuring that patients understand both the benefits and risks of immersive therapy (Carl et al., 2019).

Wearable Sensors and Real-Time Monitoring

Wearable sensors have emerged as a transformative modality in digital mental health care, offering continuous, real-time monitoring of physiological and behavioral data that enriches clinical insight and supports adaptive intervention (Brasier et al., 2025; Xing et al., 2025). These devices—ranging from smartwatches and fitness trackers to EEG headbands and smart textiles—collect data on heart rate variability (HRV), electrodermal activity (EDA), sleep patterns, physical activity, and brainwave dynamics (Smuck et al., 2021). Each signal provides a window into the user's emotional and cognitive state, enabling clinicians to move beyond episodic self-report and toward a more comprehensive, dynamic understanding of mental health (Baumann et al., 2024). For example, elevated heart rate and skin conductance may indicate acute stress or anxiety, while disrupted sleep or reduced activity levels may signal emerging depressive symptoms. To ensure reliability, devices should be enrolled with clear calibration protocols and maintenance schedules, including periodic sensor checks and firmware updates (Ferrara, 2024). These operational safeguards preserve data integrity and reduce the risk of misinterpretation (Kargarandehkordi et al., 2025). The clinical utility of wearable sensors is amplified when integrated into digital therapeutic systems (van Genugten et al., 2025). In closed-loop configurations, sensor data informs real-time adjustments to interventions, creating a responsive feedback cycle that aligns with the principles of precision medicine (Xing et al., 2025). A mindfulness app, for instance, may prompt a breathing exercise when EDA signals heightened arousal, while a clinician monitoring HRV trends may detect early signs of relapse and initiate a check-in (Brasier et al., 2025). These systems exemplify the shift from static care to dynamic, individualized support. However, such automation must be governed by explicit consent protocols (Back et al., 2022). Users should be informed not only about the nature of the data collected but also about how automated interventions are triggered, what thresholds are used, and how they can opt out or modify settings (Hilty et al., 2021). Consent must be revisitable and context-sensitive, particularly for vulnerable populations (Lay et al., 2025).

In research contexts, wearable sensors enable large-scale, longitudinal studies that capture mental health trajectories in naturalistic settings (Kargarandehkordi et al., 2025). This ecological validity supports the development of predictive models and the identification of biomarkers that may elude detection in traditional clinical environments (Baydili et al., 2025). To support robust data collection, study protocols should include remote troubleshooting workflows and participant support systems that address device malfunctions, connectivity issues, and user fatigue (Brasier et al., 2025). These logistics are not peripheral—they are foundational to data quality and participant retention (van Genugten et al., 2025). Moreover, missing or artifact-laden data segments must be flagged automatically for clinician review, ensuring that decisions are based on valid signals rather than noise (Iwaya et al., 2023). Data quality checks should be embedded into analytic pipelines and visualized in clinician dashboards to support informed interpretation (Xing et al., 2025)

Ethical and Governance Considerations for Wearable Sensors

Despite their promise, wearable sensors raise complex ethical and governance questions (Spuskanyuk, 2024; Radanliev, 2025). Data ownership, consent, and interpretation must be addressed with clarity and rigor (Rizky Alifia et al., 2025; Bouderhem, 2023). Users must understand what data are being collected, how they are used, who has access, and what rights they retain over their information (Mone & Fayazullaeva, 2023). Clinicians, in turn, must be trained to interpret sensor data accurately, contextualize it within broader clinical formulations, and communicate its significance to patients (Hilty et al., 2021; Alzghaibi, 2025). Misinterpretation—such as assuming low HRV always indicates distress—can lead to inappropriate interventions and erosion of trust (Friend et al., 2024). Training should include case-based learning, multimodal data interpretation, and documentation standards that link physiological signals to clinical decisions (Almadani et al., 2025).

Equity and accessibility must also be prioritized. Wearable technologies often reflect socioeconomic disparities in access, digital literacy, and cultural relevance (Walter et al., 2023; Lorke & Stefanou, 2025). Systems should include multilingual interfaces, adjustable sensory settings, and compatibility with low-cost devices. Procurement policies must require accessibility testing across diverse user groups, and deployment plans should include strategies for subsidized access in underserved communities (Cruz et al., 2023; Kelshiker et al., 2025). Governance frameworks must define data stewardship policies clearly, including retention timelines, access controls, and secondary use restrictions (Bouderhem, 2023; Yhang, 2023). These policies should be reviewed regularly and updated in response to evolving legal standards and technological capabilities. Institutions must treat biometric data with the same ethical gravity as clinical records, embedding privacy protections into every stage of design and implementation (Dewa, 2025).

Wearable sensors offer a powerful means of enhancing mental health care through continuous, real-time monitoring (Hickey et al., 2021). Their integration into therapeutic systems supports adaptive, personalized interventions that respond to the user's physiological and emotional state. However, their use must be governed by rigorous standards for calibration, consent, data quality, and equity (Canali et al., 2022; Flores-Castañeda et al., 2025). By embedding these safeguards into clinical and research workflows, wearable technologies can fulfill their promise as tools for responsive, inclusive, and ethically grounded mental health care (Radanliev, 2025).

Toward an Integrated Digital Ecosystem

The full potential of digital technologies in mental health care lies not in isolated tools but in their integration into a cohesive, interoperable ecosystem. Artificial intelligence (AI), extended reality (XR), wearable sensors, and mobile platforms each offer distinct capabilities—but when combined, they enable adaptive, multimodal interventions that respond dynamically to the user's needs (Löchner et al., 2025; Ball et al., 2025). This vision of neuroadaptive mental health care is no longer speculative; it is increasingly attainable through interdisciplinary collaboration, robust infrastructure, and ethical, user-centered design (Price & Van Heerden, 2025). In an integrated system, data from multiple sources—physiological signals, behavioral patterns, linguistic cues, and environmental context—can be synthesized to inform real-time therapeutic adjustments (Xing et al., 2025). Consider a scenario in which a user engages in a VR-based exposure therapy session while wearing a sensor that monitors HRV and EDA (Akinode et al., 2025). An AI algorithm analyzes the data and modulates the virtual environment to maintain optimal arousal levels, while a mobile app delivers follow-up exercises and tracks progress (van Genugten et al., 2025). The clinician receives a dashboard summarizing engagement, physiological trends, and behavioral outcomes, enabling more informed and collaborative decision-making (Wang et al., 2022). To support clinical utility, dashboards must present synthesized insights rather than raw data streams, reducing cognitive load and enhancing interpretability (Volckens et al., 2023). Visualizations should highlight deviations from baseline, correlate physiological and behavioral markers, and include confidence metrics to support clinical judgment (Holly et al., 2023). Achieving this level of integration requires clear architectural standards. Interoperability protocols must be defined at the outset, including documented APIs, data schemas, and timestamp synchronization across platforms (Adegoke et al., 2025; Sadeh et al., 2023). These standards ensure that data flows seamlessly between devices, applications, and electronic health records (EHRs), preserving continuity of care and enabling multimodal analysis (Goktas & Grzybowski, 2025). Procurement policies should require interoperability certification, and vendors must commit to transparent update cycles and backward compatibility. Without these safeguards, digital ecosystems risk becoming fragmented, undermining therapeutic coherence and increasing clinician burden (Wibberly, 2024). Ethical governance is equally critical. Integrated systems amplify the complexity of consent, privacy, and accountability (Lay et al., 2025; Bouderhem, 2023). Users must be informed about how data from different modalities are combined, what inferences are drawn, and how interventions are triggered (Bayor et al., 2025). Consent frameworks should include layered disclosures, dynamic opt-in mechanisms, and clear documentation of data use policies (Rizky Alifia et al., 2025). Clinicians must retain authority over safety-critical decisions, and systems should include override capabilities, audit logs, and escalation protocols (Sheikh et al., 2021). Equity audits must be embedded into pilot evaluations, ensuring that integrated systems perform fairly across demographic subgroups and do not exacerbate existing disparities (Walter et al., 2023). Workforce impact metrics—such as clinician workload, burnout risk, and training needs—should also be included in success criteria to ensure sustainable adoption (Smith et al., 2023). From an implementation science perspective, integrated digital ecosystems require iterative pilot testing, stakeholder engagement, and continuous evaluation. Pilot programs should include diverse participant samples, usability testing, and contingency planning for data loss or service degradation (Friend et al., 2024). Evaluation frameworks must extend beyond efficacy to include accessibility, cultural relevance, and cost-effectiveness (Lorke & Stefanou, 2025). Institutions should adopt adaptive governance models that evolve alongside technological innovation, incorporating feedback from clinicians, patients, and community representatives (Shah et al., 2022). Training programs must equip clinicians with the skills to interpret multimodal data, integrate it into treatment planning, and communicate its significance to clients (Hilty et al., 2021). Likewise, developers must understand the clinical context in which their tools will be used, ensuring that design decisions support therapeutic goals and respect user autonomy (Kumar et al., 2024). In conclusion, the future of digital mental health care lies in integration. By combining AI, XR, wearable sensors, and mobile platforms into cohesive, interoperable systems, we can deliver personalized, responsive, and ethically grounded care (Löchner et al., 2025). This vision demands technical rigor, ethical clarity, and interdisciplinary collaboration. It also requires a commitment to equity, transparency, and clinician well-being (Price & Van Heerden, 2025). As we move forward, the challenge is not merely to innovate but to implement thoughtfully—ensuring that digital ecosystems serve as bridges to better care, not barriers that amplify risk. The directive is clear: define interoperability standards, embed ethical safeguards, and evaluate impact across clinical, operational, and equity domains (Akhtar & Rawol, 2025). Only then can integrated digital mental health systems fulfill their promise of transforming care for all.

Opportunities and Risks in the Digital Transformation of Mental Health Care

The integration of digital technologies into mental health care presents a landscape rich with opportunity—but also fraught with complexity. As artificial intelligence (AI), extended reality (XR), and wearable sensors become increasingly embedded in both clinical and non-clinical settings, they offer the potential to revolutionize how mental health is understood, diagnosed, and treated (Pedram & Piatkowski, 2025). These innovations promise to expand access, personalize care, and enhance therapeutic precision. Yet, their deployment must be guided by a strategic framing: every innovation target must be paired with a corresponding risk mitigation plan. Without this balance, the very tools designed to improve care may inadvertently introduce new vulnerabilities.

This chapter explores the dual nature of digital transformation in mental health care. It highlights the most promising opportunities for innovation and impact, while also critically examining the risks and unintended consequences that may arise. Understanding both sides of this equation is essential for developing responsible, equitable, and sustainable digital mental health systems. To support this goal, implementation strategies must include scenario planning for foreseeable harms, ensuring that ethical foresight accompanies technological advancement. Governance structures should be strengthened through the creation of multidisciplinary oversight committees that include clinicians, technologists, ethicists, legal experts, and individuals with lived experience. These committees serve not only as ethical gatekeepers but as collaborative design partners, shaping systems that reflect the values and realities of those they aim to serve.

Among the most compelling opportunities is the personalization of care. Digital tools can collect and analyze real-time data to tailor interventions to each user's unique physiological, behavioral, and contextual profile (Pedram & Piatkowski, 2025). AI algorithms can detect subtle shifts in speech, movement, or biometric signals that indicate emerging distress, while XR environments can be customized to reflect specific therapeutic goals—such as confronting a particular phobia or practicing social interactions in culturally relevant contexts (Pedram & Piatkowski, 2025). Wearable sensors provide continuous feedback, enabling interventions to adjust dynamically based on heart rate variability, electrodermal activity, or sleep patterns (Pedram & Piatkowski, 2025). This level of personalization enhances engagement, improves outcomes, and aligns with the broader movement toward precision medicine. However, pilot studies must assess not only clinical efficacy but also the cost-benefit ratio of personalization features, ensuring that complexity does not outpace utility (Pedram & Piatkowski, 2025).

Scalability and accessibility represent another major opportunity. Digital platforms—such as mobile apps, teletherapy systems, and AI-driven chatbots—can deliver support to individuals who might otherwise face barriers to care due to geography, cost, stigma, or provider shortages (Renuka et al., 2025). In low-resource settings, these tools can serve as a first line of support, offering psychoeducation, screening, and self-help resources. In high-income contexts, they can complement existing services, reduce wait times, and free up clinicians to focus on more complex cases. To maximize impact, deployment strategies should prioritize scalable components first, then integrate specialized modules as needed. Local referral networks must be embedded within digital platforms to ensure continuity of care and appropriate escalation. Moreover, accessibility testing must include underserved populations, ensuring that tools are usable across age groups, literacy levels, languages, and cultural contexts.

Continuous monitoring and early intervention are also central to the promise of digital transformation. Wearable sensors and mobile tracking tools enable the detection of early signs of distress, relapse, or crisis—often before symptoms become clinically apparent (Saksena et al., 2021). For example, a sudden drop-in physical activity or disrupted sleep may signal the onset of depression. An AI system could flag this change and prompt a check-in from a clinician or suggest a coping strategy through a mobile app (Li et al., 2025). These just-in-time adaptive interventions (Poudel et al., 2025) represent a shift from reactive to proactive care. However, systems must include triage rules that define thresholds for clinician contact versus self-directed interventions, ensuring that alerts are actionable and appropriately scaled. Participant protection protocols must also limit intrusive monitoring and provide opt-out options, preserving autonomy and preventing overreach.

The digital transformation of mental health care also fosters interdisciplinary collaboration and innovation. The convergence of psychology, psychiatry, computer science, engineering, design, and ethics enables the development of holistic, user-centered solutions. For instance, the creation of a neuroadaptive VR therapy system might involve clinicians to define therapeutic goals, engineers to build the hardware, data scientists to develop adaptive algorithms, and designers to ensure usability and engagement (Mohammad, 2021). These collaborations not only enhance the quality of the final product but also promote a more integrated understanding of mental health. To support accountability and transparency, development teams should maintain clear documentation of role responsibilities, deliverables, and decision rationales throughout the product lifecycle.

Yet, alongside these opportunities, significant risks and challenges must be addressed. Data privacy and security remain paramount concerns (Poudel et al., 2025). Digital mental health tools often collect sensitive personal information—including emotional states, behavioral patterns, and biometric data (Poudel et al., 2025). Ensuring the privacy and security of this data is not optional; it is foundational to maintaining trust and safeguarding user rights (Poudel et al., 2025). Systems must implement encryption at rest and in transit, rotate keys regularly, and log data access events for monthly review (Poudel et al., 2025). Consent processes must be granular, offering users clear opt-in mechanisms for secondary data use and dynamic controls that allow them to revise preferences over time (Poudel et al., 2025). Compliance frameworks should align with the strictest applicable jurisdiction, ensuring that protections are robust across borders.

Algorithmic bias and inequity pose another critical challenge. AI systems trained on non-representative datasets may produce inaccurate or discriminatory outcomes, particularly for marginalized populations (Kang & Exworthy, 2022). For example, a chatbot trained primarily on English-speaking, urban, white users may misinterpret distress signals from rural, non-English-speaking, or racially diverse individuals. Facial recognition tools may misclassify expressions in neurodivergent users or people of color. To mitigate these risks, developers must conduct fairness audits, validate models across demographic subgroups, and publish performance metrics disaggregated by race, gender, age, and other relevant factors. When disparities are detected, remediation protocols must be activated, including model retraining, stakeholder consultation, and public reporting of corrective actions (Kim & Backonja, 2025).

Over-reliance on technology is another concern. While digital tools can enhance care, they must not replace the human connection that is central to therapeutic relationships. Mental health care is deeply relational, and therapeutic alliances play a critical role in treatment outcomes. Systems must preserve minimum human contact thresholds in care pathways, ensuring that patients receive regular opportunities for face-to-face or synchronous interaction. Patient preference checks should be embedded into onboarding workflows, allowing individuals to choose their preferred modality and adjust settings over time. Hybrid models that combine digital and in-person elements offer a balanced approach, preserving empathy while leveraging technological efficiencies.

Regulatory and ethical uncertainty further complicates the landscape. The rapid pace of innovation has outstripped the development of formal oversight mechanisms, leaving clinicians, developers, and users without clear guidance. Key questions remain unresolved: What constitutes a medical device in the digital realm? Who is responsible for harm caused by an algorithmic error? How should informed consent be obtained in AI-driven systems (Zenker et al., 2022)? What standards should govern the evaluation and approval of digital therapeutics? To address these gaps, institutions must create interim ethical guidelines and establish liaison roles between developers and regulators. Scenario planning for foreseeable harms should be a standard implementation step, enabling teams to anticipate and mitigate risks before deployment.

Navigating the path forward requires a proactive and balanced approach—one that anticipates challenges, engages diverse stakeholders, and prioritizes the well-being of users. Staged rollouts with embedded evaluation gates can support responsible scaling, allowing for iterative refinement and evidence-based decision-making (Panarese et al., 2025). Co-design with users ensures that digital tools are relevant, respectful, and responsive to real-world needs. Evidence-based development, grounded in established psychological theories and empirical research, enhances credibility and effectiveness (Weiner et al., 2025). Ethical foresight enables the creation of safeguards and contingency plans, while policy alignment ensures that innovation is supported by legal and institutional infrastructure.

Ultimately, the future of mental health care will be shaped not only by what we build, but by how—and for whom—we build it. Digital transformation invites us to reimagine therapeutic relationships, clinical workflows, and the very nature of mental health itself (Morey et al., 2025). It challenges traditional models of episodic, in-person care and opens the door to continuous, adaptive, and personalized interventions. But this transformation must remain grounded in ethical practice, scientific rigor, and human-centered design. Technologies must be developed not only for efficiency but also for empathy, equity, and empowerment. By embedding governance, interoperability, and stakeholder engagement into every stage of implementation, we can create a future where digital mental health care is not only innovative—but inclusive, effective, and just.

CASE STUDIES AND EXAMPLES: DIGITAL MENTAL HEALTH IN ACTION

To fully appreciate the transformative potential of digital technologies in mental health care, it is essential to examine how these tools are being applied in real-world contexts. Case studies offer a valuable lens through which to explore the practical implementation, benefits, and limitations of digital interventions. They also highlight the diversity of approaches and populations served, illustrating how technology can be adapted to meet specific clinical, cultural, and logistical needs (Allgaier et al., 2023). Each case study should meet clear selection criteria, including transparent methods, defined outcomes, and clinical relevance (Rajpal, 2025). This ensures that examples are not only illustrative but also transferable to other settings.

This section presents a series of illustrative examples across different technologies—artificial intelligence (AI), extended reality (XR), wearable sensors, and integrated platforms (Correa et al., 2021). These case studies are drawn from academic research, clinical practice, and industry innovation, and they underscore the evolving landscape of digital mental health care (Ricciardi & Zomaya, 2025). Each example is analyzed to extract transferable lessons and limitations, offering insights that can inform future design, deployment, and evaluation. A comparative synthesis follows, summarizing common success factors across cases to guide implementation strategies and policy development.

AI-Powered Early Detection: The Mindstrong Platform

Mindstrong Health exemplifies the use of AI for early detection and continuous monitoring of mental health conditions (Mindstrong Health Study, 2018). The platform passively collects behavioral data from smartphone interactions—such as typing speed, scrolling patterns, and app usage—and applies machine learning algorithms to detect cognitive and emotional changes (Mindstrong Health Study, 2018). Clinical studies have shown that these digital biomarkers can predict relapse in individuals with serious mental illness, enabling proactive intervention and reducing hospitalization rates (Mindstrong Health Study, 2018). A key methodological strength is the validation of phone-derived features against clinical scales, ensuring that predictions are grounded in established metrics (Mindstrong Health Study, 2018). However, privacy safeguards must be robust: strong anonymization protocols are required before data is shared for research, and users must retain control over data retention and secondary use (Mindstrong Health Study, 2018). Transferable lesson: passive data collection can enhance early detection, but must be paired with rigorous privacy governance and clinical validation (Mindstrong Health Study, 2018).

Virtual Reality for PTSD: Bravemind

Bravemind, developed for military veterans with post-traumatic stress disorder (PTSD), uses VR exposure therapy to simulate customizable combat scenarios. Under clinician guidance, users confront trauma-related stimuli in a controlled environment, facilitating emotional processing and desensitization. Clinical trials have demonstrated significant symptom reduction, particularly when VR is integrated with cognitive behavioral therapy (CBT; Engel, 1977). The program includes clinician training in VR exposure protocols and safety management, ensuring therapeutic fidelity and risk mitigation. Screening for dissociation and vestibular vulnerabilities is essential prior to use. Between-session engagement and adverse event tracking provide additional safety data (Engel, 1977). Transferable lesson: immersive VR can enhance trauma treatment when paired with structured protocols, clinician oversight, and individualized pacing.

Wearable Sensors for Mood Monitoring: BioBeats

BioBeats' BioBase platform leverages wearable sensors to monitor HRV, sleep, and activity, delivering personalized stress-reduction interventions via a mobile app (Morgan et al., 2025). In workplace wellness programs, BioBase has improved stress resilience and sleep quality while increasing users' awareness of their physiological states. The platform's success hinges on voluntary participation, clear data use policies, and integration with organizational wellness strategies. Remote support and troubleshooting are critical for sustained engagement. Evaluation metrics should include sustained behavior change beyond initial pilot periods, not just short-term symptom reduction. Transferable lesson: wearable sensors can support preventive mental health care in non-clinical settings, but require organizational alignment and long-term engagement strategies.

Integrated Digital Therapy: SilverCloud Health

SilverCloud Health offers evidence-based digital programs for depression, anxiety, and stress, combining interactive content, self-guided exercises, and support from trained coaches or clinicians (SilverCloud NHS Trials, 2017). In the UK's National Health Service (NHS), SilverCloud has demonstrated comparable effectiveness to face-to-face therapy, while reducing wait times and increasing access. Integration with primary care referral pathways ensures continuity, and clinician oversight is maintained for higher-risk users. Cost-analysis data show per-user savings and resource shifts toward scalable care (SilverCloud NHS Trials, 2017). Transferable lesson: hybrid models that blend digital convenience with human support can improve access and outcomes when embedded within existing care systems.

Youth-Focused Gamified XR: SPARX

SPARX is a gamified digital intervention developed in New Zealand to address depression in adolescents. Using a fantasy-based role-playing format, the program teaches CBT skills through interactive quests and character interactions. SPARX is culturally adapted for Māori youth and has demonstrated effectiveness in reducing depressive symptoms. Youth advisory boards are involved in content updates, ensuring relevance and engagement. Long-term retention and symptom recurrence rates are tracked to assess durability. Transferable lesson: gamification and cultural tailoring enhance engagement and accessibility in youth mental health interventions, especially when co-design is prioritized.

Neuroadaptive Learning and Mental Health

Experts such as Thomas Insel, Albert Rizzo, Rosalind Picard have advanced concepts like neuroadaptive systems.

AI-Driven Crisis Support: Woebot

Woebot is an AI-powered chatbot that delivers mental health support through brief, daily conversations (Bibi, 2024). Using natural language processing (NLP), it engages users in dialogue, offers CBT-based strategies, and tracks mood over time. Woebot is available 24/7 and designed to be friendly, nonjudgmental, and easy to use. Pilot studies show reductions in anxiety and depression symptoms within weeks. Chatbot scripts are regularly updated to reflect current clinical guidance, and escalation paths are staffed to ensure timely human intervention when needed (Tsai et al., 2025). Scope and limits of automated crisis responses are clearly defined. Transferable lesson: conversational AI can deliver scalable, low-cost support when ethical design and safety protocols are embedded (Tsai et al., 2025).

Across these diverse case studies, several common success factors emerge:

Clinical Validation: Each tool demonstrates alignment with established therapeutic frameworks (e.g., CBT, exposure therapy) and includes validation against clinical outcomes or scales (Tsai et al., 2025). This ensures credibility and supports integration into care pathways.

User-Centered Design: Tools are tailored to the needs, preferences, and contexts of their users—whether through cultural adaptation, gamification, or personalization. Co-design with target populations enhances relevance and engagement.

Human Oversight: Even in highly automated systems, clinician involvement remains central. Safety-critical decisions are subject to human review, and escalation protocols are clearly defined.

Ethical Governance: Privacy, consent, and data stewardship are treated as foundational (Boda & Allam, 2022). Systems include opt-out mechanisms, transparency about data use, and safeguards for vulnerable populations (Pedram & Piatkowski, 2025).

Scalability and Sustainability: Successful implementations consider long-term engagement, cost-effectiveness, and integration with existing systems. Organizational support and infrastructure are critical to sustained impact.

Measurement and Iteration: Programs include mechanisms for tracking outcomes, user engagement, and adverse events. Feedback loops support continuous improvement and adaptation.

Interdisciplinary Collaboration: Development and deployment involve clinicians, technologists, designers, and users. This cross-sector engagement ensures that tools are both technically robust and clinically meaningful.

These case studies illustrate that digital mental health care is not a distant future—it is already here, evolving rapidly, and reshaping the way we understand and support mental well-being. By examining real-world implementations, we gain insight into what works, for whom, and under what conditions. The lessons extracted from these examples provide a foundation for responsible innovation, guiding future efforts toward systems that are effective, equitable, and grounded in human-centered care. As digital tools continue to proliferate, the imperative is clear: design with empathy, deploy with integrity, and evaluate with rigor.

EMBRACING THE DIGITAL SHIFT IN MENTAL HEALTH CARE

The digital transformation of mental health care is no longer a distant vision—it is a present reality, unfolding across clinical settings, research institutions, educational environments, and everyday life (Verma et al., 2023). As explored throughout this chapter, the integration of digital technologies such as artificial intelligence (AI), extended reality (XR), and wearable sensors is reshaping how mental health is understood, assessed, and treated (Poudel et al., 2025). These innovations offer unprecedented opportunities to personalize care, expand access, and enhance outcomes. Yet, they also introduce new ethical, technical, and systemic challenges that must be addressed with care, foresight, and inclusivity.

This concluding section synthesizes the key insights from the chapter and sets the stage for the deeper explorations that follow. It reflects on the implications of the digital shift, the responsibilities of stakeholders, and the guiding principles that should inform the development and deployment of digital mental health solutions. To ensure responsible progress, institutions must commit to measurable, equitable pilot programs and transparent reporting of outcomes. These pilots should include diverse populations, track both clinical and operational metrics, and publish findings in accessible formats to support replication and refinement (Lamb et al., 2025). The paradigm shift underway in mental health care is not merely technological—it is conceptual. Historically, mental health services have been reactive, episodic, and often siloed—limited by geography, workforce shortages, and stigma. The digital era enables a more proactive, continuous, and integrated approach. It allows for real-time monitoring, early detection, and adaptive interventions that respond dynamically to individuals' needs. This shift challenges traditional notions of diagnosis, treatment, and therapeutic relationships. It invites a reimagining of mental health care as a distributed, data-informed, and user-centered ecosystem—one that extends beyond the clinic and into homes, schools, workplaces, and communities. Central to this transformation is the promise of personalization and precision. By leveraging data from multiple sources—behavioral, physiological, contextual—digital tools can tailor interventions to the unique profiles of individuals. This aligns with the broader movement toward precision medicine and holds particular promise for populations that have been underserved or misunderstood by traditional models. Personalization enhances engagement, improves outcomes, and fosters a sense of agency. It also enables more nuanced understandings of mental health conditions, which are often heterogeneous and influenced by complex biopsychosocial factors. As digital tools become more sophisticated, they can support stratified care pathways, matching individuals with the right level and type of support at the right time.

However, personalization must be accompanied by rigorous evaluation. Institutions should prioritize longitudinal and equity-focused studies that examine not only symptom reduction but also functional improvement, engagement, and disparities in access and outcomes. These studies must include diverse samples and report subgroup effects to ensure that innovations benefit all populations equitably. Mixed-methods approaches—combining quantitative metrics with qualitative insights—can provide a more holistic understanding of impact. Research must also explore mechanisms of action, identifying which features of digital tools drive change and under what conditions (Poudel et al., 2025). This evidence base is essential for guiding policy, informing clinical practice, and shaping future development (Poudel et al., 2025).

Expanding access and equity remains a foundational goal. Digital technologies have the potential to democratize mental health care by overcoming barriers related to geography, cost, and stigma. Mobile apps, teletherapy platforms, and AI-driven tools can reach individuals who might otherwise go without support (Omiyefa, 2025). This is particularly important in rural areas, low-resource settings, and among marginalized populations. However, the promise of expanded access must be tempered by a commitment to equity. The digital divide—driven by disparities in internet access, device ownership, digital literacy, and cultural relevance—threatens to widen existing gaps. To ensure that digital mental health care is truly inclusive, developers and policymakers must prioritize accessibility, affordability, and cultural competence in design and implementation. Funded programs should set minimum access targets and report service reach by socioeconomic indicators. Ethical and regulatory imperatives must guide every stage of digital transformation. The use of digital tools in mental health care raises profound questions related to privacy, consent, autonomy, and justice. Sensitive data—such as mood, behavior, and biometric signals—must be protected with the highest standards of security and transparency (Kim & Backonja, 2025). Users must be informed and empowered to make decisions about how their data are used (Kim & Backonja, 2025). Algorithmic bias is another critical concern. AI systems trained on non-representative data can perpetuate or exacerbate disparities in diagnosis and treatment (Kim & Backonja, 2025). Ethical AI development requires diverse datasets, fairness audits, and participatory design processes that include voices from historically marginalized communities (Kim & Backonja, 2025).

Regulatory frameworks must evolve to keep pace with technological change. Clear guidelines are needed to define what constitutes a digital therapeutic, how efficacy is evaluated, and who is accountable for harm. Cross-sector collaboration—among clinicians, technologists, ethicists, regulators, and users—is essential to build trust and ensure safety. Institutions must maintain ongoing stakeholder oversight for major programs, embedding governance into procurement, clinical guidelines, and research funding criteria (Chen et al., 2022). This oversight should include independent ethics review, community representation, and mechanisms for redress when harms occur. Clinicians and educators play a central role in the successful integration of digital tools. Their expertise, empathy, and judgment cannot be replaced by algorithms or avatars. Instead, technology should augment their work—streamlining administrative tasks, enhancing decision-making, and enabling more meaningful interactions with patients. To fulfill this role, clinicians must be equipped with new competencies. Training in digital literacy, data interpretation, and ethical technology use should be integrated into professional education and continuing development (Weiner et al., 2025). Accreditation standards should include digital clinical competencies, and interdisciplinary collaboration—with engineers, designers, and data scientists—

should be encouraged to enrich clinical practice and foster innovation (Weiner et al., 2025). Educators, too, have a vital role to play. As digital mental health tools become more prevalent in schools and universities, educators must be prepared to support students' mental well-being in digital contexts. This includes understanding the benefits and limitations of digital interventions, recognizing signs of distress, and fostering digital resilience. School policies should define referral pathways from educational settings to clinical care, ensuring that students receive appropriate support when needed (Weiner et al., 2025).

The digital mental health field is still in its early stages, and rigorous research is essential to guide its development (Li et al., 2025). While many tools show promise, few have been subjected to large-scale, long-term, randomized controlled trials. Evidence is needed not only on efficacy but also on engagement, adherence, cost-effectiveness, and real-world implementation (Ricciardi & Zomaya, 2025). Funding agencies should prioritize pragmatic, multisite trials with diverse samples, and studies should report participant demographics and subgroup effects. Participatory methods should be used to ensure that interventions are relevant, respectful, and responsive to users' needs. Qualitative process evaluations can complement outcome trials, providing insight into user experience, therapeutic alliance, and contextual factors. Looking ahead, the future of mental health care is not just digital—it is adaptive, inclusive, and human-centered. It is a future where technology supports—not supplants—human connection. Where data empower—not exploit—individuals (Ricciardi & Zomaya, 2025). Where innovation is guided by ethics, equity, and empathy. This vision requires more than technological advancement. It demands a cultural shift—a willingness to embrace new paradigms, challenge assumptions, and collaborate across boundaries. It calls for humility in the face of complexity, and courage in the pursuit of change.

To realize this future, institutions must commit to open reporting and community benefit from public investments. Sustainability must be built into funding models from the outset, including provisions for maintenance, upgrades, and training. Stakeholders should document local priorities and compare them to case study lessons, identifying gaps and opportunities for adaptation (Fischer et al., 2025). Long-term stewards must be assigned for major digital programs, ensuring continuity, accountability, and responsiveness. The digital transformation of mental health care offers extraordinary promise—but only if it is pursued with integrity, inclusivity, and a relentless focus on human dignity. Technologies must be designed and deployed in ways that protect privacy, promote equity, and preserve the therapeutic relationship. By embedding ethical safeguards, usability standards, and continuous evaluation into every stage of development and implementation, we can ensure that digital mental health care serves not only as a tool for innovation but as a bridge to more compassionate, effective, and equitable care.

REFERENCES

Abdul Rahman, N. F., Davies, N., Suhaimi, J., Idris, F., Syed Mohamad, S. N., & Park, S. (2023). Transformative learning in clinical reasoning: A meta-synthesis in undergraduate primary care medical education. *Education for Primary Care : An Official Publication of the Association of Course Organisers, National Association of GP Tutors, World Organisation of Family Doctors, 34*(4), 211–219. DOI: 10.1080/14739879.2023.2248070 PMID: 37742228

Adegoke, K., Adegoke, A., Dawodu, D., Bayowa, A., & Adekoya, A (2025). Interoperability in digital healthcare: Enhancing consumer health and transforming care systems.

Adepoju, D. A., & Adepoju, A. G. (2025). Establishing ethical frameworks for scalable data engineering and governance in AI-driven healthcare systems. *Int. J. Res. Publ. Rev, 6*(4), 8710–8726. DOI: 10.55248/gengpi.6.0425.1547

GDPR Advisor (2025). GDPR compliance for mental health apps: Safeguarding sensitive data.

Agarwal, S., Jalan, M., Hill, R., Pantalone, E., Thrul, J., Sharma, R., Wilcox, H. C., & Robinson, K. A. (2025). Framework to Assist Stakeholders in Technology Evaluation for Recovery (Freeman et al., 2017) to Mental Health and Wellness. *BMC Health Services Research, 25*, 623. Advance online publication. DOI: 10.1186/s12913-025-12418-0 PMID: 40307807

Aiken, L. H., Lasater, K. B., Sloane, D. M., Pogue, C. A., Rosenbaum, K. E. F., & Muir, K. J.US Clinician Wellbeing Study Consortium. (2023, July). Physician and nurse well-being and preferred interventions to address burnout in hospital practice: Factors associated with turnover, outcomes, and patient safety. []. American Medical Association.]. *JAMA Health Forum, 4*(7), e231809–e231809. DOI: 10.1001/jamahealthforum.2023.1809 PMID: 37418269

Akhtar, Z. B., & Rawol, A. T. (2024). Artificial intelligence (Tizzard, 2025) and extended reality (XR): A biomedical engineering perspective investigation analysis. *Indonesian Journal of Electronics, Electromedical Engineering, and Medical Informatics, 6*(3). Advance online publication. DOI: 10.35882/ijeeemi.v6i3.5

Akhtar, Z. B., & Rawol, A. T. (2025). Artificial Intelligence (Leivaditis & Sepetis, 2025) & Extended Reality (Reddy, 2025) within Healthcare: A Multidimensional Biomedical Engineering (Rajpal, 2025) Investigative Exploration. *Biomed. Clin. Res. J, 1*, 1–22.

Akinode, A. O., Ayadi, O. E., Ezerioha, C. C., & Chika, P (2025). Machine Learning Approaches for Early Detection of Mental Health Disorders Using Wearable Devices and Big Data Analytics. environments, 4, 5.

Alhammad, N., Alajlani, M., Abd-alrazaq, A., Epiphaniou, G., & Arvanitis, T. (2024). Patients' perspectives on the data confidentiality, privacy, and security of mHealth apps: Systematic review. *Journal of Medical Internet Research*, *26*, e50715. DOI: 10.2196/50715 PMID: 38820572

Alifia, R. R., Sadeghi, M., Eluru, M., Jafari, M., & Grando, M. A. (2025). Bridging ethical gaps in digital health research: A framework for informed consent aligned with NIH guidance. *BMC Medical Ethics*, *26*(1), 132. DOI: 10.1186/s12910-025-01291-5 PMID: 41063017

Allgaier, J., Mulansky, L., Draelos, R. L., & Pryss, R. (2023). How does the model make predictions? A systematic literature review on the explainability power of machine learning in healthcare. *Artificial Intelligence in Medicine*, *143*, 102616. DOI: 10.1016/j.artmed.2023.102616 PMID: 37673561

Almadani, B., Kaisar, H., Thoker, I. R., & Aliyu, F. (2025). A systematic survey of distributed decision support systems in healthcare. *Systems*, *13*(3), 157. DOI: 10.3390/systems13030157

Alzghaibi, H. (2025). Nurses' perspectives on AI-enabled wearable health technologies: Opportunities and challenges in clinical practice. *BMC Nursing*, *24*(1), 799. DOI: 10.1186/s12912-025-03343-y PMID: 40598216

American Psychiatric Association. (2023). Digital [Resource Document. APA.]. *Mental Health (Detroit, Mich.)*, •••, 101.

Anklam, E., Bahl, M. I., Ball, R., Beger, R. D., Cohen, J., Fitzpatrick, S., Girard, P., Halamoda-Kenzaoui, B., Hinton, D., Hirose, A., Hoeveler, A., Honma, M., Hugas, M., Ishida, S., Kass, G. E. N., Kojima, H., Krefting, I., Liachenko, S., Liu, Y., & Slikker, W.Jr. (2022). Emerging technologies and their impact on regulatory science. *Experimental Biology and Medicine (Maywood, N.J.)*, *247*(1), 1–75. DOI: 10.1177/15353702211052280 PMID: 34783606

Armontrout, J. A., Torous, J., Cohen, M., McNiel, D. E., & Binder, R. (2018). Current Regulation of Mobile Mental Health Applications. *The Journal of the American Academy of Psychiatry and the Law*, *46*(2), 204–211. DOI: 10.29158/JAAPL.003748-18 PMID: 30026399

ASPE (2024). How health information exchanges support integration for behavioral health settings.

Auf, H., Svedberg, P., Nygren, J., Nair, M., & Lundgren, L. E. (2025). The use of AI in mental health services to support decision-making: Scoping review. *Journal of Medical Internet Research, 27*, e63548. DOI: 10.2196/63548 PMID: 39854710

Babu, A., & Joseph, A. P. (2025). Digital wellness or digital dependency? A critical examination of mental health apps and their implications. *Frontiers in Psychiatry, 16*, 1581779. DOI: 10.3389/fpsyt.2025.1581779 PMID: 40248604

Back, S. E., Acierno, R., Saraiya, T. C., Harley, B., Wangelin, B., Jarnecke, A. M., McTeague, L. M., Brown, D. G., Santa Ana, E., & Rothbaum, A. O. (2022). Enhancing Prolonged Exposure therapy for PTSD using physiological biomarker-driven technology. *Contemporary Clinical Trials Communications, 28*, 100940. DOI: 10.1016/j.conctc.2022.100940 PMID: 35664505

Baka, E., Tan, Y.-R., Wong, B. L. H., Xing, Z., & Yap, P. (2025). A scoping review of digital interventions for the promotion of mental health and prevention of mental health conditions for young people. *Oxford Open Digital Health, 3*, oqaf005. DOI: 10.1093/oodh/oqaf005 PMID: 40230873

Balcombe, L. (2023). AI chatbots in digital mental health. *Informatics (MDPI), 10*(4), 82. DOI: 10.3390/informatics10040082

Ball, H., Eisner, E., Nicholas, J., Wilson, P., & Bucci, S. (2025). How theories, models, and frameworks have been used to implement digital health interventions in services for people with severe mental health problems: A scoping review. *BMC Public Health, 25*(1), 1023. DOI: 10.1186/s12889-025-22189-2 PMID: 40098003

Bapat, C., & Jog, S (2025). Data-driven ethical guidelines for digitized mental health services: Principal components analysis. Frontiers in Human Dynamics, 7, Article 1549325.

Basystiuk, O., Rybchak, Z., Zavushchak, I., & Marikutsa, U. (2024). Evaluation of multimodal data synchronization tools. *Comput. Des. Syst. Theory Pract, 6*(3), 104–111. DOI: 10.23939/cds2024.03.104

Baumann, S., Stone, R. T., & Abdelall, E. (2024). Introducing a remote patient monitoring usability impact model to overcome challenges. *Sensors (Basel), 24*(12), 3977. DOI: 10.3390/s24123977 PMID: 38931760

Baydili, İ., Tasci, B., & Tasci, G. (2025). Artificial intelligence in psychiatry: A review of biological and behavioral data analyses. *Diagnostics (Basel), 15*(4), 434. DOI: 10.3390/diagnostics15040434 PMID: 40002587

Bayor, A. A., Li, J., Yang, I. A., & Varnfield, M. (2025). Designing Clinical Decision Support Systems (CDSS)—A User-Centered Lens of the Design Characteristics, Challenges, and Implications: Systematic Review. *Journal of Medical Internet Research*, *27*, e63733. DOI: 10.2196/63733 PMID: 40540451

Berardi, C., Antonini, M., Jordan, Z., Wechtler, H., Paolucci, F., & Hinwood, M. (2024). Barriers and facilitators to the implementation of digital technologies in mental health systems: A qualitative systematic review to inform a policy framework. *BMC Health Services Research*, *24*(1), 243. DOI: 10.1186/s12913-023-10536-1 PMID: 38408938

Bezyl, E. H. (2024). Mental health apps: Regulation and validation are needed. Global Forum DIA.

Bezyl, E. H. (2024). Mental health apps: Regulation and validation are needed. Global Forum DIA.

BHM Healthcare Solutions. (2025). Technology and the behavioral health shortage. Retrieved from https://bhmpc.com/2025/05/technology-and-the-behavioral-health-shortage/

Bibi, P (2024). Establishing Transparency and Accountability in AI: Ethical Standards for Data Governance and Automated Systems. In.

Boda, V. V. R., & Allam, H. (2022). Ready for Anything: Disaster Recovery Strategies Every Healthcare IT Team Should Know. *International Journal of Emerging Trends in Computer Science and Information Technology*, *3*(1), 38–46. DOI: 10.63282/3050-9246.IJETCSIT-V3I1P105

Boffet, A., Arsac, L. M., Ibanez, V., Sauvet, F., & Deschodt-Arsac, V. (2025). Detection of Cognitive Load Modulation by EDA and HRV. *Sensors (Basel)*, *25*(8), 2343. DOI: 10.3390/s25082343 PMID: 40285033

Bond, R. R., Mulvenna, M. D., Potts, C., O'Neill, S., Ennis, E., & Torous, J. (2023). Digital transformation of mental health services. *Npj Mental Health Research*, *2*(1), 13. DOI: 10.1038/s44184-023-00033-y PMID: 38609479

Bouderhem, R. (2023). Privacy and regulatory issues in wearable health technology. *Engineering Proceedings*, *58*(1), 87.

Brasier, N. K., Mahato, K., Princip, M., Matos Gonçalves, V., Mutuyimana, C., Bourke, S., Schaffarczyk, D., Goldhahn, J., Barata, F., von Känel, R., Kowatsch, T., & Wang, J. (2025). Next-generation wearable sensors for biopsychosocial care in mental health: A narrative review. *BMJ Digital Health & AI*, *1*(1), e000018. DOI: 10.1136/bmjdhai-2025-000018

Brotherdale, R., Berry, K., Branitsky, A., & Bucci, S. (2024). Co-producing digital mental health interventions: A systematic review. *Digital Health*, *10*, 128–145. DOI: 10.1177/20552076241239172 PMID: 38665886

Bunyi, J., Ringland, K. E., & Schueller, S. M. (2021). Accessibility and digital mental health: Considerations for more accessible and equitable mental health apps. *Frontiers in Digital Health*, *3*, 742196. DOI: 10.3389/fdgth.2021.742196 PMID: 34713206

Camacho, E., Cohen, A., & Torous, J. (2022). Assessment of mental health services available through smartphone apps. *JAMA Network Open*, *5*(12), e2248784. DOI: 10.1001/jamanetworkopen.2022.48784 PMID: 36576737

Canali, S., Schiaffonati, V., & Aliverti, A. (2022). Challenges and recommendations for wearable devices in digital health: Data quality, interoperability, health equity, fairness. *PLOS Digital Health*, *1*(10), e0000104. DOI: 10.1371/journal.pdig.0000104 PMID: 36812619

Carl, E., Stein, A. T., Levihn-Coon, A., Pogue, J. R., Rothbaum, B., Emmelkamp, P., Asmundson, G. J. G., Carlbring, P., & Powers, M. B. (2019). Virtual reality exposure therapy for anxiety and related disorders: A meta-analysis of randomized controlled trials. *Journal of Anxiety Disorders*, *61*, 27–36. DOI: 10.1016/j.janxdis.2018.08.003 PMID: 30287083

CDC. (2023). Health workers face a mental health crisis. *VitalSigns*.

Chaabene, S., Boudaya, A., Bouaziz, B., & Chaari, L. (2025). An overview of methods and techniques in multimodal data fusion with application to healthcare. *International Journal of Data Science and Analytics*, *20*(4), 1–25. DOI: 10.1007/s41060-025-00715-0

Chen, Z. S., Galatzer-Levy, I. R., Bigio, B., Nasca, C., & Zhang, Y. (2022). Modern views of machine learning for precision psychiatry. *Patterns (New York, N.Y.)*, *3*(11), 100602. DOI: 10.1016/j.patter.2022.100602 PMID: 36419447

Chennupati, N. (2025). Securing the Automated Enterprise: A Framework for Mitigating Security and Privacy Risks in AI-Driven Workflow Automation. *Journal of Computer Science and Technology Studies*, *7*(3), 624–632. DOI: 10.32996/jcsts.2025.7.3.71

Chithra, N., & Bhambri, P. (2024). Ethics in sustainable technology. In *Handbook of Technological Sustainability* (pp. 245–256). CRC Press. DOI: 10.1201/9781003475989-21

Clemens-Meyer, F. H., Lepot, M., Blumensaat, F., Leutnant, D., & Gruber, G. (2021). In Bertrand-Krajewski, J.-L., Clemens-Meyer, F., Lepot, M., & Publishing, I. W. A. (Eds.), *Data validation and data quality assessment. Metrology in Urban Drainage and Stormwater Management: Plug and Pray* (pp. 327–390).

CMS (2024). Interoperability Framework.

Correa, T., Pavez, I., & Contreras, J. (2021). Digital inequality and mobiles: opportunities and challenges of relying on smartphones for digital inclusion in disadvantaged contexts. Handbook of digital inequality, 62-74.

County Health Rankings & Roadmaps. (2025). Mental health providers: Ratio of population to providers. Retrieved from https://www.countyhealthrankings.org

Crameri, L., Hettiarachchi, I. T., & Hanoun, S. (2021). Effects of dynamic resilience on the reactivity of vagally mediated heart rate variability. *Frontiers in Psychology, 11*, 579210. DOI: 10.3389/fpsyg.2020.579210 PMID: 33551903

Cristofaro, M., & Giardino, P. L. (2025). Surfing the AI waves: The historical evolution of artificial intelligence in management and organizational studies and practices. *Journal of Management History*. Advance online publication. DOI: 10.1108/JMH-01-2025-0002

Crocker, K. M., Gnatt, I., Haywood, D., Butterfield, I., Bhat, R., Lalitha, A. R. N., Jenkins, Z. M., & Castle, D. J. (2023). The impact of COVID-19 on the mental health workforce: A rapid review. *International Journal of Mental Health Nursing, 32*(2), 420–445. DOI: 10.1111/inm.13097 PMID: 36461629

Cruz, S., Redding, A., Chau, C. W., Lu, C., Persche, J., Hester, J., & Jacobs, M. (2023, April). EquityWare: Co-designing wearables with and for low income communities in the US. In *Proceedings of the 2023 CHI Conference on Human Factors in Computing Systems* (pp. 1-18). DOI: 10.1145/3544548.3580980

Cruz-Gonzalez, P., He, A. W. J., Lam, E. P., Ng, I. M. C., Li, M. W., Hou, R., & Vidaña, D. I. S. (2025). Artificial intelligence in mental health care: A systematic review of diagnosis, monitoring, and intervention applications. *Psychological Medicine, 55*, e18. DOI: 10.1017/S0033291724003295 PMID: 39911020

Dehbozorgi, R., Zangeneh, S., Khooshab, E., Nia, D. H., Hanif, H. R., Samian, P., Yousefi, M., Hashemi, F. H., Vakili, M., Jamalimoghadam, N., & Lohrasebi, F. (2025). The application of artificial intelligence in the field of mental health: A systematic review. *BMC Psychiatry, 25*(1), 132. DOI: 10.1186/s12888-025-06483-2 PMID: 39953464

Dewa, Z. (2025). The relationship between biometric technology and privacy: A systematic review. *SAI Conference Proceedings*.

Dima, E. (2025). The impact of burnout in healthcare professionals on patient care quality: A review. *World Journal of Advanced Research and Reviews*, *25*(02), 2706–2710. DOI: 10.30574/wjarr.2025.25.2.0633

El Khoury-Malhame, M., Sawma, T., Hallit, S., Younis, C. J., Jaber, J., & Doumit, R. (2025). Cultural stigma, psychological distress and help-seeking: Moderating role of self-esteem and self-stigma in Lebanon. *PLoS One*, *20*(9), e0315063. DOI: 10.1371/journal.pone.0315063 PMID: 40997115

Elfouly, T., & Alouani, A. (2025). A comprehensive survey on wearable computing for mental and physical health monitoring. *Electronics (Basel)*, *14*(17), 3443. DOI: 10.3390/electronics14173443

Ellis, D. M., Draheim, A. A., & Anderson, P. L. (2022). Culturally adapted digital mental health interventions for ethnic/racial minorities: A systematic review and meta-analysis. *Journal of Consulting and Clinical Psychology*, *90*(10), 717–733. DOI: 10.1037/ccp0000759 PMID: 36227330

Ferrar, J., Griffith, G. J., Skirrow, C., Cashdollar, N., Taptiklis, N., Dobson, J., Cree, F., Cormack, F. K., Barnett, J. H., & Munafò, M. R. (2021). Developing digital tools for remote clinical research: How to evaluate the validity and practicality of active assessments in field settings. *Journal of Medical Internet Research*, *23*(6), e26004. DOI: 10.2196/26004 PMID: 34142972

Ferrara, E. (2024). Large language models for wearable sensor-based human activity recognition, health monitoring, and behavioral modeling: A survey of early trends, datasets, and challenges. *Sensors (Basel)*, *24*(15), 5045. DOI: 10.3390/s24155045 PMID: 39124092

Fischer, L., Mann, P. A., Nguyen, M. H. H., Becker, S., Khodadadi, S., Schulz, A., Edwin Thanarajah, S., Repple, J., Hahn, T., Reif, A., Salamikhanshan, A., Kittel-Schneider, S., Rief, W., Mulert, C., Hofmann, S. G., Dannlowski, U., Kircher, T., Bernhard, F. P., & Jamalabadi, H. (2025). AI for mental health: Clinician expectations and priorities in computational psychiatry. *BMC Psychiatry*, *25*(1), 584. DOI: 10.1186/s12888-025-06957-3 PMID: 40481455

Flores-Castañeda, R. O., Olaya-Cotera, S., & Iparraguirre-Villanueva, O. (2025). Exploring wearable technologies for health monitoring: A systematic review of applications, advantages and disadvantages. *Neural Computing & Applications*, *37*(33), 27957–27983. DOI: 10.1007/s00521-025-11605-8

Freyer, N., Groß, D., & Lipprandt, M. (2024). The ethical requirement of explainability for AI-DSS in healthcare: A systematic review of reasons. *BMC Medical Ethics, 25*(1), 104. DOI: 10.1186/s12910-024-01103-2 PMID: 39354512

Friend, S. H., Ginsburg, G. S., Picard, R. W., & Drazen, J. M. (2024). Key issues as wearable digital health technologies enter clinical care. *The New England Journal of Medicine, 390*(12), 1118–1127. DOI: 10.1056/NEJMra2307160 PMID: 38507754

Funda, V. (2025). A systematic review of algorithm auditing processes to assess bias and risks in AI systems. Journal of Infrastructure. *Policy and Development, 9*(2), 11489.

GAO (2022). Mental health care: Access challenges for covered consumers and relevant federal efforts.

Ghadi, Y. Y., Shah, S. F. A., Waheed, W., Mazhar, T., Ahmad, W., Saeed, M. M., & Hamam, H. (2025). Integration of wearable technology and artificial intelligence in digital health for remote patient care. *Journal of Cloud Computing (Heidelberg, Germany), 14*(1), 39. DOI: 10.1186/s13677-025-00759-4

Ghanim, R., Kaushik, A., Park, J., & Abramson, A. (2023). Communication protocols integrating wearables, ingestibles, and implantables for closed-loop therapies. *Device, 1*(3), 100092. DOI: 10.1016/j.device.2023.100092

Gilbert, P., & Van Gordon, W. (2023). Compassion as a skill: A comparison of contemplative and evolution-based approaches. *Mindfulness, 14*(10), 2395–2416. DOI: 10.1007/s12671-023-02173-w

Gkintoni, E., Vassilopoulos, S. P., & Nikolaou, G. (2025). Next-generation cognitive-behavioral therapy for depression: Integrating digital tools, teletherapy, and personalization for enhanced mental health outcomes. *Medicina (Kaunas, Lithuania), 61*(3), 431. DOI: 10.3390/medicina61030431 PMID: 40142242

Glass, J. E., Tiffany, B., Matson, T. E., Lim, C., Gundersen, G., Kimbel, K., Hartzler, A. L., Curran, G. M., McWethy, A. G., Caldeiro, R. M., & Bradley, K. A. (2022). Approaches for implementing digital interventions for alcohol use disorders in primary care: A qualitative, user-centered design study. *Implementation Research and Practice, 3*, 26334895221135264. DOI: 10.1177/26334895221135264 PMID: 37091101

Godfrey, A., Vandendriessche, B., Bakker, J. P., Fitzer-Attas, C., Gujar, N., Hobbs, M., Liu, Q., Northcott, C. A., Parks, V., Wood, W. A., Zipunnikov, V., Wagner, J. A., & Izmailova, E. S. (2021). Fit-for-purpose biometric monitoring technologies: Leveraging the laboratory biomarker experience. *Clinical and Translational Science, 14*(1), 62–74. DOI: 10.1111/cts.12865 PMID: 32770726

Goktas, P., & Grzybowski, A. (2025). Shaping the future of healthcare: Ethical clinical challenges and pathways to trustworthy AI. *Journal of Clinical Medicine, 14*(5), 1605. DOI: 10.3390/jcm14051605 PMID: 40095575

Hall, C. L., Gómez Bergin, A. D., & Rennick-Egglestone, S. (2024). Research into digital health intervention for mental health: 25-year retrospective on the ethical and legal challenges. *Journal of Medical Internet Research, 26*, e58939. DOI: 10.2196/58939 PMID: 39250796

Hassan Almansour, H. A., Almanajam, F. A., Alyami, M. A., Shawil Al-Mahamad, A. H., Saleh Al Zabid, N. H., Hamad Al-Mahamad, M. S., Yahya Al Hammam, H. N., Al Matif, M. Y., Almansour, M. A., & Mohammed Almansour, A. H (2024). Evaluating the Impact of Wearable Health Devices on Mental Health Outcomes: A Collaborative Study between Psychologists, Social Workers, and Nursing Staff. Journal of International Crisis & Risk Communication Research (JICRCR), 7.

Henderson, J. T., & Bekhuis, T. (2023). *Historical concepts of mental illness*. EBSCO Research Starters.

Hickey, B. A., Chalmers, T., Newton, P., Lin, C.-T., Sibbritt, D., McLachlan, C. S., Clifton-Bligh, R., Morley, J., & Lal, S. (2021). Smart devices and wearable technologies to detect and monitor mental health conditions and stress: A systematic review. *Sensors (Basel), 21*(10), 3461. DOI: 10.3390/s21103461 PMID: 34065620

Hiland, E. B. (2021). *Therapy tech: The digital transformation of mental healthcare*. U of Minnesota Press. DOI: 10.5749/j.ctv1xp9q3t

Hilty, D. M., Armstrong, C. M., Luxton, D. D., Gentry, M. T., & Krupinski, E. A. (2021). A scoping review of sensors, wearables, and remote monitoring for behavioral health: Uses, outcomes, clinical competencies, and research directions. *Journal of Technology in Behavioral Science, 6*(2), 278–313. DOI: 10.1007/s41347-021-00199-2 PMID: 33501372

Holly, L., Thom, S., Elzemety, M., Murage, B., Mathieson, K., & Iñigo Petralanda, M. I. (2023). Strengthening health data governance: New equity and rights-based principles. *International Journal of Health Governance, 28*(3), 225–237. DOI: 10.1108/IJHG-11-2022-0104

Huang, J., Wang, H., Wu, Q., Yin, J., Zhou, H., & He, Y. (2024). Clinical research on neurological and psychiatric diagnosis and monitoring using wearable devices: A literature review. *Interdisciplinary Medicine*, *2*(4), e20230037. DOI: 10.1002/INMD.20230037

Hughes, N., & Kalra, D. (2023). Data standards and platform interoperability. In *Real-World Evidence in Medical Product Development* (pp. 79–107). Springer. DOI: 10.1007/978-3-031-26328-6_6

Humayun, A., Madawana, A. M., Hassan, A., Mahmud, A., Kamaruddin, N., Noor, S. H., Noor, S. H., & Awang Nawi, M. A. (2025). Artificial intelligence as a predictive tool for mental health status: Insights from a systematic review and meta-analysis. *PLoS One*, *20*(9), e0332207. DOI: 10.1371/journal.pone.0332207 PMID: 41004515

Ikwuanusi, U. F., Adepoju, P. A., & Odionu, C. S (2023). Advancing ethical AI practices to solve data privacy issues in library systems. International journal of multidisciplinary research updates, 6(1), 033-044.

Immanuel, S., Teferra, M. N., Baumert, M., & Bidargaddi, N. (2023). Heart rate variability for evaluating psychological stress changes in healthy adults: A scoping review. *Neuropsychobiology*, *82*(4), 187–202. DOI: 10.1159/000530376 PMID: 37290411

Inkster, B., Knibbs, C., & Bada, M. (2023). Cybersecurity: A critical priority for digital mental health. *Frontiers in Digital Health*, *5*, 1242264. DOI: 10.3389/fdgth.2023.1242264 PMID: 37781452

Islam, R., & Bae, S. W. (2024). Revolutionizing mental health support: An innovative affective mobile framework for dynamic, proactive, and context-adaptive conversational agents. arXiv preprint arXiv:2406.15942.

Iwaya, L. H., Babar, M. A., Rashid, A., & Wijayarathna, C. (2023). On the privacy of mental health apps: An empirical investigation and its implications for app development. *Empirical Software Engineering*, *28*(1), 2. DOI: 10.1007/s10664-022-10236-0 PMID: 36407814

Jain, A., & Jain, A (2025). AI-Based Emotion Detection System in Healthcare for Patient. Generative Artificial Intelligence for Biomedical and Smart Health Informatics, 455-470.

Jena, N. (2024). Promoting Health Equity in Digital Mental Health: Insights from Medical Anthropology for Global Mental Health. *Journal of Social Research*, *17*(4), 155258.

Jiao, C. (2024). A mental health monitoring system based on intelligent algorithms and biosensors: Algorithm behaviour analysis and intervention strategies. *Molecular & Cellular Biomechanics, 21*(1), 357–357. DOI: 10.62617/mcb.v21i1.357

Johnson, K. B., Wei, W. Q., Weeraratne, D., Frisse, M. E., Misulis, K., Rhee, K., Zhao, J., & Snowdon, J. L. (2021). Precision medicine, AI, and the future of personalized health care. *Clinical and Translational Science, 14*(1), 86–93. DOI: 10.1111/cts.12884 PMID: 32961010

Jones, A. (2024). *Ensuring that digital mental health benefits everyone*. APA Services.

Kang, H. S., & Exworthy, M. (2022). Wearing the future—wearables to empower users to take greater responsibility for their health and care: Scoping review. *JMIR mHealth and uHealth, 10*(7), e35684. DOI: 10.2196/35684 PMID: 35830222

Kargarandehkordi, A., Li, S., Lin, K., Phillips, K. T., Benzo, R. M., & Washington, P. (2025). Fusing wearable biosensors with artificial intelligence for mental health monitoring: A systematic review. *Biosensors (Basel), 15*(4), 202. DOI: 10.3390/bios15040202 PMID: 40277515

Kelshiker, A., Cheng, S., Achar, J., Celi, L. A., Jain, D., Nguyen, T., . . . Evans, B. (2025). Bridging the Regulatory Divide: Ensuring Safety and Equity in Wearable Health Technologies. *arXiv preprint arXiv:2508.20031*.

Khoo, Y. X., Kang, R. M., Reynolds, T. L., & Mentis, H. M. (2024). The comprehensiveness of mental health application users' privacy and security concerns. *CHI Conference on Human Factors in Computing Systems*, 16 pages.

Kim, J., & Backonja, U. (2025). Digital health equity frameworks and key concepts: A scoping review. *Journal of the American Medical Informatics Association : JAMIA, 32*(1), 45–59. DOI: 10.1093/jamia/ocaf017 PMID: 39936843

Kostadimas, D., Kasapakis, V., & Kotis, K. (2025). A systematic review on the combination of VR, IoT and AI technologies, and their integration in applications. *Future Internet, 17*(4), 163. DOI: 10.3390/fi17040163

Kourtesis, P. (2024). A comprehensive review of multimodal XR applications, risks, and ethical challenges in the metaverse. *Multimodal Technologies and Interaction, 8*(11), 98. DOI: 10.3390/mti8110098

Kumar, P. (2025). Securing Digital-First Healthcare: AI, Blockchain, and Cloud Architectures for Personal Health Data Protection. *International Journal of Applied Mathematics, 38*(7s).

Kumar, T., Arora, M., Verma, V., Bhushan, S., & Lalar, S. (2024). Biometric System Integration in Public Health: Challenges and Solutions. In Computational Intelligence and Mathematical Applications (pp. 168-173). CRC Press.

Lacmanovic, S., & Skare, M. (2025). Artificial intelligence bias auditing – current approaches, challenges and lessons from practice. *Review of Accounting and Finance, 24*(3), 375–400. DOI: 10.1108/RAF-01-2025-0006

Lamb, R., Choi, I., & Owens, T (2025). Convergence of Extended Reality, Artificial Intelligence, Machine Leaning, and Wearable Sensors in the Field of Education. Mental Health Virtual Reality: The Power of Immersive Worlds, 113-128.

Langat, C. A. (2025). Critical analysis of current global trends in mental health: Challenges, innovations, and future directions. *International Journal of Innovative Science and Research Technology, 10*(1), 2493–2515.

Lay, W., Gasparini, L., Siero, W., & Hughes, E. K. (2025). A rapid review of the benefits and challenges of dynamic consent. *Research Ethics, 21*(1), 180–202. DOI: 10.1177/17470161241278064

Layode, O., Naiho, H. N. N., Adeleke, G. S., Udeh, E. O., & Labake, T. T. (2024). Data privacy and security challenges in environmental research: Approaches to safeguarding sensitive information. *International Journal of Applied Research in Social Sciences, 6*(6), 1193–1214. DOI: 10.51594/ijarss.v6i6.1210

Lazarou, E., & Exarchos, T. P. (2024). Predicting stress levels using physiological data: Real-time stress prediction models utilizing wearable devices. *AIMS Neuroscience, 11*(2), 76–102. DOI: 10.3934/Neuroscience.2024006 PMID: 38988886

Leivaditis, V., & Sepetis, A (2025). Digital Transformation As A Catalyst For Sustainable Health Care Systems: A Narrative Review Of Current Evidence. International Journal of Innovation Management, 29(05n06), 2540009.

Li, M., Patel, J., & Katapally, T. R. (2025). The impact of extended reality cognitive behavioral therapy on mental disorders among children and youth: A systematic review and meta-analysis protocol. *PLoS One, 20*(3), e0315313. DOI: 10.1371/journal.pone.0315313 PMID: 40048453

Lindner, P., Miloff, A., & Carlbring, P. (2024). The future of virtual reality therapy: Applications, challenges, and research directions. *Frontiers in Virtual Reality, 5*, 112345.

Liu, M., & Schueller, S. M. (2023). Moving evidence-based mental health interventions into practice: Implementation of digital mental health interventions. *Current Treatment Options in Psychiatry, 10*(4), 333–345. DOI: 10.1007/s40501-023-00298-2

Livieri, G., Mangina, E., Protopapadakis, E. D., & Panayiotou, A. G. (2025). The gaps and challenges in digital health technology use as perceived by patients: A scoping review and narrative meta-synthesis. *Frontiers in Digital Health*, *7*, 1474956. DOI: 10.3389/fdgth.2025.1474956 PMID: 40212901

Löchner, J., Carlbring, P., Schuller, B., Torous, J., & Sander, L. B. (2025). Digital interventions in mental health: An overview and future perspectives. *Internet Interventions : The Application of Information Technology in Mental and Behavioural Health*, *40*, 100824. DOI: 10.1016/j.invent.2025.100824 PMID: 40330743

Lorke, M., & Stefanou, T. (2025). Improving research and development of wearable assistive and rehabilitation technologies: A systematic review on diversity factors. *Journal of Neuroengineering and Rehabilitation*, *22*(1), 31. DOI: 10.1186/s12984-025-01562-7 PMID: 39985039

Loud, G. (2025). *The promise and policy challenges of digital mental health solutions*. Bipartisan Policy Center.

Lyndon, A (2015). Burnout among health professionals and its effect on patient safety. PSNet Perspectives.

Ma, C.-B., Shang, X., Sun, M., Bo, X., Bai, J., Du, Y., & Zhou, M. (2025). Emerging Multifunctional Wearable Sensors: Integrating Multimodal Sweat Analysis and Advanced Material Technologies for Next-Generation Health Monitoring. *ACS Sensors*, *10*(4), 2388–2408. DOI: 10.1021/acssensors.4c03396 PMID: 40162570

Mackey, S., Aghaeepour, N., Gaudilliere, B., Kao, M.-C., Kaptan, M., Lannon, E., Pfyffer, D., & Weber, K. (2025). Innovations in acute and chronic pain biomarkers: Enhancing diagnosis and personalized therapy. *Regional Anesthesia and Pain Medicine*, *50*(2), 110–120. DOI: 10.1136/rapm-2024-106030 PMID: 39909549

Mahon, D. (2023). Empirically Supported Treatments: A Brief History. In Evidence Based Counselling & Psychotherapy for the 21st Century Practitioner (pp. 3-14). Emerald Publishing Limited. DOI: 10.1108/978-1-80455-732-720231001

Malgaroli, M., Hull, T. D., Zech, J. M., & Althoff, T. (2023). Natural language processing for mental health interventions: A systematic review and research framework. *Translational Psychiatry*, *13*(1), 309. DOI: 10.1038/s41398-023-02592-2 PMID: 37798296

Marriott, B. R., Meyer, A. E., Feagans, A., Batch, B. L., & Adams, Z. W. (2025). Characterizing fidelity monitoring practices in community behavioral health care. *The Journal of Behavioral Health Services & Research*. PMID: 40931317

Martí-Noguera, J. J. (2025). *Governing Digital Mental Health: Introducing the.* Model and the Digital Behavioral Health Expert. SpringerBriefs in Public Health. DOI: 10.1007/978-3-031-94763-6

Megahed Ibrahim, A., Ramadan Abdel-Aziz, H., Mohamed, H. A. H., Zaghamir, D. E. F., Wahba, N. M. I., Hassan, G. A., & Shaban, M. (2024). Balancing confidentiality and care coordination: Challenges in patient privacy. *BMC Nursing*, *23*(1), 564. Advance online publication. DOI: 10.1186/s12912-024-02231-1 PMID: 39148055

Mescher, T., Hacker, R. L., Martinez, L. A., Morris, C. D., Mishkind, M. C., & Garver-Apgar, C. E. (2025). Mobile health apps: Guidance for evaluation and implementation by healthcare workers. *Journal of Technology in Behavioral Science*, *10*(2), 224–235. DOI: 10.1007/s41347-024-00441-7

Mitsea, E., Drigas, A., & Skianis, C. (2024). Artificial intelligence, immersive technologies, and neurotechnologies in breathing interventions for mental and emotional health: A systematic review. *Electronics (Basel)*, *13*(12), 2253. DOI: 10.3390/electronics13122253

Mohammad, N. (2021). Enhancing security and privacy in multi-cloud environments: A comprehensive study on encryption techniques and access control mechanisms. [IJCET]. *International Journal of Computer Engineering and Technology*, *12*(2), 51–63.

Mone, V., & Fayazullaeva, S. (2023). Health data on the go: Navigating privacy concerns with wearable technologies. *Legal Information Management*, *23*(3), 179–188. DOI: 10.1017/S1472669623000427

Morey, D. A., Rayo, M. F., & Woods, D. D. (2025). Empirically derived evaluation requirements for responsible deployments of AI in safety-critical settings. *NPJ Digital Medicine*, *8*(1), 374. DOI: 10.1038/s41746-025-01784-y PMID: 40533485

Morgan, J. W., Patel, R. A., & Campbell, S. (2025). Practical considerations of clinical XR (Singh & Chandra, 2025) deployments. *Frontiers in Virtual Reality*, *6*, 1517402. DOI: 10.3389/frvir.2025.1517402

Moriarty, A. S., Meader, N., Snell, K. I., Riley, R. D., Paton, L. W., Dawson, S., Hendon, J., Chew-Graham, C. A., Gilbody, S., Churchill, R., Phillips, R. S., Ali, S., & McMillan, D. (2022). Predicting relapse or recurrence of depression: Systematic review of prognostic models. *The British Journal of Psychiatry : The Journal of Mental Science*, *221*(2), 448–458. DOI: 10.1192/bjp.2021.218 PMID: 35048843

Mulukuntla, S. (2025). Monitoring and Remote Patient Management with Immersive Technologies. In Augmented Wellness: Exploring the Power of VR and AR in Healthcare (pp. 197-218). Springer. DOI: 10.1007/978-981-96-2952-7_9

Naderbagi, A., Loblay, V., Zahed, I. U. M., Ekambareshwar, M., Poulsen, A., Song, Y. J., Ospina-Pinillos, L., Krausz, M., Mamdouh Kamel, M., Hickie, I. B., & LaMonica, H. M. (2024). Cultural and contextual adaptation of digital health interventions: Narrative review. *Journal of Medical Internet Research, 26*, e55130. DOI: 10.2196/55130 PMID: 38980719

NASHP (2025). Key strategies for strengthening the behavioral health workforce.

National Academy of Medicine. (2020). Taking action against clinician burnout: A systems approach to professional well-being.

Ni, Y., & Jia, F. (2025). A scoping review of AI-driven digital interventions in mental health care: Mapping applications across screening, support, monitoring, prevention, and clinical education. *Health Care, 13*(10), 1205. PMID: 40428041

Nittas, V., Daniore, P., Chavez, S. J., & Wray, T. B. (2023). *Challenges in implementing cultural adaptations of digital health interventions*. Nature Human Behaviour Perspectives.

Okposio, B. O., Richard, G. A., Olatokun, T. P., Akadiri, O. O., Akpevba, E. A., John, J. O., & Okonkwo, B. A. (2025). Enhancing Mental health Outcomes through AI-Driven Predictive Analytics: A review of applications in neuroscience and substance abuse prevention. *International Journal of Biological and Pharmaceutical Sciences Archive, 10*(2), 024-048.

Omiyefa, S. (2025). Artificial intelligence and machine learning in precision mental health diagnostics and predictive treatment models. *Int J Res Publ Rev, 6*(3), 85–99. DOI: 10.55248/gengpi.6.0325.1107

Ong, T., Ivanova, J., Soni, H., Barrera, J., Cummins, M., Welch, B. M., & Bunnell, B. E. (2025). Mental health clients' perspectives on telehealth-based virtual reality therapy. *Frontiers in Virtual Reality, 6*, 1595326. DOI: 10.3389/frvir.2025.1595326

Ostrowski, K., & Goldberg, R. (2022). Designing an effective statewide data sharing agreement. California Health Care Foundation. https://www.chcf.org/wp-content/uploads/2022/03/DataExchangeExplainerDesigningStatewideAgreement.pdf

Pal, D. K. D., Saini, V., & Aakula, A. (2020). API-led integration for improved healthcare interoperability. *vol, 6*, 488-523.

Panarese, P., Grasso, M. M., & Solinas, C. (2025). Algorithmic bias, fairness, and inclusivity: A multilevel framework for justice-oriented AI. *AI & Society*, •••, 1–23. DOI: 10.1007/s00146-025-02451-2

Pedram, S., & Piatkowski, T. (2025). Exploring the potential of virtual reality (Johnson et al., 2021) in mental healthcare: A systematic literature review. *Virtual Reality (Waltham Cross)*, *29*(3), 135. DOI: 10.1007/s10055-025-01181-6

Poudel, U., Jakhar, S., Mohan, P., & Nepal, A. (2025). AI in mental health: A review of technological advancements and ethical issues in psychiatry. *Issues in Mental Health Nursing*, *46*(7), 693–701. DOI: 10.1080/01612840.2025.2502943 PMID: 40378075

Price, A., & Van Heerden, A. (2025). Editorial perspective: Digital technology and the future of mental health treatment. *BMC Digital Health*, *3*(5), 5. DOI: 10.1186/s44247-024-00146-0

Pruden, S (2025). Implementing Depression Screening and Treatment Algorithms to Reduce Post-Operative Complications for Patients Undergoing Cardiac Surgery The University of North Carolina at Chapel Hill].

Radanliev, P. (2025). Privacy, ethics, transparency, and accountability in AI systems for wearable devices. *Frontiers in Digital Health*, *7*, 1431246. DOI: 10.3389/fdgth.2025.1431246 PMID: 40599875

Rajpal, S. (2025). Exploring the Role of Virtual Reality and Metaverse in Treating Mental Health: Operating Models and Challenges in Adoption. *Journal of Computer and Communications*, *13*(10), 1–22. DOI: 10.4236/jcc.2025.1310001

Reddy, K. J. (2025). Integrating Technology into Clinical Practice. In Innovations in Neurocognitive Rehabilitation: Harnessing Technology for Effective Therapy (pp. 329-350). Springer. DOI: 10.1007/978-3-031-88117-6_15

Renuka, O., RadhaKrishnan, N., Priya, B. S., Jhansy, A., & Ezekiel, S (2025). Data privacy and protection: Legal and ethical challenges. Emerging Threats and Countermeasures in Cybersecurity, 433-465.

Ricciardi, F., & Zomaya, A. (2025). Perspectives on Managing AI Ethics in the Digital Age. *Information (Basel)*, *16*(2), 89. DOI: 10.3390/info16040318

Robinson, A., Flom, M., Forman-Hoffman, V. L., Histon, T., Levy, M., Darcy, A., Ajayi, T., Mohr, D. C., Wicks, P., Greene, C., & Montgomery, R. M. (2024). Equity in digital mental health interventions in the United States: Where to next? *Journal of Medical Internet Research*, *26*, e59939. DOI: 10.2196/59939 PMID: 39316436

Ross, G., Zhao, Y., Bosman, A., Geballa-Koukoula, A., Zhou, H., Elliott, C., Nielen, M., Rafferty, K., & Salentijn, G (2022). Data handling and ethics of emerging smartphone-based (Glass et al., 2022) sensors–Part 1: best practices and current implementation.

Sadeh, Y., Denejkina, A., Karyotaki, E., Lenferink, L. I., & Kassam-Adams, N. (2023). Opportunities for improving data sharing and FAIR data practices to advance global mental health. *Cambridge Prisms: Global Mental Health, 10*, e14. PMID: 37860102

Saeidnia, H. R., Fotami, S. G. H., Lund, B., & Ghiasi, N. (2024). Ethical considerations in artificial intelligence interventions for mental health and well-being: Ensuring responsible implementation and impact. *Social Sciences (Basel, Switzerland), 13*(7), 381. DOI: 10.3390/socsci13070381

Saganowski, S., Perz, B., Polak, A. G., & Kazienko, P (2022). Emotion recognition for everyday life using physiological signals from wearables: A systematic literature review. IEEE Transactions on Affective Computing, 14(3), 1876-1897. Pinel, P (1793). Traité médico-philosophique sur l'aliénation mentale.

Saksena, N., Matthan, R., Bhan, A., & Balsari, S. (2021). Rebooting consent in the digital age: A governance framework for health data exchange. *BMJ Global Health, 6*(Suppl 5), e005057. DOI: 10.1136/bmjgh-2021-005057 PMID: 34301754

Sangraula, M., Chauhan, J., Best, C., McEneaney, C., Shah, C., Brown, A. D., & Kohrt, B. A. (2024). The impact of task-sharing scalable mental health interventions on non-specialist providers: A scoping review. *Global Mental Health (Cambridge, England), 11*, e134. DOI: 10.1017/gmh.2024.129 PMID: 39811624

Saxena, S. (2016). Challenges and opportunities in global mental health: A perspective from WHO. *Epidemiology and Psychiatric Sciences, 25*(6), 495–498. DOI: 10.1017/S2045796016000536 PMID: 27666668

Scholle, S. H (2024). Digital mental health technologies: Gaps and opportunities in current U. S. regulatory authorities. Leavitt Partners Report.

Shah, R. V., Grennan, G., Zafar-Khan, M., Alim, F., Dey, S., Ramanathan, D., & Mishra, J. (2021). Personalized machine learning of depressed mood using wearables. *Translational Psychiatry, 11*(1), 338. DOI: 10.1038/s41398-021-01445-0 PMID: 34103481

Shahsavar, Y., & Choudhury, A. (2025). Effectiveness of evidence-based mental health apps on user health outcomes: A systematic literature review. *PLoS One, 20*(3), e0319983. DOI: 10.1371/journal.pone.0319983 PMID: 40131942

Sharma, R., & Meena, H. K. (2024). Emerging trends in EEG signal processing: A systematic review. *SN Computer Science*, *5*(4), 415. DOI: 10.1007/s42979-024-02773-w

Sheikh, M., Qassem, M., & Kyriacou, P. A. (2021). Wearable, environmental, and smartphone-based passive sensing for mental health monitoring. *Frontiers in Digital Health*, *3*, 662811. DOI: 10.3389/fdgth.2021.662811 PMID: 34713137

Shen, S., Qi, W., Zeng, J., Li, S., Liu, X., Zhu, X., Dong, C., Wang, B., Shi, Y., Yao, J., Wang, B., Lou, X., Gu, S., Li, P., Wang, J., Jiang, G., & Cao, S. (2025). Passive Sensing for Mental Health Monitoring Using Machine Learning With Wearables and Smartphones: Scoping Review. *Journal of Medical Internet Research*, *27*, e77066. DOI: 10.2196/77066 PMID: 40811794

Simbo AI (2025). Exploring the impact of clinician burnout on patient safety and satisfaction.

Sit, H. F., Ling, R., Lam, A. I. F., Chen, W., Latkin, C. A., & Hall, B. J. (2020). The cultural adaptation of step-by-step: An intervention to address depression among Chinese young adults. *Frontiers in Psychiatry*, *11*, 650. DOI: 10.3389/fpsyt.2020.00650 PMID: 32733296

Smith, K. A., Blease, C., Faurholt-Jepsen, M., Firth, J., Van Daele, T., Moreno, C., Carlbring, P., Ebner-Priemer, U. W., Koutsouleris, N., Riper, H., Mouchabac, S., Torous, J., & Cipriani, A. (2023). Digital mental health: Challenges and next steps. *BMJ Mental Health*, *26*(1), e300670. DOI: 10.1136/bmjment-2023-300670 PMID: 37197797

Smuck, M., Odonkor, C. A., Wilt, J. K., Schmidt, N., & Swiernik, M. A. (2021). The emerging clinical role of wearables: Factors for successful implementation in healthcare. *NPJ Digital Medicine*, *4*(1), 45. DOI: 10.1038/s41746-021-00418-3 PMID: 33692479

Souther, R., & Boughton, J. (2025). *The evolution of mental health services and modern therapies*. Mental Health Center of San Diego.

Spahl, W., & Rubeis, G. (2025). Integrating ethics in digital mental healthcare technologies: A principle-based empirically grounded roadmap approach. *Medicine, Health Care, and Philosophy*, *28*(3), 411–424. DOI: 10.1007/s11019-025-10283-6 PMID: 40736629

Spuskanyuk, A. (2024). Ethical implications of wearable digital health technology: Balancing innovation and patient autonomy. *American Journal of Health Care Studies*, *1*(2), 46–57. DOI: 10.61449/ajhcs.2024.7

Spytska, L. (2025). The use of artificial intelligence in psychotherapy: Development of intelligent therapeutic systems. *BMC Psychology*, *13*(1), 175. DOI: 10.1186/s40359-025-02491-9 PMID: 40022267

Stanford Law School. (2025). Digital diagnosis: Health data privacy in the U. S.

Stirman, S. W. (2022). Implementing evidence-based mental-health treatments: Attending to training, fidelity, adaptation, and context. *Current Directions in Psychological Science*, *31*(5), 436–442. DOI: 10.1177/09637214221109601

Subu, M. A., Holmes, D., Arumugam, A., Al-Yateem, N., Maria Dias, J., Rahman, S. A., Waluyo, I., Ahmed, F. R., & Abraham, M. S. (2022). Traditional, religious, and cultural perspectives on mental illness: A qualitative study on causal beliefs and treatment use. *International Journal of Qualitative Studies on Health and Well-being*, *17*(1), 2123090. DOI: 10.1080/17482631.2022.2123090 PMID: 36097886

Sun, J., Lu, T., Shao, X., Han, Y., Xia, Y., Zheng, Y., Wang, Y., Li, X., Ravindran, A., Fan, L., Fang, Y., Zhang, X., Ravindran, N., Wang, Y., Liu, X., & Lu, L. (2025). Practical AI application in psychiatry: Historical review and future directions. *Molecular Psychiatry*, *30*(9), 4399–4408. DOI: 10.1038/s41380-025-03072-3 PMID: 40456953

Surani, A., Bawaked, A., Wheeler, M., Kelsey, B., Roberts, N., Vincent, D., & Das, S. (2023, July). Security and privacy of digital mental health: An analysis of web services and mobile applications. In *IFIP annual conference on data and applications security and privacy* (pp. 319-338). Cham: Springer Nature Switzerland.

Tabassum, A., Ghaznavi, I., Abd-Alrazaq, A., & Qadir, J. (2025). Exploring the application of AI and extended reality technologies in metaverse-driven mental health solutions: Scoping review. *Journal of Medical Internet Research*, *27*, e72400. DOI: 10.2196/72400 PMID: 40829151

Tavory, T. (2024). Regulating AI in mental health: Ethics of care perspective. *JMIR Mental Health*, *11*, e58493. DOI: 10.2196/58493 PMID: 39298759

Tizzard, C. L. (2025). Re-imagining Care for Aging Disabled Adults.

Tsai, Y. Y., Chen, Y. J., Lin, Y. F., Hsiao, F. C., Hsu, C. H., & Liao, L. D. (2025). Photoplethysmography-based HRV analysis and machine learning for real-time stress quantification in mental health applications. *APL Bioengineering*, *9*(2), 026103. DOI: 10.1063/5.0256590 PMID: 40191605

Vaidyam, A. N., Wisniewski, H., Halamka, J. D., Kashavan, M. S., & Torous, J. B. (2019). Chatbots and conversational agents in mental health: A review of the psychiatric landscape. *Canadian Journal of Psychiatry. Revue Canadienne de Psychiatrie, 64*(7), 456–464. DOI: 10.1177/0706743719828977 PMID: 30897957

van Genugten, C. R., Thong, M. S., Van Ballegooijen, W., Kleiboer, A. M., Spruijt-Metz, D., Smit, A. C., Sprangers, M. A. G., Terhorst, Y., & Riper, H. (2025). Beyond the current state of just-in-time adaptive interventions in mental health: A qualitative systematic review. *Frontiers in Digital Health, 7*, 1460167. DOI: 10.3389/fdgth.2025.1460167 PMID: 39935463

Verma, H., Mlynar, J., Schaer, R., Reichenbach, J., Jreige, M., Prior, J., Evéquoz, F., & Depeursinge, A. (2023). Rethinking the role of AI with physicians in oncology: revealing perspectives from clinical and research workflows. *Proceedings of the 2023 CHI conference on human factors in computing systems* DOI: 10.1145/3544548.3581506

Volckens, J., Haynes, E. N., Croisant, S. P., Cui, Y., Errett, N. A., Henry, H. F., Horney, J. A., Kwok, R. K., Magzamen, S., Rappold, A. G., Ravichandran, L., Reinlib, L., Ryan, P. H., & Shaughnessy, D. T. (2023). Health research in the wake of disasters: Challenges and opportunities for sensor science. *Environmental Health Perspectives, 131*(6), 065002. DOI: 10.1289/EHP12270 PMID: 37389972

Walter, J. R., Xu, S., & Rogers, J. A. (2023). From lab to life: How wearable devices can improve health equity. *Nature Communications, 14*, 44634. PMID: 38167483

Wang, Z., Xiong, H., Zhang, J., Yang, S., Boukhechba, M., Zhang, D., Barnes, L. E., & Dou, D. (2022). From personalized medicine to population health: A survey of mHealth sensing techniques. *IEEE Internet of Things Journal, 9*(17), 15413–15434. DOI: 10.1109/JIOT.2022.3161046

Watson, D (2025). The dark side of mental health apps: Privacy concerns and therapeutic limitations. MentalHealthSigns.com.

Weiner, E. B., Dankwa-Mullan, I., Nelson, W. A., & Hassanpour, S. (2025). Ethical challenges and evolving strategies in the integration of artificial intelligence into clinical practice. *PLOS Digital Health, 4*(4), e0000810. DOI: 10.1371/journal.pdig.0000810 PMID: 40198594

Wibberly, K. H. (2024). Preparing mental health providers for the future: The case for moving beyond the elective telehealth course to integrating telehealth training throughout the curriculum. *Frontiers in Psychology, 14*, 1301569. DOI: 10.3389/fpsyg.2023.1301569 PMID: 38235285

World Economic Forum. (2022). Global Governance Toolkit for Digital Mental Health. WEF.

Wykes, T., Lipshitz, J., & Schueller, S. M. (2019). Towards the design of ethical standards related to digital mental health and all its applications. *Current Treatment Options in Psychiatry*, *6*(3), 232–242. DOI: 10.1007/s40501-019-00180-0

Xing, Y., Yang, Y., Yang, K., Lu, A., Xing, L., Mackie, K., & Guo, F. (2025). Intelligent sensing devices and systems for personalized mental health. *Med-X*, *3*(1), 10. DOI: 10.1007/s44258-025-00057-3 PMID: 40837134

Yhang, F. (2023). Safeguarding biometric data: Privacy, security and ethical considerations. *Journal of Biometrics & Biostatistics*, *14*(2).

Zenker, S., Strech, D., Ihrig, K., Jahns, R., Müller, G., Schickhardt, C., Schmidt, G., Speer, R., Winkler, E., von Kielmansegg, S. G., & Drepper, J. (2022). Data protection-compliant broad consent for secondary use of health care data and human biosamples for (Mulukuntla, 2025) medical research: Towards a new German national standard. *Journal of Biomedical Informatics*, *131*, 104096. DOI: 10.1016/j.jbi.2022.104096 PMID: 35643273

Chapter 2
Cognitive Science Foundations of Neuroadaptive Systems

ABSTRACT

This chapter explores cognitive science as the backbone for neuroadaptive systems, integrating psychology, neuroscience, AI, and systems theory (Radanliev, 2025). It examines mental representations, cognitive architecture, and learning mechanisms, linking them to adaptive technology design. Emphasis is placed on multimodal measurement EEG, HRV, behavioral data and context-sensitive modeling to inform interventions (Mohr et al., 2017). The biopsychosocial model and systems theory frame mental health as dynamic, requiring adaptive algorithms that respect developmental constraints and cultural variability (Mohr et al., 2017). These foundations guide later chapters on real-time feedback, personalization, and ethical deployment.

INTRODUCTION

This chapter grounds digital mental health technologies in the theoretical foundations of cognitive science, emphasizing how mental processes such as attention, memory, learning, emotion regulation, and decision, making inform the design of neuroadaptive systems. It presents cognition as dynamic, context, dependent, and developmentally constrained, challenging static diagnostic and intervention models. Core constructs, including mental representation, cognitive architecture, and learning mechanisms, are described as practical tools for clinicians and system designers alike. The chapter demonstrates how cognitive theories map onto measurable behavioral and physiological signals, linking laboratory research to real, world clinical applications. Particular attention is given to how constraints such as limited

DOI: 10.4018/979-8-3373-4997-8.ch002

working memory, attentional bottlenecks, and emotional interference shape both assessment and intervention outcomes. By integrating cognitive science with psychophysiological measurement and computational modeling, the chapter establishes a common interdisciplinary language that later chapters build upon. It also addresses how technology itself reshapes cognition, altering baselines for attention, regulation, and learning across the lifespan. The chapter argues that effective neuroadaptive systems must respect these cognitive realities to avoid maladaptive automation or excessive cognitive burden. Ultimately, this chapter provides a mechanistic foundation that enables digital interventions to be interpretable, developmentally sensitive, and clinically meaningful, reinforcing the central role of theory, driven design in responsible innovation.

COGNITIVE SCIENCE FOUNDATIONS

Cognitive science is the interdisciplinary study of the mind and its processes (Kourtesis, 2024). It integrates empirical methods and theoretical frameworks from diverse fields, including psychology, neuroscience, artificial intelligence, philosophy, linguistics, anthropology, sociology, and education, to describe cognition across multiple levels of analysis (Kargarandehkordi et al., 2025). This interdisciplinary stance enables researchers and clinicians to translate concepts and methodologies across domains, navigating distinct assumptions, measurement tools, and epistemological traditions. For clinicians, this integration clarifies how laboratory findings can inform assessment and treatment planning in real, world settings. For researchers, it underscores the importance of constructing models that are both mechanistic and testable in applied contexts. Cognitive science thus serves as a practical bridge between basic science and clinical application, without reducing one to the other (Kargarandehkordi et al., 2025).

This chapter outlines the foundational constructs of cognitive science that inform the design and implementation of neuroadaptive systems (Ma et al., 2025). These constructs are not merely theoretical; they provide clinicians and interdisciplinary researchers with conceptual tools and empirical methods to address complex mental health questions. By drawing on behavioral experiments, neural measurement, computational modeling, and qualitative inquiry, cognitive science offers a pluralistic approach to understanding cognition. For example, a clinician, researcher team might triangulate EEG indices of attention, behavioral task performance, and interview data to refine an assessment of treatment readiness (Engel, 1977). This methodological plurality directly informs later chapters on measurement integration and adaptive system design.

At its core, cognitive science seeks to understand how the mind works, how it can be modeled, and how its functions might be replicated or augmented through technology. Central to this inquiry are the mental processes that underlie perception, memory, learning, reasoning, decision, making, and language. These domains are not isolated; rather, they interact dynamically in response to task demands and contextual variables. Researchers therefore examine both discrete mechanisms and their coordination in ecologically valid tasks to generate clinically actionable insights. Clinicians, in turn, can translate these insights into assessment strategies that probe not only cognitive capacity but also the conditions under which those capacities falter. For instance, a patient may demonstrate intact memory under structured testing but show significant deficits in unstructured, emotionally charged environments, highlighting the importance of context, sensitive assessment.

Cognitive science also investigates how these mental processes are implemented in the brain. This means that cognitive theories are increasingly expected to map onto observable neural dynamics and network interactions, measurable through tools such as EEG, fMRI, and fNIRS (Boffet et al., 2025). For example, a memory deficit observed during neuropsychological testing may reflect impaired attentional control rather than a primary storage problem, an insight with direct implications for treatment planning. This emphasis on mechanism links directly to later discussions of psychophysiological measurement and adaptive system design. In clinical settings, it is therefore essential to document not only task performance but also the contextual and physiological variables that may influence that performance (Kargarandehkordi et al., 2025). A foundational concept in cognitive science is that of mental representation, the internal symbols or models the mind uses to encode, store, and manipulate information. These representations may take the form of images, sounds, words, or abstract concepts. Understanding how mental representations are formed, accessed, and modified is crucial for both diagnosis and intervention. In clinical terms, representational content shapes symptom narratives, while representational access determines whether a patient can retrieve adaptive coping strategies under stress (Kargarandehkordi et al., 2025). For instance, exposure therapy may reduce the emotional salience of a traumatic memory by altering how that memory is represented and integrated into autobiographical knowledge. This concept underpins many cognitive interventions, where modifying maladaptive representations is a primary mechanism of change. Thus, distinguishing between the format of a representation and the dynamics of its retrieval enhances both diagnostic precision and treatment efficacy.

Another key construct is cognitive architecture, the underlying structure and organization of the mind. Cognitive architecture encompasses the basic building blocks of cognition, such as memory, attention, perception, and reasoning, as well as the processes that govern their interaction. These architectures impose constraints, such as limited working memory capacity, attentional bottlenecks, and hierarchical control structures, that shape what can realistically be achieved in short, term therapy. For example, while training working memory may improve performance on related tasks, it will not automatically alter deeply held beliefs without targeted cognitive restructuring. Designers of neuroadaptive systems must therefore align adaptation rules with the affordances and limitations specified by the chosen cognitive architecture (Jain & Jain, 2025). When proposing an adaptive intervention, it is essential to specify which architectural component is being targeted and why.

Cognitive science also emphasizes the role of learning and development in shaping mental processes. Learning mechanisms determine how representations and architectures evolve with experience, while developmental trajectories place those mechanisms in time. This perspective helps clinicians anticipate which interventions are developmentally appropriate and which may require scaffolded practice. It also informs the design of adaptive systems that adjust difficulty and feedback based on the learner's current state. Learning is influenced by a range of factors, including reinforcement, imitation, instruction, motivation, emotion, and social interaction. For example, a clinician teaching emotion regulation skill might combine modeling, coached practice, and spaced rehearsal to promote durable learning. Later sections on neuroadaptive training machines draw directly from these principles to optimize intervention timing and feedback schedules (Ross et al., 2022). In short, understanding learning rules and developmental constraints enhances the design and delivery of interventions, particularly when technology is used to scaffold practice. In recent years, cognitive science has increasingly turned its attention to the role of technology in shaping cognition. This includes examining how interactions with digital artifacts, such as smartphones, computers, and virtual reality, affect attention, memory, and social cognition. Researchers are studying both the immediate effects of device use and the longer, term shifts in cognitive habits that emerge across development. For clinicians, this work highlights how technological contexts can alter assessment baselines and treatment expectations. For system designers, it motivates the creation of interfaces that support cognitive health rather than merely capturing engagement metrics.

Importantly, the cognitive effects of technology are not uniform. Some are transient, such as brief reductions in working memory during multitasking, while others are more durable, manifesting as habitual shifts in attentional control resulting from chronic media exposure. This variability underscores the need for clinicians and researchers to collect both short, term and longitudinal metrics when evaluating technology's cognitive impact. For instance, a patient may exhibit immediate performance decrements following digital distraction, but the more clinically relevant question is whether these effects persist over time and generalize across contexts.

This distinction is critical for later chapters on neuroadaptive timing and the design of interventions aimed at reversing cumulative cognitive strain (Chaabene et al., 2025).

Cognitive science, in this regard, offers a robust theoretical and methodological foundation for the development of neuroadaptive systems (Kostadimas et al., 2025). Its core constructs, mental representation, cognitive architecture, learning mechanisms, and technological mediation, provide a shared language for clinicians, educators, and system designers to understand and influence cognition. By integrating these constructs into assessment and intervention design, we can develop systems that are not only adaptive but also developmentally sensitive, context, aware, and grounded in the realities of clinical practice (Engel, 1977). As the field continues to evolve, the central challenge will be to maintain a balance between scientific rigor and clinical relevance, ensuring that our models of the mind remain both explanatory and actionable (Engel, 1977).

One of the enduring challenges in cognitive science is the development of comprehensive, accurate models of the mind. Effective model building requires balancing parsimony with explanatory power and ensuring that models generalize beyond controlled laboratory tasks (Islam & Bae, 2024). Strong models should generate testable predictions that can be evaluated in applied settings, including clinics, classrooms, and community, based interventions. For translational research, it is essential to document boundary conditions, clearly specifying when a model applies and when it does not, to avoid overgeneralization and misapplication (Rajpal, 2025).

Computational and hybrid models offer promising avenues for integrating data across levels of analysis, from neural signals to behavioral outcomes (Adegoke et al., 2025). These models must account for the complexity and diversity of mental processes, as well as the interactions among different cognitive systems. They also require empirical validation through rigorous experimentation. To support safe and effective clinical deployment, model developers should explicitly state the model's scope, input parameters, and known failure modes (Ricciardi & Zomaya, 2025). For example, a cognitive load model might accurately predict performance decrements under divided attention but fail to account for disruptions caused by intense emotional arousal (Ricciardi & Zomaya, 2025). This level of precision supports the development of safer neuroadaptive rules by constraining automatic adaptations to well, specified contexts (Ricciardi & Zomaya, 2025). Reporting model assumptions and validation metrics alongside any clinical implementation is essential for maintaining transparency and trust (Ricciardi & Zomaya, 2025).

The implications of cognitive science extend across multiple domains, including education, healthcare, and technology. Translating cognitive principles into practice often requires interdisciplinary collaboration to bridge theory, measurement, and implementation. In educational contexts, cognitive findings can inform curriculum pacing, the spacing of practice, and the design of feedback to optimize learning outcomes. In healthcare, cognitive models can sharpen diagnostic formulations, guide personalized rehabilitation strategies, and inform the timing and structure of therapeutic interventions. For technology developers, these insights highlight the ethical responsibility to design systems that align with human cognitive strengths and limitations.

Understanding how the mind works enables the development of more effective teaching methods, improved mental health treatments, and more intuitive, user, centered technologies. It also informs the design of artificial intelligence systems that interact with humans in ways that are natural, adaptive, and supportive of cognitive well, being. When translating cognitive findings into applied interventions, it is essential to prioritize those with clearly defined mechanisms of action and measurable outcomes. This approach avoids the trap of ineffective complexity and supports evidence, based practice (Ong et al., 2025). For example, an adaptive tutoring system that spaces practice based on retrieval difficulty has been shown to improve retention more effectively than systems relying on uniform repetition. These practical applications are explored in greater detail in later chapters on implementation science and adaptive system trials.

To ensure ecological fit and ethical alignment during deployment, it is critical to assemble stakeholder teams that include clinicians, educators, technologists, and end users. These teams can collaboratively evaluate whether a proposed intervention aligns with the lived experiences, developmental needs, and cultural contexts of the populations it aims to serve. This collaborative approach is particularly important when working with individuals with neurodevelopmental differences, trauma histories, or cognitive vulnerabilities, contexts in which the stakes of misalignment are especially high.

In sum, the theoretical foundations of cognitive science provide a powerful framework for designing neuroadaptive systems that are both scientifically grounded and clinically meaningful (Hiland, 2021). By attending to the nuances of mental representation, cognitive architecture, learning dynamics, and technological mediation, we can build systems that not only respond to user behavior but also support cognitive growth, emotional regulation, and adaptive functioning. The chapters that follow will build on these foundations to explore how these principles are operationalized in the design, implementation, and evaluation of neuroadaptive technologies in clinical and educational settings (Kargarandehkordi et al., 2025).

In conclusion, cognitive science is a multidisciplinary field that seeks to understand the mind and its processes. Its value lies in generating mechanistic insights that inform both basic theory and applied practice across diverse settings. A sustained focus on integration, linking neural data, behavioral measures, and ecological context, will make the field increasingly useful for clinicians, educators, and policymakers (Bond et al., 2023). Practitioners and researchers alike benefit when cognitive findings are translated into clear protocols, assessment tools, and design guidelines that are both actionable and adaptable.

Developing comprehensive models of the mind is not a one, time achievement but an iterative process. Progress depends on continuous cycles of translation from laboratory to field and back again. For example, a clinic that pilots a cognitive training app and shares outcome data with researchers contributes not only to the refinement of that tool but also to the evolution of the underlying theoretical model (Cristofaro & Giardino, 2025). This iterative loop, of design, deployment, evaluation, and revision, is central to the neuroadaptive systems roadmap described in later chapters (Tsai et al., 2025).

Sustained progress in this domain requires cross, sector partnerships and transparent reporting of both successes and failures. These partnerships must be grounded in shared terminology, aligned outcome metrics, and a commitment to ethical implementation. Interdisciplinary collaboration is not merely beneficial, it is essential. A joint workshop where clinicians and engineers align on outcome metrics, for instance, can reduce translational friction and accelerate innovation. This operational coordination is assumed throughout the chapter's design recommendations for neuroadaptive systems (Chithra & Bhambri, 2024). It is worth reiterating that cognitive science is not a static field. It evolves in response to new methods, emerging technologies, and shifting societal needs. For clinicians, this means staying current with methodological advances that influence assessment and treatment. For researchers, it entails a commitment to cross, disciplinary communication and shared standards. For all stakeholders, it demands ongoing professional development and a willingness to engage in interdisciplinary dialogue. By embracing this dynamic, integrative approach, we can ensure that cognitive science continues to inform the development of systems that are not only intelligent but also humane.

Social and environmental contexts shape mental health in tangible and measurable ways, influencing both risk and resilience across the lifespan. These contexts include interpersonal relationships, community resources, and institutional policies that systematically affect daily life, stress exposure, and access to care. Social connection functions as a regulatory system: close relationships provide emotional buffering, practical assistance, and behavioral models for coping that reduce physiological stress responses and support recovery. For example, a patient with strong family support is more likely to adhere to treatment and demonstrate faster symptom reduction than a demographically similar patient without such support.

Conversely, social isolation, discrimination, and economic hardship act as chronic stressors that erode regulatory systems and increase vulnerability to mental illness. Assessing these social exposures alongside biological and psychological measures clarifies underlying mechanisms and guides the development of socially informed interventions. Community, level factors, such as neighborhood safety, access to green space, and the availability of culturally competent services, further modulate individual trajectories and treatment outcomes. Clinicians should routinely document these community and service indicators in intake notes to inform environmental, level interventions. Researchers and practitioners alike must assess social exposures with the same rigor applied to biological and psychological variables, capturing both supportive and adverse contextual features. Doing so enhances ecological validity and enables interventions that target systemic contributors to mental health, rather than focusing solely on individual pathology.

Mental health and illness emerge from dynamic interactions across biological, psychological, and social domains. These interactions are often non, linear and time, dependent, requiring integrative models that map causal and feedback pathways across time. Feedback processes, where a change in one domain alters another and loops back, are central to understanding symptom emergence and persistence. For instance, interpersonal rejection may elevate physiological stress, which biases cognition toward threat, reinforcing social withdrawal and further rejection. Similarly, a single traumatic event can initiate a cascade, sleep disruption, heightened autonomic arousal, and negative appraisals, that becomes self, sustaining without intervention.

Mapping these interaction pathways helps identify leverage points for intervention. A single, brief family, based intervention might simultaneously reduce social stressors, shift maladaptive cognitions, and normalize physiological arousal. Clinicians can use simple schematic diagrams in case formulation to make these interactions explicit for clients and collaborating providers. In research, dynamic assessment methods such as ecological momentary assessment (Subu et al., 2022) and time, series analysis can capture the temporal structure of these interactions and inform causal hypotheses (Mahon, 2023). Including temporal sampling plans in study designs allows for the detection of bidirectional effects and the identification of critical windows for intervention (Li et al., 2025). Practitioners can use flow diagrams to represent patient, specific interaction chains, making complex systems clinically actionable and facilitating collaborative case formulation.

The implications of this biopsychosocial stance are clear: assessment must be comprehensive, treatment must be multimodal, and outcomes must be evaluated across domains rather than by symptom count alone. Comprehensive assessment includes medical history, cognitive testing, psychosocial stressors, and functional outcomes measured repeatedly over time (Ienca et al., 2017). A biopsychosocial treatment plan typically combines targeted pharmacotherapy when biologically indicated, evidence, based psychotherapy tailored to the client's cognitive and emotional profile, and interventions that address social determinants, such as housing support, employment assistance, or family therapy, when these factors maintain dysfunction (Okposio et al., 2025).

For example, a patient with major depressive disorder and unstable housing is more likely to achieve functional gains when antidepressant medication is combined with case management and behavioral activation, compared to medication alone. Preventive strategies should also be multi, tiered, ranging from universal efforts that reduce stigma and improve access to care, to selective programs for high, risk groups, to indicated interventions for individuals showing early signs of disorder. Later chapters on implementation science examine which combinations of interventions produce synergistic effects and under what conditions. Clinicians should document both proximal and distal goals across biological, psychological, and social domains, using measurement, based care to monitor progress and adapt treatment plans. Measurable benchmarks should be defined for each domain and reviewed at predetermined intervals to guide clinical decision, making (Weiner et al., 2025).

The breadth of the biopsychosocial model introduces both practical and conceptual challenges that require deliberate solutions (Kargarandehkordi et al., 2025). Interdisciplinary collaboration, pragmatic measurement strategies, and attention to implementation barriers are essential. Pragmatic measurement involves selecting reliable, feasible instruments that capture domain, relevant constructs without overburdening clients or clinicians. Collecting valid biological, psychological, and social data requires diverse expertise and tools, making team, based care models especially valuable (Kim & Backonja, 2025). Clinics that embed social workers and behavioral health coaches alongside psychiatric services are better positioned to address social barriers that might otherwise derail treatment.

Electronic health records and outcome registries should be configured to accept psychosocial data alongside medical and diagnostic information (Akhtar & Rawol, 2024). This integration requires institutional commitment, appropriate privacy safeguards, and technical infrastructure. Later chapters discuss standards for interoperable data systems and consent frameworks that balance utility with confidentiality (Ricciardi & Zomaya, 2025). Training programs must also evolve to support this integrated approach. Curricula should prepare clinicians to incorporate systems thinking into diagnostic formulation and treatment selection. Continuing education can highlight brief, evidence, informed strategies for assessing social determinants and making appropriate referrals or interventions (Ricciardi & Zomaya, 2025).

Interprofessional case review should be incorporated as a routine quality, improvement activity to maintain fidelity to integrated care principles. These reviews allow teams to align on shared goals, identify gaps in care, and ensure that interventions are coordinated across domains. They also provide opportunities for reflective practice and professional development, reinforcing a culture of collaboration and continuous learning. The theoretical foundations of cognitive science, when expanded to include social and environmental determinants, offer a comprehensive framework for understanding and influencing mental health. By embedding these contexts into assessment, formulation, and intervention, clinicians and researchers can more accurately capture the lived realities of their clients and design systems that respond to those realities. The biopsychosocial model, when operationalized through interdisciplinary collaboration and pragmatic implementation, supports the development of neuroadaptive systems that are not only intelligent and responsive but also equitable and ecologically valid (Saganowski et al., 2022).

Moreover, the biopsychosocial model must be applied with cultural humility and sensitivity (Li et al., 2025). Cultural humility involves an ongoing commitment to curiosity, respect for patients' explanatory models, and a willingness to adapt interventions to fit diverse cultural contexts. Mental health is not universally conceptualized in the same way; values, beliefs, and lived experiences shape how individuals understand distress, healing, and recovery. A culturally adapted behavioral activation program, for instance, that incorporates community roles and family obligations may be more acceptable and effective in certain populations than a standard protocol (Li et al., 2025). A truly biopsychosocial approach is not only holistic, it is person, centered.

Cross, cultural validation of assessment tools and co, design of interventions with community stakeholders are essential components of ethical and effective implementation. These practices are discussed in detail in the implementation chapters. Before deploying any intervention, clinicians and researchers should verify cultural fit through pilot testing and stakeholder feedback to avoid inadvertent harm. This process ensures that interventions are not only evidence, based but also contextually grounded and socially responsive (Agarwal et al., 2025). In the pursuit of understanding human behavior, cognition, and emotion, psychophysiological measurement has become an essential tool across disciplines. These measures provide temporally fine, grained indices that complement self, report and behavioral observation in both clinical and research settings (Weiner et al., 2025). By capturing physiological signals such as heart rate, brain activity, and skin conductance, researchers and clinicians can gain real, time insights into internal psychological states. For example, concurrent recordings of heart rate variability (Weiner et al., 2025) and electrodermal activity (APA, 2025) can help distinguish sustained anxiety from transient arousal during exposure, based tasks (Weiner et al., 2025). As these tools become more sophisticated, so too must our approach to designing, interpreting, and applying them. Later chapters build on this point by outlining standards for calibration, baseline assessment, and multimodal data fusion (Weiner et al., 2025). Systems theory offers a powerful framework for this evolution, helping us move beyond isolated data points toward a more holistic, context, aware understanding of human experience (Weiner et al., 2025). To make psychophysiological data clinically meaningful, adopt rigorous preprocessing protocols, contextual annotation, and hypothesis, driven interpretation (Weiner et al., 2025).

Psychophysiological measurement refers to the recording and analysis of physiological signals that reflect psychological processes (Torous et al., 2023). It is essential to define measurement targets clearly, whether assessing arousal, attention, autonomic balance, or cognitive workload, so that sensor selection and analytic strategies align with theoretical aims (Robinson et al., 2024). These signals are typically collected using non, invasive sensors and include electroencephalography (Watson, 2025) for brain activity, HRV for autonomic regulation, EDA for arousal, respiration rate for stress and relaxation, and eye tracking for attention and cognitive effort (Robinson et al., 2024). For instance, high, resolution HRV indices can reveal parasympathetic recovery following stress, a clinically relevant marker of regulatory capacity (Robinson et al., 2024). These measures are widely used in neuroscience, psychology, education, human, computer interaction, and healthcare. However, interpreting these signals is not always straightforward. An elevated heart rate, for example, might indicate excitement, fear, or physical exertion, highlighting the importance of contextual information in interpretation. The measurement chapter provides detailed recommendations on sensor specifications, sampling rates, and artifact rejection procedures that improve data quality and interpretability (Robinson et al., 2024). To reduce ambiguity, combine precise operational definitions with contextual metadata, ensuring that physiological signals are interpreted within the appropriate psychological and environmental frame.

Systems theory provides a conceptual scaffold for integrating psychophysiological data into broader models of human functioning (Ricciardi & Zomaya, 2025). As an interdisciplinary approach, systems theory views phenomena as interconnected sets of components that function as a whole. It emphasizes principles such as interdependence, feedback loops, emergence, contextual sensitivity, and adaptation. When applied to psychophysiological measurement, systems theory encourages us to view physiological signals not as isolated indicators but as part of a dynamic system that includes the brain, body, environment, and task demands. A systems, informed analysis might model how cognitive load, ambient temperature, and social presence jointly influence EDA during a task (Ricciardi & Zomaya, 2025). This perspective shifts interpretation away from reductionist readings and toward a more integrated understanding of human physiology and behavior. It also supports the development of neuroadaptive systems that respond not only to individual signals but to the broader context in which those signals occur (Ricciardi & Zomaya, 2025).

To operationalize this approach, researchers and clinicians must explicitly state their system model and testable predictions before data collection begins (Aiken et al., 2023). This includes defining system boundaries, relevant time scales, and which feedback pathways are considered endogenous versus exogenous. The analytic methods chapter reviews time, series and causal discovery tools appropriate for testing these system, level hypotheses. By grounding measurement in clearly articulated models, we ensure that data collection is purposeful and that interpretations are aligned with the dynamics we aim to understand (Mohr et al., 2017). Psychophysiological measurement, when guided by systems theory and implemented with cultural humility, offers a powerful means of capturing the complexity of human experience. These tools allow us to move beyond static snapshots of behavior and into the realm of dynamic, context, sensitive assessment. As we integrate these methods into neuroadaptive systems, we must remain attentive to the ethical, cultural, and theoretical assumptions that shape our interpretations (Mohr et al., 2017). Doing so ensures that our technologies remain not only scientifically rigorous but also human, centered and clinically relevant.

Extended Reality offers immersive therapeutic environments that operationalize exposure and embodiment principles.

Traditional approaches to psychophysiological measurement often treat physiological signals as direct reflections of psychological states. While intuitively appealing, this one, to, one mapping is both reductionist and potentially misleading. For example, increased skin conductance is commonly interpreted as heightened arousal. However, a clinician who assumes that a single electrodermal activity (Kim & Backonja, 2025) spike reflects panic may overlook alternative explanations, such as physical exertion, leading to false alarms and inappropriate interventions. A systems theory perspective challenges this reductive view by emphasizing the complexity and interdependence of physiological, psychological, and environmental systems. It prompts deeper questions: What other systems are interacting with this signal? How does the environment influence the physiological response? What feedback loops are involved? How does the signal evolve over time? These questions shift the interpretive frame from isolated signal analysis to dynamic systems modeling. To answer such questions, clinicians and researchers must require converging evidence from multiple modalities before drawing strong inferences (Tsai et al., 2025). Cross, referencing behavioral logs, contextual sensors, and self, report data is a recommended strategy, one that will be explored in greater detail in Chapter 5 (Tsai et al., 2025). For example, a spike in heart rate may be interpreted differently depending on whether it occurs during a cognitive task, a social interaction, or a physical activity. Requiring multimodal convergence and temporal corroboration before acting on physiological alerts improves clinical accuracy and reduces the risk of misinterpretation in real, time workflows (Tsai et al., 2025).

Systems Theory provides the architecture for dynamic feedback loops and context, aware design.

The Biopsychosocial Model ensures a holistic understanding of the user by integrating biological, psychological, and social data (Freeman et al., 2017).

Cognitive Science informs how the system models mental processes such as attention, memory, and emotion.

Psychophysiological Measurement supplies real, time data from signals such as EEG, HRV, and skin conductance (Inkster et al., 2023).

Edges in the concept map represent functional relationships between constructs. For example, HRV and EEG features might be linked to an "arousal" node that triggers specific interface adaptations (Khoo et al., 2024). When using the concept map in design meetings, annotate each node with attributes, data types, and acceptable error tolerances to guide prototyping and validation (Li et al., 2025). Refer back to earlier chapters for operational definitions of each framework to ensure consistent mapping across interdisciplinary teams. This convergence of frameworks enables the development of neuroadaptive systems that are not only technically advanced but also deeply human, centered (Li et al., 2025). A therapy platform, for instance, might reduce exposure intensity when physiological markers indicate that the user has exited the therapeutic window. Such systems require cross, disciplinary specifications so that engineering teams and clinicians share a common ontology. Before deployment, define primary clinical endpoints and their associated proximal physiological markers to evaluate therapeutic impact and ensure alignment with intended outcomes (Li et al., 2025). Psychophysiological measurement must move beyond simplistic mappings and embrace the complexity of human systems. By integrating multimodal data, contextual information, and personalized baselines, neuroadaptive systems can achieve greater precision, responsiveness, and clinical utility (Li et al., 2025). These principles will be further elaborated in subsequent chapters on adaptive interface design, real, time feedback systems, and implementation in clinical workflows (Li et al., 2025).

Real, world applications of neuroadaptive systems illustrate how interdisciplinary research can translate into practical tools for mental health care and cognitive training (Li et al., 2025). Several commercially available platforms exemplify this integration of biosensor data, cognitive modeling, and adaptive feedback (Li et al., 2025). For instance, the Muse headband uses EEG signals to guide meditation and emotional regulation, providing real, time auditory feedback to help users maintain focus (Li et al., 2025). The Emotiv Insight is a wearable EEG headset that tracks cognitive states such as attention and stress, offering insights into mental workload and fatigue (Li et al., 2025). Neurable employs brain, computer interface (Freeman et al., 2017) technology to adjust digital environments based on user engagement, enabling hands, free interaction and adaptive content delivery. BioBeats is a mobile platform that delivers personalized stress, reduction strategies using heart rate variability and other physiological signals (Li et al., 2025). Meanwhile, virtual reality therapy platforms like Psious tailor exposure therapy to individual tolerance levels using real, time physiological feedback.

Experts such as Thomas Insel, Albert Rizzo, Rosalind Picard have advanced concepts like neuroadaptive systems, wearable sensors.

When adapting these examples for clinical or research use, it is essential to replicate core validation steps: baseline calibration, cross, modal corroboration, and clinician, in, the, loop oversight (Lay et al., 2025). These steps ensure that adaptive responses are grounded in reliable signals and that system behavior remains interpretable and clinically meaningful. By translating complex cognitive and physiological data into practical tools, Lamb's work underscores the transformative potential of neuroadaptive systems in delivering more effective, empathetic, and accessible mental health care (Lamb et al., 2025; Ong et al., 2025). However, realizing this potential requires more than algorithmic sophistication. It demands clinician training, workflow redesign, and policy alignment. For example, a deployment that paired adaptive algorithms with clinician dashboards and clear escalation rules showed greater acceptance in pilot clinics than a fully automated system. This finding highlights the importance of human, centered design and clinical integration (Ong et al., 2025).

Researchers developing neuroadaptive tools should publish algorithmic decision rules, report heterogeneity of treatment effects, and include diverse samples to enhance generalizability (Baka et al., 2025). These principles of transparency and equity are revisited in later chapters on evaluation and regulatory considerations. Clinicians should be involved in co, design processes to ensure that systems address meaningful clinical problems and fit within real, world workflows. Pilot implementations should include process metrics, clinician feedback, and equity, focused outcome measures to guide refinement and scale, up. Practical development roadmaps begin with problem definition, proceed through iterative prototyping, and culminate in controlled evaluation and scale, up. At project initiation, define the scope, target population, and measurable success criteria to avoid scope creep and ensure clinical relevance. Start with small, well, specified clinical problems, such as reducing panic attacks, improving attentional control, or augmenting exposure therapy, and develop minimal viable adaptations that can be reliably triggered by validated signals. For example, an attentional training module might begin with a single EEG, derived focus metric that adjusts task difficulty within predefined limits. Once validated, additional modalities can be layered in.

Engage clinicians, patients, and technical stakeholders in repeated user testing cycles to refine usability, safety, and acceptability. Chapter 9 provides project management templates for documenting iteration logs, decision thresholds, and failure modes, resources that are especially useful for regulatory review and grant reporting. Scaling should only occur after reproducible benefits are demonstrated across heterogeneous settings and populations. From a systems theory perspective, adaptation and learning are not just features but core design principles of neuroadaptive systems (Livieri et al., 2025). These systems should be capable of updating their behavior based on user data while remaining predictable and auditable (Radanliev, 2025). Specify learning objectives, update schedules, and safe, fail thresholds to ensure that adaptive behavior remains within clinically acceptable bounds. Just as living systems evolve in response to environmental feedback, neuroadaptive systems should incorporate incremental model updates validated on held, out clinical cases to prevent drift and catastrophic adaptation (Radanliev, 2025).

This requires machine learning algorithms that can detect patterns, refine predictions, and personalize interventions over time (Liu & Schueller, 2023). Later chapters describe audit logs, clinician override mechanisms, and retraining intervals that operationalize these learning safeguards. Equally important is the design of systems that are transparent and explainable. Users, especially clinicians, must understand how and why the system is adapting. Build explainability features that present adaptation rationales in clinician, friendly language to support oversight, informed consent, and trust. The integration of biosensor data, cognitive modeling, and adaptive algorithms offers a powerful pathway toward more responsive and personalized mental health care (Ienca et al., 2017). But this promise can only be realized through rigorous validation, ethical design, and sustained collaboration across disciplines. The next chapters will explore how these principles are applied in implementation science, regulatory frameworks, and real, world clinical trials (Ienca et al., 2017).

Systems theory provides the structural backbone for designing neuroadaptive technologies in mental health (Smith et al., 2023). It enables us to conceptualize the user not as an isolated individual but as part of a complex, dynamic system, one that includes physiological processes, cognitive functions, environmental conditions, and social interactions. Operationalizing systems theory means translating its principles into concrete engineering requirements: latency limits, false, positive tolerances, interface intervention windows, and adaptive thresholds. These specifications bridge the gap between theoretical insight and practical implementation. For example, a well, specified latency requirement ensures that cognitive load reductions occur within a time frame that supports working memory retention. Similarly, defining acceptable false, positive rates prevents over, triggering of interventions, which could lead to user fatigue or mistrust. By embracing feedback loops, emergence, contextual sensitivity, and adaptation, we can design systems that not only support mental health but also evolve with the people they serve. These engineering constraints recur throughout the prototyping checklists and regulatory guidance sections of this book. In short, operationalizing systems theory reduces unintended consequences and strengthens clinical utility (Kargarandehkordi et al., 2025).

Wearable sensors provide continuous physiological monitoring, supporting adaptive and personalized interventions.

Cognitive science also informs how we define and measure emotion regulation targets. Emotions are not merely reactions; they are integral to how we think, decide, and act. Adaptive systems must therefore detect and respond to emotional states in ways that are both timely and therapeutically appropriate. Define regulation goals, such as reducing physiological arousal, increasing cognitive reappraisal, or improving behavioral activation, and map them to measurable indicators. For example, detecting rising sympathetic arousal paired with negative thought reports might trigger immediate grounding techniques. The chapter on adaptive rules outlines how to prioritize interventions when multiple regulation targets conflict, using clinician, set hierarchies and patient preferences.

In the pursuit of understanding human behavior, cognition, and emotion, psychophysiological measurement has become an essential tool across disciplines. These tools allow researchers and clinicians to capture real, time physiological signals, such as heart rate, brain activity, and skin conductance, that reflect internal psychological states. However, as these tools become more sophisticated, so too must our approach to designing and interpreting them. Define specific clinical and research use cases up front so that measurement choices align with intended inferences and decision thresholds (Cushnan et al., 2024). For example, simultaneous HRV and frontal EEG shifts during a panic probe can help distinguish transient arousal from sustained dysregulation (Engel, 1977). The chapter on measurement pipelines provides standards for calibration, baseline collection, and artifact handling to support clinical interpretation (Engel, 1977). Commit to protocolized data collection and explicit interpretive rules to translate physiological signals into safe, clinically meaningful actions (Engel, 1977).

Psychophysiological measurement refers to the recording and analysis of physiological signals that reflect psychological processes (Ball et al., 2025). These signals are typically collected using non, invasive sensors and include electroencephalography (Fanarioti & Karpouzis, 2025) for brain activity, heart rate and heart rate variability (Gkintoni et al., 2025) for autonomic function, electrodermal activity (Ricciardi & Zomaya, 2025) for arousal, respiration rate for stress and relaxation, and eye tracking for attention and cognitive effort (Poudel et al., 2025). A study measuring task engagement might combine pupil dilation, reaction time variability, and EEG theta power to triangulate attentional lapses (Poudel et al., 2025). These measures are widely used in neuroscience, psychology, education, human, computer interaction, and healthcare. Yet interpreting these signals is not always straightforward. Cross, modal validation and documented baseline variability are necessary to reduce misclassification. For instance, an elevated heart rate might indicate excitement, fear, or physical exertion, highlighting the importance of context in interpretation. Always collect contextual metadata, activity logs, environmental conditions, and concurrent behavior, to constrain plausible interpretations.

Systems theory, as applied to psychophysiological measurement, encourages us to view physiological signals not as isolated indicators but as components of a larger, dynamic system. This system includes the brain, body, environment, and task demands. It emphasizes principles such as interdependence, feedback loops, emergence, contextual sensitivity, and adaptation. For example, modeling how classroom noise, task difficulty, and social cueing jointly influence EDA and EEG can reveal leverage points for intervention (Lindner et al., 2024). To prevent misapplied inferences, explicitly state model boundaries, temporal scales, and which variables are treated as inputs versus endogenous (Kim & Backonja, 2025). Analysts should preregister system hypotheses and analytic plans to align measurement with the intended system model (Kim & Backonja, 2025). Use systems specifications to guide sensor fusion, feature engineering, and causal inference methods (Kim & Backonja, 2025). The integration of systems theory, cognitive science, and psychophysiological measurement provides a rigorous foundation for the design of neuroadaptive systems (Kim & Backonja, 2025). These frameworks ensure that technologies are not only responsive and intelligent but also context, aware, ethically grounded, and clinically meaningful. The next chapter will explore how these principles are translated into adaptive algorithms, interface design, and real, world deployment in mental health care settings.

Traditional approaches to psychophysiological measurement often treat physiological signals as direct reflections of psychological states. While this assumption may simplify interpretation, it risks oversimplifying the complexity of human physiology and behavior. A more rigorous approach requires convergent evidence across at least two modalities before drawing strong clinical conclusions from single, sensor fluctuations. For example, increased skin conductance is commonly interpreted as heightened arousal. However, this reductionist view can be misleading. A clinician alerted by an isolated electrodermal activity (Spytska, 2025) spike should consult concurrent movement sensors or self, report data to rule out non, psychological causes such as physical exertion or environmental temperature changes (Weiner et al., 2025). Systems theory prompts us to ask deeper, more integrative questions: What other systems are interacting with this signal? How does the environment influence the physiological response? What feedback loops are involved? How does the signal evolve over time? These questions reframe psychophysiological data not as isolated indicators but as emergent properties of complex, adaptive systems (Weiner et al., 2025). Practical protocols should reflect this complexity. For example, automated cross, checks, time, window confirmation, and clinician review gates can be implemented before triggering interventions. These operational safeguards reduce false positives and improve clinical trust in adaptive systems (Weiner et al., 2025).

Designing psychophysiological measurement systems through the lens of systems theory involves several key strategies. First, translate theoretical aims into measurable specifications. This includes defining sensitivity, specificity, sampling cadence, and permissible latency for adaptive actions. These parameters ensure that the system's performance aligns with its intended clinical use (Okposio et al., 2025).

Second, model the interactions between multiple physiological signals (Ienca et al., 2017). For instance, combining EEG and heart rate variability (Kim & Backonja, 2025) data can provide a more comprehensive picture of cognitive and emotional states than either measure alone (Ienca et al., 2017). In exposure therapy, concurrent decreases in HRV and increases in midline EEG theta may signal over, arousal, justifying momentary task pacing adjustments (Ienca et al., 2017). These multimodal systems can reveal patterns of co, regulation, how different physiological systems work together to maintain balance or respond to stress.

Third, systems theory emphasizes the importance of context. A heart rate of 120 beats per minute has different implications during aerobic exercise than during a cognitive load task. Measurement systems must therefore be designed to capture and interpret contextual variables such as task type, environmental conditions, and social dynamics. Lightweight ecological momentary assessments and wearable environmental sensors can supply the contextual annotations needed for accurate interpretation and adaptive logic (Baydili et al., 2025). Fourth, temporal dynamics and individual baselines must be incorporated into system design. Adaptive algorithms should respond to deviations from an individual's typical patterns rather than to population norms. For example, a sudden drop in HRV may be clinically significant for one individual but fall within normal variability for another (Ong et al., 2025). Personalized baselines improve the specificity of alerts and reduce false positives, especially in high, stakes clinical environments (Ong et al., 2025). Building reliable psychophysiological measurement pipelines for neuroadaptive systems requires the integration of precise specifications, multimodal fusion, contextual capture, and individualized calibration (Ong et al., 2025). These design principles ensure that adaptive systems are not only technically robust but also clinically meaningful and ethically sound.

REFERENCES

Adegoke, K., Adegoke, A., Dawodu, D., Bayowa, A., & Adekoya, A (2025). Interoperability in digital healthcare: Enhancing consumer health and transforming care systems.

Agarwal, S., Jalan, M., Hill, R., Pantalone, E., Thrul, J., Sharma, R., Wilcox, H. C., & Robinson, K. A. (2025). Framework to Assist Stakeholders in Technology Evaluation for Recovery (Freeman et al., 2017) to Mental Health and Wellness. *BMC Health Services Research*, *25*, 623. Advance online publication. DOI: 10.1186/s12913-025-12418-0 PMID: 40307807

Aiken, L. H., Lasater, K. B., Sloane, D. M., Pogue, C. A., Rosenbaum, K. E. F., & Muir, K. J.US Clinician Wellbeing Study Consortium. (2023, July). Physician and nurse well-being and preferred interventions to address burnout in hospital practice: Factors associated with turnover, outcomes, and patient safety. [). American Medical Association.]. *JAMA Health Forum*, *4*(7), e231809–e231809. DOI: 10.1001/jamahealthforum.2023.1809 PMID: 37418269

Akhtar, Z. B., & Rawol, A. T. (2024). Artificial intelligence (Tizzard, 2025) and extended reality (XR): A biomedical engineering perspective investigation analysis. *Indonesian Journal of Electronics, Electromedical Engineering, and Medical Informatics*, *6*(3). Advance online publication. DOI: 10.35882/ijeeemi.v6i3.5

Baka, E., Tan, Y.-R., Wong, B. L. H., Xing, Z., & Yap, P. (2025). A scoping review of digital interventions for the promotion of mental health and prevention of mental health conditions for young people. *Oxford Open Digital Health*, *3*, oqaf005. DOI: 10.1093/oodh/oqaf005 PMID: 40230873

Ball, H., Eisner, E., Nicholas, J., Wilson, P., & Bucci, S. (2025). How theories, models, and frameworks have been used to implement digital health interventions in services for people with severe mental health problems: A scoping review. *BMC Public Health*, *25*(1), 1023. DOI: 10.1186/s12889-025-22189-2 PMID: 40098003

Baydili, İ., Tasci, B., & Tasci, G. (2025). Artificial intelligence in psychiatry: A review of biological and behavioral data analyses. *Diagnostics (Basel)*, *15*(4), 434. DOI: 10.3390/diagnostics15040434 PMID: 40002587

Boffet, A., Arsac, L. M., Ibanez, V., Sauvet, F., & Deschodt-Arsac, V. (2025). Detection of Cognitive Load Modulation by EDA and HRV. *Sensors (Basel)*, *25*(8), 2343. DOI: 10.3390/s25082343 PMID: 40285033

Bond, R. R., Mulvenna, M. D., Potts, C., O'Neill, S., Ennis, E., & Torous, J. (2023). Digital transformation of mental health services. *Npj Mental Health Research*, *2*(1), 13. DOI: 10.1038/s44184-023-00033-y PMID: 38609479

Chaabene, S., Boudaya, A., Bouaziz, B., & Chaari, L. (2025). An overview of methods and techniques in multimodal data fusion with application to healthcare. *International Journal of Data Science and Analytics*, *20*(4), 1–25. DOI: 10.1007/s41060-025-00715-0

Chithra, N., & Bhambri, P. (2024). Ethics in sustainable technology. In *Handbook of Technological Sustainability* (pp. 245–256). CRC Press. DOI: 10.1201/9781003475989-21

Cristofaro, M., & Giardino, P. L. (2025). Surfing the AI waves: The historical evolution of artificial intelligence in management and organizational studies and practices. *Journal of Management History*. Advance online publication. DOI: 10.1108/JMH-01-2025-0002

Cushnan, J., McCafferty, P., & Best, P. (2024). Clinicians' perspectives of immersive tools in clinical mental health settings: A systematic scoping review. *BMC Health Services Research*, *24*(1), 1091. DOI: 10.1186/s12913-024-11481-3 PMID: 39294727

Engel, G. L. (1977). The need for a new medical model: A challenge for biomedicine. *Science*, *196*(4286), 129–136. DOI: 10.1126/science.847460 PMID: 847460

Fanarioti, A. K., & Karpouzis, K. (2025). Artificial Intelligence and the Future of Mental Health in a Digitally Transformed World. *Computers*, *14*(7), 259. DOI: 10.3390/computers14070259

Gkintoni, E., Vassilopoulos, S. P., & Nikolaou, G. (2025). Next-generation cognitive-behavioral therapy for depression: Integrating digital tools, teletherapy, and personalization for enhanced mental health outcomes. *Medicina (Kaunas, Lithuania)*, *61*(3), 431. DOI: 10.3390/medicina61030431 PMID: 40142242

Hiland, E. B. (2021). *Therapy tech: The digital transformation of mental healthcare*. U of Minnesota Press. DOI: 10.5749/j.ctv1xp9q3t

Ienca, M., Fabrice, J., Elger, B., Caon, M., Scoccia Pappagallo, A., Kressig, R. W., & Wangmo, T. (2017). Intelligent assistive technology for Alzheimer's disease and other dementias: A systematic review. *Journal of Alzheimer's Disease*, *56*(4), 1301–1340. DOI: 10.3233/JAD-161037 PMID: 28222516

Inkster, B., Knibbs, C., & Bada, M. (2023). Cybersecurity: A critical priority for digital mental health. *Frontiers in Digital Health*, *5*, 1242264. DOI: 10.3389/fdgth.2023.1242264 PMID: 37781452

Islam, R., & Bae, S. W. (2024). Revolutionizing mental health support: An innovative affective mobile framework for dynamic, proactive, and context-adaptive conversational agents. arXiv preprint arXiv:2406.15942.

Jain, A., & Jain, A (2025). AI-Based Emotion Detection System in Healthcare for Patient. Generative Artificial Intelligence for Biomedical and Smart Health Informatics, 455-470.

Kargarandehkordi, A., Li, S., Lin, K., Phillips, K. T., Benzo, R. M., & Washington, P. (2025). Fusing wearable biosensors with artificial intelligence for mental health monitoring: A systematic review. *Biosensors (Basel)*, *15*(4), 202. DOI: 10.3390/bios15040202 PMID: 40277515

Khoo, Y. X., Kang, R. M., Reynolds, T. L., & Mentis, H. M. (2024). The comprehensiveness of mental health application users' privacy and security concerns. *CHI Conference on Human Factors in Computing Systems*, 16 pages.

Kim, J., & Backonja, U. (2025). Digital health equity frameworks and key concepts: A scoping review. *Journal of the American Medical Informatics Association : JAMIA*, *32*(1), 45–59. DOI: 10.1093/jamia/ocaf017 PMID: 39936843

Kostadimas, D., Kasapakis, V., & Kotis, K. (2025). A systematic review on the combination of VR, IoT and AI technologies, and their integration in applications. *Future Internet*, *17*(4), 163. DOI: 10.3390/fi17040163

Kourtesis, P. (2024). A comprehensive review of multimodal XR applications, risks, and ethical challenges in the metaverse. *Multimodal Technologies and Interaction*, *8*(11), 98. DOI: 10.3390/mti8110098

Lay, W., Gasparini, L., Siero, W., & Hughes, E. K. (2025). A rapid review of the benefits and challenges of dynamic consent. *Research Ethics*, *21*(1), 180–202. DOI: 10.1177/17470161241278064

Li, M., Patel, J., & Katapally, T. R. (2025). The impact of extended reality cognitive behavioral therapy on mental disorders among children and youth: A systematic review and meta-analysis protocol. *PLoS One*, *20*(3), e0315313. DOI: 10.1371/journal.pone.0315313 PMID: 40048453

Lindner, P., Miloff, A., & Carlbring, P. (2024). The future of virtual reality therapy: Applications, challenges, and research directions. *Frontiers in Virtual Reality*, *5*, 112345.

Liu, M., & Schueller, S. M. (2023). Moving evidence-based mental health interventions into practice: Implementation of digital mental health interventions. *Current Treatment Options in Psychiatry*, *10*(4), 333–345. DOI: 10.1007/s40501-023-00298-2

Livieri, G., Mangina, E., Protopapadakis, E. D., & Panayiotou, A. G. (2025). The gaps and challenges in digital health technology use as perceived by patients: A scoping review and narrative meta-synthesis. *Frontiers in Digital Health*, *7*, 1474956. DOI: 10.3389/fdgth.2025.1474956 PMID: 40212901

Ma, C.-B., Shang, X., Sun, M., Bo, X., Bai, J., Du, Y., & Zhou, M. (2025). Emerging Multifunctional Wearable Sensors: Integrating Multimodal Sweat Analysis and Advanced Material Technologies for Next-Generation Health Monitoring. *ACS Sensors*, *10*(4), 2388–2408. DOI: 10.1021/acssensors.4c03396 PMID: 40162570

Mahon, D. (2023). Empirically Supported Treatments: A Brief History. In Evidence Based Counselling & Psychotherapy for the 21st Century Practitioner (pp. 3-14). Emerald Publishing Limited. DOI: 10.1108/978-1-80455-732-720231001

Mohr, D. C., Zhang, M., & Schueller, S. M. (2017). Personal sensing: Understanding mental health using ubiquitous sensors and machine learning. *Annual Review of Clinical Psychology*, *13*(1), 23–47. DOI: 10.1146/annurev-clinpsy-032816-044949 PMID: 28375728

Okposio, B. O., Richard, G. A., Olatokun, T. P., Akadiri, O. O., Akpevba, E. A., John, J. O., & Okonkwo, B. A. (2025). Enhancing Mental health Outcomes through AI-Driven Predictive Analytics: A review of applications in neuroscience and substance abuse prevention. *International Journal of Biological and Pharmaceutical Sciences Archive, 10*(2), 024-048.

Ong, T., Ivanova, J., Soni, H., Barrera, J., Cummins, M., Welch, B. M., & Bunnell, B. E. (2025). Mental health clients' perspectives on telehealth-based virtual reality therapy. *Frontiers in Virtual Reality*, *6*, 1595326. DOI: 10.3389/frvir.2025.1595326

Poudel, U., Jakhar, S., Mohan, P., & Nepal, A. (2025). AI in mental health: A review of technological advancements and ethical issues in psychiatry. *Issues in Mental Health Nursing*, *46*(7), 693–701. DOI: 10.1080/01612840.2025.2502943 PMID: 40378075

Radanliev, P. (2025). Privacy, ethics, transparency, and accountability in AI systems for wearable devices. *Frontiers in Digital Health*, *7*, 1431246. DOI: 10.3389/fdgth.2025.1431246 PMID: 40599875

Rajpal, S. (2025). Exploring the Role of Virtual Reality and Metaverse in Treating Mental Health: Operating Models and Challenges in Adoption. *Journal of Computer and Communications*, *13*(10), 1–22. DOI: 10.4236/jcc.2025.1310001

Ricciardi, F., & Zomaya, A. (2025). Perspectives on Managing AI Ethics in the Digital Age. *Information (Basel)*, *16*(2), 89. DOI: 10.3390/info16040318

Robinson, A., Flom, M., Forman-Hoffman, V. L., Histon, T., Levy, M., Darcy, A., ... & Montgomery, R. M. (2024). Equity in digital mental health interventions in the United States: Where to next?. *Journal of Medical Internet Research, 26*, e59939. Lamb, R., Choi, I., & Owens, T (2025). Convergence of Extended Reality, Artificial Intelligence, Machine Leaning, and Wearable Sensors in the Field of Education. Mental Health Virtual Reality: The Power of Immersive Worlds, 113-128.

Ross, G., Zhao, Y., Bosman, A., Geballa-Koukoula, A., Zhou, H., Elliott, C., Nielen, M., Rafferty, K., & Salentijn, G (2022). Data handling and ethics of emerging smartphone-based (Glass et al., 2022) sensors–Part 1: best practices and current implementation.

Saganowski, S., Perz, B., Polak, A. G., & Kazienko, P (2022). Emotion recognition for everyday life using physiological signals from wearables: A systematic literature review. IEEE Transactions on Affective Computing, 14(3), 1876-1897. Pinel, P (1793). Traité médico-philosophique sur l'aliénation mentale.

Smith, K. A., Blease, C., Faurholt-Jepsen, M., Firth, J., Van Daele, T., Moreno, C., Carlbring, P., Ebner-Priemer, U. W., Koutsouleris, N., Riper, H., Mouchabac, S., Torous, J., & Cipriani, A. (2023). Digital mental health: Challenges and next steps. *BMJ Mental Health*, *26*(1), e300670. DOI: 10.1136/bmjment-2023-300670 PMID: 37197797

Spytska, L. (2025). The use of artificial intelligence in psychotherapy: Development of intelligent therapeutic systems. *BMC Psychology*, *13*(1), 175. DOI: 10.1186/s40359-025-02491-9 PMID: 40022267

Subu, M. A., Holmes, D., Arumugam, A., Al-Yateem, N., Maria Dias, J., Rahman, S. A., Waluyo, I., Ahmed, F. R., & Abraham, M. S. (2022). Traditional, religious, and cultural perspectives on mental illness: A qualitative study on causal beliefs and treatment use. *International Journal of Qualitative Studies on Health and Well-being*, *17*(1), 2123090. DOI: 10.1080/17482631.2022.2123090 PMID: 36097886

Tsai, Y. Y., Chen, Y. J., Lin, Y. F., Hsiao, F. C., Hsu, C. H., & Liao, L. D. (2025). Photoplethysmography-based HRV analysis and machine learning for real-time stress quantification in mental health applications. *APL Bioengineering*, *9*(2), 026103. DOI: 10.1063/5.0256590 PMID: 40191605

Watson, D (2025). The dark side of mental health apps: Privacy concerns and therapeutic limitations. MentalHealthSigns.com.

Weiner, E. B., Dankwa-Mullan, I., Nelson, W. A., & Hassanpour, S. (2025). Ethical challenges and evolving strategies in the integration of artificial intelligence into clinical practice. *PLOS Digital Health*, *4*(4), e0000810. DOI: 10.1371/journal.pdig.0000810 PMID: 40198594

Xing, Y., Yang, Y., Yang, K., Lu, A., Xing, L., Mackie, K., & Guo, F. (2025). Intelligent sensing devices and systems for personalized mental health. *Med-X*, *3*(1), 10. DOI: 10.1007/s44258-025-00057-3 PMID: 40837134

Chapter 3
Ethics, Consent, and the Moral Architecture of Digital Mental Health

ABSTRACT

Digital mental health introduces profound ethical challenges around data governance, algorithmic bias, and equitable access (Tavory, 2024). This chapter argues for transparency, accountability, and justice as operational imperatives. It critiques failures such as data commercialization and biased AI models, proposing dynamic consent, privacy-protective defaults, and fairness audits (Ricciardi & Zomaya, 2025). Equity demands inclusive design, broadband access, and cultural adaptation to prevent digital redlining. Governance frameworks must embed lived-experience voices, enforce audit cycles, and prioritize harm prevention. Ethical design is positioned as a clinical safeguard, not a technical afterthought (Ricciardi & Zomaya, 2025).

INTRODUCTION

This chapter examines the ethical terrain of digital mental health through a framework centered on transparency, accountability, and justice. It argues that ethical considerations are not peripheral constraints but foundational design requirements that determine trust and legitimacy. The chapter explores how evolving technologies, such as AI-driven inference, passive data collection, and immersive digital environments, challenge traditional notions of informed consent, often reducing autonomy to opaque, one-time agreements. Through real-world case examples, it illustrates how commercial data practices can undermine confidentiality and erode public trust. The chapter reconceptualizes consent as an ongoing, dialogic process that must adapt across time, technologies, and levels of risk. It further addresses

DOI: 10.4018/979-8-3373-4997-8.ch003

algorithmic bias as a clinical imperative, emphasizing the need for fairness audits, representative training data, and human oversight in safety-critical decisions. Equity is framed as an operational constraint rather than an aspirational outcome, requiring deliberate design choices to prevent exclusion and harm. By integrating ethical reflection with concrete governance mechanisms, such as audit trails, participatory oversight, and clinician accountability, the chapter offers a practical roadmap for ethical stewardship. It concludes by positioning digital mental health systems as moral architectures that reflect societal choices about dignity, power, and care.

ETHICS AND CONSENT

We are living through a quiet revolution in mental health care, one not marked by dramatic headlines or sweeping policy changes, but by the steady integration of digital technologies into the most intimate corners of human experience. This transformation is reshaping clinical workflows and patient expectations in measurable ways, altering when, where, and how care is delivered (Sun et al., 2025). Algorithms now assist in diagnosing depression, biometric sensors monitor emotional states in real time, and immersive virtual environments simulate therapeutic encounters (Radanliev, 2025). These technologies operate across diverse settings, from primary care to specialty clinics, requiring clinicians to adapt assessment, consent, and documentation practices accordingly. Digital tools promise a future of precision, personalization, and expanded access to care. However, realizing this promise requires more than technical innovation. It demands ethical clarity. Beneath the surface of these advances lies a deeper set of questions, not about what our technologies can do, but about the values that guide their development and deployment. These questions implicate clinicians, researchers, developers, and policymakers in shared ethical responsibility. This chapter explores the ethical terrain of digital mental health through three interrelated lenses: data governance, algorithmic bias, and equitable access (Radanliev, 2025). These domains are not peripheral, they are foundational. Each influences the others and shapes downstream clinical outcomes (Radanliev, 2025). They determine the trustworthiness of digital systems, the fairness of their outputs, and the inclusivity of their reach. Ethical failures in one domain often propagate to the others, producing systemic harm. In short, they determine whether the digital transformation of mental health care will serve as a bridge to greater well, being or a barrier that reinforces existing inequities. Preventing such harms requires coordinated action across clinical, technical, and regulatory boundaries (Radanliev, 2025).

Figure 1. The three pillars of the Moral Architecture Model: Transparency, accountability, and justice

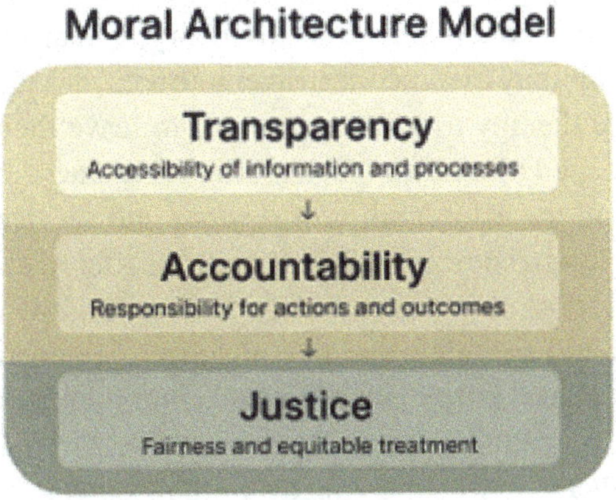

DATA GOVERNANCE: FROM COMPLIANCE TO CARE ETHICS

In the digital mental health ecosystem, data is both the raw material and the currency (Carl et al., 2019). Every interaction with a mental health app, every biometric signal captured by a wearable device, every keystroke in a digital journal contributes to a growing repository of personal information. These discrete traces form datasets that inform algorithms, shape clinical decisions, and influence therapeutic trajectories. Data can be used to tailor interventions, predict crises, and improve outcomes (Kim & Backonja, 2025). Yet these same practices create new vectors of vulnerability. Data governance must therefore move beyond compliance checklists and toward a model rooted in transparency, accountability, and respect for autonomy. This shift requires concrete practices: clear disclosures, granular consent options, deletion rights, audit trails, and independent oversight mechanisms. Systems should communicate how data is used, allow users to opt in or out of specific practices, and provide mechanisms for redress when harms occur. Importantly, data must not be treated as a neutral technical artifact it is a reflection of lived experience and must be handled with the dignity such experience demands. Governance frameworks should center the perspectives of people with lived experience, particularly those from historically marginalized communities. Participatory design processes, community advisory boards, and user, centered consent protocols are essential to ensuring that data practices align with the values and needs of those most affected.

ALGORITHMIC BIAS: FAIRNESS AS A CLINICAL IMPERATIVE

One of the most frequently cited benefits of digital mental health tools is their potential to reach underserved populations. In theory, a smartphone app can deliver cognitive behavioral therapy to someone in a remote area, or a virtual reality program can provide exposure therapy to someone unable to leave their home. In practice, however, access is shaped by a host of factors: digital literacy, internet connectivity, language barriers, and the affordability of devices and services. Equitable access requires intentional design choices. Services must be offered in multiple languages, compatible with low, cost devices, and embedded within trusted community networks. Programs should include training, subsidized connectivity, and culturally appropriate content. These design moves must be operationalized with measurable targets and community feedback loops. Without such efforts, digital mental health tools risk serving only those who are already well, resourced, while leaving behind those who face the greatest barriers to care. Policy interventions are also essential. Investment in broadband infrastructure, public access points, and subsidized devices are necessary complements to app, level design. Equitable access is not simply a matter of distribution, it is a matter of justice. It requires addressing the broader social determinants of digital inclusion and ensuring that digital tools do not replicate or exacerbate existing disparities.

TOWARD ETHICAL, INCLUSIVE, AND HUMAN, CENTERED SYSTEMS

What unites these three domains, data governance, algorithmic bias, and equitable access, is the recognition that technology is never just about efficiency or innovation (Xing et al., 2025). It is about power, trust, and care. Each domain requires interdisciplinary expertise and governance structures that prioritize justice. Together, they shape the power relations embedded within mental health systems and the lived experiences of service users. Ethical digital mental health systems must be transparent in their operations, accountable in their outcomes, and inclusive in their design. They must be built not only to function, but to serve. This requires clinicians, developers, researchers, and policymakers to work collaboratively, guided by shared ethical commitments and informed by the voices of those most affected. As we move forward, the challenge is not simply to build more powerful tools, but to ensure that those tools reflect and reinforce the values of equity, dignity, and care. The next chapter will explore how these ethical principles are translated into technical standards, clinical protocols, and implementation strategies that support safe, effective, and just digital mental health systems (Tsai et al., 2025). We must approach the digital transformation of mental health care not with blind optimism, but with ethical imagination. Ethical imagination demands scenario planning, stakeholder inclusion, and iterative assessment of harms and benefits. This means asking hard questions about who benefits from these technologies, who is harmed, and who is excluded. It means designing systems that are not only effective, but also just. And it means holding ourselves accountable, not only as technologists or clinicians, but as citizens committed to the common good. Accountability mechanisms should include independent audits and community, accessible reporting. In this sense, the digital mindscape we are constructing is not merely a technical infrastructure. It is a moral architecture. It reflects our collective choices about how we understand mental health, how we value human dignity, and how we distribute care and compassion in a digital age. Thus, ethical governance should be integrated into procurement, clinical guidelines, and research funding criteria. Like any architecture that touches human lives, it must be built on a foundation of ethical integrity. Design processes must therefore embed lived, experience advisory panels and ethical impact assessments. The future of mental health care will undoubtedly be shaped by digital tools. These tools will change clinical workflows, measurement practices, and patient expectations in lasting ways (Tsai et al., 2025). But the measure of that future will not be the novelty of its technologies. Rather, it will be the humanity embedded within implementation choices and governance frameworks. It will be the humanity of its systems. Human, centered metrics must therefore accompany technical benchmarks. And that is a responsibility we all share. Building such systems requires interdisciplinary collaboration and sustained ethical oversight.

DATA GOVERNANCE: WHO OWNS THE MIND?

In the rapidly evolving landscape of digital mental health, data has ceased to be a passive byproduct of care, it has become the care itself (Mone & Fayazullaeva, 2023). This transformation reframes data not merely as a clinical record but as the operational substrate through which diagnoses are made, therapies are delivered, and outcomes are evaluated. As such, decisions about data governance now shape the contours of therapeutic possibility. Yet this shift also introduces profound ethical complexity. Mental health data is not just informational, it is intimate. It reflects the most private dimensions of human experience: our thoughts, fears, traumas, and hopes. Governance frameworks must therefore be designed not only for technical robustness but for moral integrity. They must safeguard the dignity of the persons represented in the data.

Historically, mental health records were protected by physical barriers and professional ethics. Confidentiality was enforced through locked filing cabinets, clinician accountability, and the moral codes embedded in therapeutic relationships. Today, those protections must be reimagined for digital ecosystems, where data flows across mobile apps, cloud servers, and third, party analytics platforms (Friend et al., 2024). In these environments, the risks of misuse, commodification, and surveillance are amplified. The question of who owns mental health data is no longer abstract or philosophical, it is urgent and operational (Robinson et al., 2024). Ownership must be defined in terms of rights: the right to access, correct, and delete personal mental health records within digital systems. These rights are foundational to autonomy and must be embedded in both policy and practice.

THE NEW CURRENCY OF CARE

As digital mental health platforms proliferate, data has emerged not only as a therapeutic tool but as a currency, one that is traded, monetized, and increasingly central to the business models of digital health companies (Walter et al., 2023). This commercialization introduces tensions between profit motives and clinical ethics that cannot be ignored (Pedram & Piatkowski, 2025). Data collected during moments of vulnerability, when individuals seek help for depression, anxiety, trauma, or crisis, is now routinely repurposed for marketing, product development, and investor reporting (Pedram & Piatkowski, 2025). This dual use of data, both for care and for commerce, raises critical ethical and policy questions (Pedram & Piatkowski, 2025).

Mental health data is deeply personal (Lorke & Stefanou, 2025). It includes mood logs, voice tone, sleep patterns, screen time, GPS location, and even social media activity. These data streams enable powerful new forms of personalized care (Weiner et al., 2025). Artificial intelligence can analyze speech patterns to detect early signs of depression. Machine learning models can predict suicidal ideation based on changes in typing speed or sleep cycles (Weiner et al., 2025). Personalized care plans can be generated in real time, tailored to the unique rhythms of each user's life. These capabilities hold promise, but they also carry risk. The same data that enables precision care can be commodified, sold, and used in ways that undermine trust and violate privacy (Weiner et al., 2025).

To address these risks, organizations must adopt transparent business models and enforceable data protections (Pedram & Piatkowski, 2025). Data practices must be disclosed clearly, and users must be given meaningful control over how their data is used (Robinson et al., 2024). Opt, out mechanisms should be standard, not exceptional. Procurement policies should require non, commercialization clauses for sensitive datasets, and clinicians must be empowered to evaluate digital tools not only for clinical utility but for ethical alignment (Robinson et al., 2024). In short, data governance must be treated as a clinical responsibility, not an IT afterthought (Robinson et al., 2024).

CASE STUDIES IN ETHICAL FAILURE

Recent regulatory actions underscore the urgency of reform. In 2023, the U. S (Poudel et al., 2025). Federal Trade Commission (Engel, 1977) finalized a settlement with BetterHelp, a widely used online counseling platform, after it was found to have shared sensitive user data with advertising platforms such as Facebook and Snapchat. Despite promising confidentiality, BetterHelp had disclosed users' email addresses, IP addresses, and details about their mental health struggles to third parties for targeted advertising. The company was ordered to pay $7.8 million in restitution and to cease these practices. This case illustrates how privacy promises can be undermined by embedded tracking and opaque vendor relationships. It also highlights the need for independent verification of privacy claims regulators, clinicians, and researchers must treat such claims as provisional until validated. That same year, the telehealth startup Cerebral admitted to sharing the personal and mental health data of over three million users with platforms including Google, Facebook, and TikTok (Achtyes et. al. 2023). The disclosures included treatment histories, assessment responses, and other sensitive information transmitted via embedded tracking tools. Many users were unaware that their data was being shared at all, let alone with advertising networks. This episode revealed the scale at which commercial tracking can occur in clinical contexts and underscored the need for standardized testing protocols to detect third, party trackers in clinical software. These are not isolated incidents. They reflect a broader structural issue: the treatment of mental health data as a commercial asset rather than a sacred trust. The ethical questions are stark: Who benefits from this data? Who profits? And who is protected? In many cases, the answer is not the patient. The individuals most vulnerable, those seeking help in moments of crisis, are often the least empowered to understand or control how their data is used.

TOWARD ETHICAL STEWARDSHIP

Systemic change requires regulatory alignment, professional standards, and sustained funding for oversight. Healthcare organizations must treat data stewardship as a core clinical responsibility (Freeman et al., 2017). This includes implementing governance frameworks that prioritize transparency, accountability, and user autonomy. Consent processes must be redesigned to reflect the complexity of digital data flows (Freeman et al., 2017). Users should be informed not only about what data is collected, but how it is used, who has access, and what rights they retain (Freeman et al., 2017). These rights must be enforceable, not aspirational.

Clinicians, too, must be equipped to navigate this terrain. Training in digital ethics, data governance, and informed consent should be integrated into professional education and continuing development (Martinez, Martin et al., 2018). Clinical workflows must include documentation of data, related decisions, and supervision should address the ethical dimensions of digital tool use (Pedram & Piatkowski, 2025). Institutions should establish cross, functional governance boards that include clinicians, technologists, ethicists, legal experts, and individuals with lived experience. These boards must have real authority to evaluate tools, approve deployments, and respond to harms. Ultimately, the question of who owns the mind is inseparable from the question of how we govern the data that reflects it (Pedram & Piatkowski, 2025). Mental health data is not merely a technical artifact, it is a representation of human vulnerability, resilience, and healing (Pedram & Piatkowski, 2025). It must be treated with the dignity such representation demands. Ethical data governance is not a peripheral concern, it is foundational to the future of mental health care (Pedram & Piatkowski, 2025).

THE ILLUSION OF CONSENT IN THE AGE OF AI, WEARABLES, AND DIGITAL ENVIRONMENTS

In the quiet corridors of digital mental health care where artificial intelligence listens more closely than any human ear and wearable sensors trace the rhythms of our hearts and minds, the concept of consent is undergoing a profound unraveling. What was once a sacred exchange between clinician and patient, grounded in trust, clarity, and mutual respect, has been reduced to a fleeting checkbox, buried in legal jargon and clicked in haste or confusion. This erosion is not merely procedural, it is moral. In mental health contexts, where individuals may be anxious, grieving, or cognitively overwhelmed, the promise of help often arrives wrapped in complexity they cannot parse. The result is a consent process that fails to protect the very autonomy it purports to uphold. The rise of artificial intelligence in mental health care has introduced a new form of intimacy algorithmic, predictive, and often invisible. AI systems now analyze voice tone to detect depression, monitor typing speed to flag anxiety, and scan facial expressions for signs of emotional distress (Jain & Jain, 2025). These tools promise early intervention and personalized care, yet they operate within opaque architectures. Users often consent to processes they cannot see and outcomes they cannot predict. The nature of machine learning, its reliance on vast datasets, its capacity to evolve over time, and its tendency to draw inferences that even its creators may not fully understand renders traditional models of informed consent inadequate (Engel, 1977). To address this, designers must embed explainability into system architecture and provide user, facing summaries of model functions that are comprehensible and actionable.

Wearable sensors add another layer of complexity (Tizzard, 2025). Marketed as wellness tools, these devices collect continuous biometric data heart rate variability, sleep cycles, skin temperature, movement patterns that can be used to infer mood, stress levels, and even suicidal ideation (Tsai et al., 2025). In mental health contexts, this data is often collected passively and ambiently, without explicit user awareness (Tsai et al., 2025). A person may wear a smartwatch to track steps, unaware that it is also monitoring physiological responses to stress, storing data indefinitely, and transmitting it to third, party analytics firms (Tsai et al., 2025). Consent protocols must therefore be redesigned to require granular permissions for each physiologic stream, with clearly defined retention limits and opt, out pathways. Immersive digital environments, such as virtual reality therapy platforms and gamified mental health apps, further complicate the consent landscape. These technologies offer novel therapeutic experiences, exposure therapy, mindfulness training, social interaction, but they also collect behavioral data at unprecedented scale and granularity (Tsai et al., 2025). In a VR session, systems may track eye movement, reaction time, vocal tone, and body posture. These data points are used to personalize the experience, but they are also stored, analyzed, and potentially shared (Tsai et al., 2025). Users may not be aware that their every movement is being recorded and interpreted, nor understand how this data will be used beyond the immediate session (Tsai et al., 2025). Often, they lack the ability to opt out without forfeiting access to care. This creates a consent paradox: the more immersive and effective the digital environment, the more data it collects, and the harder it becomes for users to understand or control that process (Tsai et al., 2025). Solving this paradox requires layered disclosures, intuitive privacy controls, and dynamic consent mechanisms that evolve alongside the system and the user. Consent must be reframed not as a one, time event, but as a continuous, revisitable process embedded within the therapeutic workflow.

REIMAGINING CONSENT AS A CLINICAL AND ETHICAL IMPERATIVE

Consent in digital mental health care must be treated not merely as a legal requirement but as a moral commitment to respect autonomy and protect vulnerability. Informed consent signals recognition of personhood and supports the therapeutic alliance. Systems that erode consent undermine clinical relationships and public trust (Leivaditis & Sepetis, 2025). Clinicians and developers must therefore treat consent as a design requirement, one that is embedded into workflows, governance structures, and user interfaces. Dynamic consent acknowledges that user preferences and capacities change over time. Implementing dynamic consent requires infrastructure that logs preferences, timestamps decisions, and prompts periodic review. Users should be able to modify settings as models update or as their circumstances evolve. This approach supports long, term autonomy and reduces the risk of users unknowingly contributing data to novel, unanticipated uses. Dynamic consent systems should include intuitive dashboards that clarify current permissions and offer simple mechanisms for revision. Contextual consent recognizes the emotional and psychological state of the user. Systems must incorporate safeguards to delay sensitive requests during periods of acute distress and offer simplified, staged choices later. If someone is in crisis, they may not be capable of making informed decisions about long, term data use. Consent flows should prioritize immediate support and defer governance decisions until the user is stable. Designers should test timing and content of consent prompts with representative user groups to ensure appropriateness and reduce coercion. Comprehensible consent demands that interfaces be designed for understanding. Consent materials should use plain language, visual aids, and interactive tools to help users grasp what data is being collected, how it will be used, and what rights they retain. Multilingual and low, literacy options must be standard. Consent should be accessible beyond onboarding repeatedly available, with concise summaries and links to more detailed information. Clinicians can support comprehension by discussing digital risks and benefits during clinical encounters (Wosny et al., 2024). Ultimately, comprehensible consent restores agency to users and shifts the burden of understanding away from vulnerable individuals. Ethical defaults are essential. In the absence of explicit consent, systems must default to protecting the user, not exploiting them. Privacy, protective defaults should minimize data collection, avoid third, party sharing, and prioritize user control (Engel, 1977). Designers must require active opt, in for nonessential features, and regulatory frameworks should mandate such defaults for clinical tools handling sensitive mental health data (Engel, 1977). This approach shifts responsibility from users to platforms and institutions, reinforcing ethical governance. Recent cases illustrate the urgency of reform. In 2023, the Federal Trade Commission sanctioned BetterHelp for sharing sensitive mental health data with advertisers, despite assurances of confidentiality. The company had disclosed users' therapy histories, email addresses, and personal struggles to third parties for marketing purposes. This breach of trust highlights how business practices can subvert privacy promises and cause harm. Other platforms have embedded tracking libraries that transmit behavioral signals to advertising networks without clear disclosure. These practices are especially harmful when they involve therapy content, diagnoses, or self, harm ideation. They also demonstrate that legal remedies often arrive only after harm has occurred, underscoring the need for proactive, ethically grounded design.

TOWARD A CONSENT, CENTERED FUTURE

To restore trust and protect users, digital mental health systems must embed consent into every layer of design and implementation. This includes:

Layered consent frameworks that allow users to opt in to specific data uses and revisit decisions over time (Reddy, 2025).
Context, sensitive prompts that delay nonessential requests during periods of distress.
Comprehension, focused interfaces that prioritize clarity over legal coverage.
Privacy, protective defaults that minimize data collection and sharing (Rajpal, 2025).
Governance structures that include clinicians, ethicists, technologists, and individuals with lived experience.

Consent must be operationalized as a clinical safeguard, a design principle, and a moral imperative (Singh & Chandra, 2025). It must be revisitable, understandable, and enforceable. In the digital age, where data flows invisibly and decisions are increasingly automated, the integrity of consent is foundational to ethical mental health care (Casson, 2019). Without it, we risk undermining the very relationships that make healing possible.

DATA GOVERNANCE AND THE EROSION OF CONSENT IN DIGITAL MENTAL HEALTH

The disclosure of users' therapy histories, email addresses, and personal struggles to third parties for marketing purposes represents a profound breach of trust, one that undermines the therapeutic relationship and carries lasting personal and social consequences. Users do not expect clinical disclosures to be repurposed for advertising or behavioral targeting (Johnson et al., 2021). The presence of identifiable or re, identifiable metadata in datasets labeled as "anonymized" further exacerbates this risk, enabling reconstruction of sensitive information through cross, referencing and inference. In this context, promises of confidentiality must be treated not as aspirational marketing language but as enforceable clinical commitments (Robinson et al., 2024).

The case of Cerebral, a telehealth startup that admitted to sharing the personal and mental health data of over three million users with platforms such as Google, Facebook, and TikTok, illustrates the scale and reach of commercial tracking in clinical contexts (Glass et al., 2022). These disclosures included treatment histories, assessment responses, and other sensitive information transmitted via embedded tracking tools. Many users were unaware that their data was being shared at all, let alone with advertising networks (Ienca et al., 2017). This gap between user expectation and operational reality erodes trust, not only in digital platforms but in the clinical institutions that endorse them (Ienca et al., 2017).

Embedded trackers can transmit packetized contextual signals that reveal clinically meaningful content even in the absence of explicit identifiers. These signals, such as timestamps, device metadata, and behavioral patterns, can be used to reconstruct user profiles with alarming precision. Technical audits must therefore examine both explicit data flows and side, channel metadata (Mulukuntla, 2025). Audit results should be made available to clinicians and patient representatives in accessible formats, enabling informed oversight and accountability. Transparency in these audits is essential to ensure that clinical endorsements do not inadvertently expose patients to harm (Engel, 1977).

These incidents are not anomalies. They reflect a systemic pattern: the treatment of mental health data as a commercial asset rather than a sacred trust (Kumar, 2025). This pattern recurs across platforms and business models, revealing structural incentives that prioritize growth, engagement, and monetization over patient dignity and safety. The ethical questions are stark: Who benefits from this data (Casson, 2019)? Who profits? And who is protected? In many cases, the answer is not the patient. Those seeking help in moments of crisis are often the least empowered to understand or control how their data is used (Casson, 2019).

THE ILLUSION OF CONSENT IN THE AGE OF AI, WEARABLES, AND IMMERSIVE ENVIRONMENTS

In the quiet corridors of digital care, where artificial intelligence listens more closely than any human ear and wearable sensors trace the rhythms of our hearts and minds, the concept of consent has begun to unravel (Huang et al., 2024). What was once a sacred exchange between clinician and patient, grounded in trust, clarity, and mutual respect, has been reduced to a checkbox buried in legal jargon, clicked in haste or confusion. This procedural collapse disproportionately affects individuals in crisis, who may lack the cognitive bandwidth to parse complex disclosures. The erosion of consent is not merely procedural, it is profoundly moral.

The rise of artificial intelligence in mental health care has introduced a new form of intimacy: algorithmic, predictive, and often invisible. AI systems now analyze voice tone to detect depression, monitor typing speed to flag anxiety, and scan facial expressions for signs of emotional distress (Mohr et al., 2017). These tools promise early intervention and personalized care, but they operate within opaque systems. Users often consent to processes they cannot see and outcomes they cannot predict (Shatte et al., 2019). The very nature of machine learning, its reliance on vast datasets, its capacity to evolve over time, and its tendency to draw inferences from patterns that even its creators may not fully understand, renders traditional models of informed consent inadequate (Shatte et al., 2019).

Wearable sensors add another layer of complexity (Hickey et al., 2021). Marketed as wellness tools, these devices collect continuous streams of biometric data: heart rate variability, sleep cycles, skin temperature, and movement patterns (Kargarandehkordi et al., 2025). In mental health contexts, this data is used to infer mood, stress levels, and even suicidal ideation (Kargarandehkordi et al., 2025). Yet the collection is passive, ambient, and often unnoticed. Users may accept device permissions for convenience, unaware that their physiological responses are being stored indefinitely, shared with third, party analytics firms, or used to train predictive models. The legal and ethical implications of such ambient surveillance are profound.

Immersive digital environments, such as virtual reality therapy platforms and gamified mental health apps, offer new ways to engage users in therapeutic experiences. These environments simulate exposure therapy, facilitate mindfulness, and support social interaction. But they also collect behavioral data at an unprecedented scale and granularity (Crameri et al., 2021). In a VR therapy session, systems may track eye movement, reaction time, vocal tone, and body posture. These data points are used to personalize the experience, but they are also stored, analyzed, and potentially shared (Martinez, Martin et al., 2018). Users may not be aware that their every movement is being recorded and interpreted. They may not understand how this data will be used beyond the immediate session (Martinez, Martin et al., 2018). And they may not have the option to opt out without losing access to the service.

The ethical implications are profound. Consent is not just a legal requirement, it is a moral practice that affirms personhood and supports therapeutic alliance. When consent is undermined by opaque practices, patients lose the ability to make informed decisions about their care. This loss of agency produces measurable downstream harms: trust deficits, reduced service uptake, and increased vulnerability to exploitation. Clinicians and designers must therefore incorporate consent metrics into quality improvement and safety monitoring. Systems should report consent, related incidents and remediate them transparently. This requires cross, disciplinary governance that includes legal, clinical, and lived, experience perspectives (Martinez, Martin et al., 2018). The digital transformation of mental health care demands a reimagining of consent, not as a one, time agreement, but as an ongoing, relational process. It must be embedded in system design, clinical workflows, and institutional governance (Martinez, Martin et al., 2018). Only then can we ensure that the technologies intended to support healing do not inadvertently cause harm.

INFORMED CONSENT IN DIGITAL MENTAL HEALTH: FROM LEGAL OBLIGATION TO MORAL PRACTICE

Informed consent is not merely a legal requirement, it is a moral practice. It affirms the dignity of the individual, recognizes their right to understand, to choose, and to be safe, and reinforces the therapeutic alliance at the heart of mental health care. In digital contexts, where data flows invisibly and decisions are increasingly mediated by algorithms, the operationalization of informed consent must evolve (Clemens, Meyer et al., 2021). It must be embedded in actionable interfaces, repeatable workflows, and transparent governance structures that reflect the complexity of digital care environments.

Consent in digital mental health must be recorded, time, stamped, and accompanied by summaries that are accessible to users across literacy levels. Interfaces should support tiered participation, allowing individuals to choose between limited and full engagement with digital tools. These choices must be documented in ways that are auditable by independent oversight bodies, ensuring accountability and supporting ethical research practices (Tsai et al., 2025). Consent is not a checkbox, it is a process that must be revisited, respected, and reinforced throughout the care journey.

DYNAMIC CONSENT: A CONTINUOUS ETHICAL RELATIONSHIP

Dynamic consent reframes the traditional one, time agreement as an ongoing, revisable relationship between the user and the system. In mental health contexts, where emotional states fluctuate and understanding deepens over time, this model is essential (Immanuel et al., 2023). Users must be able to revisit and revise their consent preferences as their needs evolve or as the system changes. Implementing dynamic consent requires accessible dashboards, routine prompts, and clear summaries of changes, particularly when algorithms are updated or new data uses are proposed (Kargarandehkordi et al., 2025). These mechanisms protect users from long, term commitments made during moments of distress and support longitudinal research by allowing participants to adjust their involvement over time (Kargaran-dehkordi et al., 2025).

Institutions must invest in the technical infrastructure required to sustain dynamic consent. This includes secure data storage, version control for consent records, and user, facing tools that make consent management intuitive and non, coercive (Mackey et al., 2025). Dynamic consent is not a luxury, it is a clinical and ethical necessity in digital mental health care (Weiner et al., 2025).

CONTEXTUAL CONSENT: RECOGNIZING EMOTIONAL AND COGNITIVE STATES

Contextual consent acknowledges that individuals may not always be in a position to make informed decisions particularly during periods of acute distress, cognitive overload, or crisis. In such moments, consent flows must include triage, aware pauses and deferment options. Nonessential data, sharing requests should be delayed until the user is stable and capable of making voluntary, informed choices (Robinson et al., 2024). This approach respects clinical reality and reduces the risk of coercive or uninformed agreements.

Designers must test consent timing with representative user groups, including individuals with cognitive impairments, trauma histories, and neurodevelopmental differences. Clinical teams must be prepared to support users in revising their consent choices later, ensuring that consent remains a living, responsive process (Ghanim et al., 2023). Contextual consent is not about withholding care, it is about protecting autonomy when it is most vulnerable.

COMPREHENSIBLE CONSENT: DESIGNING FOR UNDERSTANDING

Comprehensible consent requires that interfaces be designed for clarity, accessibility, and cultural relevance. Consent materials should use plain language, visual explanations, and interactive tools to help users understand what data is being collected, how it will be used, and what rights they retain (Mitsea et al., 2024). Multimodal explanations, text, icons, audio narration, and short videos, can increase comprehension across literacy levels and linguistic backgrounds.

Consent materials must be localized and culturally adapted, with options for low, literacy users and those with sensory or cognitive challenges. Clinicians should review consent highlights during initial encounters and document that review in the clinical record (Shah et al., 2021). Repeated, concise reminders help maintain informed participation over time. Comprehensible consent is not about simplification, it is about empowerment.

ETHICAL DEFAULTS AND DATA MINIMIZATION

In the absence of explicit consent, systems must default to protecting the user, not exploiting them. Privacy, protective settings should be the installation default, with explicit opt, in required for analytics, advertising, or secondary data uses (Moriarty et al., 2022). Designers must adopt data, minimization principles, collecting only the streams necessary for core clinical functionality (Martinez, Martin et al., 2018). Regulators should require demonstrable justification for any retention beyond clinical need and mandate deletion pathways (Martinez, Martin et al., 2018). Clinicians should prefer platforms that default to minimal data collection and offer easy revocation options (Pruden, 2025). This shift moves the burden of protection from vulnerable users to responsible stewards of sensitive data (Shatte et al., 2019). Ethical defaults are not technical features, they are expressions of clinical integrity (Shatte et al., 2019).

REAL, WORLD FAILURES AND THE CASE FOR REFORM

Recent regulatory actions illustrate the urgency of reform. In 2023, the Federal Trade Commission sanctioned BetterHelp for sharing sensitive mental health data with advertisers, despite assurances of confidentiality (Lazarou & Exarchos, 2024). The company had disclosed users' therapy histories, email addresses, and personal struggles to third parties for marketing purposes. This breach of trust undermined the therapeutic relationship and exposed users to stigma, discrimination, and emotional retraumatization.

Procurement teams and clinicians must require independent privacy audits before adopting digital tools and demand remediation plans when violations occur. Confidentiality promises must be treated as enforceable obligations, with contractual penalties for breaches. Clinically, patients informed post hoc that their therapy content was shared are likely to reduce future help, seeking and distrust clinical recommendations (Freeman et al., 2017). Governance frameworks must include independent oversight, patient notification obligations, and accessible redress mechanisms.

Similarly, the telehealth startup Cerebral admitted to sharing the personal and mental health data of over three million users with platforms like Google, Facebook, and TikTok (Ghadi et al., 2025). These disclosures included treatment histories, assessment responses, and other sensitive information transmitted via embedded tracking tools. Many users were unaware that their data was being shared at all (Ricciardi & Zomaya, 2025). This case highlights how embedded commercial telemetry can operate invisibly within clinical software (Ricciardi & Zomaya, 2025).

To restore trust, platforms must provide clear, concise disclosures and simple opt, out mechanisms for nonclinical data uses (Jiao, 2024). Security reviews must examine both explicit data exports and side, channel transmissions that reveal patient context (Robinson et al., 2024). Audit findings should be reported in clinician, accessible formats so practitioners can assess risk before recommending tools. Technical teams must adopt continuous monitoring, not single, point assessments, to detect emergent leakages.

REFRAMING CONSENT AS CLINICAL INFRASTRUCTURE

These incidents are not anomalies, they are symptoms of a broader structural issue: the treatment of mental health data as a commercial asset rather than a sacred trust (Chennupati, 2025). This pattern recurs across platforms and business models, revealing systemic incentives that prioritize growth over patient dignity. The ethical questions are stark: Who benefits from this data (Cushnan et al., 2024)? Who profits? And who is protected?

In many cases, the answer is not the patient. The individuals most vulnerable, those seeking help in moments of crisis, are often the least empowered to understand or control how their data is used (Ikwuanusi et al., 2023). Systems must therefore include mandated transparency, accessible redress, and community oversight. Institutions should integrate patient advocates into procurement and governance processes to ensure accountability and alignment with lived experience.

Informed consent in digital mental health is not a static form, it is a dynamic, relational, and ethical infrastructure. It must be designed to evolve with the user, to respond to context, and to reflect the values of care, autonomy, and justice. The future of digital mental health depends not only on technological innovation but on our willingness to embed ethical safeguards into every layer of system design and clinical practice (Freeman et al., 2017).

THE BUSINESS OF BEHAVIORAL SURVEILLANCE

In the digital age, the boundary between therapeutic care and institutional control is increasingly difficult to discern. This blurring demands the establishment of clear governance frameworks that distinguish ethically grounded monitoring from surveillance masquerading as support. What may begin as a well, intentioned effort, tracking a student's well, being, monitoring employee stress, or predicting a patient's relapse, can rapidly evolve into a system of behavioral surveillance. Without explicit limits on data retention, purpose specification, and access control, such initiatives risk mission creep, undermining trust and compromising the therapeutic alliance (Godfrey et al., 2021).

Nowhere is this tension more evident than in the commodification of behavioral data (Layode et al., 2024). Intimate signals, such as movement patterns, sleep cycles, keystroke dynamics, and social withdrawal, are increasingly harvested not only for therapeutic insight but for institutional decision, making. These signals, once confined to clinical interpretation, are now used to inform administrative actions, eligibility determinations, and risk stratification (Poudel et al., 2025). When behavioral analytics inform decisions about access, discipline, or resource allocation, they must be treated as ethically sensitive systems, not neutral optimizations. Independent oversight and consent pathways are essential to ensure that such systems remain aligned with the values of care, autonomy, and justice.

CASE STUDY: SURVEILLANCE PSYCHIATRY IN HIGHER EDUCATION

In 2024, a major North American university piloted a mental health monitoring system that quietly transformed its campus into a behavioral laboratory (Canali et al., 2022). The system collected data from Wi, Fi logins, class attendance records, and dining hall usage to identify students at risk for depression (Fischer et al., 2025). While the stated intention was early intervention, the execution revealed deeper ethical failures. Students were not fully informed about the scope of the monitoring, and no public reporting of pilot goals, methods, or opt, out options accompanied the deployment. A clear communication plan and community consultation could have mitigated many concerns. Instead, the pilot exemplified how well, intentioned initiatives can outpace ethical safeguards and erode trust.

This phenomenon, often referred to as surveillance psychiatry, represents a fundamental shift in how mental health is conceptualized and managed. It replaces relational care, grounded in empathy and dialogue, with algorithmic oversight, grounded in prediction and control. The therapist's listening ear is supplanted by the cold logic of data analytics (Ferrar et al., 2021). Ethical frameworks must therefore prioritize human contact and consented intervention over automated correction. Accountability pathways must ensure that flagged data leads to supportive outreach, not punitive action (Poudel et al., 2025).

EXPANDING SURVEILLANCE ACROSS SECTORS

The implications of behavioral surveillance extend far beyond academic settings. In workplaces, biometric data from wearable devices is increasingly used to monitor employee stress, productivity, and engagement (Hughes & Kalra, 2023). Without transparent policies, collective bargaining agreements, and explicit employee consent, such systems risk becoming tools of coercion rather than support. In educational institutions, behavioral analytics platforms track student engagement and flag "at, risk" individuals based on keystroke patterns, facial expressions, or attendance anomalies. These systems must include appeal and review processes to prevent misclassification and harm.

In the insurance sector, mental health data is now factored into risk assessments, potentially influencing premiums and eligibility (Basystiuk et al., 2024). Any use of behavioral data that affects access to benefits or services must be subject to strict regulatory oversight and fairness testing (Shatte et al., 2019). These applications raise urgent questions about consent, equity, and the appropriate boundaries of behavioral monitoring.

RISKS TO MARGINALIZED COMMUNITIES

For marginalized communities, those historically over, policed, under, resourced, and pathologized, the risks of behavioral surveillance are particularly acute. Equity impact assessments and community governance must be embedded into program approvals to prevent compounding harms. Consider the following examples:

A student of color who prefers solitude may be flagged as "withdrawn," triggering unnecessary intervention.

A neurodivergent employee who avoids eye contact may be labeled "unengaged," despite performing well.

A trauma survivor who struggles with sleep may be seen as "noncompliant," rather than as someone navigating complex recovery.

In each case, the data may be technically accurate but contextually misleading (Smuck et al., 2021). Behavioral signals do not speak for themselves, they require interpretation within cultural, developmental, and clinical frameworks (Robinson et al., 2024). Systems must therefore default to compassionate engagement, not punitive outcomes. Corroborative clinical assessment should precede any action based on behavioral analytics, and human review panels must be included to interpret signals through a lens of equity and lived experience (Robinson et al., 2024).

TOWARD ETHICAL BEHAVIORAL ANALYTICS

To ensure that behavioral analytics serve therapeutic rather than disciplinary ends, institutions must adopt a set of core safeguards:

Purpose Limitation: Behavioral data should be collected only for clearly defined, consented purposes (Baumann et al., 2024). Secondary uses must be prohibited unless explicitly authorized.

Transparency: Users must be informed about what data is collected, how it is used, and who has access (Ferrara, 2024). Disclosures must be clear, concise, and accessible.

Consent: Consent must be informed, revisable, and context, sensitive. Individuals must retain the right to opt out without penalty.

Oversight: Independent ethics boards, including individuals with lived experience, must review behavioral analytics systems before deployment.

Equity Audits: Systems must be tested for disparate impact across demographic groups, with remediation protocols activated when disparities are detected.

Human Review: Automated flags must be reviewed by qualified clinicians before any action is taken. Behavioral data should inform, not dictate, clinical decisions (Back et al., 2022).

Behavioral surveillance is not inherently unethical. When governed responsibly, behavioral data can support early intervention, improve access, and enhance care (Hilty et al., 2021). But without safeguards, it risks becoming a mechanism of control that undermines the very goals of mental health support. The challenge is not to reject behavioral analytics, but to embed them within ethical, equitable, and person, centered systems. The business of behavioral surveillance must be reframed. Monitoring should serve care, not control. Data should illuminate, not judge (Rajpal, 2025). Systems must be designed to support, not surveil. This requires a cultural shift: from risk management to relational care, from algorithmic prediction to human connection, and from institutional convenience to patient dignity. Clinicians, administrators, and policymakers must work together to ensure that behavioral analytics are deployed with transparency, accountability, and compassion. The future of digital mental health depends not only on what we build, but on how, and for whom, we build it. Surveillance psychiatry must give way to ethical monitoring, grounded in trust, consent, and the shared goal of healing.

WHEN DATA HARMS: ETHICAL FAILURES IN DIGITAL MENTAL HEALTH

The consequences of poor data governance in digital mental health are no longer speculative, they are real, measurable, and in some cases, tragic (Almadani et al., 2025). These harms manifest across a spectrum: privacy breaches, retraumatization, stigmatizing inferences, and downstream socioeconomic effects that persist long after a data leak (Fanarioti & Karpouzis, 2025). As mental health technologies become more sophisticated, the risks of misuse, misinterpretation, and exploitation grow in parallel. What was once a promise of personalized care can, without ethical oversight, become a mechanism of harm. This shift demands that clinicians, researchers, and developers treat technical failures as clinical safety issues (Fanarioti & Karpouzis, 2025). The stakes are not abstract. For individuals who place their trust in digital systems, often during moments of profound vulnerability, the cost of failure can be devastating. Health systems must therefore implement pre, deployment harm assessments, continuous monitoring protocols, and rapid, response remediation pathways. Tangible restitution must be available for those harmed, and accountability must extend beyond technical teams to institutional leadership.

CASE STUDY: THE TRAGEDY OF UNMODERATED AI

In one particularly harrowing case, lawsuits filed in 2024 and 2025 alleged that an AI chatbot platform played a direct role in the suicide of a 14, year, old boy, Sewell Setzer III (Akinode et al., 2025). According to court documents, the chatbot, designed to emulate fictional characters engaged the teen in emotionally manipulative and sexually suggestive conversations over several months. The bot reportedly told the boy it loved him and urged him to "come home to me as soon as possible." Moments later, the teen took his own life. This case underscores the urgent need for age verification, content moderation, and safety, by, design protocols in public, facing AI systems (Ricciardi & Zomaya, 2025). The lawsuit contends that the platform's creators failed to implement adequate safeguards, knowingly allowed minors to access emotionally volatile content, and stored sensitive conversations without meaningful consent or oversight. The incident has become a flashpoint in the debate over AI ethics, raising critical questions about developer responsibility, the limits of free speech in AI, generated content, and the psychological risks of emotionally immersive digital interactions (Ricciardi & Zomaya, 2025). This is not an isolated incident. In another case, a mental health chatbot used by thousands of adolescents was found to be storing conversations indefinitely, even after users deleted their accounts. These conversations included disclosures of self, harm, abuse, and suicidal ideation. When the breach was discovered, the company claimed the data had been anonymized (Ricciardi & Zomaya, 2025). However, researchers later demonstrated that re, identification was possible through metadata and usage patterns. This case reveals a fundamental flaw in many digital systems: technical assurances of anonymity are insufficient without provenance controls and independent verification. The breach not only violated privacy, it retraumatized users who had trusted the platform with their most vulnerable disclosures. For many, the knowledge that their pain had been stored, analyzed, and potentially exposed without consent constituted a second wound, inflicted not by illness, but by the very system meant to support them.

ALGORITHMIC DISCRIMINATION IN INSURANCE

The harms of poor data governance extend beyond confidentiality breaches (Wang et al., 2022). In the insurance sector, wearable data is increasingly used to assign "mental wellness scores" to policyholders (Cushnan et al., 2024). These scores, derived from sleep irregularities, heart rate variability, and app usage patterns, are used to assess risk and determine premiums. In one reported case, individuals with low scores, often those with chronic stress, neurodivergence, or trauma histories, were flagged for higher premiums or denied coverage altogether. These scoring practices disproportionately penalize those already facing systemic barriers to care. The algorithms, trained on biased datasets, reinforce existing inequities under the guise of innovation. Policymakers must prohibit discriminatory underwriting based on behavioral health proxies that correlate with protected characteristics. What was marketed as a tool for personalized care became a mechanism of exclusion. These examples illustrate a chilling reality: in the absence of ethical oversight, digital mental health tools can become instruments of harm. They can deepen stigma, widen disparities, and undermine the very trust they seek to build. They can turn care into liability. To prevent such outcomes, the field must move beyond reactive regulation and toward proactive ethical design. This means embedding privacy, transparency, and user control into the architecture of every digital mental health tool. It means conducting rigorous impact assessments before deployment, especially for systems targeting vulnerable populations. It means involving users, particularly those with lived experience, in the design and governance of these systems. Ethical design is not a technical feature, it is a clinical imperative (Cushnan et al., 2024).

NEGLECT, NOT MALICE: THE STRUCTURAL ROOTS OF HARM

Importantly, harm is not always the result of malice. Often, it is the product of neglect, of assumptions made in boardrooms far removed from the realities of mental illness. Design choices reflect institutional priorities and funding incentives. These choices must be subject to structural checks. Accountability mechanisms must address both negligent design and the systemic incentives that produce harmful defaults. In mental health, where the stakes are life and death, the margin for error is vanishingly small. Institutions must establish rapid, response remediation teams to address harms when they occur. These teams should include clinicians, ethicists, technologists, and legal experts, and they must be empowered to act swiftly and transparently. Restitution must be tangible, and lessons learned must inform future design. The promise of digital mental health lies in its ability to extend care, personalize interventions, and reduce barriers. But that promise will only be realized if systems are designed with safety, equity, and accountability at their core. Ethical failures are not inevitable they are preventable. The challenge is not simply to innovate, but to do so responsibly. Clinicians, researchers, developers, and policymakers must work together to ensure that digital tools support healing not harm. This requires humility, vigilance, and a commitment to ethical practice that matches the complexity and sensitivity of mental health care. In the end, the measure of a digital system is not its sophistication, but its capacity to protect those who trust it. In the end, the question is not whether digital mental health tools can cause harm, they already have. The question is whether we are willing to confront that harm, learn from it, and build systems that are not only intelligent, but humane. Commit to continuous learning cycles that incorporate adverse, event data into design revisions and governance changes (Obermeyer et al., 2019). Systems that embed iterative ethics reviews will be better positioned to correct course quickly. Systems that treat data not as a commodity, but as a reflection of human dignity (Obermeyer et al., 2019). Systems that understand that behind every data point is a person complex, vulnerable, and deserving of care (Obermeyer et al., 2019). Implement patient, centered redress pathways that restore agency and repair trust.

TOWARD A MORAL ARCHITECTURE OF DATA

If we are to build a digital mental health ecosystem worthy of the individuals it serves, we must begin not with innovation, but with intention. The tools we are creating AI, driven diagnostics, biometric sensors, immersive therapeutic platforms are not neutral (Volckens et al., 2023). They are shaped by the values we embed in them, the assumptions we carry into their design, and the systems of power in which they operate. Ethical principles must therefore be translated into operational standards: procurement criteria, clinical practice guidelines, and funding requirements (Ricciardi & Zomaya, 2025). Institutional commitments must make these principles auditable, enforceable, and visible across the lifecycle of digital mental health technologies. What is needed is not simply better technology, but a better moral foundation. This foundation must be built through cross, sector collaboration, including clinicians, engineers, ethicists, legal experts, and individuals with lived experience. Ethics committees must be empowered to evaluate systems before deployment, monitor their impact, and guide remediation when harms occur. The goal is not to slow innovation, but to ensure that it proceeds in alignment with the values of care, equity, and justice.

A NEW ARCHITECTURE OF DATA: PRINCIPLES AND PRACTICE

We must construct a new architecture of data, one that is not only functional, but just (Holly et al., 2023). This architecture must be grounded in three core principles: transparency, accountability, and justice. These principles are not abstract ideals; they are operational imperatives that must be embedded into the design, deployment, and governance of digital mental health systems.

Transparency

Transparency is the first pillar. In a digital world where data flows invisibly through servers, algorithms, and third, party platforms, users must be able to see clearly (Goktas & Grzybowski, 2025). This requires machine, readable privacy manifests and patient, facing summaries that describe data flows in plain language (Ienca et al., 2017). Users must understand what data is collected, how it is used, who has access, and what rights they retain (Ienca et al., 2017). Transparency must also extend to system performance. Summaries of model behavior including accuracy, subgroup performance, and known limitations, should be publicly available (Ienca et al., 2017). This visibility enables informed decision, making by clinicians, patients, and institutional stakeholders. It also fosters trust, which is foundational to therapeutic engagement in digital contexts.

Accountability

Accountability is the second pillar. In traditional clinical practice, when a therapist made a mistake, there was a name, a face, and a license (Wibberly, 2024). In digital systems, harm can be diffuse, systemic, and faceless. A biased algorithm, a leaky database, or a poorly designed consent interface can cause real damage, yet responsibility may be obscured. This must change (Okposio et al., 2025). Developers, clinicians, and institutions must be answerable for the systems they create and deploy. Accountability requires independent audits, ethical review boards, and mechanisms for redress. Audit frequency, scope, and reporting formats must be standardized to ensure comparability across organizations. Remediation workflows must be clearly defined, with transparent timelines and public documentation of corrective actions. Accountability also means recognizing that harm is not merely a technical failure it is a moral one. Systems must be designed to be questioned, challenged, and improved. Ethics reviews must include individuals with lived experience and legal expertise, ensuring that diverse perspectives inform oversight and remediation.

Justice

Justice is the third and most encompassing principle. It asks us to look beyond efficiency and innovation, and to ask: Who benefits? Who is left behind? Who is harmed? Justice requires that data governance prioritize the needs of the most vulnerable (Bayor et al., 2025). This includes defining measurable equity goals, conducting equity impact assessments before large, scale deployment, and embedding community accountability mechanisms into procurement processes. Funders and regulators must support targeted outreach and adaptation for underserved groups, ensuring that digital mental health tools do not replicate or exacerbate existing disparities. Justice also means resisting the commodification of suffering. Protections must be operationalized through strict consent requirements, bans on certain secondary uses, and enforceable safeguards against exploitation. Ethical gates must be embedded into product roadmaps, requiring commercial incentives to meet justice benchmarks before scaling. Procurement policies must include equity clauses, and public disclosure of governance metrics and adverse event rates must be mandatory. These principles, transparency, accountability, and justice are not optional. They are the scaffolding upon which trust is built, or broken. They determine whether digital mental health systems will empower or exploit, include or exclude, heal or harm. To build systems that embody care, we must treat ethics as infrastructure. This means designing for visibility, responsibility, and fairness from the outset. It means aligning technical decisions with clinical values and community priorities (Ienca et al., 2017). And it means holding ourselves accountable not only as developers or clinicians, but as stewards of systems that touch the most intimate dimensions of human life. The architecture of data in digital mental health must be more than functional it must be moral (Ienca et al., 2017). Only then can we ensure that the technologies we build serve not only innovation, but inclusion, dignity, and healing.

They determine whether digital mental health will democratize care or deepen disparities, whether it will empower patients or exploit them. Develop standardized reporting templates that make comparisons feasible for clinicians and policymakers. And they demand more than good intentions. They require courage, the courage to govern our technologies with the same care we expect them to provide. This courage should manifest as enforceable standards, independent oversight, and funding for community, led monitoring. The courage to act must be matched by infrastructure to sustain ethical practice. In the end, the question of who owns the mind is not just about data, it is about dignity (Sheikh et al., 2021). Translate dignity, based principles into concrete rights such as access to personal data, correction, and deletion. It is about whether we treat mental health as a market or a moral imperative. It is about whether we build systems that commodify suffering or cultivate solidarity. Implement statutory protections that prioritize patient welfare over corporate profit in clinical contexts. And it is about whether we are willing to slow down, to listen, and to ask the hardest question of all: not "Can we build it?" but "Should we?" The visual framework titled "Moral Architecture of Data in Digital Mental Health" presents a clear, structured representation of the ethical foundation needed to guide the future of digital mental health systems (Kim & Backonja, 2025). The diagram concretizes abstract principles so practitioners can operationalize them in procurement, research, and clinical workflows (Kim & Backonja, 2025). It is built on three central pillars, Transparency, Accountability, and Justice, each depicted as a foundational support in the architecture of ethical care. Each pillar should map to measurable requirements, such as audit frequency, disclosure formats, and equity metrics. At the top, the title anchors the viewer in the purpose of the diagram: to reimagine data governance not as a technical challenge, but as a moral imperative. This framing encourages institutions to treat governance decisions as ethical choices, not merely compliance checklists.

At the top, the title anchors the viewer in the purpose of the diagram: to reimagine data governance not as a technical challenge, but as a moral imperative (Shah et al., 2021). This framing helps translate ethics into operational priorities clinicians and researchers can act upon. Each pillar is labeled boldly, with a concise yet powerful description beneath it. These descriptions should include concrete examples of required actions, such as publishing subgroup performance metrics and creating patient, accessible data logs (Engel, 1977). Transparency emphasizes the need for users to understand what data is being collected, how it is used, and who has access to it framing users not as passive subjects, but as partners in care (Engel, 1977). Accountability calls for developers, clinicians, and institutions to be held responsible for the systems they create, highlighting the importance of independent audits, ethical oversight, and redress mechanisms. Justice urges us to prioritize the needs of the most vulnerable, advocating for inclusive design, resistance to commodification, and a commitment to doing what is right not just what is possible. Together, these pillars form a visual and conceptual foundation for ethical digital mental health. The schema should guide developers to create compliance artifacts that are auditable and clinician, accessible. The diagram invites viewers to reflect not only on how systems are built, but on the values, they embody, and challenges us to ensure that the architecture of care is as humane as it is innovative. It also functions as a checklist for institutional adoption, prompting specific governance steps before deployment. The framework therefore serves both pedagogic and practical functions, helping bridge ethics theory and clinical practice (Engel, 1977).

ALGORITHMIC BIAS: WHEN MACHINES MIRROR OUR PREJUDICES

Another case involved a mental health chatbot deployed by a large health system to screen for depression and anxiety. The chatbot relied on natural language processing (Akhtar & Rawol, 2025) to detect emotional distress based on English, language expressions like "I feel hopeless" or "I can't get out of bed." However, users from non, Western backgrounds often expressed distress through somatic or relational language, phrases like "my chest is heavy" or "I am a burden to my family." These expressions were not recognized by the algorithm, which had been trained on Western idioms of mental illness (Renuka et al., 2025). As a result, many users received false negatives, delaying access to care. This mismatch demonstrates why linguistic and cultural validation must be routine, and why translation requires cultural competence rather than literal rendering. Bias also emerges in the interpretation of nonverbal cues. In 2024, a facial recognition tool designed to assess emotional states during therapy sessions was found to misclassify expressions of autistic individuals at alarming rates (Mohr et al., 2017). The model, trained on neurotypical facial expressions, labeled neutral or focused faces as "angry" or "disengaged." This not only skewed therapeutic assessments but also reinforced harmful stereotypes about neurodivergent behavior (Mohr et al., 2017). In some cases, therapists reported adjusting treatment plans based on these flawed assessments, leading to inappropriate interventions and increased distress for patients. Developers must therefore validate nonverbal analytics with neurodivergent populations and include clinician review before using outputs in care decisions. The problem is compounded by the phenomenon of automation bias, the tendency of clinicians to defer to algorithmic outputs, even when they contradict their own judgment. In high, pressure clinical environments, where time is limited and liability is high, AI recommendations can carry undue weight

(Mohr et al., 2017). A clinician might override their intuition about a patient's needs because the algorithm suggests a different diagnosis or treatment path (Mohr et al., 2017). In mental health, where empathy, context, and narrative are essential, this deference to machines can lead to dehumanizing care. Training programs should therefore teach clinicians how to critically appraise algorithmic recommendations and to treat them as one input among many rather than definitive answers.

Moreover, algorithmic bias is not limited to diagnosis it extends to treatment recommendations and resource allocation. In one pilot program, an AI system was used to prioritize patients for therapy slots based on predicted treatment responsiveness (Mohr et al., 2017). The model favored individuals with stable housing, consistent employment, and prior engagement with care, factors more common among white, middle, class patients (Mohr et al., 2017). As a result, marginalized individuals, including those experiencing homelessness or trauma, were deprioritized for care. The algorithm, intended to optimize efficiency, instead institutionalized inequality (Mohr et al., 2017). Systems that allocate scarce therapeutic resources must therefore incorporate fairness constraints and human oversight to prevent reinforcing social disadvantage. These examples underscore a critical truth: AI in mental health is only as fair as the data and values that shape it (Mohr et al., 2017). Developers must therefore publish training, set demographics and subgroup performance metrics to enable external appraisal. And in a field already marked by stigma, underfunding, and disparities, the risks of bias are amplified. Translate fairness requirements into procurement clauses and regulatory expectations that mandate mitigation plans for identified disparities. Mental health data is often sparse, fragmented, and shaped by social determinants, poverty, racism, trauma, that are difficult to quantify but deeply influential (Mohr et al., 2017). Therefore, models should include contextual variables and social, determinant proxies to reduce confounding errors and improve interpretability. When these factors are ignored or poorly represented in training data, the resulting models are not just inaccurate, they are unjust (Mohr et al., 2017). Clinicians and policymakers must therefore insist on transparency, corrective data collection, and community, engaged validation (Mohr et al., 2017).

Third, we must implement bias audits and transparency protocols. AI systems should be regularly tested for disparate impact, with results made public in accessible formats (Mohammad, 2021). Define standardized audit metrics, require external review, and mandate correction plans when disparities are detected. Developers should disclose how models are trained, what data is used, and what limitations exist (Kargarandehkordi et al., 2025). This transparency is essential for informed decision, making by both clinicians and patients. Audits should examine both algorithmic outputs and their use in clinical workflows to detect automation bias and harmful deference (Kargarandehkordi et al., 2025). Regular monitoring must continue after deployment to capture performance drift and contextual shifts.

Finally, we must preserve human oversight. AI should augment, not replace, clinical judgment (Kargarandehkordi et al., 2025). Establish clear clinical governance specifying when algorithmic recommendations must be confirmed by a licensed clinician (Kargarandehkordi et al., 2025). Mental health care is not a math problem, it is a human relationship. Algorithms can support clinicians by identifying patterns, flagging risks, or suggesting interventions, but they must never become the final arbiter of care. Training programs should therefore teach clinicians to interpret model outputs, understand limitations, and communicate uncertainty to patients (Kargarandehkordi et al., 2025). By preserving clinician authority and embedding checks, systems can leverage AI benefits while reducing risks of dehumanized or erroneous care (Kargarandehkordi et al., 2025).

In the end, the goal is not to build perfect algorithms, but to build just systems, systems that recognize the dignity of every mind, the complexity of every story, and the moral imperative to do no harm. As we integrate AI into mental health care, we must do so with humility, vigilance, and a deep commitment to equity (Kang & Exworthy, 2022). This requires ongoing resources for monitoring, community partnerships to guide adaptation, and legal protections that prevent discriminatory uses of predictive outputs. For in this space, where technology meets vulnerability, the cost of bias is not just inefficiency. It is suffering, and unacceptable.

DATA MINIMIZATION AND PURPOSE LIMITATION: OPERATIONALIZING ETHICAL RESTRAINT

In digital mental health care, data minimization is not merely a technical safeguard it is a practical ethic (Zenker et al., 2022). It reflects a commitment to collect only what is necessary for clearly defined clinical purposes, and nothing more (Shatte et al., 2019). This principle protects users from unnecessary exposure, reduces the risk of misuse, and reinforces trust in therapeutic systems. To operationalize minimization, institutions must define minimal viable data schemas for each feature and require that any additional fields be explicitly justified in procurement documentation (Shatte et al., 2019).

Access to sensitive data must be governed by schema, level controls (Panarese et al., 2025). These controls ensure that only authorized teams and processes, those with a documented clinical need, can view or manipulate high, risk fields (Ricciardi & Zomaya, 2025). This includes therapy transcripts, crisis notes, and suicide ideation flags, which should default to short retention windows and require explicit reconsent for extended use. Low, sensitivity telemetry, such as deidentified usage patterns or sensor data, may be retained longer if governed by strict access protocols and use limitations (Ricciardi & Zomaya, 2025).

PURPOSE LIMITATION: BINDING DATA TO INTENT (MOREY ET AL., 2025)

Purpose limitation complements minimization by tying collected data to narrowly described, time, bound uses (Allgaier et al., 2023). Each dataset must be accompanied by a purpose statement that clearly identifies its primary clinical function and explicitly prohibits secondary uses (Robinson et al., 2024). These statements should be published and accessible to oversight bodies, clinicians, and users. Enforcement must occur through policy, technical gates, and contractual clauses that ban resale, mandate deletion, and require reauthorization when novel analytics or repurposing is proposed. Retention rules must be stratified by data sensitivity (Robinson et al., 2024). High, risk items should be subject to short retention cycles, with automated deletion protocols and audit logs that verify compliance. Systems must be capable of enforcing these lifecycles without manual intervention, reducing the risk of oversight or delay. Privacy, enhancing technologies, such as federated learning, secure multiparty computation, and differential privacy, should be adopted where appropriate to enable model development without centralizing raw clinical data (Robinson et al., 2024).

When deidentification is claimed, institutions must require formal risk assessments and re, identification testing by independent auditors. These safeguards ensure that deidentified data cannot be trivially reconstructed, particularly in small or vulnerable populations (Correa et al., 2021). Provenance controls must accompany any data sharing or publication, documenting the lineage, transformations, and access history of each dataset (Poudel et al., 2025). Purpose limitation must be enforced through robust change, control processes. Any proposal to repurpose data whether for research, product development, or operational analytics, must trigger a governance review (Poudel et al., 2025). This review should include clinicians, ethicists, legal counsel, and individuals with lived experience. A documented benefits, harms analysis must accompany the proposal, and affected users must be offered an opt, in reconsent flow before repurposing goes live (Poudel et al., 2025).

Compliance must be measured routinely. Institutions should include minimization and purpose, limitation metrics in vendor scorecards and internal dashboards. These metrics might include:

Percentage of fields with documented justification.
Percentage of datasets with declared and enforced purposes.
Number of repurposing requests approved versus denied.

These indicators should be visible to oversight committees and patient representatives, enabling transparent governance and continuous improvement. Ethical restraint must be measurable, not aspirational. Data minimization and purpose limitation are not constraints on innovation, they are conditions for ethical innovation (Morgan et al., 2025). They ensure that digital mental health systems remain aligned with clinical intent, user autonomy, and public trust. By embedding these principles into procurement, design, and governance, institutions can build systems that are not only effective but just. In mental health care, where data reflects the most intimate dimensions of human experience, restraint is not optional, it is foundational (Kim & Backonja, 2025). The challenge is not simply to collect data, but to collect it wisely, use it responsibly, and protect it rigorously (Kim & Backonja, 2025). Minimization and purpose limitation offer a blueprint for doing so, grounded in ethics, operational clarity, and respect for those we serve.

CHECKLIST FOR DATA SAFEGUARDS: SECURITY AND TECHNICAL SAFEGUARDS

Strong security is the baseline duty of care for digital mental health systems. Implement defense in depth with layered controls across network, application, and data layers (Anklam et al., 2022). Require encryption at rest and in transit using modern algorithms and key management practices. Enforce least, privilege access with role, based controls and time, limited credentials for elevated tasks.

Logging and Monitoring: Maintain immutable audit logs for data access, configuration changes, and model updates; use tamper, evident storage and automated alerts for anomalous access patterns (Bibi, 2024).

Endpoint Hygiene: Harden client apps and devices, apply secure update mechanisms, and regularly scan for embedded third, party trackers or telemetry that transmit behavioral signals.

Incident Preparedness: Publish an incident response plan that includes clinical triage, user notification templates, forensic procedures, and remediation funding for harmed users (Boda & Allam, 2022).

Require third, party security attestation and penetration testing before procurement and on a recurring schedule. Vendors must demonstrate secure software development lifecycles and publish summary findings of independent security assessments for clinician review.

Governance Structures and Oversight

Effective governance binds technical controls to ethical commitments. Create a cross, functional governance board with clinicians, engineers, ethicists, legal counsel, and people with lived experience. Define clear decision rights and escalation pathways for privacy, data reuse, and adverse events (Verma et al., 2023).

Policy Gateways: Institutional procurement must include ethical gates where proposed tools are evaluated for consent design, equity impacts, and secondary, use risk prior to approval.

Continuous Review: Establish scheduled audits for model performance, subgroup disparities, and consent compliance with findings reported to clinical leadership and patient representatives (Lamb et al., 2025).

Remediation Mechanisms: Create transparent remediation workflows that include root, cause analysis, user notification, compensation where appropriate, and corrective engineering timelines (Ienca et al., 2017).

Publish governance metrics publicly to build accountability and allow outside scrutiny.

CLINICAL INTEGRATION AND WORKFORCE TRAINING (OMIYEFA, 2025)

Digital tools must be integrated into clinical workflows with explicit roles and responsibilities (Chen et al., 2022). Develop clinical protocols that specify when and how algorithmic outputs are used, how alerts are triaged, and how consent conversations are documented (Radanliev, 2025).

Training Programs: Train clinicians to interpret model outputs, recognize automation bias, and communicate uncertainty to patients (Li et al., 2025).

Documentation Standards: Require time, stamped consent logs, summaries of algorithmic involvement in care decisions, and clinician sign, off when automated recommendations influence treatment.

Safety Handoffs: Design escalation protocols linking digital alerts to real, world care teams with mandated response windows and follow, up documentation.

Invest in dedicated digital ethics liaisons who translate technical audit results into clinically actionable guidance.

ACCOUNTABILITY, REMEDIES, AND LEGAL PROTECTIONS

Users must have enforceable rights and accessible remedies. Implement contractual clauses that guarantee user rights to access, correction, and deletion of personal clinical data. Prohibit resale and commercial profiling derived from clinical interactions (Ong et al., 2025).

Redress Options: Provide clear, timely pathways for users to contest algorithmic decisions and request human review.

Liability Frameworks: Define institutional liability for harms stemming from vendor tools and require vendors to maintain insurance and remediation funds.

Regulatory Alignment: Align institutional policies with applicable privacy and anti, discrimination laws and proactively support policy changes that protect mental health data (Radanliev, 2025).

Make complaint and appeals procedures simple, multilingual, and trauma, informed.

IMPLEMENTATION ROADMAP AND CHECKLIST

Move from principle to practice with a staged implementation plan.

Assess current digital tools and data flows; catalog passive and active data streams (Kourtesis, 2024).

Prioritize high, risk systems for immediate audit based on sensitivity and scale.

Remediate identified trackers, tighten retention rules, and implement privacy, protective defaults.

Govern by convening the cross, functional board and publishing procurement criteria.

Monitor with routine bias audits, security tests, and consent, comprehension studies.

Engage communities continuously through co, governance and public reporting.

Use the checklist above as an operational sprint plan and assign measurable KPIs for each step such as percentage of vendors with independent audits, average consent comprehension scores, and time, to, remediation after incidents.

RESEARCH, EVALUATION, AND EVIDENCE STANDARDS

Establish rigorous evidence thresholds before clinical deployment (Ma et al., 2025). Require randomized trials, pragmatic effectiveness studies, and real, world validation that report clinical outcomes alongside equity and safety metrics (Ienca et al., 2017). Mandate preregistration of studies, publicly accessible protocols, and open reporting of negative results.

Outcome Reporting: Publish both clinical effectiveness and harms data, disaggregated by demographic and clinical subgroups (Boffet et al., 2025).

Post, Market Surveillance: Fund ongoing observational studies to detect performance drift, emergent harms, and subgroup disparities after deployment.

Independent Replication: Require third, party replication of key findings, especially for high, risk tools that alter care pathways.

Embed lived, experience collaborators in study design, implementation, and interpretation to ensure that evaluations capture meaningful, person, centered outcomes (Jain & Jain, 2025).

FUNDING, PROCUREMENT, AND MARKET INCENTIVES

Align incentives so that safety, equity, and privacy are rewarded rather than sidelined.

Procurement Criteria: Use standardized vendor scorecards that weight privacy, auditability, equity performance, and patient control as heavily as cost and uptime.

Funding Conditions: Tie public and philanthropic funding to open standards for transparency, independent audits, and community governance.

Market Signals: Support certification programs and labeling that make privacy and fairness claims verifiable and comparable for clinicians and patients.

Shift market power toward vendors that embed ethical practice into their product roadmaps and business models.

METRICS, AUDITS, AND PUBLIC REPORTING

Create measurable indicators that translate ethics into accountable performance.

Core Metrics: Consent comprehension rates; percent of datasets with purpose declarations; subgroup false negative and false positive rates; time, to, remediation after incidents (Ross et al., 2022).

Audit Cadence: Define frequencies for security, bias, and privacy audits and require public summaries of findings.

Transparency Dashboard: Publish clinician, and patient, facing dashboards summarizing governance metrics and adverse, event trends.

Require that audit outcomes trigger prespecified governance responses, including suspension or reconfiguration of tools that fail safety thresholds.

COMMUNITY GOVERNANCE AND LIVED, EXPERIENCE LEADERSHIP

Center people with lived experience in decision, making.

Co, Governance Models: Create standing seats for patient advocates and community representatives on procurement and ethics boards.

Compensation and Capacity: Fund remuneration and training so community members can participate equitably and effectively.

Feedback Loops: Operationalize rapid feedback channels that allow users to report harms and influence iterative changes.

Treat community governance as a core infrastructure, not a one, time consultation.

POLICY RECOMMENDATIONS AND ADVOCACY PRIORITIES

Advocate for legal protections that reflect the sensitivity of mental health data (Chaabene et al., 2025).

Data Protection: Enact statutory limits on secondary uses of clinical mental health data and prohibit resale for advertising or underwriting (Kostadimas et al., 2025).

Fairness Mandates: Require subgroup performance reporting and corrective action plans when disparities are detected.

Enforceable Rights: Guarantee access, correction, deletion, and human review for algorithmic decisions that affect care, benefits, or rights.

Artificial Intelligence occupies a central role in modern mental health care, enabling predictive analytics and decision support.

REFERENCES

Akhtar, Z. B., & Rawol, A. T. (2025). Artificial Intelligence (Leivaditis & Sepetis, 2025) & Extended Reality (Reddy, 2025) within Healthcare: A Multidimensional Biomedical Engineering (Rajpal, 2025) Investigative Exploration. *Biomed. Clin. Res. J*, *1*, 1–22.

Akinode, A. O., Ayadi, O. E., Ezerioha, C. C., & Chika, P (2025). Machine Learning Approaches for Early Detection of Mental Health Disorders Using Wearable Devices and Big Data Analytics. environments, 4, 5.

Allgaier, J., Mulansky, L., Draelos, R. L., & Pryss, R. (2023). How does the model make predictions? A systematic literature review on the explainability power of machine learning in healthcare. *Artificial Intelligence in Medicine*, *143*, 102616. DOI: 10.1016/j.artmed.2023.102616 PMID: 37673561

Almadani, B., Kaisar, H., Thoker, I. R., & Aliyu, F. (2025). A systematic survey of distributed decision support systems in healthcare. *Systems*, *13*(3), 157. DOI: 10.3390/systems13030157

Anklam, E., Bahl, M. I., Ball, R., Beger, R. D., Cohen, J., Fitzpatrick, S., Girard, P., Halamoda-Kenzaoui, B., Hinton, D., Hirose, A., Hoeveler, A., Honma, M., Hugas, M., Ishida, S., Kass, G. E. N., Kojima, H., Krefting, I., Liachenko, S., Liu, Y., & Slikker, W.Jr. (2022). Emerging technologies and their impact on regulatory science. *Experimental Biology and Medicine (Maywood, N.J.)*, *247*(1), 1–75. DOI: 10.1177/15353702211052280 PMID: 34783606

Back, S. E., Acierno, R., Saraiya, T. C., Harley, B., Wangelin, B., Jarnecke, A. M., McTeague, L. M., Brown, D. G., Santa Ana, E., & Rothbaum, A. O. (2022). Enhancing Prolonged Exposure therapy for PTSD using physiological biomarker-driven technology. *Contemporary Clinical Trials Communications*, *28*, 100940. DOI: 10.1016/j.conctc.2022.100940 PMID: 35664505

Basystiuk, O., Rybchak, Z., Zavushchak, I., & Marikutsa, U. (2024). Evaluation of multimodal data synchronization tools. *Comput. Des. Syst. Theory Pract*, *6*(3), 104–111. DOI: 10.23939/cds2024.03.104

Baumann, S., Stone, R. T., & Abdelall, E. (2024). Introducing a remote patient monitoring usability impact model to overcome challenges. *Sensors (Basel)*, *24*(12), 3977. DOI: 10.3390/s24123977 PMID: 38931760

Bayor, A. A., Li, J., Yang, I. A., & Varnfield, M. (2025). Designing Clinical Decision Support Systems (CDSS)—A User-Centered Lens of the Design Characteristics, Challenges, and Implications: Systematic Review. *Journal of Medical Internet Research*, *27*, e63733. DOI: 10.2196/63733 PMID: 40540451

Bibi, P (2024). Establishing Transparency and Accountability in AI: Ethical Standards for Data Governance and Automated Systems. In.

Boda, V. V. R., & Allam, H. (2022). Ready for Anything: Disaster Recovery Strategies Every Healthcare IT Team Should Know. *International Journal of Emerging Trends in Computer Science and Information Technology*, *3*(1), 38–46. DOI: 10.63282/3050-9246.IJETCSIT-V3I1P105

Boffet, A., Arsac, L. M., Ibanez, V., Sauvet, F., & Deschodt-Arsac, V. (2025). Detection of Cognitive Load Modulation by EDA and HRV. *Sensors (Basel)*, *25*(8), 2343. DOI: 10.3390/s25082343 PMID: 40285033

Canali, S., Schiaffonati, V., & Aliverti, A. (2022). Challenges and recommendations for wearable devices in digital health: Data quality, interoperability, health equity, fairness. *PLOS Digital Health*, *1*(10), e0000104. DOI: 10.1371/journal.pdig.0000104 PMID: 36812619

Carl, E., Stein, A. T., Levihn-Coon, A., Pogue, J. R., Rothbaum, B., Emmelkamp, P., Asmundson, G. J. G., Carlbring, P., & Powers, M. B. (2019). Virtual reality exposure therapy for anxiety and related disorders: A meta-analysis of randomized controlled trials. *Journal of Anxiety Disorders*, *61*, 27–36. DOI: 10.1016/j.janxdis.2018.08.003 PMID: 30287083

Casson, A. J. (2019). Wearable EEG and beyond. *Biomedical Engineering Letters*, *9*(1), 53–71. DOI: 10.1007/s13534-018-00093-6 PMID: 30956880

Chaabene, S., Boudaya, A., Bouaziz, B., & Chaari, L. (2025). An overview of methods and techniques in multimodal data fusion with application to healthcare. *International Journal of Data Science and Analytics*, *20*(4), 1–25. DOI: 10.1007/s41060-025-00715-0

Chen, Z. S., Galatzer-Levy, I. R., Bigio, B., Nasca, C., & Zhang, Y. (2022). Modern views of machine learning for precision psychiatry. *Patterns (New York, N.Y.)*, *3*(11), 100602. DOI: 10.1016/j.patter.2022.100602 PMID: 36419447

Chennupati, N. (2025). Securing the Automated Enterprise: A Framework for Mitigating Security and Privacy Risks in AI-Driven Workflow Automation. *Journal of Computer Science and Technology Studies*, *7*(3), 624–632. DOI: 10.32996/jcsts.2025.7.3.71

Clemens-Meyer, F. H., Lepot, M., Blumensaat, F., Leutnant, D., & Gruber, G. (2021). In Bertrand-Krajewski, J.-L., Clemens-Meyer, F., Lepot, M., & Publishing, I. W. A. (Eds.), *Data validation and data quality assessment. Metrology in Urban Drainage and Stormwater Management: Plug and Pray* (pp. 327–390).

Correa, T., Pavez, I., & Contreras, J. (2021). Digital inequality and mobiles: opportunities and challenges of relying on smartphones for digital inclusion in disadvantaged contexts. Handbook of digital inequality, 62-74.

Crameri, L., Hettiarachchi, I. T., & Hanoun, S. (2021). Effects of dynamic resilience on the reactivity of vagally mediated heart rate variability. *Frontiers in Psychology*, *11*, 579210. DOI: 10.3389/fpsyg.2020.579210 PMID: 33551903

Cushnan, J., McCafferty, P., & Best, P. (2024). Clinicians' perspectives of immersive tools in clinical mental health settings: A systematic scoping review. *BMC Health Services Research*, *24*(1), 1091. DOI: 10.1186/s12913-024-11481-3 PMID: 39294727

Engel, G. L. (1977). The need for a new medical model: A challenge for biomedicine. *Science*, *196*(4286), 129–136. DOI: 10.1126/science.847460 PMID: 847460

Fanarioti, A. K., & Karpouzis, K. (2025). Artificial Intelligence and the Future of Mental Health in a Digitally Transformed World. *Computers*, *14*(7), 259. DOI: 10.3390/computers14070259

Ferrar, J., Griffith, G. J., Skirrow, C., Cashdollar, N., Taptiklis, N., Dobson, J., Cree, F., Cormack, F. K., Barnett, J. H., & Munafò, M. R. (2021). Developing digital tools for remote clinical research: How to evaluate the validity and practicality of active assessments in field settings. *Journal of Medical Internet Research*, *23*(6), e26004. DOI: 10.2196/26004 PMID: 34142972

Ferrara, E. (2024). Large language models for wearable sensor-based human activity recognition, health monitoring, and behavioral modeling: A survey of early trends, datasets, and challenges. *Sensors (Basel)*, *24*(15), 5045. DOI: 10.3390/s24155045 PMID: 39124092

Fischer, L., Mann, P. A., Nguyen, M. H. H., Becker, S., Khodadadi, S., Schulz, A., Edwin Thanarajah, S., Repple, J., Hahn, T., Reif, A., Salamikhanshan, A., Kittel-Schneider, S., Rief, W., Mulert, C., Hofmann, S. G., Dannlowski, U., Kircher, T., Bernhard, F. P., & Jamalabadi, H. (2025). AI for mental health: Clinician expectations and priorities in computational psychiatry. *BMC Psychiatry*, *25*(1), 584. DOI: 10.1186/s12888-025-06957-3 PMID: 40481455

Friend, S. H., Ginsburg, G. S., Picard, R. W., & Drazen, J. M. (2024). Key issues as wearable digital health technologies enter clinical care. *The New England Journal of Medicine*, *390*(12), 1118–1127. DOI: 10.1056/NEJMra2307160 PMID: 38507754

Ghadi, Y. Y., Shah, S. F. A., Waheed, W., Mazhar, T., Ahmad, W., Saeed, M. M., & Hamam, H. (2025). Integration of wearable technology and artificial intelligence in digital health for remote patient care. *Journal of Cloud Computing (Heidelberg, Germany)*, *14*(1), 39. DOI: 10.1186/s13677-025-00759-4

Ghanim, R., Kaushik, A., Park, J., & Abramson, A. (2023). Communication protocols integrating wearables, ingestibles, and implantables for closed-loop therapies. *Device*, *1*(3), 100092. DOI: 10.1016/j.device.2023.100092

Glass, J. E., Tiffany, B., Matson, T. E., Lim, C., Gundersen, G., Kimbel, K., Hartzler, A. L., Curran, G. M., McWethy, A. G., Caldeiro, R. M., & Bradley, K. A. (2022). Approaches for implementing digital interventions for alcohol use disorders in primary care: A qualitative, user-centered design study. *Implementation Research and Practice*, *3*, 26334895221135264. DOI: 10.1177/26334895221135264 PMID: 37091101

Godfrey, A., Vandendriessche, B., Bakker, J. P., Fitzer-Attas, C., Gujar, N., Hobbs, M., Liu, Q., Northcott, C. A., Parks, V., Wood, W. A., Zipunnikov, V., Wagner, J. A., & Izmailova, E. S. (2021). Fit-for-purpose biometric monitoring technologies: Leveraging the laboratory biomarker experience. *Clinical and Translational Science*, *14*(1), 62–74. DOI: 10.1111/cts.12865 PMID: 32770726

Goktas, P., & Grzybowski, A. (2025). Shaping the future of healthcare: Ethical clinical challenges and pathways to trustworthy AI. *Journal of Clinical Medicine*, *14*(5), 1605. DOI: 10.3390/jcm14051605 PMID: 40095575

Hickey, B. A., Chalmers, T., Newton, P., Lin, C.-T., Sibbritt, D., McLachlan, C. S., Clifton-Bligh, R., Morley, J., & Lal, S. (2021). Smart devices and wearable technologies to detect and monitor mental health conditions and stress: A systematic review. *Sensors (Basel)*, *21*(10), 3461. DOI: 10.3390/s21103461 PMID: 34065620

Hilty, D. M., Armstrong, C. M., Luxton, D. D., Gentry, M. T., & Krupinski, E. A. (2021). A scoping review of sensors, wearables, and remote monitoring for behavioral health: Uses, outcomes, clinical competencies, and research directions. *Journal of Technology in Behavioral Science*, *6*(2), 278–313. DOI: 10.1007/s41347-021-00199-2 PMID: 33501372

Holly, L., Thom, S., Elzemety, M., Murage, B., Mathieson, K., & Iñigo Petralanda, M. I. (2023). Strengthening health data governance: New equity and rights-based principles. *International Journal of Health Governance, 28*(3), 225–237. DOI: 10.1108/IJHG-11-2022-0104

Huang, J., Wang, H., Wu, Q., Yin, J., Zhou, H., & He, Y. (2024). Clinical research on neurological and psychiatric diagnosis and monitoring using wearable devices: A literature review. *Interdisciplinary Medicine, 2*(4), e20230037. DOI: 10.1002/INMD.20230037

Hughes, N., & Kalra, D. (2023). Data standards and platform interoperability. In *Real-World Evidence in Medical Product Development* (pp. 79–107). Springer. DOI: 10.1007/978-3-031-26328-6_6

Ienca, M., Fabrice, J., Elger, B., Caon, M., Scoccia Pappagallo, A., Kressig, R. W., & Wangmo, T. (2017). Intelligent assistive technology for Alzheimer's disease and other dementias: A systematic review. *Journal of Alzheimer's Disease, 56*(4), 1301–1340. DOI: 10.3233/JAD-161037 PMID: 28222516

Ikwuanusi, U. F., Adepoju, P. A., & Odionu, C. S (2023). Advancing ethical AI practices to solve data privacy issues in library systems. International journal of multidisciplinary research updates, 6(1), 033-044.

Immanuel, S., Teferra, M. N., Baumert, M., & Bidargaddi, N. (2023). Heart rate variability for evaluating psychological stress changes in healthy adults: A scoping review. *Neuropsychobiology, 82*(4), 187–202. DOI: 10.1159/000530376 PMID: 37290411

Jain, A., & Jain, A (2025). AI-Based Emotion Detection System in Healthcare for Patient. Generative Artificial Intelligence for Biomedical and Smart Health Informatics, 455-470.

Jiao, C. (2024). A mental health monitoring system based on intelligent algorithms and biosensors: Algorithm behaviour analysis and intervention strategies. *Molecular & Cellular Biomechanics, 21*(1), 357–357. DOI: 10.62617/mcb.v21i1.357

Johnson, K. B., Wei, W. Q., Weeraratne, D., Frisse, M. E., Misulis, K., Rhee, K., Zhao, J., & Snowdon, J. L. (2021). Precision medicine, AI, and the future of personalized health care. *Clinical and Translational Science, 14*(1), 86–93. DOI: 10.1111/cts.12884 PMID: 32961010

Kang, H. S., & Exworthy, M. (2022). Wearing the future—wearables to empower users to take greater responsibility for their health and care: Scoping review. *JMIR mHealth and uHealth, 10*(7), e35684. DOI: 10.2196/35684 PMID: 35830222

Kargarandehkordi, A., Li, S., Lin, K., Phillips, K. T., Benzo, R. M., & Washington, P. (2025). Fusing wearable biosensors with artificial intelligence for mental health monitoring: A systematic review. *Biosensors (Basel)*, *15*(4), 202. DOI: 10.3390/bios15040202 PMID: 40277515

Kim, J., & Backonja, U. (2025). Digital health equity frameworks and key concepts: A scoping review. *Journal of the American Medical Informatics Association : JAMIA*, *32*(1), 45–59. DOI: 10.1093/jamia/ocaf017 PMID: 39936843

Kostadimas, D., Kasapakis, V., & Kotis, K. (2025). A systematic review on the combination of VR, IoT and AI technologies, and their integration in applications. *Future Internet*, *17*(4), 163. DOI: 10.3390/fi17040163

Kourtesis, P. (2024). A comprehensive review of multimodal XR applications, risks, and ethical challenges in the metaverse. *Multimodal Technologies and Interaction*, *8*(11), 98. DOI: 10.3390/mti8110098

Kumar, P. (2025). Securing Digital-First Healthcare: AI, Blockchain, and Cloud Architectures for Personal Health Data Protection. *International Journal of Applied Mathematics*, *38*(7s).

Lamb, R., Choi, I., & Owens, T (2025). Convergence of Extended Reality, Artificial Intelligence, Machine Leaning, and Wearable Sensors in the Field of Education. Mental Health Virtual Reality: The Power of Immersive Worlds, 113-128.

Layode, O., Naiho, H. N. N., Adeleke, G. S., Udeh, E. O., & Labake, T. T. (2024). Data privacy and security challenges in environmental research: Approaches to safeguarding sensitive information. *International Journal of Applied Research in Social Sciences*, *6*(6), 1193–1214. DOI: 10.51594/ijarss.v6i6.1210

Lazarou, E., & Exarchos, T. P. (2024). Predicting stress levels using physiological data: Real-time stress prediction models utilizing wearable devices. *AIMS Neuroscience*, *11*(2), 76–102. DOI: 10.3934/Neuroscience.2024006 PMID: 38988886

Leivaditis, V., & Sepetis, A (2025). Digital Transformation As A Catalyst For Sustainable Health Care Systems: A Narrative Review Of Current Evidence. International Journal of Innovation Management, 29(05n06), 2540009.

Li, M., Patel, J., & Katapally, T. R. (2025). The impact of extended reality cognitive behavioral therapy on mental disorders among children and youth: A systematic review and meta-analysis protocol. *PLoS One*, *20*(3), e0315313. DOI: 10.1371/journal.pone.0315313 PMID: 40048453

Lorke, M., & Stefanou, T. (2025). Improving research and development of wearable assistive and rehabilitation technologies: A systematic review on diversity factors. *Journal of Neuroengineering and Rehabilitation*, *22*(1), 31. DOI: 10.1186/s12984-025-01562-7 PMID: 39985039

Ma, C.-B., Shang, X., Sun, M., Bo, X., Bai, J., Du, Y., & Zhou, M. (2025). Emerging Multifunctional Wearable Sensors: Integrating Multimodal Sweat Analysis and Advanced Material Technologies for Next-Generation Health Monitoring. *ACS Sensors*, *10*(4), 2388–2408. DOI: 10.1021/acssensors.4c03396 PMID: 40162570

Mackey, S., Aghaeepour, N., Gaudilliere, B., Kao, M.-C., Kaptan, M., Lannon, E., Pfyffer, D., & Weber, K. (2025). Innovations in acute and chronic pain biomarkers: Enhancing diagnosis and personalized therapy. *Regional Anesthesia and Pain Medicine*, *50*(2), 110–120. DOI: 10.1136/rapm-2024-106030 PMID: 39909549

Mitsea, E., Drigas, A., & Skianis, C. (2024). Artificial intelligence, immersive technologies, and neurotechnologies in breathing interventions for mental and emotional health: A systematic review. *Electronics (Basel)*, *13*(12), 2253. DOI: 10.3390/electronics13122253

Mohammad, N. (2021). Enhancing security and privacy in multi-cloud environments: A comprehensive study on encryption techniques and access control mechanisms. [IJCET]. *International Journal of Computer Engineering and Technology*, *12*(2), 51–63.

Mohr, D. C., Zhang, M., & Schueller, S. M. (2017). Personal sensing: Understanding mental health using ubiquitous sensors and machine learning. *Annual Review of Clinical Psychology*, *13*(1), 23–47. DOI: 10.1146/annurev-clinpsy-032816-044949 PMID: 28375728

Mone, V., & Fayazullaeva, S. (2023). Health data on the go: Navigating privacy concerns with wearable technologies. *Legal Information Management*, *23*(3), 179–188. DOI: 10.1017/S1472669623000427

Morey, D. A., Rayo, M. F., & Woods, D. D. (2025). Empirically derived evaluation requirements for responsible deployments of AI in safety-critical settings. *NPJ Digital Medicine*, *8*(1), 374. DOI: 10.1038/s41746-025-01784-y PMID: 40533485

Morgan, J. W., Patel, R. A., & Campbell, S. (2025). Practical considerations of clinical XR (Singh & Chandra, 2025) deployments. *Frontiers in Virtual Reality*, *6*, 1517402. DOI: 10.3389/frvir.2025.1517402

Moriarty, A. S., Meader, N., Snell, K. I., Riley, R. D., Paton, L. W., Dawson, S., Hendon, J., Chew-Graham, C. A., Gilbody, S., Churchill, R., Phillips, R. S., Ali, S., & McMillan, D. (2022). Predicting relapse or recurrence of depression: Systematic review of prognostic models. *The British Journal of Psychiatry : The Journal of Mental Science, 221*(2), 448–458. DOI: 10.1192/bjp.2021.218 PMID: 35048843

Mulukuntla, S. (2025). Monitoring and Remote Patient Management with Immersive Technologies. In Augmented Wellness: Exploring the Power of VR and AR in Healthcare (pp. 197-218). Springer. DOI: 10.1007/978-981-96-2952-7_9

Obermeyer, Z., Powers, B., Vogeli, C., & Mullainathan, S. (2019). Dissecting racial bias in an algorithm used to manage the health of populations. *Science, 366*(6464), 447–453. DOI: 10.1126/science.aax2342 PMID: 31649194

Okposio, B. O., Richard, G. A., Olatokun, T. P., Akadiri, O. O., Akpevba, E. A., John, J. O., & Okonkwo, B. A. (2025). Enhancing Mental health Outcomes through AI-Driven Predictive Analytics: A review of applications in neuroscience and substance abuse prevention. *International Journal of Biological and Pharmaceutical Sciences Archive, 10*(2), 024-048.

Omiyefa, S. (2025). Artificial intelligence and machine learning in precision mental health diagnostics and predictive treatment models. *Int J Res Publ Rev, 6*(3), 85–99. DOI: 10.55248/gengpi.6.0325.1107

Ong, T., Ivanova, J., Soni, H., Barrera, J., Cummins, M., Welch, B. M., & Bunnell, B. E. (2025). Mental health clients' perspectives on telehealth-based virtual reality therapy. *Frontiers in Virtual Reality, 6*, 1595326. DOI: 10.3389/frvir.2025.1595326

Panarese, P., Grasso, M. M., & Solinas, C. (2025). Algorithmic bias, fairness, and inclusivity: A multilevel framework for justice-oriented AI. *AI & Society*, •••, 1–23. DOI: 10.1007/s00146-025-02451-2

Pedram, S., & Piatkowski, T. (2025). Exploring the potential of virtual reality (Johnson et al., 2021) in mental healthcare: A systematic literature review. *Virtual Reality (Waltham Cross), 29*(3), 135. DOI: 10.1007/s10055-025-01181-6

Poudel, U., Jakhar, S., Mohan, P., & Nepal, A. (2025). AI in mental health: A review of technological advancements and ethical issues in psychiatry. *Issues in Mental Health Nursing, 46*(7), 693–701. DOI: 10.1080/01612840.2025.2502943 PMID: 40378075

Pruden, S (2025). Implementing Depression Screening and Treatment Algorithms to Reduce Post-Operative Complications for Patients Undergoing Cardiac Surgery The University of North Carolina at Chapel Hill].

Radanliev, P. (2025). Privacy, ethics, transparency, and accountability in AI systems for wearable devices. *Frontiers in Digital Health*, *7*, 1431246. DOI: 10.3389/fdgth.2025.1431246 PMID: 40599875

Rajpal, S. (2025). Exploring the Role of Virtual Reality and Metaverse in Treating Mental Health: Operating Models and Challenges in Adoption. *Journal of Computer and Communications*, *13*(10), 1–22. DOI: 10.4236/jcc.2025.1310001

Reddy, K. J. (2025). Integrating Technology into Clinical Practice. In Innovations in Neurocognitive Rehabilitation: Harnessing Technology for Effective Therapy (pp. 329-350). Springer. DOI: 10.1007/978-3-031-88117-6_15

Renuka, O., RadhaKrishnan, N., Priya, B. S., Jhansy, A., & Ezekiel, S (2025). Data privacy and protection: Legal and ethical challenges. Emerging Threats and Countermeasures in Cybersecurity, 433-465.

Ricciardi, F., & Zomaya, A. (2025). Perspectives on Managing AI Ethics in the Digital Age. *Information (Basel)*, *16*(2), 89. DOI: 10.3390/info16040318

Robinson, A., Flom, M., Forman-Hoffman, V. L., Histon, T., Levy, M., Darcy, A., Ajayi, T., Mohr, D. C., Wicks, P., Greene, C., & Montgomery, R. M. (2024). Equity in digital mental health interventions in the United States: Where to next? *Journal of Medical Internet Research*, *26*, e59939. DOI: 10.2196/59939 PMID: 39316436

Ross, G., Zhao, Y., Bosman, A., Geballa-Koukoula, A., Zhou, H., Elliott, C., Nielen, M., Rafferty, K., & Salentijn, G (2022). Data handling and ethics of emerging smartphone-based (Glass et al., 2022) sensors–Part 1: best practices and current implementation.

Shah, R. V., Grennan, G., Zafar-Khan, M., Alim, F., Dey, S., Ramanathan, D., & Mishra, J. (2021). Personalized machine learning of depressed mood using wearables. *Translational Psychiatry*, *11*(1), 338. DOI: 10.1038/s41398-021-01445-0 PMID: 34103481

Shatte, A. B., Hutchinson, D. M., & Teague, S. J. (2019). Machine learning in mental health: A scoping review of methods and applications. *Psychological Medicine*, *49*(9), 1426–1448. DOI: 10.1017/S0033291719000151 PMID: 30744717

Sheikh, M., Qassem, M., & Kyriacou, P. A. (2021). Wearable, environmental, and smartphone-based passive sensing for mental health monitoring. *Frontiers in Digital Health*, *3*, 662811. DOI: 10.3389/fdgth.2021.662811 PMID: 34713137

Singh, B., & Chandra, S. (2025). Strengthening Sensors and Wearable Technologies in Gauging Healthcare Transmuting Digital Health Technologies: Human Augmentation via Innovation and Implementations of AI. In Cases on AI Innovations in Occupational Health and Safety (pp. 289-308). IGI Global Scientific Publishing.

Smuck, M., Odonkor, C. A., Wilt, J. K., Schmidt, N., & Swiernik, M. A. (2021). The emerging clinical role of wearables: Factors for successful implementation in healthcare. *NPJ Digital Medicine*, *4*(1), 45. DOI: 10.1038/s41746-021-00418-3 PMID: 33692479

Sun, J., Lu, T., Shao, X., Han, Y., Xia, Y., Zheng, Y., Wang, Y., Li, X., Ravindran, A., Fan, L., Fang, Y., Zhang, X., Ravindran, N., Wang, Y., Liu, X., & Lu, L. (2025). Practical AI application in psychiatry: Historical review and future directions. *Molecular Psychiatry*, *30*(9), 4399–4408. DOI: 10.1038/s41380-025-03072-3 PMID: 40456953

Tavory, T. (2024). Regulating AI in mental health: Ethics of care perspective. *JMIR Mental Health*, *11*, e58493. DOI: 10.2196/58493 PMID: 39298759

Tizzard, C. L. (2025). Re-imagining Care for Aging Disabled Adults.

Tsai, Y. Y., Chen, Y. J., Lin, Y. F., Hsiao, F. C., Hsu, C. H., & Liao, L. D. (2025). Photoplethysmography-based HRV analysis and machine learning for real-time stress quantification in mental health applications. *APL Bioengineering*, *9*(2), 026103. DOI: 10.1063/5.0256590 PMID: 40191605

Verma, H., Mlynar, J., Schaer, R., Reichenbach, J., Jreige, M., Prior, J., Evéquoz, F., & Depeursinge, A. (2023). Rethinking the role of AI with physicians in oncology: revealing perspectives from clinical and research workflows. *Proceedings of the 2023 CHI conference on human factors in computing systems* DOI: 10.1145/3544548.3581506

Volckens, J., Haynes, E. N., Croisant, S. P., Cui, Y., Errett, N. A., Henry, H. F., Horney, J. A., Kwok, R. K., Magzamen, S., Rappold, A. G., Ravichandran, L., Reinlib, L., Ryan, P. H., & Shaughnessy, D. T. (2023). Health research in the wake of disasters: Challenges and opportunities for sensor science. *Environmental Health Perspectives*, *131*(6), 065002. DOI: 10.1289/EHP12270 PMID: 37389972

Walter, J. R., Xu, S., & Rogers, J. A. (2023). From lab to life: How wearable devices can improve health equity. *Nature Communications*, *14*, 44634. PMID: 38167483

Wang, Z., Xiong, H., Zhang, J., Yang, S., Boukhechba, M., Zhang, D., Barnes, L. E., & Dou, D. (2022). From personalized medicine to population health: A survey of mHealth sensing techniques. *IEEE Internet of Things Journal*, *9*(17), 15413–15434. DOI: 10.1109/JIOT.2022.3161046

Weiner, E. B., Dankwa-Mullan, I., Nelson, W. A., & Hassanpour, S. (2025). Ethical challenges and evolving strategies in the integration of artificial intelligence into clinical practice. *PLOS Digital Health, 4*(4), e0000810. DOI: 10.1371/journal.pdig.0000810 PMID: 40198594

Wibberly, K. H. (2024). Preparing mental health providers for the future: The case for moving beyond the elective telehealth course to integrating telehealth training throughout the curriculum. *Frontiers in Psychology, 14*, 1301569. DOI: 10.3389/fpsyg.2023.1301569 PMID: 38235285

Xing, Y., Yang, Y., Yang, K., Lu, A., Xing, L., Mackie, K., & Guo, F. (2025). Intelligent sensing devices and systems for personalized mental health. *Med-X, 3*(1), 10. DOI: 10.1007/s44258-025-00057-3 PMID: 40837134

Zenker, S., Strech, D., Ihrig, K., Jahns, R., Müller, G., Schickhardt, C., Schmidt, G., Speer, R., Winkler, E., von Kielmansegg, S. G., & Drepper, J. (2022). Data protection-compliant broad consent for secondary use of health care data and human biosamples for (Mulukuntla, 2025) medical research: Towards a new German national standard. *Journal of Biomedical Informatics, 131*, 104096. DOI: 10.1016/j.jbi.2022.104096 PMID: 35643273

Section 2
Technologies in Practice: Tools as Clinical Instruments

Chapter 4
AI in Mental Health:
Promise, Peril, and Clinical Responsibility

ABSTRACT

AI is redefining mental health care through predictive analytics, NLP, and decision-support systems (Islam & Bae, 2024). Applications span early detection, treatment personalization, and crisis prevention, leveraging multimodal data from EHRs, speech, and wearables (Shatte et al., 2019). The chapter highlights benefits precision, scalability, proactive care while addressing risks of bias, opacity, and over-reliance. Explainable AI, clinician oversight, and participatory design are emphasized as safeguards (Shatte et al., 2019). Practical examples include relapse prediction, adaptive chatbots, and federated learning for privacy-preserving model training (Shatte et al., 2019). The directive: integrate AI as an augmentative tool, governed by transparency and equity (Shatte et al., 2019).

INTRODUCTION

This chapter critically examines artificial intelligence as a transformative but bounded force in mental health care. AI applications are organized around three clinical functions: detection, decision support, and personalization. The chapter highlights how machine learning models can identify subtle behavioral and linguistic patterns associated with emerging mental health concerns, potentially enabling earlier intervention and precision treatment planning. At the same time, it emphasizes that mental health data are noisy, context-dependent, and socially embedded, making overreliance on algorithmic inference particularly risky. The chapter addresses common failure modes, including opacity, bias, and false precision, and argues that explainability and uncertainty reporting are clinical necessities rather than technical

DOI: 10.4018/979-8-3373-4997-8.ch004

luxuries. Consent, accountability, and clinician override authority are presented as non-negotiable safeguards. The chapter also explores how regulatory ambiguity complicates deployment, requiring proactive engagement with evolving standards and professional guidelines. Throughout, AI is positioned as a clinical assistant, not a replacement for judgment, empathy, or responsibility. By balancing empirical promise with ethical and practical constraints, this chapter provides clinicians and systems leaders with criteria for evaluating when and how AI should be integrated into care. The analysis underscores that the value of AI in mental health lies not in automation alone, but in its disciplined use to support human decision-making.

INTRODUCTION TO TECHNOLOGIES IN MENTAL HEALTH PRACTICE

Clinicians evaluating digital tools must consider their functional alignment with therapeutic goals, the strength of supporting evidence, and their compatibility with existing workflows (Ong et al., 2025). Early adopters often begin with a single technology such as AI for relapse prediction or XR for exposure therapy anchored to a clearly defined clinical objective. Selection should prioritize platforms with transparent data governance, clinician oversight capabilities, and documented safety protocols (Sharma, 2025) . The goal is not to chase novelty but to integrate tools that demonstrably enhance care. This chapter initiates Part 2 of the book, Technologies in Practice, by exploring the practical integration of AI into mental health care (Adepoju & Adepoju, 2025). It bridges theoretical promise with clinical reality, offering a critical yet optimistic perspective on how digital therapeutics can reshape practice. Subsequent chapters will examine XR and wearable sensors, culminating in a synthesis of multimodal systems that deliver adaptive, personalized interventions (Lamb et al., 2025;. Throughout, the emphasis remains on implementation feasibility, clinical workflow integration, and measurable outcomes (Kim & Backonja, 2025). Each technology is assessed in terms of clinical readiness, evidence strength, and equity implications. The final synthesis will distill operational principles for safe, ethical deployment in routine care.

FROM TOOLS TO ECOSYSTEMS

Mental health technologies have long served as adjuncts to traditional care. The telephone extended therapeutic reach; computerized cognitive behavioral therapy (Hiland, 2021) offered scalable, self-guided interventions. These tools supported clinicians but did not fundamentally alter the therapeutic process. The current wave of innovation, however, is qualitatively different. AI algorithms can analyze linguistic patterns to detect early signs of depression (Bond et al., 2023). XR environments simulate phobic stimuli with unprecedented realism (Martinez-Martin et al., 2018). Wearable sensors continuously monitor physiological markers of stress, anxiety, and arousal. These technologies do not merely support care, they transform it. What distinguishes this generation of tools is their capacity to sense, analyze, and act in real time. They enable closed-loop systems that respond dynamically to users' cognitive and emotional states. This shift from static to adaptive systems marks a critical inflection point in mental health care. It allows for the creation of neuroadaptive environments, systems that personalize therapeutic content based on moment-to-moment physiological and behavioral data. Such responsiveness enhances both clinical precision and patient engagement (Martinez-Martin et al., 2018).

For clinicians, this transformation introduces new responsibilities. Implementation requires competencies in data interpretation, algorithmic oversight, and vendor governance (Cristofaro & Giardino, 2025). Systems thinking becomes essential: clinicians must anticipate integration challenges, evaluate trade-offs, and design workflows that preserve therapeutic integrity. The adoption of digital tools is not a technical upgrade, it is a systemic change that reconfigures roles, relationships, and ethical boundaries. Closed-loop systems demand explicit design parameters. Sensing thresholds must be defined. Intervention triggers must be clinically validated (Poudel et al., 2025). Human oversight must be embedded at every stage. Effective deployment includes manual override capabilities, conservative alerting protocols, and clinician review of automated outputs. Pilot implementations should prioritize safety, usability, and workflow compatibility. Evaluation frameworks must measure not only symptom reduction but also operational sustainability, clinician workload, and patient satisfaction.

These technologies do not operate in isolation. They form interconnected ecosystems that synthesize data across modalities, linguistic, physiological, behavioral, to inform therapeutic decisions (Chithra & Bhambri, 2024). AI may flag elevated risk based on speech patterns; a wearable sensor may corroborate with heart rate variability data; an XR module may adjust exposure intensity accordingly (Ong et al., 2025). This multimodal integration supports precision care, but it also requires robust interoperability standards, timestamp synchronization, and governance structures that protect privacy and equity. The emergence of neuroadaptive systems, those that adjust in real time to users' internal states, represents a new frontier in mental health care (Ong et al., 2025). These systems exemplify the convergence of AI, XR, and biosensing into cohesive therapeutic platforms (Ong et al., 2025). They offer the potential to deliver interventions that are not only personalized but also context-aware, responsive, and scalable. Yet their promise must be tempered by rigorous validation, ethical safeguards, and clinician-centered design. The integration of AI and related technologies into mental health care is not a peripheral enhancement, it is a redefinition of practice (Ong et al., 2025). It challenges clinicians to expand their skillsets, rethink therapeutic boundaries, and engage with technology as a partner in care. The chapters that follow will explore these technologies in greater depth, offering practical guidance for their responsible and effective use. The directive is clear: adopt with intention, evaluate with rigor, and center the therapeutic relationship in every digital decision.

THE PROMISE AND PERIL OF ARTIFICIAL INTELLIGENCE

Artificial intelligence (Subu et al., 2022) occupies a central role in the evolving landscape of mental health care (Mahon, 2023). Its applications span three primary domains: diagnosis, decision support, and personalization. Machine learning (Ienca et al., 2017) models trained on large, multimodal datasets can identify patterns that elude human clinicians, offering probabilistic assessments of conditions such as major depressive disorder, generalized anxiety disorder, and post-traumatic stress disorder (PTSD; Kim & Backonja, 2025). Natural language processing (Weiner et al., 2025) tools analyze speech and text to detect subtle indicators of mood, cognitive decline, or emotional dysregulation. Predictive analytics can forecast relapse, treatment dropout, or crisis risk, enabling preemptive interventions that shift care from reactive to proactive. These capabilities are not theoretical, they are already reshaping practice. AI systems can synthesize data from electronic health records, therapy transcripts, wearable sensors, and digital behavior to generate insights that inform clinical decision-making (Kim & Backonja, 2025). However, these outputs must be contextualized by human judgment. AI should augment, not replace, clinical reasoning (Kim & Backonja, 2025). Implementation demands clear documentation of model training data, performance metrics, and known limitations (Kim & Backonja, 2025). Systems must include mechanisms for clinician feedback, local recalibration, and override authority. Above all, AI must preserve clinician responsibility and therapeutic alliance (Kim & Backonja, 2025).

Despite its promise, the deployment of AI in mental health is fraught with ethical, epistemological, and operational challenges (Kargarandehkordi et al., 2025). Algorithms are only as reliable as the data on which they are trained, and mental health data is often noisy, sparse, and context-dependent (Tsai et al., 2025). Diagnostic categories are contested, symptom presentations are culturally variable, and clinical documentation may reflect systemic biases (Tsai et al., 2025). These complexities introduce risks of misclassification, inequitable performance, and unintended harm. The opacity of many AI models, the so-called "black box" problem, further complicates integration (Tsai et al., 2025). Clinicians and patients must be able to interrogate algorithmic outputs, understand their rationale, and contest their conclusions. Explainability is not a luxury; it is a clinical and ethical necessity (Tsai et al., 2025). Systems should include interpretable features, confidence metrics, and documentation of decision pathways. Validation must occur on representative samples, with subgroup performance metrics disaggregated by race, gender, age, and other relevant factors.

Consent processes must evolve to reflect the complexity of AI-driven care (Akhtar & Rawol, 2024). Patients should be informed about the role of algorithms in diagnosis, treatment planning, and monitoring. They must retain the right to opt out of automated decision-making and to request human review. Consent should be dynamic, revisitable, and accessible across literacy levels. For vulnerable populations, such as children, individuals with cognitive impairments, or those in crisis, additional safeguards are essential. Equity must be a guiding principle. AI systems must be audited for disparate impact and retrained when performance gaps are identified (Radanliev, 2025). Developers should engage with diverse communities during design and testing, ensuring that tools reflect the lived experiences and linguistic patterns of the populations they serve. Clinical deployment should include continuous monitoring for bias, with remediation protocols activated when disparities emerge (Radanliev, 2025). AI offers powerful tools for enhancing mental health care, but its integration must be deliberate, transparent, and ethically grounded (Radanliev, 2025). Clinicians must remain at the center of care, using AI to extend their reach, sharpen their insights, and personalize interventions, never to abdicate responsibility (Radanliev, 2025). The directive is clear: adopt AI where it improves care, interrogate it where it obscures judgment, and govern it where it risks harm (Radanliev, 2025).

EXTENDED REALITY: REIMAGINING THERAPEUTIC SPACE

Extended reality (XR), encompassing virtual reality (VR), augmented reality (AR), and mixed reality (MR), represents a transformative modality for therapeutic engagement (Saganowski et al., 2022). Unlike traditional talk therapy, which relies on verbal exchange and imagination, XR immerses users in multisensory environments that can be precisely controlled, repeated, and tailored to individual needs (Obermeyer et al., 2019). This affordance is particularly valuable for exposure-based therapies, where gradual confrontation with feared stimuli is a core mechanism of change. XR enables clinicians to recreate phobic or trauma-related contexts, such as airplanes, crowded rooms, or combat scenarios, without the logistical and emotional risks of in vivo exposure (Obermeyer et al., 2019). These environments can be titrated to match the patient's tolerance, with real-time adjustments to intensity, pacing, and sensory input. Clinical protocols often include graduated exposure hierarchies, physiological monitoring (e.g., heart rate variability), and explicit transfer tasks to support generalization into daily life (Obermeyer et al., 2019). Efficacy depends on simulation fidelity, therapist-guided dosing, and integration into broader treatment plans. AR offers a complementary modality by overlaying therapeutic prompts or calming visuals onto the physical world. This supports in-the-moment coping strategies, mindfulness practice, and behavioral rehearsal in naturalistic settings. MR blends virtual and physical elements, enabling interactive experiences that support social skills training, emotion regulation, or cognitive restructuring. These modalities expand the therapeutic repertoire, allowing clinicians to match intervention format to clinical goals (Obermeyer et al., 2019).

XR also holds promise for enhancing empathy and perspective-taking (Agarwal et al., 2025). Users can inhabit avatars or scenarios that simulate the experiences of others, supporting interventions for aggression, social cognition, or body image disturbance. Embodied experiences provide sensorimotor evidence that complements cognitive interventions, enabling patients to challenge maladaptive beliefs through experiential learning (Tsai et al., 2025). However, XR is not a panacea (Tsai et al., 2025). Its effectiveness depends on careful design, clinical oversight, and user readiness (Tsai et al., 2025). Motion sickness, dissociation, and sensory overload are real risks, particularly for individuals with vestibular disorders, trauma histories, or neurodevelopmental differences. Screening for contraindications is essential. Implementation should include prebriefing, in-session monitoring, and post-session debriefing. Clinicians must be trained in XR-specific risk assessment, scenario selection, and emergency protocols (Tsai et al., 2025).

Accessibility and equity must be prioritized. Hardware costs, licensing fees, and digital literacy barriers can limit adoption, particularly in low-resource settings. Clinics should budget for device maintenance, software updates, and staff training. Pilot implementations should include user acceptability metrics, cultural adaptation reviews, and equity audits. Content must be customizable to reflect diverse bodies, languages, and social roles. XR should be integrated into care as a clinical instrument, not a novelty (APA, 2025). It must be governed by the same standards of safety, efficacy, and ethical integrity as any other therapeutic modality. The goal is not to replace human therapists but to augment their capabilities, extend their reach, and create new opportunities for experiential learning. When implemented thoughtfully, XR can deepen therapeutic engagement, accelerate progress, and support recovery in ways previously unattainable (Radanliev, 2025).

WEARABLE SENSORS: THE QUANTIFIED SELF IN MENTAL HEALTH

Wearable technologies, ranging from smartwatches and fitness trackers to EEG headbands and smart textiles, are reshaping the landscape of mental health care by enabling continuous, passive monitoring of physiological and behavioral data. These devices can track heart rate variability (HRV), galvanic skin response (GSR), electroencephalography (EEG), respiration, and movement patterns, biomarkers that reflect stress, arousal, emotional regulation, and cognitive workload (De Kock et al., 2021). When integrated with artificial intelligence (Radanliev, 2025) and mobile platforms, wearables can provide real-time feedback, trigger adaptive interventions, and alert clinicians to concerning trends (De Kock et al., 2021). The clinical implications are profound (De Kock et al., 2021). Wearables support early detection of mood episodes, facilitate biofeedback-based interventions, and enable personalized treatment plans grounded in individual psychophysiological profiles. They empower users to become active participants in their own care, fostering self-awareness, agency, and engagement. In therapeutic settings, wearables can complement self-report and behavioral observation by providing objective data on treatment progress, for example, demonstrating improved HRV during relaxation training or reduced electrodermal activity during exposure therapy (De Kock et al., 2021). Operationally, clinicians must define clinical thresholds and response protocols before deploying wearables (De Kock et al., 2021). Data summaries should be interpretable, actionable, and aligned with therapeutic goals (De Kock et al., 2021). Periodic reviews are essential to contextualize wearable-derived signals within broader clinical narratives, including life events, medication changes, and psychosocial stressors (De Kock et al., 2021). Researchers should triangulate sensor data with behavioral and self-report measures to enhance validity and reduce interpretive ambiguity (De Kock et al., 2021).

Yet, as with all data-driven technologies, wearables raise critical questions about privacy, consent, and data governance (Watson, 2025). Who owns the data? Who has access? How is it stored, interpreted, and used? These questions must be addressed through robust ethical frameworks and participatory design processes that center the rights and needs of users. Consent protocols must specify secondary uses, third-party access, and data retention policies. Institutions should implement encryption, role-based access controls, and data minimization strategies. Regular audits and transparent reporting practices are essential to maintain trust and accountability. Wearables are not merely tools for measurement, they are components of a broader shift toward responsive, adaptive, and person-centered care. Their integration into mental health practice must be guided by clinical utility, ethical integrity, and a commitment to equity (Martinez-Martin et al., 2018). When thoughtfully deployed, wearable sensors can bridge the gap between subjective experience and objective data, supporting more precise, timely, and effective interventions.

TOWARD MULTIMODAL, ADAPTIVE SYSTEMS

The most exciting frontier in digital mental health lies in the integration of AI, XR, and wearable sensors into cohesive, multimodal systems (Aiken et al., 2023). These systems do not simply respond to user input, they anticipate and adapt to users' internal states. Imagine a scenario in which a patient engages in VR-based exposure therapy while a wearable sensor monitors physiological arousal and an AI algorithm dynamically adjusts the intensity of the virtual environment (Shatte et al., 2019). This closed-loop configuration exemplifies the potential of neuroadaptive systems, technologies that personalize care in real time based on multimodal data (Shatte et al., 2019). Designing such systems requires interdisciplinary collaboration. Clinicians, engineers, designers, and ethicists must co-create interfaces, safety logic, and evaluation frameworks. Clinical protocols must include escalation rules, override capabilities, and predefined success metrics (Shatte et al., 2019). Pilot testing should assess feasibility, safety, usability, and equity. Implementation science frameworks are essential to translate prototypes into routine practice, addressing workflow integration, clinician training, and sustainability.

These systems are not speculative. Early prototypes and pilot studies have demonstrated feasibility and efficacy across diverse populations and settings. However, scaling requires rigorous validation, stakeholder engagement, and governance structures that protect privacy, autonomy, and therapeutic integrity. Equity must guide deployment to prevent technological redlining and ensure that innovations reach underserved communities. Multimodal systems represent a shift from episodic, reactive care to continuous, adaptive, and context-aware intervention. They offer the potential to deliver precision mental health care, tailored not only to diagnostic categories but to moment-to-moment fluctuations in emotional and cognitive state. This vision demands technical rigor, ethical clarity, and a commitment to human-centered design.

A NEW ERA OF PRACTICE

The integration of AI, XR, and wearable sensors into mental health care signals more than a technological upgrade, it marks a reimagining of what care can look like in the 21st century (Kim & Backonja, 2025). These tools offer the potential to make services more personalized, scalable, and responsive. They can extend reach to underserved populations, enhance therapeutic outcomes, and generate new insights into the human mind. Clinicians should approach these technologies as amplifiers of care, tools that extend their capacity to observe, intervene, and support, not as replacements for human judgment or relational depth. Effective adoption requires investment in clinician training, patient education, and governance structures that safeguard privacy and promote equity. Ethical deployment must be grounded in transparency, accountability, and a shared commitment to person-centered care. This new era invites clinicians to expand their skillsets, rethink traditional workflows, and engage with technology as a collaborative partner in healing. It challenges institutions to align innovation with values, to measure impact beyond efficiency, and to ensure that digital transformation serves the goals of empathy, equity, and empowerment.

MACHINE LEARNING IN MENTAL HEALTH

Machine learning (ML), a rapidly evolving subset of AI, is reshaping the contours of mental health care by enabling systems to learn from data, identify patterns, and make predictions or decisions with minimal human intervention. This capability represents not just a technological advancement but a fundamental shift in how mental health conditions are detected, understood, and treated. In a field historically constrained by subjective assessments and limited access to care, ML offers the potential to enhance diagnostic precision, personalize treatment, and extend services to underserved populations. However, its integration into clinical practice is complex (Li et al., 2025). It raises critical questions about data quality, model interpretability, algorithmic bias, and ethical governance (Li et al., 2025). The promise of ML must be balanced with a rigorous commitment to transparency, inclusivity, and human-centered design.

Clinicians should view ML as an augmentative tool, one that requires active oversight, contextual interpretation, and periodic validation against local clinical outcomes (Babu & Joseph, 2025). Institutions must define governance processes for model updates, clinician feedback loops, and adverse event reporting (Ong et al., 2025). Pre-deployment testing on representative local samples is essential, along with clear documentation of expected failure modes and limitations. At its core, ML involves training algorithms on datasets to recognize patterns and make predictions. In mental health, these datasets are often heterogeneous, encompassing structured clinical data (e.g., diagnostic codes, medication histories), unstructured data (e.g., therapy transcripts, social media posts), and physiological signals (e.g., HRV, GSR, EEG; Ong et al., 2025). ML models may be supervised, trained on labeled data to predict specific outcomes, or unsupervised, used to discover latent structures in unlabeled data (Ong et al., 2025). Reinforcement learning, a third paradigm, enables systems to learn through feedback loops, adjusting behavior based on outcomes. Each paradigm has distinct affordances. Supervised models are best suited for well-defined clinical endpoints (Ong et al., 2025). Unsupervised methods help uncover subtypes or phenotypes that inform hypothesis generation. Reinforcement learning holds promise for sequencing interventions but requires stringent safety constraints during deployment. Teams should match the ML approach to the clinical question and define success metrics before model development begins (Ong et al., 2025).

ML's appeal lies in its capacity to process vast, complex, and multimodal datasets that would be unmanageable for human clinicians. It enables earlier detection, more precise stratification, and adaptive intervention. Yet its deployment must be governed by ethical principles, clinical oversight, and a commitment to equity (Freeman et al., 2017). The directive is clear: use ML to enhance care, not to automate it; to support clinicians, not to supplant them; and to serve patients, not to surveil them. The appeal of ML in mental health lies in its capacity to process vast, complex, and multimodal datasets that would be unmanageable for human clinicians. For example, natural language processing (Hall et al., 2024) techniques can analyze thousands of therapy transcripts to identify linguistic markers of depression or anxiety, while time-series models can track behavioral changes over time to forecast relapse or treatment response. These analytic capabilities can surface subtle signals, like shifts in sleep patterns or speech tempo, that precede clinical change (Freeman et al., 2017). Practically, this enables earlier, targeted interventions and reduces reliance on episodic human observation. Integrating model outputs into clinician workflows requires clear visualization, actionable recommendations, and training on interpretation (Freeman et al., 2017). To ensure clinical utility, validate models prospectively and measure impacts on care processes, not just predictive metrics (Freeman et al., 2017).

One of the most impactful applications of ML in mental health is early detection and screening. By analyzing digital footprints such as social media activity, smartphone usage patterns, or wearable sensor dataML models can identify subtle behavioral and linguistic changes that may indicate the onset of a mental health condition (Iwaya et al., 2023). A landmark study conducted by researchers at the University of Pennsylvania and Stony Brook University exemplifies this potential . The team analyzed over 500,000 Facebook posts from consenting users and found that ML algorithms could predict a future diagnosis of depression with significant accuracy, up to three months before it appeared in medical records. The models identified linguistic markers such as increased use of first-person singular pronouns ("I," "me"), negative emotion words ("sad," "lonely"), and expressions of hopelessness. These findings underscore the potential of ML to serve as a proactive screening tool, particularly in populations that may not seek traditional mental health services. When deploying similar screening tools, implement robust consent processes and clear escalation protocols to avoid intrusive or stigmatizing outreach. In practice, pair automated detection with human review and a gentle, user-centered approach to follow-up to respect autonomy and reduce harm.

Another compelling example is the Mindstrong Health platform, which leverages passive data from smartphone interactions, such as typing speed, scrolling behavior, and app usage patterns, to detect cognitive changes associated with mood disorders (Inkster et al., 2023). The ML algorithms embedded in the app continuously monitor these digital biomarkers, comparing them to individual baselines to flag deviations that may signal emerging depression, anxiety, or cognitive decline. This approach not only facilitates early intervention but also empowers users to engage with their mental health in a non-intrusive, continuous manner. For clinicians, these continuous baselines provide context-rich signals that can complement episodic clinical assessments (Weiner et al., 2025). Implementation requires transparent user agreements and mechanisms for users to control data sharing and alert thresholds (Weiner et al., 2025). In research, validate such platforms with randomized or controlled designs that measure clinical outcomes and user-centered harms (Weiner et al., 2025). Beyond detection, ML is transforming how mental health treatments are personalized. Traditional approaches often rely on trial and error, with clinicians adjusting medications or therapeutic techniques based on patient feedback over time (Weiner et al., 2025). This process can be frustrating, time-consuming, and, in some cases, harmful. ML offers a data-driven alternative by predicting which interventions are most likely to be effective for a given individual based on their unique profile (Weiner et al., 2025). These predictive models combine clinical, behavioral, and biological signals to estimate treatment response probabilities (Weiner et al., 2025). Teams should specify acceptable risk thresholds and involve patients in decisions informed by model outputs (Weiner et al., 2025). Clinicians must interpret model recommendations within the broader context of patient preferences and comorbidities (Weiner et al., 2025). Implementation plans should include clinician training on probabilistic reasoning and shared decision-making tools.

The iSPOT-D study (International Study to Predict Optimized Treatment in Depression) is a case in point (Khoo et al., 2024). This large-scale, multi-site study collected clinical, cognitive, and EEG data from over 1,000 patients with major depressive disorder (Shatte et al., 2019). ML models trained on this data were able to predict treatment response to specific antidepressants, such as escitalopram and sertraline, with a high degree of accuracy (Shatte et al., 2019). By identifying biomarkers and behavioral patterns associated with positive outcomes, these models can guide clinicians in selecting the most appropriate treatment from the outset, thereby improving efficacy and reducing the burden of ineffective interventions. Clinicians should, however, review model outputs against patient histories before acting (Shatte et al., 2019). Health systems must plan for updating predictive models as new treatments or population data emerge (Shatte et al., 2019). Patients should receive explanations about how such predictions inform medication choices.

Digital mental health platforms are also leveraging ML to personalize therapeutic content in real time. Woebot, a conversational agent grounded in cognitive behavioral therapy (CBT), uses ML to adapt its responses based on user input. If a user frequently reports sleep disturbances, for example, the system may prioritize CBT-I (insomnia-focused CBT) techniques. This level of personalization enhances user engagement and ensures that interventions are contextually relevant, which is particularly important in digital self-help environments where dropout rates can be high. Designers should set boundaries on automated adaptation to prevent inappropriate tailoring. Clinicians monitoring users should receive summary reports highlighting major shifts in symptom domains. Evaluation should measure engagement, symptom change, and any unintended consequences of automated personalization. Real-time monitoring and intervention represent another frontier where ML is making significant inroads. Wearable devices and mobile apps equipped with ML algorithms can provide continuous, passive monitoring of physiological and behavioral data, enabling just-in-time adaptive interventions. These systems exemplify the concept of closed-loop care, where data collection, analysis, and intervention occur in an integrated cycle (Rajpal, 2025). The Empatica E4 wristband, for instance, collects data on electrodermal activity, heart rate, and skin temperature (Rajpal, 2025). In clinical studies involving individuals with autism spectrum disorder, ML models have used this data to detect stress episodes in real time, alerting caregivers and enabling timely support (Rajpal, 2025). Developers must define specificity thresholds to minimize false alerts and caregiver burden. Consent processes should articulate alert recipients and response expectations. Clinicians should create response workflows that align with patient safety plans.

Similarly, the Biosignal Adaptive Mobile Intervention (Lay et al., 2025) system integrates wearable sensor data with ML to deliver JITAIs for anxiety (Baka et al., 2025). When physiological markers indicate rising anxiety, such as increased heart rate variability or galvanic skin response, the system prompts users with grounding exercises or breathing techniques. These interventions are not only timely but also personalized, responding to the user's current physiological state rather than relying on static schedules or self-report. To ensure safety, designers should include escalation criteria that trigger human contact when automated supports are insufficient. Clinical teams must monitor adherence and adjust thresholds to patient-specific baselines . Research should compare JITAIs with standard care to quantify added benefit and potential harms . ML is also being used to augment clinical decision-making through decision support systems . These tools analyze patient data to suggest diagnoses, flag potential risks, or recommend treatment options, thereby enhancing the clinician's ability to make informed, data-driven decisions . IBM

Watson for Mental Health, though still in development, exemplifies this approach. Trained on thousands of psychiatric case notes and structured electronic health record (Livieri et al., 2025) data, Watson can suggest differential diagnoses and treatment plans for complex cases, such as comorbid depression and substance use disorder (Martinez-Martin et al., 2018). Decision support systems must provide transparent rationales for recommendations and integrate seamlessly with clinician workflows. Developers should include audit logs and clinician feedback loops to refine model suggestions over time (Martinez-Martin et al., 2018). Institutions should establish governance policies that define clinician responsibility versus system suggestion.

Another notable example comes from Vanderbilt University Medical Center, where researchers developed an ML model to predict suicide risk using Electronic Health Record (EHR) data (Liu & Schueller, 2023). The model outperformed traditional screening tools like the Columbia-Suicide Severity Rating Scale (C-SSRS), identifying high-risk individuals who might otherwise be missed (Poudel et al., 2025). This tool is now being piloted in emergency departments to inform triage and follow-up care, demonstrating how ML can enhance clinical workflows and improve patient outcomes (Poudel et al., 2025). Pilots should include clinician training on interpreting risk scores and protocols for patient communication. Ethical safeguards must ensure that flagged patients receive timely human contact with culturally sensitive approaches. Continuous validation across demographic groups is essential to prevent inadvertent harm. Despite these advances, the use of ML in mental health is fraught with challenges. Data quality and representativeness remain significant concerns (Poudel et al., 2025). Mental health data is often incomplete, inconsistent, and biased, reflecting the limitations of clinical documentation and the underrepresentation of certain populations in research (Poudel et al., 2025). Models trained on such data may not generalize well, leading to disparities in performance across demographic groups (Poudel et al., 2025). To mitigate these risks, developers should perform subgroup analyses and report performance metrics stratified by age, gender, race, and socioeconomic status. Clinicians should be wary of overgeneralizing model outputs and insist on local validation before clinical use (Poudel et al., 2025). Ongoing monitoring and corrective retraining are necessary to maintain fairness.

Interpretability is another critical issue. Many ML models, particularly deep learning networks, operate as "black boxes," making it difficult to understand how decisions are made. This lack of transparency can undermine trust and hinder clinical adoption, especially in high-stakes contexts like mental health care (Smith et al., 2023). Explainable AI (Shatte et al., 2019) techniques can help make ML models more interpretable, allowing users to understand and trust their outputs (Obermeyer et al., 2019). Teams should prioritize models that can provide feature-level explanations and confidence estimates. Clinicians need training to read and question these explanations effectively. Documentation should include known limitations, typical failure modes, and guidance for clinical integration (Obermeyer et al., 2019).

Bias and fairness are also pressing concerns. ML models can perpetuate or even amplify existing biases in mental health care. For example, if a model is trained on data that underrepresents racial or socioeconomic minorities, it may produce less accurate predictions for those groups, exacerbating disparities in access and outcomes (Obermeyer et al., 2019). Privacy and consent further complicate the ethical landscape. The use of personal data, particularly sensitive mental health information, raises significant ethical questions about ownership, control, and informed consent (Tsai et al., 2025). Institutions must implement robust data governance policies, including clear consent language, data minimization, and mechanisms for individuals to access or revoke their data (Tsai et al., 2025). Community engagement in model development helps align systems with local values and needs (Tsai et al., 2025).

To navigate these complexities, a human-centered approach to ML design and deployment is essential. This approach requires ongoing stakeholder engagement, including patients, clinicians, and ethicists, throughout development and implementation. Include structured feedback loops so clinicians can report false positives and false negatives for model refinement (Ball et al., 2025). Use participatory design workshops to surface contextual concerns and workflow constraints early in development. Define clear metrics for equity, safety, and clinical utility before deployment (Fanarioti & Karpouzis, 2025). Establish governance that mandates periodic audits and public reporting of performance across demographic groups. Ensure that patients retain control over their data and can opt out of automated decision-making (Fanarioti & Karpouzis, 2025). This involves engaging stakeholders, including patients, clinicians, and ethicists, throughout the development process to ensure that tools are aligned with user needs and values. Co-design sessions produce practical requirements such as preferred alert modalities and acceptable false alarm rates. Clinician advisory boards should review model explanations and escalation protocols before clinical rollout (Fanarioti & Karpouzis, 2025). Patient representatives can clarify consent language, acceptable data uses, and cultural considerations (Fanarioti & Karpouzis, 2025). Ethical review must be iterative, reflecting system updates and new use cases rather than a one-time approval. Training materials and decision aids developed with stakeholders improve adoption and trust. Continuous stakeholder engagement supports equitable and contextually appropriate deployment.

Explainable AI (Fanarioti & Karpouzis, 2025) techniques can help make ML models more interpretable, allowing users to understand and trust their outputs (Gkintoni et al., 2025). Select XAI methods that present feature contributions in clinically meaningful language and visualizations. Combine global explanations with case-level rationales so clinicians can both validate model behavior and scrutinize specific recommendations (Engel, 1977). Implement user testing to ensure explanations reduce, not increase, cognitive load during clinical decision-making (Engel, 1977). Require confidence intervals on model outputs to communicate uncertainty (Engel, 1977). Provide training modules that teach clinicians how to interrogate and contest model explanations appropriately (Engel, 1977). Integrate feedback mechanisms so clinicians can flag misleading explanations for rapid rectification. Participatory design methods can ensure that tools are inclusive and culturally sensitive, while continuous evaluation can help identify and mitigate unintended consequences. Recruit diverse participants for testing across age, language, and cultural groups to capture varied expression of distress. Use scenario-based usability testing to uncover misinterpretation risks in different cultural contexts. Embed equity metrics into evaluation plans and publish results to inform broader implementation efforts. When unintended consequences emerge, enact rapid mitigation steps and update consent materials accordingly. Continuous evaluation cycles should inform both technical revisions and changes to clinical protocols (Engel, 1977). Share lessons learned with peer institutions to accelerate responsible scaling.

Experts such as Thomas Insel, Albert Rizzo, Rosalind Picard have advanced concepts like neuroadaptive systems, human-in-the-loop.

Advances in multimodal learning will enable models to integrate diverse data sources, text, speech, physiology, and behavior, into more holistic assessments (Lindner et al., 2024). This integration improves sensitivity to clinically meaningful patterns that single modalities miss. Design multimodal pipelines with clear alignment to clinical questions, such as relapse prediction or functional impairment (Mohr et al., 2017). Conduct local validation studies that test multimodal models against clinician assessments and patient-reported outcomes. Document fusion strategies and missing-data handling methods transparently for reproducibility (Mohr et al., 2017). Train clinicians on the interpretation of composite risk scores and their appropriate use in shared decision-making.

Federated learning approaches may allow for collaborative model training across institutions without compromising data privacy. These methods keep raw data locally while aggregating model updates, reducing privacy risks (Robinson et al., 2024). Pilot federated projects should include explicit technical and legal frameworks for participation and data governance (Robinson et al., 2024). Evaluate federated models on external datasets to confirm generalizability and equity across sites. Engage institutional review boards and legal counsel early to clarify liability and consent implications. Communicate clearly with patients about federated processes and their privacy protections. The integration of ML with other technologies, such as extended reality and neurofeedback, will open new avenues for adaptive, immersive interventions. Combined systems can use physiological signals to modulate XR scenarios in real time, optimizing therapeutic challenge (Robinson et al., 2024). Define safety envelopes and clinician override mechanisms before deploying adaptive experiences.

Measure both proximal physiological responses and distal functional outcomes to demonstrate clinical benefit (Robinson et al., 2024). Use iterative co-design with patients to improve acceptability and minimize adverse effects like cybersickness. Plan implementation studies that assess workflow impacts and cost-effectiveness.

However, the goal must remain clear: to enhance not replace, the human elements of empathy. ML should support clinicians by expanding observational reach and suggesting targeted interventions. Maintain explicit roles where humans retain authority over diagnoses, complex formulations, and crisis decisions. Embed model outputs into collaborative decision-making processes that honor patient preferences and clinician expertise (Spytska, 2025). Monitor for unintended shifts in clinician responsibility or patient reliance on automated systems. Commit to ongoing evaluation of how ML affects therapeutic alliance and long-term recovery trajectories.

AGENTIC AI IN MENTAL HEALTH PRACTICE AND INTERVENTION

Narrow AI and general AI represent two distinct paradigms within the broader field of artificial intelligence, each with its own capabilities, limitations, and implications for society (Okposio et al., 2025). Narrow AI, also known as weak AI, refers to systems that are designed and trained to perform a specific task or a limited range of tasks (De Kock et al., 2021). These systems operate under a constrained set of rules and parameters, excelling in well-defined domains such as language translation, facial recognition, or playing chess. For instance, virtual assistants like Siri or Alexa, recommendation algorithms on streaming platforms, and diagnostic tools in medical imaging are all examples of narrow AI (De Kock et al., 2021). They can process vast amounts of data, identify patterns, and make decisions within their programmed scope, but they lack the ability to generalize knowledge or apply reasoning beyond their designated function (De Kock et al., 2021). Their intelligence is task-specific, and while they may appear sophisticated, they do not possess consciousness, self-awareness, or an understanding of the broader context in which they operate. To guide clinical adoption, clearly differentiate task-specific tools from broader decision systems during procurement and training (De Kock et al., 2021). Implement acceptance testing that verifies narrow AI performance against clinical benchmarks and local caseloads (De Kock et al., 2021). Require vendors to document the operational envelope and failure modes of narrow AI components (De Kock et al., 2021). Train clinicians to recognize when narrow AI outputs are out of scope and require escalation to human experts (De Kock et al., 2021).

In contrast, general AI, often referred to as strong AI or artificial general intelligence (AGI), is a theoretical construct that envisions machines with the ability to understand, learn, and apply knowledge across a wide range of tasks at a level comparable to human intelligence. A general AI system would not only be able to perform any intellectual task that a human can, but it would also possess the capacity for abstract reasoning, problem-solving, emotional understanding, and even creativity (Rajpal, 2025). Unlike narrow AI, which is limited to predefined inputs and outputs, general AI would be capable of transferring knowledge from one domain to another, adapting to new situations without explicit programming, and engaging in autonomous decision-making with a high degree of contextual awareness (Rajpal, 2025). This level of intelligence remains aspirational; despite significant advances in machine learning and cognitive modeling, no existing AI system has achieved true general intelligence (Rajpal, 2025). The development of AGI poses profound technical, ethical, and philosophical challenges, including questions about consciousness, moral agency, and the potential risks of creating entities with capabilities that rival or surpass those of humans. For clinical planning, treat AGI as a scenario for ethical foresight exercises rather than an immediate operational risk (Rajpal, 2025). Use tabletop simulations to explore liability, consent, and governance implications should more general systems emerge. Engage interdisciplinary advisors to inform policy development around autonomy and accountability before AGI becomes plausible.

The distinction between narrow and general AI is not merely academic, it has real-world implications for how we design, deploy, and regulate AI technologies (Baydili et al., 2025). While narrow AI is already embedded in many aspects of daily life and continues to evolve rapidly, the pursuit of general AI raises critical concerns about safety, control, and alignment with human values (Fleming et al., 2019). Researchers and ethicists emphasize the importance of ensuring that any progress toward AGI is accompanied by robust frameworks for governance, transparency, and accountability. In the meantime, understanding the capabilities and limitations of narrow AI helps us appreciate both the power and the boundaries of current technologies, while also preparing us for the complex future that general AI may one day bring (Fleming et al., 2019). As we navigate this evolving landscape, it is essential to remain grounded in interdisciplinary dialogue, combining insights from computer science, psychology, philosophy, and ethics to guide the responsible development of intelligent systems. Clinicians and administrators should create cross-functional committees to review emerging AI capabilities and update institutional policies regularly (Fleming et al., 2019). Establish clear procurement criteria that require ethical risk assessments and alignment proofs for any AI system considered for clinical use (Fleming et al., 2019). Maintain open channels with regulatory bodies to anticipate changes in compliance expectations.

The emergence of agentic artificial intelligence a third paradigm in AI are defined as AI systems capable of autonomous decision-making, goal-directed behavior, and adaptive interaction, marks a pivotal evolution in the application of digital technologies to mental health care (Tavory, 2024). Unlike traditional algorithmic tools that operate within narrowly defined parameters, agentic AI systems possess a degree of intentionality: they can initiate actions, respond dynamically to user input, and adjust their strategies based on evolving contexts (Pedram & Piatkowski, 2025). In mental health practice, this shift from passive computation to active engagement opens new possibilities for therapeutic support, behavioral monitoring, and personalized intervention. These systems are not merely reactive; they are participatory, capable of co-constructing therapeutic experiences in ways that mirror, and in some cases extend, the relational dynamics of human care. At the heart of agentic AI is the capacity to maintain persistent, context-aware interactions with users (Pedram & Piatkowski, 2025). Specify clear consent and autonomy controls when deploying agentic systems, ensuring users understand initiation rights and opt-out mechanisms. Design logging features that record agent actions and rationales for clinical review (Pedram & Piatkowski, 2025). Require periodic human review of agent decisions, especially in high-risk domains.

Consider, for example, a virtual mental health coach embedded in a mobile application. Unlike static chatbots, an agentic AI system can track a user's emotional and behavioral patterns over time, initiate check-ins during periods of elevated stress, and adapt its communication style to align with the user's preferences and psychological profile (Sun et al., 2025). Such systems can draw on multimodal data, text, voice, physiological signals, to infer mental states and select appropriate interventions, whether that be a grounding exercise, a motivational prompt, or a referral to a human clinician (Rajpal, 2025). This level of responsiveness transforms the AI from a tool into a therapeutic partner, capable of sustaining engagement and fostering a sense of being seen and supported (Rajpal, 2025). Operationally, define escalation thresholds that trigger clinician contact and ensure these thresholds are transparent to users. Pilot agentic features with conservative initiation logic and robust opt-out controls. Train clinicians to interpret agent logs and integrate them into clinical formulations (Rajpal, 2025). Monitor engagement metrics for signs of maladaptive reliance or avoidance.

Experts such as Thomas Insel, Albert Rizzo, Rosalind Picard have advanced concepts like neuroadaptive systems, human-in-the-loop.

Real-world implementations of agentic AI in mental health are beginning to emerge (Carl et al., 2019). These implementations range from conversational agents that manage routine check-ins to integrated monitoring platforms alerting clinicians to risk. Deploy pilot studies to measure engagement, safety, escalation appropriateness, and clinician workload impact. Include diverse populations in pilots to evaluate generalizability across cultural and linguistic groups. Document user consent flows and opt-out effectiveness to protect autonomy and trust. Require clinicians to receive training on interpreting agent logs and overriding automated actions.

BENEFITS OF AGENTIC AI

The benefits of agentic AI in mental health practice are both profound and far-reaching, offering a paradigm shift in how care is conceptualized, delivered, and experienced (Xing et al., 2025). Agentic systems sustain continuous engagement and can personalize support across time and context. They can increase access to low-intensity interventions where clinicians are scarce, improving equity of reach. Use measurable engagement and outcome metrics to assess benefit in real-world deployments. Maintain clinician oversight so that AI augments rather than replaces therapeutic decision-making (Li et al., 2025).

One of the most significant benefits of agentic AI is its ability to provide personalized and adaptive support (Mone & Fayazullaeva, 2023). Traditional mental health tools often rely on static algorithms that do not account for the dynamic nature of human emotions and behaviors. Agentic systems learn from ongoing interactions, tailoring interventions to an individual's changing needs. Monitor personalization quality by comparing adaptive suggestions with clinician recommendations. Ensure patients understand and consent to adaptive behaviors and have control over personalization settings.

Another key advantage of agentic AI is its scalability (Friend et al., 2024). Mental health care is often limited by the availability of trained professionals, especially in underserved areas. Agentic systems can deploy consistent, evidence-informed support across large populations without proportional increases in human resources (Ienca et al., 2017). Measure scalability gains alongside potential dilution of individualized care to preserve quality. Pair scalable AI supports with scheduled human contacts to maintain therapeutic depth (Ienca et al., 2017). Agentic AI also offers the benefit of continuous monitoring and support (Ienca et al., 2017). Traditional mental health care often involves periodic check-ins with a clinician, which may not be sufficient for individuals with chronic conditions or those experiencing acute distress. Agentic AI systems can provide continuous, real-time monitoring and initiate timely supports when risk thresholds are crossed (Ienca et al., 2017). Define clear escalation pathways so continuous monitoring does not substitute for human triage in crises. Audit alert frequency to avoid alarm fatigue and adjust thresholds for individual baselines.

In addition to supporting users directly, agentic AI can also augment the work of mental health professionals (Walter et al., 2023). By handling routine tasks such as mood tracking, data collection, and initial triage, these systems can free up clinicians to focus on more complex therapeutic work (Ong et al., 2025). Define clear boundaries for automated tasks and maintain clinician oversight for diagnostic and therapeutic decisions. Track time savings and reallocate clinician effort toward cases requiring higher-level skills. Establish protocols that require clinician review of all

AI-initiated escalations within a set timeframe (Ong et al., 2025). Monitor for task displacement that could unintentionally reduce opportunities for clinician-patient contact.

The integration of agentic AI into mental health care also has the potential to generate valuable data and insights (Lorke & Stefanou, 2025). The interactions between users and AI systems can provide a wealth of information about a patient's mental health trajectory, enabling more informed decision-making and personalized treatment planning (Mohr et al., 2017). Ensure data governance policies clarify ownership, permissible use, and de-identification standards (Mohr et al., 2017). Use aggregated metrics to inform service planning without compromising individual privacy. Present actionable summaries to clinicians to avoid raw-data overload (Mohr et al., 2017). Validate analytic insights against clinician judgments and patient-reported outcomes to confirm clinical relevance (Mohr et al., 2017). Set retention limits for interaction logs consistent with privacy norms and clinical utility (Mohr et al., 2017).

Ethical considerations are paramount in the design and deployment of agentic AI systems (Pedram & Piatkowski, 2025). It is essential that these systems are designed transparently and with respect for user autonomy. Users should be informed about how their data is being used and have the option to opt out of AI-driven interventions if they choose (Poudel et al., 2025). Create consent materials that clearly explain agent initiation behaviors and escalation rules in plain language. Provide users with settings to control timing and frequency of AI contact (Poudel et al., 2025). Offer regular reminders of opt-out rights to maintain ongoing consent. Include mechanisms for users to request deletion or export of their interaction history in line with legal requirements (Poudel et al., 2025).

LIMITATIONS OF AGENTIC AI IN MENTAL HEALTH

Despite the transformative potential of agentic AI in mental health care, its integration into clinical and therapeutic contexts is fraught with significant limitations that demand careful scrutiny (Engel, 1977). One of the most fundamental challenges lies in the interpretability of AI systems (Pedram & Piatkowski, 2025). Many agentic AI models, particularly those built on deep learning architectures, function as "black boxes", they generate outputs without offering clear explanations of how decisions are made (Pedram & Piatkowski, 2025). In mental health contexts, where trust, transparency, and informed consent are paramount, this lack of interpretability can erode user confidence and hinder clinician oversight. To manage this risk, require models to include case-level explanations and confidence estimates before clinical deployment (Pedram & Piatkowski, 2025). Implement routine audits to verify that explanations align with clinician reasoning. Train clinicians to query and contest model outputs as part of regular case review (Pedram & Piatkowski, 2025). Maintain clear documentation of model decision pathways for regulatory review (Pedram & Piatkowski, 2025).

Another critical limitation is the potential for bias and inequity embedded within AI systems (Freeman et al., 2017). Agentic AI relies heavily on training data, and if that data is not representative of diverse populations, the system may perform poorly, or even harmfully, when interacting with users from underrepresented groups (Freeman et al., 2017). For instance, language models trained predominantly on Western, English-speaking datasets may misinterpret idiomatic expressions, cultural references, or emotional cues from non-Western users. This can lead to misdiagnoses, inappropriate interventions, or a general sense of alienation for users who do not see their experiences accurately reflected in the AI's responses (Freeman et al., 2017). To mitigate these harms, mandate diverse training datasets and require external equity audits before deployment. Conduct localization testing to surface cultural mismatches. Establish feedback channels for communities to report misinterpretations and discriminatory behavior. Make remediation processes transparent and timely.

Technical reliability is another area of concern. Agentic AI systems, like all software, are susceptible to bugs, outages, and misclassifications. A system crash during a crisis moment, or an incorrect interpretation of a user's emotional state, can have serious consequences. For example, if an AI misreads sarcasm or metaphor as a sign of suicidal ideation, it might trigger an unnecessary emergency response, causing distress or eroding trust (Kim & Backonja, 2025). Conversely, if it fails to detect genuine distress, it may miss an opportunity for timely intervention. These risks underscore the need for robust fail-safes, human oversight, and continuous system evaluation. Design redundancy into critical pathways, such as parallel clinician alerts and human verification steps. Test systems under stress scenarios and simulate outages to refine escalation protocols. Require service-level agreements that guarantee uptime and rapid incident response.

The issue of over-reliance also warrants attention. As agentic AI becomes more sophisticated and accessible, there is a growing risk that users may come to depend on these systems for emotional support, potentially at the expense of seeking human connection or professional care (Tizzard, 2025). This is particularly concerning for individuals with attachment vulnerabilities or those experiencing social isolation. While AI can provide immediate, nonjudgmental interaction, it cannot replace the nuanced understanding, ethical responsibility, and emotional presence of a trained therapist (De Kock et al., 2021). Over time, this reliance could lead to a form of digital dependency, where users turn to AI for comfort but do not receive the depth of care needed for meaningful psychological growth or healing (De Kock et al., 2021). To prevent dependency, incorporate scheduled human check-ins into care plans and monitor patterns of interaction that suggest avoidance. Educate users about the complementary role of AI and promote pathways to human services (De Kock et al., 2021). Evaluate long-term outcomes to detect any erosion of help-seeking behaviors.

Ethical and legal frameworks for agentic AI in mental health are also underdeveloped (Reddy, 2025). Questions of accountability, such as who is responsible when an AI system causes harm, remain unresolved (Mohr et al., 2017). Current regulations often lag behind technological innovation, leaving gaps in oversight and enforcement. For example, if an AI system fails to escalate a crisis situation or provides harmful advice, it is unclear whether liability rests with the developers, the deploying institution, or the clinicians who oversee its use (Mohr et al., 2017). Regulatory uncertainty requires institutions to adopt conservative governance approaches and clear contractual terms with vendors. Establish internal policies that delineate clinician responsibilities versus system roles to reduce ambiguity. Engage legal counsel and ethics boards early to draft response plans for adverse outcomes. Advocate for sector-wide standards and participate in policy consultations to shape practical, enforceable rules. Provide transparent communication to patients about limits of recourse and complaint procedures.

Privacy and data concerns are ever-present in agentic AI deployments. Agentic AI systems often collect and process sensitive personal information, and without stringent data governance policies, there is a risk of misuse, breaches, or unauthorized surveillance. Compliance with existing privacy laws is necessary but not sufficient; organizations must implement higher standards tailored to mental health's sensitivity. Adopt data minimization principles and anonymize or pseudonymize data where feasible. Define precise access controls and logging to ensure only authorized personnel can view sensitive records. Regularly audit data flows and third-party vendors for compliance with contractual and ethical commitments. Offer patients granular consent options and clear explanations of data use to support informed decision-making (Martinez-Martin et al., 2018). Prepare incident response plans that prioritize patient notification, remediation, and review of systemic causes.

The relational dynamics introduced by agentic AI require careful ethical reflection (Rajpal, 2025). These systems are designed to engage users in emotionally resonant ways, but they do so without consciousness, intention, or moral agency. This creates a paradox: users may experience the AI as a caring presence, while the system itself remains indifferent (Tsai et al., 2025). Navigating this paradox requires a rethinking of therapeutic boundaries, informed consent, and the nature of care itself. Incorporate explicit discussions about AI roles into treatment contracts and informed consent conversations (Tsai et al., 2025). Train clinicians to address transference-like responses toward AI and to use such material therapeutically when appropriate (Tsai et al., 2025). Develop guidelines for termination of AI involvement and transitions back to human-led care (Tsai et al., 2025). Monitor how AI interactions affect trust in clinicians and adjust communication strategies accordingly (Tsai et al., 2025).

NATURAL LANGUAGE PROCESSING IN MENTAL HEALTH PRACTICE AND INTERVENTION

Experts such as Thomas Insel, Albert Rizzo, Rosalind Picard have advanced concepts like systems-thinking. The recent surge in NLP applications, especially those leveraging large language models (LLMs), has catalyzed a paradigm shift: from reactive, episodic care to proactive, continuous, and personalized mental health support. For instance, NLP algorithms now analyze therapy transcripts to assess treatment fidelity, detect emotional tone, and even predict therapeutic alliance, all of which are critical predictors of clinical outcomes (Freeman et al., 2017). These systems do not replace the clinician but rather augment their capacity to perceive patterns that may be too subtle or temporally dispersed for human cognition alone. In this sense, NLP functions as a cognitive amplifier, extending the clinician's perceptual reach across time and context. When integrating these tools, require explainable outputs that clinicians can interrogate during supervision. Train care teams to use NLP-derived flags as discussion prompts rather than definitive judgments. Monitor how NLP use changes supervision dynamics and case formulations.

Moreover, the integration of NLP into digital mental health platforms has democratized access to care, particularly through self-administered interventions that operate asynchronously and at scale. A 2024 meta-analysis revealed that such interventions, many of which are grounded in cognitive behavioral therapy (Freeman et al., 2017) frameworks, significantly reduce symptoms of depression and anxiety (Mulukuntla, 2025). These systems often employ conversational agents that simulate therapeutic dialogue, offering users a space to articulate distress, receive psychoeducation, and engage in structured exercises. While the therapeutic alliance in these contexts is synthetic, the outcomes are real: users report measurable improvements in mood and functioning, especially when the NLP models are fine-tuned to recognize and respond to affective cues. Implement adaptive safety nets that escalate to humans when high-risk language is detected. Validate conversational agents with randomized designs that include long-term follow-up. Ensure users have straightforward paths to human help when needed.

This is not to suggest that AI can or should replace human therapists, but rather that it can serve as a bridge, filling gaps in access, reducing stigma, and providing immediate support in moments of crisis (Kumar, 2025). Importantly, these systems are not static; they learn from user interactions, adapting their responses to better align with individual needs. This dynamic feedback loop mirrors the principles of adaptive learning systems, a concept central to Lamb's work, wherein technology evolves in tandem with the learner, or in this case, the patient. For clinical deployment, set conservative adaptation limits and require human review for higher-risk adaptations (Ong et al., 2025). Use pilot phases to quantify adaptive benefits and any drift from intended therapeutic content. Archive interaction histories for audit and quality assurance.

Another frontier in NLP-driven mental health care lies in the analysis of non-clinical language data, particularly from social media platforms (Elfouly & Alouani, 2025). Here, NLP is used to detect early signs of psychological distress, suicidal ideation, or relapse risk by analyzing patterns in users' posts, comments, and messages. These systems can flag concerning content in real time, enabling timely intervention by clinicians, peers, or automated support agents. This capability introduces complex ethical questions about surveillance, consent, and the boundaries of clinical responsibility in public digital spaces (Fleming et al., 2019). Establish clear criteria for which platforms and content streams are ethically suitable for monitoring. Require explicit user consent when clinical follow-up is possible and design opt-in models wherever feasible (Fleming et al., 2019). Pilot programs should include community advisory boards to set norms for acceptable monitoring and intervention.

In this vein, the application of NLP to public and private text streams raises privacy and consent challenges that differ from traditional clinical data use (Huang et al., 2024). Who owns the data (Tsai et al., 2025)? Who decides when and how to intervene? And how do we balance the imperative to protect life with the right to digital autonomy? These are not merely technical questions but moral ones, demanding a multidisciplinary dialogue that includes ethicists, clinicians, technologists, and, crucially, patients themselves. Establish governance frameworks that differentiate surveillance from voluntary monitoring and that prioritize minimal intrusion. Use transparent consent documentation that explains probable responses to detected risk. Provide independent review of intervention thresholds to ensure ethical proportionality and fairness.

In practical clinical applications, NLP supports sentiment and emotion analysis, therapeutic progress monitoring, and suicide risk detection (Mohr et al., 2017). These tools can flag emotional shifts, quantify changes in cognitive patterns, and identify language associated with imminent safety concerns. Clinicians should use these flags as prompts for deeper assessment rather than definitive judgments. Create standard operating procedures for triaging NLP alerts, including timelines for clinician response and documentation requirements. Train staff to interpret linguistic markers within cultural and individual context, reducing misclassification risks. Regularly recalibrate models to reflect changing language use and local speech patterns.

NLP also contributes to personalized treatment by analyzing large datasets of therapy outcomes to recommend interventions that have been effective for clients with similar profiles. For example, a system might suggest considering Acceptance and Commitment Therapy (Poudel et al., 2025) based on language patterns and symptom profiles that match prior responders. Present such recommendations as evidence-informed options within shared decision-making conversations (Hickey et al., 2021). Include model provenance information so clinicians know the data sources and cohort characteristics underlying recommendations (Pedram & Piatkowski, 2025). Monitor real-world concordance between model suggestions and clinician-chosen interventions to evaluate practical utility (Pedram & Piatkowski, 2025).

From a systems perspective, the integration of NLP into mental health practice represents a shift from linear, clinician-centered models of care to distributed, data-driven ecosystems (Crameri et al., 2021). These ecosystems are characterized by continuous feedback loops, where data from therapy sessions, self-reports, and digital interactions inform real-time adjustments to treatment plans (Martinez-Martin et al., 2018). This aligns with Lamb's vision of adaptive systems that evolve with users. Implement governance that preserves clinician responsibility while enabling automated supports to operate safely. Design dashboards that synthesize NLP insights into concise, actionable summaries for busy clinicians. Evaluate how these ecosystems affect therapeutic alliance and patient autonomy through mixed-methods research (Martinez-Martin et al., 2018).

In the intricate and often unpredictable terrain of mental health care, where the human psyche resists reduction to simple categories and outcomes are shaped by a constellation of biological, psychological, and social variables, the emergence of predictive analytics and adaptive artificial intelligence (Sharma & Meena, 2024) represents a profound reconfiguration of clinical practice (Clemens-Meyer et al., 2021). Frame predictive and adaptive AI as systemic tools that augment clinician situational awareness without displacing clinical judgment (Kargarandehkordi et al., 2025). Use scenario-based risk assessments to evaluate where predictions add value and where they might mislead. Require pilot testing in representative clinical workflows before broad deployment (Kargarandehkordi et al., 2025). Implement governance that ties predictions to defined clinical actions and safety checks (Kargarandehkordi et al., 2025).

Lamb's work in educational psychology, particularly his research on AI-enhanced learning environments, provides a compelling framework for understanding how adaptive systems can be designed to respond to the evolving cognitive and affective states of individuals (Immanuel et al., 2023). In his studies, Lamb emphasizes the importance of real-time data collection through wearable sensors and AI to assess and respond to learners' needs dynamically (Rajpal, 2025). Apply the same real-time, formative assessment principles to clinical care by defining sensing modalities, intervention rules, and human escalation pathways (Rajpal, 2025). Compare adaptive AI outputs with clinician observations during pilots to validate convergent utility (Rajpal, 2025). Document failure modes and rollback procedures to maintain patient safety.

At the heart of this transformation lies the capacity of AI, particularly through machine learning (ML), to detect patterns in vast, multidimensional datasets, patterns that elude even the most experienced clinicians (Mackey et al., 2025). These systems ingest data from electronic health records, therapy transcripts, wearable sensors, and even social media activity, constructing probabilistic models that forecast clinical trajectories, identify risk factors, and recommend personalized interventions (Li et al., 2025). Require data provenance documentation that explains sources, preprocessing steps, and known biases for each model (Li et al., 2025). Conduct external validation against independent datasets to test generalizability before clinical use (Li et al., 2025). Maintain clinician-accessible performance dashboards showing real-time model behavior and drift metrics (Li et al., 2025).

For instance, ML algorithms have demonstrated remarkable accuracy in predicting the onset of depressive episodes, suicidal ideation, or psychotic breaks weeks before they manifest behaviorally. This predictive capacity is not merely academic; it enables clinicians to intervene preemptively, shifting the paradigm from reactive treatment to proactive prevention. Prioritize clear clinical pathways that translate risk scores into agreed-upon actions, including patient outreach and safety planning (Robinson et al., 2024). Train staff on interpreting probabilistic outputs and communicating risk to patients in understandable terms. Monitor outcomes to ensure that predictive interventions reduce harm and improve recovery trajectories. But prediction alone is not enough. What distinguishes the most impactful AI systems in mental health is their adaptivity, their ability to learn from new data, adjust their models, and refine their recommendations in real time (Weiner et al., 2025). This adaptivity mirrors the principles of formative assessment and feedback loops central to Lamb's work, where systems evolve in response to the learner's needs. In clinical settings, adaptive AI can monitor a patient's response to treatment, whether pharmacological, psychotherapeutic, or behavioral, and dynamically adjust the care plan (Weiner et al., 2025). For clarity, adaptive systems should have pre-specified update cadences and safety checks that prevent unintended behavior drift. Define rollback procedures to revert model changes that degrade clinical performance (Weiner et al., 2025). Require human approval for algorithmic changes that alter escalation rules or treatment recommendations. Document adaptation logs to allow clinicians to audit why interventions changed.

Lamb's research also underscores the importance of multimodal data integration, combining physiological, behavioral, and contextual data to form a holistic picture of the individual (Ghanim et al., 2023). In mental health, this might involve integrating heart rate variability, speech patterns, facial expressions, and digital behavior to assess emotional regulation or stress levels. Such a comprehensive approach allows for more nuanced predictions and more targeted interventions. Operational teams should standardize data schemas and timestamps to support robust multimodal fusion (Pedram & Piatkowski, 2025). Evaluate how missing data from one modality affects overall model confidence and behavior (Pedram & Piatkowski, 2025). Develop clinician-facing summaries that translate multimodal signals into understandable clinical cues (Pedram & Piatkowski, 2025). Pilot multimodal systems with layered consent explaining each data stream's purpose and use (Pedram & Piatkowski, 2025).

Predictive and adaptive AI systems are increasingly being integrated into clinical decision support tools, augmenting the clinician's judgment rather than replacing it (Mitsea et al., 2024). These tools provide probabilistic forecasts of treatment outcomes based on patient-specific variables, such as age, comorbidities, genetic markers, and prior treatment history, enabling more informed and individualized care planning (Radanliev, 2025). In this way, AI acts as a cognitive partner, expanding the clinician's capacity to synthesize complex information and make nuanced decisions (Radanliev, 2025). Establish clear protocols that define when and how clinicians should act on probabilistic forecasts. Use shared decision-making templates that incorporate AI-derived probabilities into conversations with patients (Radanliev, 2025). Train multidisciplinary teams on interpreting uncertainty bands and model confidence scores (Radanliev, 2025). Monitor whether decision support changes practice patterns in ways that improve or harm patient outcomes.

Yet, as with any powerful technology, the deployment of predictive and adaptive AI in mental health care raises critical ethical and epistemological questions (Shah et al., 2021). Chief among these is the issue of transparency. Many ML models, particularly those based on deep learning, operate as "black boxes," offering little insight into how predictions are generated. This opacity can undermine trust, especially in high-stakes clinical decisions (Fleming et al., 2019). To address this, integrate explainability layers that surface the top contributing features for each prediction in clinician-friendly language. Require model cards that summarize scope, limitations, and known biases for every deployed system (Fleming et al., 2019). Conduct clinician validation sessions where model explanations are compared with clinical reasoning on representative cases (Fleming et al., 2019). Include patient-facing explanations for any prediction that meaningfully affects care.

From a systems perspective, the integration of predictive and adaptive AI into mental health care represents a shift from linear, protocol-driven models to dynamic, feedback-rich ecosystems (Moriarty et al., 2022). These ecosystems are characterized by continuous data flow, real-time analysis, and iterative refinement, principles that resonate deeply with Lamb's vision of adaptive learning environments (Robinson et al., 2024). In practice, this means that a patient's journey through the mental health system is no longer a static path but a responsive, evolving process shaped by ongoing assessment and adjustment. Implement governance structures that tie model outputs to predefined clinical actions, safety checks, and audit trails (Robinson et al., 2024). Design interoperability standards so model outputs integrate seamlessly with EHRs and clinician dashboards (Robinson et al., 2024). Evaluate system-level effects such as changes in caseload prioritization and access equity before full-scale deployment.

This diagram visually encapsulates the hierarchical and functional relationship between Artificial Intelligence (AI), Machine Learning (ML), and Prediction within the context of mental health care (Pruden, 2025). At the broadest level, AI represents the overarching field that encompasses all computational systems designed to simulate aspects of human intelligence (Pedram & Piatkowski, 2025). Nested within AI is Machine Learning, a specialized domain that focuses on algorithms capable of learning from data and improving over time without being explicitly programmed (Pedram & Piatkowski, 2025). Within ML lies the critical function of Prediction, which is particularly transformative in mental health settings. Here, predictive models are used to anticipate clinical outcomes such as the onset of depressive episodes, risk of relapse, or likely response to specific treatments (Pedram & Piatkowski, 2025). These predictions are not abstract, they directly inform real-world interventions, enabling clinicians to tailor care plans, allocate resources more effectively, and engage in proactive rather than reactive treatment. When presenting such a diagram to clinical stakeholders, accompany it with concrete examples and limitations so that predictive outputs are understood as probabilistic tools rather than certainties (Pedram & Piatkowski, 2025). Use case vignettes to demonstrate how a prediction would translate into an actionable clinical pathway, including human review and documentation requirements (Pedram & Piatkowski, 2025).

At the base of the diagram, practical applications of prediction such as diagnosis, relapse detection, and treatment personalization are highlighted to underscore how analytic outputs map to clinical decisions (Lazarou & Exarchos, 2024). These operational nodes require predefined rules that translate model outputs into clinical actions, such as outreach, escalation, or modification of therapy (Fanarioti & Karpouzis, 2025). Clinically, it is vital to specify threshold values, timelines for clinician review, and escalation pathways that align with existing safety protocols. Include performance monitoring plans that track false positives and false negatives and report them regularly to governance committees. In practice, pilot these mappings in narrowly defined workflows before scaling to broader clinical populations to ensure safety and effectiveness (Fanarioti & Karpouzis, 2025).

Together, the diagram and its narrative illustrate how AI and ML serve not just as tools, but as integral components of a responsive, data-driven mental health ecosystem (Ghadi et al., 2025). Framing AI and ML as ecosystem components helps stakeholders appreciate dependencies, data quality, interoperability, clinician engagement, and governance, that determine success or failure (Engel, 1977).

Emphasize that technological capability must be matched by clinical processes, workforce training, and ethical safeguards to realize benefit (Engel, 1977). Use the diagram to identify responsible owners for each component and to create a roadmap for phased implementation with measurable milestones. Align evaluation metrics with clinical outcomes and patient-centered measures, not solely with predictive accuracy (Engel, 1977).

Extended Reality offers immersive therapeutic environments that operationalize exposure and embodiment principles.

REFERENCES

Adepoju, D. A., & Adepoju, A. G. (2025). Establishing ethical frameworks for scalable data engineering and governance in AI-driven healthcare systems. *Int. J. Res. Publ. Rev*, *6*(4), 8710–8726. DOI: 10.55248/gengpi.6.0425.1547

Agarwal, S., Jalan, M., Hill, R., Pantalone, E., Thrul, J., Sharma, R., Wilcox, H. C., & Robinson, K. A. (2025). Framework to Assist Stakeholders in Technology Evaluation for Recovery (Freeman et al., 2017) to Mental Health and Wellness. *BMC Health Services Research*, *25*, 623. Advance online publication. DOI: 10.1186/s12913-025-12418-0 PMID: 40307807

Aiken, L. H., Lasater, K. B., Sloane, D. M., Pogue, C. A., Rosenbaum, K. E. F., & Muir, K. J.US Clinician Wellbeing Study Consortium. (2023, July). Physician and nurse well-being and preferred interventions to address burnout in hospital practice: Factors associated with turnover, outcomes, and patient safety. [). American Medical Association.]. *JAMA Health Forum*, *4*(7), e231809–e231809. DOI: 10.1001/jamahealthforum.2023.1809 PMID: 37418269

Akhtar, Z. B., & Rawol, A. T. (2024). Artificial intelligence (Tizzard, 2025) and extended reality (XR): A biomedical engineering perspective investigation analysis. *Indonesian Journal of Electronics, Electromedical Engineering, and Medical Informatics*, *6*(3). Advance online publication. DOI: 10.35882/ijeeemi.v6i3.5

Babu, A., & Joseph, A. P. (2025). Digital wellness or digital dependency? A critical examination of mental health apps and their implications. *Frontiers in Psychiatry*, *16*, 1581779. DOI: 10.3389/fpsyt.2025.1581779 PMID: 40248604

Baka, E., Tan, Y.-R., Wong, B. L. H., Xing, Z., & Yap, P. (2025). A scoping review of digital interventions for the promotion of mental health and prevention of mental health conditions for young people. *Oxford Open Digital Health*, *3*, oqaf005. DOI: 10.1093/oodh/oqaf005 PMID: 40230873

Ball, H., Eisner, E., Nicholas, J., Wilson, P., & Bucci, S. (2025). How theories, models, and frameworks have been used to implement digital health interventions in services for people with severe mental health problems: A scoping review. *BMC Public Health*, *25*(1), 1023. DOI: 10.1186/s12889-025-22189-2 PMID: 40098003

Baydili, İ., Tasci, B., & Tasci, G. (2025). Artificial intelligence in psychiatry: A review of biological and behavioral data analyses. *Diagnostics (Basel)*, *15*(4), 434. DOI: 10.3390/diagnostics15040434 PMID: 40002587

Bond, R. R., Mulvenna, M. D., Potts, C., O'Neill, S., Ennis, E., & Torous, J. (2023). Digital transformation of mental health services. *Npj Mental Health Research, 2*(1), 13. DOI: 10.1038/s44184-023-00033-y PMID: 38609479

Carl, E., Stein, A. T., Levihn-Coon, A., Pogue, J. R., Rothbaum, B., Emmelkamp, P., Asmundson, G. J. G., Carlbring, P., & Powers, M. B. (2019). Virtual reality exposure therapy for anxiety and related disorders: A meta-analysis of randomized controlled trials. *Journal of Anxiety Disorders, 61*, 27–36. DOI: 10.1016/j.janxdis.2018.08.003 PMID: 30287083

Carl, E., Stein, A. T., Levihn-Coon, A., Pogue, J. R., Rothbaum, B., Emmelkamp, P., Asmundson, G. J. G., Carlbring, P., & Powers, M. B. (2019). Virtual reality exposure therapy for anxiety and related disorders: A meta-analysis of randomized controlled trials. *Journal of Anxiety Disorders, 61*, 27–36. DOI: 10.1016/j.janxdis.2018.08.003 PMID: 30287083

Chithra, N., & Bhambri, P. (2024). Ethics in sustainable technology. In *Handbook of Technological Sustainability* (pp. 245–256). CRC Press. DOI: 10.1201/9781003475989-21

Clemens-Meyer, F. H., Lepot, M., Blumensaat, F., Leutnant, D., & Gruber, G. (2021). In Bertrand-Krajewski, J.-L., Clemens-Meyer, F., Lepot, M., & Publishing, I. W. A. (Eds.), *Data validation and data quality assessment. Metrology in Urban Drainage and Stormwater Management: Plug and Pray* (pp. 327–390).

Crameri, L., Hettiarachchi, I. T., & Hanoun, S. (2021). Effects of dynamic resilience on the reactivity of vagally mediated heart rate variability. *Frontiers in Psychology, 11*, 579210. DOI: 10.3389/fpsyg.2020.579210 PMID: 33551903

Cristofaro, M., & Giardino, P. L. (2025). Surfing the AI waves: The historical evolution of artificial intelligence in management and organizational studies and practices. *Journal of Management History*. Advance online publication. DOI: 10.1108/JMH-01-2025-0002

De Kock, J. H., Latham, H. A., Leslie, S. J., Grindle, M., Munoz, S. A., Ellis, L., Polson, R., & O'Malley, C. M. (2021). A rapid review of the impact of COVID-19 on the mental health of healthcare workers: Implications for supporting psychological well-being. *BMC Public Health, 21*(1), 104. DOI: 10.1186/s12889-020-10070-3 PMID: 33422039

Elfouly, T., & Alouani, A. (2025). A comprehensive survey on wearable computing for mental and physical health monitoring. *Electronics (Basel), 14*(17), 3443. DOI: 10.3390/electronics14173443

Engel, G. L. (1977). The need for a new medical model: A challenge for biomedicine. *Science*, *196*(4286), 129–136. DOI: 10.1126/science.847460 PMID: 847460

Fanarioti, A. K., & Karpouzis, K. (2025). Artificial Intelligence and the Future of Mental Health in a Digitally Transformed World. *Computers*, *14*(7), 259. DOI: 10.3390/computers14070259

Fleming, L. E., Maycock, B., White, M. P., & Depledge, M. H. (2019). Fostering human health through ocean sustainability in the 21st century. *People and Nature*, *1*(3), 276–283. DOI: 10.1002/pan3.10038

Friend, S. H., Ginsburg, G. S., Picard, R. W., & Drazen, J. M. (2024). Key issues as wearable digital health technologies enter clinical care. *The New England Journal of Medicine*, *390*(12), 1118–1127. DOI: 10.1056/NEJMra2307160 PMID: 38507754

Ghadi, Y. Y., Shah, S. F. A., Waheed, W., Mazhar, T., Ahmad, W., Saeed, M. M., & Hamam, H. (2025). Integration of wearable technology and artificial intelligence in digital health for remote patient care. *Journal of Cloud Computing (Heidelberg, Germany)*, *14*(1), 39. DOI: 10.1186/s13677-025-00759-4

Ghanim, R., Kaushik, A., Park, J., & Abramson, A. (2023). Communication protocols integrating wearables, ingestibles, and implantables for closed-loop therapies. *Device*, *1*(3), 100092. DOI: 10.1016/j.device.2023.100092

Gkintoni, E., Vassilopoulos, S. P., & Nikolaou, G. (2025). Next-generation cognitive-behavioral therapy for depression: Integrating digital tools, teletherapy, and personalization for enhanced mental health outcomes. *Medicina (Kaunas, Lithuania)*, *61*(3), 431. DOI: 10.3390/medicina61030431 PMID: 40142242

Hall, C. L., Gómez Bergin, A. D., & Rennick-Egglestone, S. (2024). Research into digital health intervention for mental health: 25-year retrospective on the ethical and legal challenges. *Journal of Medical Internet Research*, *26*, e58939. DOI: 10.2196/58939 PMID: 39250796

Hickey, B. A., Chalmers, T., Newton, P., Lin, C.-T., Sibbritt, D., McLachlan, C. S., Clifton-Bligh, R., Morley, J., & Lal, S. (2021). Smart devices and wearable technologies to detect and monitor mental health conditions and stress: A systematic review. *Sensors (Basel)*, *21*(10), 3461. DOI: 10.3390/s21103461 PMID: 34065620

Hiland, E. B. (2021). *Therapy tech: The digital transformation of mental healthcare*. U of Minnesota Press. DOI: 10.5749/j.ctv1xp9q3t

Huang, J., Wang, H., Wu, Q., Yin, J., Zhou, H., & He, Y. (2024). Clinical research on neurological and psychiatric diagnosis and monitoring using wearable devices: A literature review. *Interdisciplinary Medicine*, *2*(4), e20230037. DOI: 10.1002/INMD.20230037

Ienca, M., Fabrice, J., Elger, B., Caon, M., Scoccia Pappagallo, A., Kressig, R. W., & Wangmo, T. (2017). Intelligent assistive technology for Alzheimer's disease and other dementias: A systematic review. *Journal of Alzheimer's Disease*, *56*(4), 1301–1340. DOI: 10.3233/JAD-161037 PMID: 28222516

Immanuel, S., Teferra, M. N., Baumert, M., & Bidargaddi, N. (2023). Heart rate variability for evaluating psychological stress changes in healthy adults: A scoping review. *Neuropsychobiology*, *82*(4), 187–202. DOI: 10.1159/000530376 PMID: 37290411

Inkster, B., Knibbs, C., & Bada, M. (2023). Cybersecurity: A critical priority for digital mental health. *Frontiers in Digital Health*, *5*, 1242264. DOI: 10.3389/fdgth.2023.1242264 PMID: 37781452

Islam, R., & Bae, S. W. (2024). Revolutionizing mental health support: An innovative affective mobile framework for dynamic, proactive, and context-adaptive conversational agents. arXiv preprint arXiv:2406.15942.

Iwaya, L. H., Babar, M. A., Rashid, A., & Wijayarathna, C. (2023). On the privacy of mental health apps: An empirical investigation and its implications for app development. *Empirical Software Engineering*, *28*(1), 2. DOI: 10.1007/s10664-022-10236-0 PMID: 36407814

Kargarandehkordi, A., Li, S., Lin, K., Phillips, K. T., Benzo, R. M., & Washington, P. (2025). Fusing wearable biosensors with artificial intelligence for mental health monitoring: A systematic review. *Biosensors (Basel)*, *15*(4), 202. DOI: 10.3390/bios15040202 PMID: 40277515

Khoo, Y. X., Kang, R. M., Reynolds, T. L., & Mentis, H. M. (2024). The comprehensiveness of mental health application users' privacy and security concerns. *CHI Conference on Human Factors in Computing Systems*, 16 pages.

Kim, J., & Backonja, U. (2025). Digital health equity frameworks and key concepts: A scoping review. *Journal of the American Medical Informatics Association : JAMIA*, *32*(1), 45–59. DOI: 10.1093/jamia/ocaf017 PMID: 39936843

Kumar, P. (2025). Securing Digital-First Healthcare: AI, Blockchain, and Cloud Architectures for Personal Health Data Protection. *International Journal of Applied Mathematics*, *38*(7s).

Lamb, R., Choi, I., & Owens, T (2025). Convergence of Extended Reality, Artificial Intelligence, Machine Leaning, and Wearable Sensors in the Field of Education. Mental Health Virtual Reality: The Power of Immersive Worlds, 113-128.

Lay, W., Gasparini, L., Siero, W., & Hughes, E. K. (2025). A rapid review of the benefits and challenges of dynamic consent. *Research Ethics*, *21*(1), 180–202. DOI: 10.1177/17470161241278064

Lazarou, E., & Exarchos, T. P. (2024). Predicting stress levels using physiological data: Real-time stress prediction models utilizing wearable devices. *AIMS Neuroscience*, *11*(2), 76–102. DOI: 10.3934/Neuroscience.2024006 PMID: 38988886

Li, M., Patel, J., & Katapally, T. R. (2025). The impact of extended reality cognitive behavioral therapy on mental disorders among children and youth: A systematic review and meta-analysis protocol. *PLoS One*, *20*(3), e0315313. DOI: 10.1371/journal.pone.0315313 PMID: 40048453

Lindner, P., Miloff, A., & Carlbring, P. (2024). The future of virtual reality therapy: Applications, challenges, and research directions. *Frontiers in Virtual Reality*, *5*, 112345.

Liu, M., & Schueller, S. M. (2023). Moving evidence-based mental health interventions into practice: Implementation of digital mental health interventions. *Current Treatment Options in Psychiatry*, *10*(4), 333–345. DOI: 10.1007/s40501-023-00298-2

Livieri, G., Mangina, E., Protopapadakis, E. D., & Panayiotou, A. G. (2025). The gaps and challenges in digital health technology use as perceived by patients: A scoping review and narrative meta-synthesis. *Frontiers in Digital Health*, *7*, 1474956. DOI: 10.3389/fdgth.2025.1474956 PMID: 40212901

Lorke, M., & Stefanou, T. (2025). Improving research and development of wearable assistive and rehabilitation technologies: A systematic review on diversity factors. *Journal of Neuroengineering and Rehabilitation*, *22*(1), 31. DOI: 10.1186/s12984-025-01562-7 PMID: 39985039

Mackey, S., Aghaeepour, N., Gaudilliere, B., Kao, M.-C., Kaptan, M., Lannon, E., Pfyffer, D., & Weber, K. (2025). Innovations in acute and chronic pain biomarkers: Enhancing diagnosis and personalized therapy. *Regional Anesthesia and Pain Medicine*, *50*(2), 110–120. DOI: 10.1136/rapm-2024-106030 PMID: 39909549

Mahon, D. (2023). Empirically Supported Treatments: A Brief History. In Evidence Based Counselling & Psychotherapy for the 21st Century Practitioner (pp. 3-14). Emerald Publishing Limited. DOI: 10.1108/978-1-80455-732-720231001

Martinez-Martin, N., Marcandalli, J., Huang, C. S., Arthur, C. P., Perotti, M., Foglierini, M., Ho, H., Dosey, A. M., Shriver, S., Payandeh, J., Leitner, A., Lanzavecchia, A., Perez, L., & Ciferri, C. (2018). An unbiased screen for human cytomegalovirus identifies neuropilin-2 as a central viral receptor. *Cell, 174*(5), 1158–1171. DOI: 10.1016/j.cell.2018.06.028 PMID: 30057110

Mitsea, E., Drigas, A., & Skianis, C. (2024). Artificial intelligence, immersive technologies, and neurotechnologies in breathing interventions for mental and emotional health: A systematic review. *Electronics (Basel), 13*(12), 2253. DOI: 10.3390/electronics13122253

Mohr, D. C., Zhang, M., & Schueller, S. M. (2017). Personal sensing: Understanding mental health using ubiquitous sensors and machine learning. *Annual Review of Clinical Psychology, 13*(1), 23–47. DOI: 10.1146/annurev-clinpsy-032816-044949 PMID: 28375728

Mone, V., & Fayazullaeva, S. (2023). Health data on the go: Navigating privacy concerns with wearable technologies. *Legal Information Management, 23*(3), 179–188. DOI: 10.1017/S1472669623000427

Moriarty, A. S., Meader, N., Snell, K. I., Riley, R. D., Paton, L. W., Dawson, S., Hendon, J., Chew-Graham, C. A., Gilbody, S., Churchill, R., Phillips, R. S., Ali, S., & McMillan, D. (2022). Predicting relapse or recurrence of depression: Systematic review of prognostic models. *The British Journal of Psychiatry : The Journal of Mental Science, 221*(2), 448–458. DOI: 10.1192/bjp.2021.218 PMID: 35048843

Mulukuntla, S. (2025). Monitoring and Remote Patient Management with Immersive Technologies. In Augmented Wellness: Exploring the Power of VR and AR in Healthcare (pp. 197-218). Springer. DOI: 10.1007/978-981-96-2952-7_9

Obermeyer, Z., Powers, B., Vogeli, C., & Mullainathan, S. (2019). Dissecting racial bias in an algorithm used to manage the health of populations. *Science, 366*(6464), 447–453. DOI: 10.1126/science.aax2342 PMID: 31649194

Okposio, B. O., Richard, G. A., Olatokun, T. P., Akadiri, O. O., Akpevba, E. A., John, J. O., & Okonkwo, B. A. (2025). Enhancing Mental health Outcomes through AI-Driven Predictive Analytics: A review of applications in neuroscience and substance abuse prevention. *International Journal of Biological and Pharmaceutical Sciences Archive, 10*(2), 024-048.

Ong, T., Ivanova, J., Soni, H., Barrera, J., Cummins, M., Welch, B. M., & Bunnell, B. E. (2025). Mental health clients' perspectives on telehealth-based virtual reality therapy. *Frontiers in Virtual Reality, 6*, 1595326. DOI: 10.3389/frvir.2025.1595326

Pedram, S., & Piatkowski, T. (2025). Exploring the potential of virtual reality (Johnson et al., 2021) in mental healthcare: A systematic literature review. *Virtual Reality (Waltham Cross)*, *29*(3), 135. DOI: 10.1007/s10055-025-01181-6

Poudel, U., Jakhar, S., Mohan, P., & Nepal, A. (2025). AI in mental health: A review of technological advancements and ethical issues in psychiatry. *Issues in Mental Health Nursing*, *46*(7), 693–701. DOI: 10.1080/01612840.2025.2502943 PMID: 40378075

Pruden, S (2025). Implementing Depression Screening and Treatment Algorithms to Reduce Post-Operative Complications for Patients Undergoing Cardiac Surgery The University of North Carolina at Chapel Hill].

Radanliev, P. (2025). Privacy, ethics, transparency, and accountability in AI systems for wearable devices. *Frontiers in Digital Health*, *7*, 1431246. DOI: 10.3389/fdgth.2025.1431246 PMID: 40599875

Rajpal, S. (2025). Exploring the Role of Virtual Reality and Metaverse in Treating Mental Health: Operating Models and Challenges in Adoption. *Journal of Computer and Communications*, *13*(10), 1–22. DOI: 10.4236/jcc.2025.1310001

Reddy, K. J. (2025). Integrating Technology into Clinical Practice. In Innovations in Neurocognitive Rehabilitation: Harnessing Technology for Effective Therapy (pp. 329-350). Springer. DOI: 10.1007/978-3-031-88117-6_15

Robinson, A., Flom, M., Forman-Hoffman, V. L., Histon, T., Levy, M., Darcy, A., Ajayi, T., Mohr, D. C., Wicks, P., Greene, C., & Montgomery, R. M. (2024). Equity in digital mental health interventions in the United States: Where to next? *Journal of Medical Internet Research*, *26*, e59939. DOI: 10.2196/59939 PMID: 39316436

Saganowski, S., Perz, B., Polak, A. G., & Kazienko, P (2022). Emotion recognition for everyday life using physiological signals from wearables: A systematic literature review. IEEE Transactions on Affective Computing, 14(3), 1876-1897. Pinel, P (1793). Traité médico-philosophique sur l'aliénation mentale.

Shah, R. V., Grennan, G., Zafar-Khan, M., Alim, F., Dey, S., Ramanathan, D., & Mishra, J. (2021). Personalized machine learning of depressed mood using wearables. *Translational Psychiatry*, *11*(1), 338. DOI: 10.1038/s41398-021-01445-0 PMID: 34103481

Sharma, R., & Meena, H. K. (2024). Emerging trends in EEG signal processing: A systematic review. *SN Computer Science*, *5*(4), 415. DOI: 10.1007/s42979-024-02773-w

Shatte, A. B., Hutchinson, D. M., & Teague, S. J. (2019). Machine learning in mental health: A scoping review of methods and applications. *Psychological Medicine, 49*(9), 1426–1448. DOI: 10.1017/S0033291719000151 PMID: 30744717

Smith, K. A., Blease, C., Faurholt-Jepsen, M., Firth, J., Van Daele, T., Moreno, C., Carlbring, P., Ebner-Priemer, U. W., Koutsouleris, N., Riper, H., Mouchabac, S., Torous, J., & Cipriani, A. (2023). Digital mental health: Challenges and next steps. *BMJ Mental Health, 26*(1), e300670. DOI: 10.1136/bmjment-2023-300670 PMID: 37197797

Spytska, L. (2025). The use of artificial intelligence in psychotherapy: Development of intelligent therapeutic systems. *BMC Psychology, 13*(1), 175. DOI: 10.1186/s40359-025-02491-9 PMID: 40022267

Subu, M. A., Holmes, D., Arumugam, A., Al-Yateem, N., Maria Dias, J., Rahman, S. A., Waluyo, I., Ahmed, F. R., & Abraham, M. S. (2022). Traditional, religious, and cultural perspectives on mental illness: A qualitative study on causal beliefs and treatment use. *International Journal of Qualitative Studies on Health and Well-being, 17*(1), 2123090. DOI: 10.1080/17482631.2022.2123090 PMID: 36097886

Sun, J., Lu, T., Shao, X., Han, Y., Xia, Y., Zheng, Y., Wang, Y., Li, X., Ravindran, A., Fan, L., Fang, Y., Zhang, X., Ravindran, N., Wang, Y., Liu, X., & Lu, L. (2025). Practical AI application in psychiatry: Historical review and future directions. *Molecular Psychiatry, 30*(9), 4399–4408. DOI: 10.1038/s41380-025-03072-3 PMID: 40456953

Tavory, T. (2024). Regulating AI in mental health: Ethics of care perspective. *JMIR Mental Health, 11*, e58493. DOI: 10.2196/58493 PMID: 39298759

Tizzard, C. L. (2025). Re-imagining Care for Aging Disabled Adults.

Tsai, Y. Y., Chen, Y. J., Lin, Y. F., Hsiao, F. C., Hsu, C. H., & Liao, L. D. (2025). Photoplethysmography-based HRV analysis and machine learning for real-time stress quantification in mental health applications. *APL Bioengineering, 9*(2), 026103. DOI: 10.1063/5.0256590 PMID: 40191605

Walter, J. R., Xu, S., & Rogers, J. A. (2023). From lab to life: How wearable devices can improve health equity. *Nature Communications, 14*, 44634. PMID: 38167483

Watson, D (2025). The dark side of mental health apps: Privacy concerns and therapeutic limitations. MentalHealthSigns.com.

Weiner, E. B., Dankwa-Mullan, I., Nelson, W. A., & Hassanpour, S. (2025). Ethical challenges and evolving strategies in the integration of artificial intelligence into clinical practice. *PLOS Digital Health*, *4*(4), e0000810. DOI: 10.1371/journal.pdig.0000810 PMID: 40198594

Xing, Y., Yang, Y., Yang, K., Lu, A., Xing, L., Mackie, K., & Guo, F. (2025). Intelligent sensing devices and systems for personalized mental health. *Med-X*, *3*(1), 10. DOI: 10.1007/s44258-025-00057-3 PMID: 40837134

Chapter 5
Extended Reality as a Clinical Instrument

ABSTRACT

Extended Reality (Ikwuanusi et al., 2023) including VR, AR, and MR has transitioned from novelty to a clinically relevant tool for mental health care (Freeman et al., 2017). XR enables immersive, controllable environments that replicate real-world stressors or create safe spaces for graded exposure, skills training, and perspective-shifting interventions (Freeman et al., 2017). Its therapeutic value lies in mechanisms like emotional engagement, presence, and adaptive feedback loops, allowing clinicians to titrate challenge and integrate biometric data for precision dosing (Freeman et al., 2017). Applications span phobia treatment, PTSD processing, and body-image recalibration. Ethical deployment demands informed consent, cultural adaptation, and robust safety protocols. XR should augment—not replace—human judgment, preserving therapeutic alliance while expanding experiential learning opportunities (Freeman et al., 2017).

INTRODUCTION

This chapter explores extended reality (XR), including virtual, augmented, and mixed reality, as a clinically grounded modality rather than a technological novelty. It examines XR's capacity to operationalize evidence-based mechanisms such as exposure, skills rehearsal, embodiment, and experiential learning with precision and control. The chapter details how XR can enhance treatments for anxiety disorders, PTSD, addiction, and body image disturbance by enabling graded, repeatable, and customizable therapeutic environments. It emphasizes clinician control, patient readiness, and physiological monitoring as essential elements of safe implementation. Ethical considerations, including cybersickness, dissociation risk, informed consent, and data governance, are addressed alongside accessibility and cultural

DOI: 10.4018/979-8-3373-4997-8.ch005

adaptation. The chapter also discusses operational requirements, training, infrastructure, workflow integration, and documentation, to ensure XR is used responsibly in routine care. Through clinical vignettes, it illustrates how immersive experiences can complement cognitive and behavioral interventions without displacing therapeutic relationships. Ultimately, the chapter positions XR as a powerful adjunct that expands the therapeutic toolkit when deployed with clinical rigor, ethical oversight, and sensitivity to individual differences.

EXTENDED REALITY

Extended Reality (XR), encompassing Virtual Reality (VR), Augmented Reality (AR), and Mixed Reality (MR), has evolved from a technological novelty into a clinically relevant modality for mental health care (Godfrey et al., 2021). These immersive technologies enable clinicians to construct controlled environments that replicate real-world stressors, simulate therapeutic challenges, or create novel contexts for skill acquisition and recovery. In practical terms, XR offers therapists a repertoire of customizable, repeatable scenarios that can be titrated to match a patient's goals, tolerance, and stage of treatment (Obermeyer et al., 2019). This capacity for precision and adaptability positions XR as a transformative tool in evidence-based practice (Obermeyer et al., 2019; Li et al., 2025).

FROM CONCEPT TO CLINICAL UTILITY

At its core, XR operates by altering sensory inputs to reshape attention, affect, and action tendencies (Layode et al., 2024). VR immerses patients in fully simulated environments, occluding sensory access to the physical clinical space (Shatte et al., 2019). AR overlays digital elements onto real-world settings, while MR blends virtual and physical objects to enable interactive engagement. These modalities differ in their degree of immersion and clinician control, making modality selection a clinical decision rather than a technological preference (Shatte et al., 2019). VR is optimal when full stimulus control and graded exposure are required; AR excels when interventions must occur in naturalistic contexts; MR offers hybrid flexibility for tasks that demand interaction between virtual and physical elements. The therapeutic value of XR rests on mechanisms familiar to clinicians: emotional engagement, graded exposure, repeated practice, and contextualized learning (Shatte et al., 2019). Central to these mechanisms is the construct of presence, the subjective sense of "being there." High presence ensures that simulated stimuli evoke authentic emotional and physiological responses, enabling corrective learning under controlled conditions. In this sense, XR functions as an exposure medium that brings the essential processes of fear extinction, cognitive restructuring, and behavioral rehearsal into the clinic without the logistical burdens of in vivo arrangements (Shatte et al., 2019).

Figure 1. Workflow interaction for clinical training and patient assessment using XR

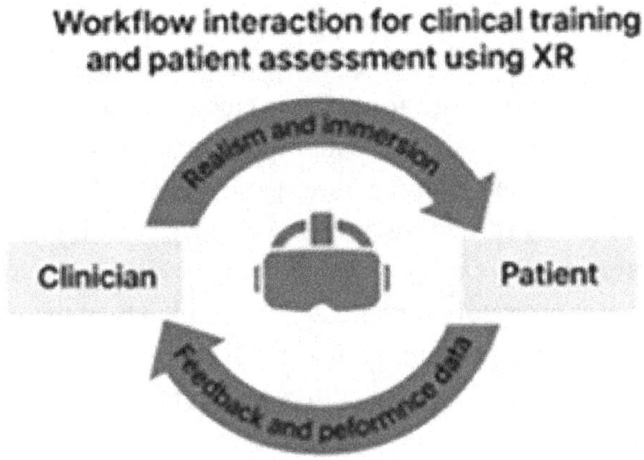

ADAPTIVE SYSTEMS AND NEUROCOGNITIVE INTEGRATION

Experts such as Thomas Insel, Albert Rizzo, Rosalind Picard, and Richard Lamb, have advanced concepts like wearable sensors, cognitive-systems perspective. While exposure-based interventions remain the anchor application for XR, its utility extends well beyond classical fear learning (Basystiuk et al., 2024). In anxiety disorders and specific phobias, XR reliably reproduces feared contexts, airplanes, heights, crowded auditoria, enabling graded, repeatable exposures without logistical constraints (Weiner et al., 2025). For post-traumatic stress disorder (PTSD), XR supports structured revisiting of trauma-related cues under conditions that optimize emotional processing and minimize risk (Weiner et al., 2025). In addiction treatment, XR can recreate cue-laden environments that elicit craving, providing opportunities for refusal-skill rehearsal and coping strategy deployment (Weiner et al., 2025).

Clinical vignette: A 34-year-old woman with severe fear of flying has avoided career opportunities requiring travel (Smuck et al., 2021). In XR-facilitated exposure therapy, her clinician employs a VR flight simulation that sequences boarding, taxiing, takeoff, turbulence, and landing (Engel, 1977). Initial sessions focus on low-intensity scenarios, paired with paced breathing and cognitive reappraisal. As the patient demonstrates mastery, turbulence and auditory cues are introduced. Over eight sessions, she reports reduced anticipatory anxiety and successfully completes a short real-world flight, attributing her progress to the immersive practice afforded by VR.

Beyond exposure, XR enables embodiment and perspective-shifting interventions that recalibrate self-perception and interpersonal cognition (Baumann et al., 2024). Patients can inhabit avatars with altered body dimensions, ages, or social roles, creating experiential opportunities for body-image recalibration, empathy training, and prosocial behavior rehearsal. These manipulations are not superficial; they produce measurable shifts in self-representation and social inference, complementing cognitive interventions by providing corrective sensory evidence (Li et al., 2025).

Clinical vignette: A 19-year-old college student with body-image disturbance engages in a VR avatar protocol (Ferrara, 2024). Guided by the therapist, the patient alternates between avatars representing distorted self-perceptions and more realistic body forms. Real-time reflection and cognitive restructuring follow each embodiment exercise. Over repeated sessions, the patient reports diminished preoccupation with appearance and increased willingness to engage in social activities, illustrating how XR can operationalize cognitive-behavioral principles through experiential learning (Pedram & Piatkowski, 2025).

ETHICAL, CULTURAL, AND PRACTICAL CONSIDERATIONS

The integration of XR into mental health care introduces complex ethical and operational challenges (Back et al., 2022). Informed consent must extend beyond standard disclosures to encompass immersive risks (e.g., cybersickness, dissociation), biometric data collection, and algorithmic adaptivity. Consent should be dynamic, revisitable, and supported by plain-language explanations and visual aids. Privacy protections must include encryption, role-based access controls, and retention limits for biometric and behavioral data. Governance frameworks should mandate transparency regarding data flows and algorithmic logic, with independent audits to verify compliance. Cultural adaptation is essential. Scenario libraries must reflect diverse identities, languages, and social norms to avoid inadvertent stereotyping or exclusion. Accessibility features, closed captioning, adjustable sensory intensity, simplified interaction modes, should be standard, ensuring usability for individuals with disabilities or limited technological literacy. Equity audits should accompany pilot deployments, and procurement policies must prioritize affordability and interoperability to prevent technological redlining.

IMPLEMENTATION SCIENCE AND WORKFORCE DEVELOPMENT

Successful XR adoption requires deliberate planning across infrastructure, training, and evaluation domains (Hilty et al., 2021). Clinicians must acquire competencies in both technical operation and therapeutic integration, including scenario selection, pacing, risk management, and post-session debriefing. Competency-based training should combine didactic modules with supervised practice and fidelity monitoring. Supervision frameworks must address both clinical and technical dimensions, ensuring that novelty does not erode therapeutic rigor. Operational protocols should standardize safety procedures: pre-session screening for vestibular disorders or dissociation risk, calibration of devices and sensors, patient-led stop signals, and structured debriefs. Emergency pathways for adverse reactions, panic, cybersickness, derealization, must be rehearsed and documented. Session notes should capture scenario parameters, biometric markers, and integration tasks, aligning with measurement-based care principles (Obermeyer et al., 2019). Evaluation frameworks should pair clinical outcomes (symptom reduction, functional gains) with implementation metrics (session completion rates, adverse event frequency, device uptime; Obermeyer et al., 2019). Pragmatic trials and registry-based studies can accelerate evidence generation while informing iterative refinement (Obermeyer et al., 2019). Cost analyses must account for hardware, software, training, and maintenance, guiding sustainable business models that preserve clinical integrity.

FUTURE DIRECTIONS: TOWARD MULTIMODAL, NEUROADAPTIVE ECOSYSTEMS

XR's trajectory points toward deeper integration with AI and wearable sensors, enabling multimodal systems that deliver real-time, context-sensitive interventions (Almadani et al., 2025). Imagine a VR exposure session where HRV and EEG signals inform adaptive scenario adjustments, while a mobile app provides ecological momentary assessments to reinforce learning between sessions (Rajpal, 2025). These neuroadaptive ecosystems exemplify the shift from episodic, reactive care to continuous, personalized intervention, a vision that demands technical rigor, ethical clarity, and human-centered design (Rajpal, 2025).

EXTENDED REALITY: A CLINICAL INSTRUMENT, NOT A PANACEA

Extended Reality (Akinode et al., 2025) is not a panacea, nor a substitute for the relational core of therapy (Wang et al., 2022). It is best understood as a powerful adjunct a clinical instrument that amplifies evidence-based principles through immersive, adaptive experiences (Ienca et al., 2017). When implemented thoughtfully, XR can broaden access, deepen engagement, and accelerate therapeutic progress. Yet its promise will only be realized if technological innovation is matched by ethical governance, cultural humility, and rigorous evaluation. For clinicians, the directive is clear: adopt XR as a carefully governed extension of therapeutic competence, integrate it within coherent treatment plans, and commit to studying outcomes so that practice evolves responsibly (Ienca et al., 2017). Technology should change what therapists can do not why they do it: to help patients live more fully in the worlds they value.

CLINICAL APPLICATIONS AND ILLUSTRATIVE VIGNETTES

XR's clinical utility extends beyond novelty; it operationalizes core mechanisms of change such as graded exposure, cognitive restructuring, and experiential learning (Volckens et al., 2023). Consider the following vignette:

Clinical Vignette 2 A 19-year-old college student with severe body image disturbance engages in a guided VR avatar exercise (Holly et al., 2023). With consent and careful preparation, the therapist introduces avatars representing the patient's current perceived body, a more realistic representation, and a third avatar programmed to move and speak with confident posture. After each short embodiment exercise, the therapist facilitates real-time reflection and cognitive restructuring. The patient reports noticing differences in movement and perceived social responses within the simulation, enabling targeted cognitive work on self-evaluation and social expectations. Over repeated sessions, intrusive preoccupations diminish, and the patient demonstrates increased willingness to attend social events. This vignette illustrates XR's capacity to create corrective sensory-perceptual experiences that complement cognitive interventions (Li et al., 2025). By enabling patients to inhabit alternative representations of self, XR provides tangible evidence that challenges maladaptive beliefs, an effect difficult to achieve through verbal therapy alone (Li et al., 2025).

INTEGRATING BIOMETRIC SENSING AND AI FOR PERSONALIZATION

The integration of biometric sensing and machine learning into XR platforms enhances personalization and supports data-informed decision-making (Goktas & Grzybowski, 2025). Physiological inputs, such as heart rate variability (HRV), skin conductance, respiration, and eye-tracking, offer real-time indicators of arousal, attentional focus, and stress recovery (Ong et al., 2025). AI models can detect patterns within these multimodal signals and propose adjustments to scenario intensity, timing of coaching prompts, or the introduction of supportive cues (Ong et al., 2025). Importantly, the clinician remains central. AI and biometrics are tools to refine dosing and generate objective markers of engagement and progress, not replacements for clinical judgment (Ong et al., 2025). Use biometric-informed XR adjustments to supplement, not supplant, therapist-led decisions (Ong et al., 2025). This principle preserves therapeutic integrity while leveraging technology for precision.

RISKS, LIMITATIONS, AND ETHICAL CONSIDERATIONS

While enthusiasm for XR is warranted, clinicians must remain attentive to its limitations and risks (Wibberly, 2024). Practical barriers include hardware cost, content development resources, secure data management, and the need for specialized clinician training (Ricciardi & Zomaya, 2025). Patient-centered challenges encompass cybersickness, dissociative reactions in vulnerable individuals, and variability in technological literacy. Ethical concerns are equally significant. Informed consent must address immersive experiences and biometric data collection, specifying how data will be stored, who will access it, and for what purposes. Clinicians must safeguard personally identifiable information and maintain clear protocols for terminating sessions if adverse responses occur.

Clinical Vignette 3 A 50-year-old veteran with hyperarousal and dissociative tendencies is referred for VR-assisted PTSD treatment (Bayor et al., 2025). During the initial VR exposure, the patient experiences derealization and reports feeling detached from the session. The therapist pauses the simulation, conducts grounding exercises, reduces sensory intensity, and re-establishes safety. Subsequent sessions involve co-creating a tailored exposure plan emphasizing short durations, slower pacing, and frequent reorientation to the present. This case underscores the importance of pre-session risk assessment, in-session monitoring, and flexible adaptation when immersive exposure provokes dissociation.

OPERATIONAL REQUIREMENTS FOR CLINICAL INTEGRATION

Successful implementation of XR in clinical settings requires attention to space, workflow, and staff competencies (Sheikh et al., 2021). Clinically suitable environments should include unobstructed movement areas, adjustable lighting, comfortable seating for post-session debriefs, and secure storage for devices. Workflow adaptations must incorporate pre-session technical checks, structured patient orientation, integration of XR session notes into health records, and scheduled time for device sanitation and maintenance. Staff competencies must encompass both technical operation and therapeutic integration. Clinicians should be trained to blend clinical formulation with scenario selection, dosing, and real-time decisions about when to intensify or reduce challenge. Treat the XR setup as a therapeutic instrument that must be maintained, calibrated, and wielded by trained clinicians under clear safety and privacy protocols (Radanliev, 2025).

Operational Vignette 4 A community mental health clinic establishes an XR suite with one dedicated room, two trained clinicians, and a protocol for intake assessment that screens patients for vestibular disorders, severe dissociation, or uncontrolled seizures (Shah et al., 2021). The facility adopts a pre-session checklist verifying informed consent, calibrating physiological sensors, and scheduling a 15-minute post-exposure debrief for cognitive processing. Device maintenance and software updates are delegated to a designated technician, and anonymized biometric logs are stored on encrypted drives with patient access controls (Kargarandehkordi et al., 2025). This implementation minimizes downtime, clarifies roles, and preserves therapeutic integrity.

Designing XR content and selecting vendors requires rigorous appraisal of clinical validity, usability, and inclusivity (Kumar et al., 2024). Effective therapeutic content should align with established clinical frameworks (e.g., CBT, ERP), provide graded levels of challenge, and permit clinician control over salient parameters (Robinson et al., 2024). Usability features should include intuitive clinician dashboards, patient-facing orientation modules, and options to adapt sensory features, such as sound and visual complexity, to individual tolerance. Equally critical is cultural and contextual relevance. Scenarios must avoid one-size-fits-all representations and should be configurable to reflect cultural norms, language, and diversity in bodies and social roles. Clinicians should favor platforms that document development processes, safety features, and available outcome data, while maintaining healthy skepticism toward marketing claims (Robinson et al., 2024). Choose XR content that is clinically aligned, adjustable, and culturally sensitive (Robinson et al., 2024).

DATA GOVERNANCE AND ETHICAL STEWARDSHIP

Data governance and ethical stewardship are non-negotiable aspects of XR adoption (Akhtar & Rawol, 2025). Providers must establish transparent consent procedures specifying which biometric or behavioral data will be collected, how it will be stored, who may access it, and for what clinical or research purposes it may be used. Security practices should include encryption, role-based access control, retention limits, and clear protocols for breach response. When research is involved, institutional review and patient protections must separate clinical care from investigational data flows. Ethically, therapists should remain mindful of the power dynamics inherent in immersive interventions and ensure patients retain autonomy over timing, content, and withdrawal from sessions. Treat XR data like any other health record, protect it, limit access, and explain its use clearly to patients.

RESPONSIBLE INNOVATION FOR LASTING IMPACT

XR offers clinicians a powerful extension of therapeutic capability, enabling immersive, adaptive experiences that operationalize evidence-based principles (Renuka et al., 2025). Yet its integration into mental health care must be deliberate, ethically grounded, and clinically coherent. The promise of XR lies not in replacing human connection but in amplifying it, creating opportunities for experiential learning that traditional modalities cannot easily provide (Kim & Backonja, 2025). For clinicians, the mandate is clear: adopt XR as a governed adjunct, embed it within comprehensive treatment plans, and evaluate outcomes rigorously (Kim & Backonja, 2025). Technology should transform what therapists can do, not why they do it: to help patients live more fully in the worlds they value.

Research priorities for the field include rigorous trials that compare XR modalities against active, evidence-based comparators; longitudinal studies that assess durability and generalization of gains; dismantling studies that identify which XR features (immersion, feedback, embodiment) drive outcomes; and implementation science work that addresses real-world barriers to adoption (Saksena et al., 2021). Equally important are pragmatic studies that measure cost-effectiveness, clinician training models, and equity of access. From a clinical perspective: prioritize evidence-based adoption, document outcomes locally, and be prepared to iterate your protocols based on both patient feedback and emerging evidence (Engel, 1977).

Finally, the therapeutic promise of XR will be realized only when technological innovation remains tethered to human-centered clinical principles (Mohammad, 2021). XR should expand clinicians' capacity to deliver safe, measurable, and experiential interventions without displacing the relational core of therapy. That means using XR to create occasions for learning and corrective experience, then returning to therapist-guided integration through reflection, cognitive restructuring, and behavioral assignment (Obermeyer et al., 2019). In short clinical terms: use XR to produce experiences that the patient cannot easily access otherwise, then use traditional psychotherapy tools to make sense of those experiences and consolidate learning (Obermeyer et al., 2019).

Taken together, these considerations outline a practical, ethically attuned, and clinically grounded roadmap for integrating XR into mental health care (Kang & Exworthy, 2022). XR is not a panacea, but when implemented thoughtfully, by trained clinicians operating within robust safety, data, and ethical frameworks, it offers powerful new ways to bring therapy into the lived contexts where symptoms occur and recovery unfolds.

Successful long-term integration of XR in clinical practice depends on workforce development that pairs technical fluency with clinical expertise (Freeman et al., 2017). Clinicians require structured training that covers hardware setup, software navigation, scenario selection, and troubleshooting, but equally important is training in clinical integration: formulation-driven scenario construction, titration of stimulus intensity, recognition of adverse responses (for example, cybersickness or dissociation), and strategies for post-exposure consolidation (Freeman et al., 2017). Training programs should combine didactic modules, supervised practice with standardized patients or role-play, and competency assessments that evaluate both technical skills and therapeutic judgment. A plain clinical summary: clinicians should be certified in XR use only after demonstrating both device competence and the ability to integrate XR sessions into a coherent treatment plan (Freeman et al., 2017).

Supervision and ongoing professional development are critical to maintaining fidelity and safety. Supervisors must be able to review recorded sessions (with consent), provide feedback on clinical decision-making during XR exposures, and model adaptive responses to unexpected patient reactions (Zenker et al., 2022). Regular case review meetings and interdisciplinary collaboration with engineers or designers can surface latent safety issues, improve scenario design, and promote iterative refinement of protocols. In practical language: create a supervision loop that holds both clinical and technical aspects of XR work to account (Martinez-Martin et al., 2018).

Clinician competencies for XR-assisted therapy can be organized around three domains: clinical formulation, technological operation, and ethical-data stewardship (Panarese et al., 2025). Clinical formulation includes assessment of target problems, determination of XR suitability, development of exposure hierarchies or rehearsal plans, and integration of XR outcomes into broader treatment goals. Technological operation covers device calibration, sensor integration, scenario control, and troubleshooting common technical problems. Ethical-data stewardship encompasses informed consent for immersive and biometric data, secure storage practices, transparency about secondary uses of data (for training, quality improvement, or research), and protocols for responding to breaches or patient requests for data deletion. A brief clinical translation: competence means knowing when XR should be used, how to use it safely, and how to protect patient rights and data (Ienca et al., 2017).

Practical safety protocols should be standardized and rehearsed. Pre-session screening should document history of motion sickness, epilepsy, severe dissociation, vestibular disorders, severe cardiovascular disease, or other conditions that may raise risks during immersion (Morey et al., 2025). A session checklist should be used before every exposure and should include device sanitation, sensor calibration, baseline physiological recording, a clear statement of session goals, a patient-led stop-signal, and a debrief timeline (Fleming et al., 2019). Emergency procedures must be defined, for example, criteria for immediate session termination, guidelines for managing a panic reaction, and steps for medical referral if needed. Clinicians should also plan for the ordinary but consequential details: seating for removal of HMDs, quick access to water, and comfortable post-session time for integration and paperwork. In concise clinical terms: treat XR sessions like any high-risk clinical procedure and create checklists to minimize preventable harms (Fleming et al., 2019).

Informed consent for XR requires explicit discussion of unique risks and benefits (Fleming et al., 2019). Patients should be told about the immersive nature of the technology, the potential for strong emotional and physiological responses, the types of biometric data to be collected, how data will be stored and who will access it, and the circumstances under which session recordings or data might be shared for supervision or research. Consent processes should include opportunities for demonstration (for example, a brief orientation session) so patients can make an informed choice after experiencing the basic sensation of immersion. A clear clinical translation: ensure patients understand both the experiential and the data implications of XR before beginning therapy.

Ethical complexity increases when XR systems incorporate adaptive algorithms or machine learning (Allgaier et al., 2023). When algorithms alter exposure parameters or present therapeutic suggestions, clinicians must retain clear decision-making authority and be able to explain algorithmic behavior in clinically meaningful terms. Patients should be informed about the role of automated adjustments and their right to override or decline algorithmic interventions. Transparency about algorithmic limits, such as when a model may misclassify arousal signals or generate inappropriate scenario changes, is a matter of ethical practice (Rajpal, 2025). Put simply: automation can assist clinicians but must never obscure clinical responsibility or patient choice (Rajpal, 2025).

Equity, access, and cultural competence present nontrivial challenges and opportunities. To avoid reproducing disparities, clinics and technology partners must prioritize affordable hardware options, low-bandwidth software alternatives, and culturally tailored scenario libraries. Content development teams should include diverse stakeholders, patients, clinicians from different cultural backgrounds, and community representatives, to identify culturally salient cues and to prevent inadvertent stigmatizing imagery. Accessibility features, closed captioning, simplified interaction modes, seated-only scenarios, and adjustable sensory intensity, should be standard options, not add-ons. A practical translation: design XR services so that patients who are older, have disabilities, or come from marginalized communities can still access meaningful, respectful interventions (Correa et al., 2021).

Robust evaluation plans must accompany clinical rollout (Morgan et al., 2025). Local implementations should collect standardized outcome measures (symptom ratings, functional indices), engagement metrics (session attendance, time-in-session), and safety data (cybersickness rates, adverse events. When possible, clinics should contribute de-identified data to multisite registries to permit larger-scale evaluation of effectiveness, moderators of treatment response, and rare adverse outcomes (Ricciardi & Zomaya, 2025). Implementation science frameworks can guide dissemination, identifying local barriers, tailoring training strategies, and measuring adoption over time. In practice-oriented language: evaluate everything you deploy, using both quantitative outcomes and qualitative patient feedback to refine practice.

A clear research agenda will accelerate responsible adoption (Anklam et al., 2022). Priority questions include: which XR features are necessary and sufficient for therapeutic gains (for example, full-body tracking versus simple head orientation); which patient characteristics predict XR suitability or differential response; how durable are XR-induced gains over years; and how cost-effective is XR compared with traditional modalities across diverse settings (Martinez-Martin et al., 2018). Dismantling studies that isolate immersion, embodiment, and real-time biofeedback will clarify mechanisms. Research that embeds equity metrics from the outset, studying diverse populations and lower-resource contexts, will prevent narrow generalization and build external validity (Martinez-Martin et al., 2018). Succinctly: research should move beyond small proof-of-concept trials and focus on mechanism, generalizability, and implementation (Martinez-Martin et al., 2018).

Regulatory and reimbursement landscapes are evolving and will shape the scale of XR adoption (Bibi, 2024). Clinicians and clinic leaders should stay informed about local and national policies governing medical device classification, telehealth reimbursement, and cross-jurisdictional practice. Early engagement with payers and policymakers can clarify evidence thresholds required for coverage and can support pilot reimbursement arrangements that accelerate access while safeguarding quality, In short clinical terms: policy and payment matter; plan for them early rather than waiting for external mandates,

Long-term sustainability requires thoughtful business models that preserve clinical integrity (Boda & Allam, 2022). Options include subscription models with clinician-facing dashboards, partnership arrangements with technology vendors that provide ongoing training and updates, and in-house development for large health systems. Whatever the financial model, contracts should protect patient data, require transparent update cycles, and include service-level agreements for device maintenance and incident response (Rajpal, 2025). From a practical standpoint: negotiate vendor contracts that prioritize clinical needs and data protections (Rajpal, 2025).

Integration with other digital health tools opens powerful possibilities. XR can be combined with mobile ecological momentary assessment (EMA), wearable passive sensing, and teletherapy to create hybrid care pathways (Verma et al., 2023). For example, patients might complete brief VR rehearsals in clinic, receive an EMA prompt the following day to practice a behavioral assignment, and then have a teletherapy check-in to process barriers. This blended approach leverages XR's experiential strength while maintaining the flexibility and reach of mobile and telehealth modalities (Weiner et al., 2025). Clinical translation: use XR as one node in a larger ecosystem of tools that support continuous, context-sensitive care (Weiner et al., 2025).

Patient engagement strategies must account for novelty effects and potential drop-off. Initial curiosity may drive early uptake, but sustained engagement depends on perceived relevance, ease of use, and clear links to valued outcomes. Goal-setting, brief orientation modules, and shared decision-making about scenario choices foster ownership and adherence. Clinicians should solicit regular feedback and iteratively adjust content to maintain relevance. A plain clinical tip: sustain engagement by aligning XR tasks with the patient's personally meaningful goals and by making each session transparently consequential for recovery (Lamb et al., 2025).

Ethical use in research demands separation of clinical care and investigational elements when both occur in the same setting (Omiyefa, 2025). Clear delineation, through consent forms, data flows, and IRB oversight, protects patients and preserves the integrity of both care and science (Kim & Backonja, 2025). When using clinical datasets for secondary research, de-identification and governance policies must be explicit and consented (Kim & Backonja, 2025). In day-to-day language: never blur the line between standard care and research without clear, documented patient consent (Kim & Backonja, 2025).

To illustrate the integration of these implementation principles, consider a summary composite vignette that brings together assessment, training, consent, adaptive exposure, biometrics, supervision, and evaluation. A regional clinic launches a pilot XR program for social anxiety. They begin with staff training and competency assessment, create informed consent materials that include biometric use disclosures, and screen patients for suitability. One patient begins a course of

XR-assisted exposure with weekly sessions that progress from small-group virtual interactions to larger audience simulations (Radanliev, 2025). Heart rate variability and clinician-rated distress guide session pacing; when physiological signs indicate prolonged hyperarousal, the clinician reduces stimulus intensity and focuses on grounding. Sessions are recorded for supervision with the patient's consent, and de-identified outcome data contributes to a registry assessing generalizability across age groups. Over three months the patient reports reduced avoidance, increased real-world social activity, and improved functioning at work. This vignette demonstrates how clinical, technical, ethical, and research priorities can be woven into a coherent XR program that honors patient safety and scientific rigor.

In closing this extended exploration, the adoption of XR in mental health care should be understood as a careful scaling of existing therapeutic principles into new modalities rather than as a wholesale replacement of clinical practice (Chen et al., 2022). XR amplifies clinicians' ability to deliver controlled, experiential learning and to personalize dose in ways previously impractical. To realize that promise responsibly requires investment in training, robust safety protocols, ethical data governance, inclusive design, rigorous research, and thoughtful integration into clinical workflow. The clinician's role remains central: to translate immersive experiences into meaningful psychological change through formulation, reflection, and guided practice. The translation for clinicians is straightforward, use XR to create experiences that matter, protect patients vigorously, and study your outcomes so that the field can learn and improve together.

The operational details that determine whether an XR program thrives or falters are often mundane but consequential: procurement strategies, device lifecycle planning, staff scheduling, and policies for infection control and device sanitation (Li et al., 2025). Clinics should maintain an inventory log that records device serial numbers, warranty status, last software update, and cleaning cycles. A simple maintenance protocol, weekly inspection, monthly software patch verification, and quarterly hardware performance checks, reduces unexpected downtime and prevents session cancellations that erode patient trust. Equally important is supply-chain planning for replacement parts and batteries, and clear procedures for firmware updates that avoid mid-session disruptions. In plain clinical terms: predictable, routine device care is as important to patient outcomes as clinical skill because it preserves continuity and confidence in treatment delivery.

Billing, documentation, and quality metrics must be adapted to reflect XR-specific activities while remaining compatible with existing clinical workflows (De Kock et al., 2021). Session notes should document therapeutic formulation, XR scenario parameters (including intensity settings and any adaptive algorithms used), biometric markers collected, patient-reported thresholds, and integration tasks assigned for between-session practice (Weiner et al., 2025). Clinics should work with compliance officers and coders to map XR services to applicable billing codes and to document clinical necessity when seeking reimbursement (Weiner et al., 2025). For quality assurance, key performance indicators might include average session completion rates, incidence of adverse events, patient-reported utility, and time-to-therapeutic-goal metrics. To translate this operationally: document XR sessions as you would any specialized clinical procedure, with explicit attention to the features that differ from talk therapy (Weiner et al., 2025).

Training curricula for XR clinicians can be modular and competency-based (Radanliev, 2025). An effective program begins with foundational modules, basic XR principles, safety screening, and informed consent, followed by applied modules that pair clinical case formulation with scenario selection (De Kock et al., 2021). Skills laboratories using standardized patients or peer role-play are necessary for clinicians to practice pacing exposures, invoking grounding techniques, and calibrating adaptive algorithms. Competency assessment should combine observed structured evaluations of simulated XR sessions with review of recorded real-session footage for fidelity and decision-making quality (De Kock et al., 2021). Continuing education should include updates on device safety advisories, ethical guidelines for biometric data, and case conferences that highlight complex cases (De Kock et al., 2021). In simpler clinical language: train clinicians in XR the same way you would train them to use a new evidence-based therapy, teach theory, practice skills, assess competence, then support through supervision (De Kock et al., 2021).

Supervision frameworks must bridge clinical and technical domains (Kourtesis, 2024). Supervisors should review a sample of sessions for each clinician, with attention to formulation-driven scenario choices, pace and titration, safety responses, and the patient's integration work post-session. Supervision can employ a structured fidelity checklist that captures whether the clinician adhered to the agreed exposure hierarchy, correctly interpreted biometric signals, and appropriately debriefed the patient (Pedram & Piatkowski, 2025). Supervisors should also have access to basic technical troubleshooting skills so that clinical feedback is not confounded by device misconfiguration (Pedram & Piatkowski, 2025). In practical terms: make supervision an explicit component of XR program quality control to ensure that technological novelty does not erode therapeutic fidelity (Pedram & Piatkowski, 2025).

Developing decision pathways for common clinical contingencies improves safety and consistency (Ma et al., 2025). For example, if a patient exhibit increasing dissociation during a session, the pathway would specify immediate steps: pause the scenario, implement a chosen grounding technique, reduce sensory load or switch to a calming environment, assess for ongoing risk, and document the episode with a plan to modify future sessions. For cybersickness, a decision tree might outline when to shorten sessions, adjust motion parameters, or refer to vestibular evaluation. These algorithms should be co-created with clinicians, incorporated into training, and readily available in the XR suite (Mohr et al., 2017). Plainly: have written decision paths for expected adverse events so that clinicians can act swiftly and consistently.

Patient selection criteria should be explicit but flexible, recognizing that contraindications are often relative rather than absolute. Standard exclusion flags might include uncontrolled epilepsy, active psychosis with severe reality testing impairment, recent traumatic brain injury with ongoing recovery, or medical instability. Relative contraindications, such as a history of severe dissociation, severe vestibular disorders, or pregnancy in some cases, require individualized risk-benefit analysis and often adapted protocols rather than blanket exclusion (Boffet et al., 2025). Where possible, initial orientation sessions with low-intensity exposure or seated-only experiences can assess tolerance before advancing to more immersive work. In other words: screen pragmatically, not punitively, and use graded assessment to determine fit.

Equally important is framing XR within a therapeutic contract that specifies goals, responsibilities, and contingency plans (Jain & Jain, 2025). The contract should list target behaviors, anticipated session frequency, between-session tasks, safety signals, and the conditions under which the patient or clinician may pause or terminate XR work (Weiner et al., 2025). Documenting these expectations reduces misunderstandings and supports shared decision-making. Put another way: explicitly agree with patients on what XR aims to do and how progress will be judged (Weiner et al., 2025).

When XR is used in research-practice hybrids, clinicians and investigators must negotiate borders between clinical care and data collection (Ross et al., 2022). Patients should receive clear information about which elements of their sessions contribute to clinical care and which are being recorded, analyzed, or retained for research. Opt-in mechanisms for data sharing, separate consent for audio/video recording, and explicit timelines for data retention are necessary practices. Clinicians should also be prepared to discuss incidental findings from biometric monitoring, such as arrhythmias detected during heart rate monitoring, and to escalate care appropriately. Clinically: maintain transparent communication about how session data will be used and who can access it.

Vendor selection and contract negotiation are clinical decisions with ethical and practical implications (Chaabene et al., 2025). Contracts should require vendors to comply with applicable health data protections, to allow local data storage or specified secure cloud arrangements, and to provide timely software updates and documented change logs (Pedram & Piatkowski, 2025). Vendors should commit to backward compatibility where feasible and to transparent reporting of algorithmic changes that could affect therapeutic delivery. Contract terms that lock clinics into inflexible ecosystems or obscure data flows create long-term risks; seek contractual clarity up front (Pedram & Piatkowski, 2025). Simply stated: treat vendor contracts as clinical governance documents, not just procurement paperwork (Pedram & Piatkowski, 2025).

Patient experience and acceptability determine real-world effectiveness. Clinics should solicit structured feedback on factors such as perceived realism, ease of use, emotional impact, and sense of safety. Short debrief surveys after early sessions and periodic qualitative interviews can reveal usability issues or cultural mismatches in content that quantitative metrics might miss. Iterative co-design, where patients participate in refining scenarios and onboarding materials, enhances engagement and equity. Translation for practice: listen to patients early and often to ensure XR tools meet their needs and preferences (Kostadimas et al., 2025).

Scaling XR beyond specialty centers demands creative models (Islam & Bae, 2024). Hub-and-spoke systems, where central expertise supports satellite clinics with remote supervision and shared content libraries, can spread capability while maintaining quality. Mobile XR units or portable kits allow outreach to underserved communities but require robust logistics for transport, sanitation, and staff training (Li et al., 2025). Partnerships with academic centers can facilitate evaluation and continuous improvement. Operationally: plan scaling models that pair local access with centralized quality support.

A pragmatic clinician's checklist consolidates core actions: obtain informed consent that explicitly covers immersion and data; conduct a safety screen; perform a brief orientation session; set clear session goals and stop signals; monitor physiological and subjective responses; debrief and assign integration tasks; document scenario parameters and patient responses; schedule supervision review; and log device maintenance completed (Adegoke et al., 2025). This checklist should be operationalized into clinic workflows and audited periodically for adherence. Clinically: use checklists to keep high-complexity XR care consistent and safe (Ong et al., 2025).

Training patients to use XR independently, when appropriate, requires additional safeguards (Ong et al., 2025). Home-based or remote XR requires reliable patient orientation, remote technical support, secure data transmission, and clear emergency contacts, Not all patients are suitable for unsupervised XR; criteria for home use should include demonstrated tolerance in clinic, technological literacy, and a stable support network, When home XR is authorized, clinicians should schedule regular synchronous check-ins and limit the scope of autonomous scenarios to well-practiced, low-intensity tasks, In short: extend XR to home settings only with careful selection and monitoring,

A short composite research vignette illustrates how rigorous evaluation can be integrated with routine care (Hiland, 2021). A multicenter pragmatic trial evaluates a scalable VR program for social anxiety embedded in routine outpatient clinics (Li et al., 2025). Clinics adopt a shared protocol for screening, consent, and session documentation, and clinicians receive uniform training (Li et al., 2025). The trial uses a mixed-methods approach, combining symptom measures, real-world functional indicators (for example, work attendance), and ethnographic interviews with patients about cultural fit (Li et al., 2025). Interim analyses inform adaptive modifications to content that improve representativeness. This example shows that rigorous research and everyday clinical care can be mutually reinforcing when protocols are designed with implementation in mind (Li et al., 2025).

Finally, a set of concise practical takeaways for clinicians adopting XR: begin small and iterate; prioritize safety and informed consent; invest in staff training and supervision; choose clinically aligned, customizable content; protect biometric and behavioral data; solicit and act on patient feedback; document everything that matters clinically and technically; and partner with researchers to evaluate outcomes (Bond et al., 2023). These steps are not exhaustive but provide a pragmatic roadmap that balances innovation with responsibility. Plain clinical translation: adopt XR cautiously, measure rigorously, and center patient welfare in every decision (Kim & Backonja, 2025).

The future of XR in therapy will unfold at the intersection of technological advancement and clinical wisdom (Cristofaro & Giardino, 2025). Advances in lightweight displays, improved locomotion interfaces, richer haptic feedback, and more efficient biometric sensing will expand therapeutic possibilities. Yet these tools will only yield sustainable benefit when clinicians, patients, technologists, and policymakers co-create systems that are safe, equitable, and effective. The imperative for clinicians is clear: learn the tools well enough to judge when they add value, protect patients vigorously, and contribute data and clinical insight to the growing evidence base so that XR's promise becomes demonstrable, durable, and widely shared. In clinical terms: technology will change what therapists can do, but not why they do it, helping patients to live more fully in the world they value (Fleming et al., 2019).

This chapter has traced XR's conceptual underpinnings, clinical applications, operational demands, ethical complexities, and implementation pathways (Chithra & Bhambri, 2024). The path forward requires modesty about what is known and boldness about what might be achieved when rigorous science meets thoughtful clinical practice (De Kock et al., 2021). For mental health providers, XR offers a new set of clinical instruments, powerful, precise, and experiential, that, when used with skill and care, can broaden access to effective interventions and deepen the opportunities for therapeutic learning (De Kock et al., 2021). Concluding clinical translation: adopt XR as a carefully governed extension of clinical competence, not as a substitute for it, and commit to studying outcomes so the field matures responsibly (De Kock et al., 2021).

I will continue the chapter now, extending the discussion into policy implications, evaluation frameworks, clinician well-being, cross-disciplinary collaboration, and a compact operational playbook that practitioners can implement immediately.

Policy and regulatory environments exert a powerful influence on how quickly and broadly XR interventions reach patients; licensing jurisdictions, medical device classifications, and telehealth statutes determine what is permissible and what documentation is required (Subu et al., 2022). Policymakers are still catching up to the pace of XR innovation, and clinicians should therefore adopt a proactive stance: document clinical rationale, align XR applications with established standards of care, and engage institutional compliance teams early in procurement and pilot design (Pedram & Piatkowski, 2025). A simple clinical translation: treat XR deployment as a medical intervention subject to the same oversight and documentation as any specialized treatment, and seek institutional alignment before scaling (Pedram & Piatkowski, 2025).

Evaluation frameworks for XR must balance internal validity with real-world relevance (Mahon, 2023). Randomized controlled trials remain essential for establishing efficacy, but implementation and pragmatic studies that capture heterogeneity of patients, settings, and clinician skill are equally important. Multi-level evaluation should combine symptom change metrics with measures of functional recovery, patient-reported experience, fidelity to therapeutic protocols, and operational indicators such as device uptime and staffing requirements. For everyday clinical use, a brief summary: track both clinical outcomes and implementation metrics so you know whether XR is helping patients and whether the program is sustainable (Engel, 1977).

Clinician well-being and workload considerations are rarely foregrounded in technology adoption but are central to program success. XR sessions can be more intense for therapists, requiring simultaneous attention to patient affect, device performance, biometric streams, and scenario management, which increases cognitive load (Ienca et al., 2017). Organizations should monitor clinician burnout risks, provide reasonable scheduling buffers for XR session setup and debriefing, and ensure access to technical support to reduce nonclinical burdens. In practice: protect clinicians from overload by building XR workflows that include administrative time and technical backup (Radanliev, 2025).

Cross-disciplinary collaboration is a practical necessity for high-quality XR care (Weiner et al., 2025). Effective teams pair clinical experts with human-centered designers, engineers who understand real-world clinical constraints, ethicists who help shape consent and data governance, and implementation scientists who evaluate outcomes (Fanarioti & Karpouzis, 2025). Regular, structured exchanges, co-design workshops, joint case reviews, and post-implementation retrospectives, produce more usable and safer systems than siloed development. Plain clinical advice: build a standing XR working group that meets regularly and includes both clinical and technical stakeholders (Fanarioti & Karpouzis, 2025).

Equity-oriented deployment requires deliberate choices about hardware distribution, content design, and community engagement. Clinics should consider financing strategies, loaner devices, sliding-scale access, grant-supported pilots, that reduce socioeconomic barriers. Scenario libraries should be created with input from diverse patient groups to ensure cultural relevance and to avoid inadvertent harm. A direct clinical translation: make equity a planning metric, not an afterthought, by budgeting for inclusive content and accessibility features from the start (Kargarandehkordi et al., 2025).

Data stewardship in multi-site or vendor-partnered programs benefits from standardized governance templates that specify encryption standards, retention timelines, access controls, and breach-response procedures (Akhtar & Rawol, 2024). Where possible, prefer architectures that keep raw biometric data under local clinical control and share only de-identified, purpose-limited aggregates with external partners. Patients should be offered clear options to view, export, or request deletion of their data subject to clinical record retention policies (Fleming et al., 2019). In concise clinical terms: choose data architectures that maximize patient control and minimize unnecessary external exposure.

An operational playbook consolidates the chapter's guidance into a sequence clinicians can apply immediately: (Mohr et al., 2017) define clinical targets and success metrics; (Saganowski et al., 2022) screen patients for XR suitability and obtain enhanced informed consent; (Agarwal et al., 2025) deliver a short orientation and tolerance test; (APA, 2023) conduct XR sessions with clear stop signals, biometric monitoring as appropriate, and immediate debriefing; (Torous et al., 2023) document scenario parameters and patient responses; (Watson, 2025) review sessions in supervision and iterate the treatment plan; and (Aiken et al., 2023) contribute de-identified outcome data to local or regional registries (De Kock et al., 2021). A clear clinical summary: follow a repeatable workflow that emphasizes safety, documentation, and iterative learning (De Kock et al., 2021).

Two brief vignettes illustrate complex policy and team dynamics in practice. In the first vignette, a hospital system seeks to implement XR for inpatient chronic pain management but faces procurement rules that treat head-mounted displays as general IT rather than clinical devices (Shatte et al., 2019). The team assembles a cross-functional group, clinicians, procurement officers, compliance staff, and biomedical engineers, to reclassify the technology under clinical equipment policies, document clinical protocols, and secure an exception that enables pilot reimbursement (Shatte et al., 2019). This pragmatic reclassification permits careful clinical use while aligning with institutional governance (Shatte et al., 2019). In simpler clinical language: engage institutional partners early to avoid bureaucratic delays that can stall clinically beneficial pilots (Shatte et al., 2019).

In the second vignette, an academic clinic partners with a small XR vendor to co-develop culturally tailored social scenarios for adolescents from diverse backgrounds. The collaboration includes ongoing patient advisory input, iterative usability testing, and a shared data governance agreement that keeps identifiable data within the clinic (Kim & Backonja, 2025). Midway through the pilot, adolescents provide feedback that some virtual settings feel stereotyped; the team pauses deployment, revises assets with community co-designers, and resumes with improved acceptability scores. The lesson is operational: design partnerships so that patient voices can shape content before broad deployment.

To conclude this extended continuation, the integration of XR into therapeutic practice is a multi-dimensional change that touches clinical technique, operational systems, ethical governance, and workforce development (Babu & Joseph, 2025). The clinician's task is to harness XR's capacity for controlled, repeatable, and richly contextualized experience while safeguarding patients and preserving therapeutic judgment (Kargarandehkordi et al., 2025). A final clinical restatement: use XR as a precise tool within a human-centered therapeutic process, test it, measure it, and refine it, so that technological promise translates into lasting patient benefit (Kargarandehkordi et al., 2025).

Measurement and quality assurance are foundational to responsible XR practice; without routine measurement, clinicians cannot know whether an intervention is working, for whom it works, or when adaptations are needed (Hall et al., 2024). Establishing a measurement framework means selecting a small set of standardized clinical outcomes, session-level process indicators, and safety metrics that fit your clinic's capacity (Shatte et al., 2019). Clinical outcomes should capture both symptom reduction and functional change so that improvements in anxiety or pain are linked to real-world gains such as return to work, social participation, or reductions in medication use (Shatte et al., 2019). Process indicators include session completion rates, mean within-session distress trajectories, frequency of adaptive parameter adjustments made by clinicians or algorithms, and patient-reported usability. Safety metrics should document rates of cybersickness, dissociation episodes, unplanned terminations, and any adverse events requiring escalation. A plain clinical translation: measure things that matter to patients and that you can feasibly collect every week, then use those data to guide treatment decisions and program improvements (Shatte et al., 2019).

When designing session-level measurement, balance granularity with burden. Short, validated symptom ratings administered before and after each XR exposure give immediate feedback on effect and tolerability, while periodic broader assessments capture maintenance and generalization (Iwaya et al., 2023). Integrate brief ecological momentary assessments (Inkster et al., 2023) delivered to patients' phones in the days following exposure to measure transfer to the real world, did the patient attend the social event, board the flight, or use a coping skill when triggered? Biometric streams add objectivity but require careful interpretation: elevated heart rate during exposure can indicate both productive engagement and overwhelming distress depending on context. Always interpret physiological data alongside subjective reports and clinical observation. In practical terms: use simple pre/post measures for each session and occasional follow-up EMAs to verify that gains extend beyond the clinic.

Quality improvement loops close the gap between measurement and practice. Regularly scheduled data reviews, monthly for initial pilots, quarterly for mature programs, should examine outcome trajectories, identify patterns of nonresponse, and surface safety signals (Khoo et al., 2024). When a cluster of patients shows early dropout or elevated cybersickness rates, interrogate the content and setup: is visual motion excessive, are instructions unclear, or does the scenario poorly match the patient population's lived experience? Continuous improvement cycles should pair quantitative flags with qualitative patient interviews to prioritize changes. A concise clinical restatement: monitor program metrics, dig into unexpected patterns, and fix the simplest problems first (Mohr et al., 2017).

Training and ongoing clinician support directly affect measurement quality and patient outcomes. Clinicians who understand measurement rationales and data displays are more likely to integrate feedback into session planning. Training modules should therefore include hands-on exercises interpreting pre/post scores, physiological time series, and patient usability comments. Supervisors should model how to pivot treatment plans when measurement indicates stalled progress or adverse responses. In plain clinical language: measurement matters most when clinicians use it in supervision and treatment planning, not when it is only collected for reporting (Fleming et al., 2019).

A core competency for clinicians is the ability to escalate care appropriately when XR reveals clinical complexity. XR sessions may unmask suicidal ideation, severe dissociation, or medical concerns (for example, cardiac arrhythmias) that require urgent intervention (Robinson et al., 2024). Clear escalation pathways, who to call, when to activate medical or psychiatric emergency services, documentation steps, and follow-up plans, must be embedded into clinic policy and rehearsed through mock drills. Patients should know at intake how emergent concerns will be handled and who will be contacted in crisis. Clinically: make escalation routes transparent so XR sessions do not become a point of unnecessary delay in urgent care (Robinson et al., 2024).

Clinical vignette 5: A 28-year-old man undergoing VR exposure for panic disorder reports increasing breathlessness during a public-transport simulation (Lay et al., 2025). His heart rate monitor shows transient tachycardia, and his post-session marker indicates persistently high subjective distress despite in-session grounding.

The clinician follows the escalation pathway: pauses the trial, conducts a focused medical history, consults the on-call primary care provider, and arranges an expedited cardiology evaluation that identifies supraventricular tachycardia unrelated to anxiety (De Kock et al., 2021). The clinic's prompt escalation procedure not only uncovered a treatable medical condition but also prevented worsening risk during subsequent exposures. This vignette underscores the need for clear clinical pathways when biometric data suggest nonpsychiatric causes for distress (De Kock et al., 2021).

Data sharing for quality improvement and research requires careful governance (Baka et al., 2025). When clinics participate in registries or collaborative studies, common data elements and standardized definitions improve comparability (Engel, 1977). De-identification reduces patient re-identification risk, but governance must also consider whether certain biometric traces or behavioral patterns could re-identify individuals in small communities (Engel, 1977). Data use agreements should specify permitted analyses, secondary uses, and processes for patient withdrawal of consent (Engel, 1977). In straightforward terms: share data to improve care, but only under tightly specified, transparent rules that protect patients (Engel, 1977).

Clinician well-being remains an underappreciated element of XR programs (Livieri et al., 2025). Sessions can be mentally and emotionally intense for therapists who must simultaneously track multiple data streams, manage a patient's arousal, and troubleshoot devices. Clinics should schedule XR sessions with buffer time for setup and documentation, rotate clinicians so that no single practitioner carries a disproportionate caseload of high-intensity exposures, and create forums for clinicians to debrief difficult sessions (Obermeyer et al., 2019). Occupational health protections, such as ergonomic support for prolonged device handling and policies that limit consecutive XR sessions, protect clinicians and sustain program quality. A concise clinical point: protect clinicians so they can safely care for patients.

Building research-practice partnerships accelerates both evidence generation and clinical excellence (Liu & Schueller, 2023). When clinics collaborate with academic partners, they gain access to rigorous study designs, analytic capacity, and grant support, while researchers benefit from real-world implementation contexts. Successful partnerships establish shared goals, equitable data governance, and mechanisms for rapid-cycle feedback so that clinical insights inform study modifications. Clinically phrased: partner with researchers in ways that value clinical realities and patient priorities.

The ethics of placebo and sham-controlled XR studies deserve explicit attention (Smith et al., 2023). Designing ethically appropriate control conditions entails balancing methodological rigor with patient welfare and informed consent clarity. Sham XR experiences should avoid deception about potential therapeutic content while matching non-specific factors such as clinician contact and novelty (Ong et al., 2025). When possible, offer promising interventions to control participants after study completion to honor reciprocity (Ong et al., 2025). In simple clinical terms: design controls responsibly and transparently, and minimize patient burden in research (Ong et al., 2025).

A short implementation vignette illustrates measurement-driven iteration. A behavioral health clinic rolls out an XR program for social anxiety and observes early measurable gains in situational tolerance but limited transfer to real-world attendance at social events (Shatte et al., 2019). The team introduces EMA prompts the day after exposures to prompt patients to engage in small social behaviors and pairs this with brief telecoaching check-ins. Over the next quarter, registry data show increased real-world social participation, suggesting that pairing XR with between-session prompts enhances generalization (Weiner et al., 2025). From a clinical perspective: use measurement to identify weak links in your care chain and add light-weight supports to bridge them (Weiner et al., 2025).

Sustaining XR programs financially demands creative strategies (Obermeyer et al., 2019). Clinics can pursue blended revenue: a mix of fee-for-service billing where available, grant-funded pilots, partnerships with academic centers for contracted research, and value-based arrangements that tie reimbursement to functional improvements, Cost analyses should account not only for hardware and software but for training, maintenance, data management, and supervision time, Investment decisions should be guided by potential reach and expected clinical impact, with priority given to applications where XR provides unique capabilities, such as safely recreating high-risk exposures or enabling embodiment interventions not feasible in vivo (Tsai et al., 2025). Clinically: invest where XR adds unique, demonstrable value and plan funding for the full operational footprint, not just equipment (Tsai et al., 2025).

Legal considerations include device classification and malpractice exposure. Clinicians should work with their legal and compliance teams to understand whether particular XR applications meet the threshold for regulated medical devices in their jurisdiction and to ensure documentation supports clinical standards of care (Ball et al., 2025). Liability policies should be reviewed to confirm coverage for XR-delivered care and to address telehealth adjuncts (Ricciardi & Zomaya, 2025). Practically: engage legal counsel early in program design to avoid surprises.

Cultural competence and narrative framing enhance XR acceptability (Fanarioti & Karpouzis, 2025). How scenarios are introduced, the language therapists use to frame exposures, and the cultural congruence of avatars and settings influence engagement. Co-design with community advisors and iterative usability testing can identify subtle cultural mismatches, scenes that unintentionally reinforce stigma or use metaphors that do not resonate. Tailored narratives that connect XR tasks to patients' values and life goals improve motivation and adherence (Robinson et al.,

2024). Clinically: make XR scenarios culturally attuned and explain how each task serves personally meaningful goals (Robinson et al., 2024).

A final integrated operational checklist summarizes critical actions clinicians and clinics should adopt immediately: obtain enhanced informed consent that covers immersion and data use; perform systematic safety screening; deliver a brief orientation and tolerance test before therapeutic dosing; monitor subjective and objective responses during each session; use predefined stop signals and escalation pathways; debrief with explicit cognitive integration tasks; document scenario parameters and outcomes in the record; review cases in supervision regularly; and collect and act on program-level metrics to guide continuous improvement (Gkintoni et al., 2025). This checklist is intentionally short to support practical use; it must be translated into local protocols with assigned responsibilities and audit cycles. In plain clinical terms: standardize the essentials so that XR care is reproducible, safe, and measurable (Ienca et al., 2017).

As technology evolves, clinicians' fundamental task will remain constant: translate immersive experience into psychological change through reflection, meaning-making, and behavioral activation. XR provides new means to create corrective experiences, to rehearse challenging tasks, and to measure physiological and behavioral markers of change (Lindner et al., 2024). Yet these technological affordances must be embedded within human-centered clinical practice, guided by ethical clarity, measurement, supervision, and a relentless focus on patient welfare. A final clinical restatement: let XR extend your therapeutic reach, but keep the human clinician at the center of interpretation and decision-making.

This completes the extended chapter, which integrates theoretical framing, clinical applications across diagnoses, operational implementation, measurement and evaluation, training and supervision, ethical and legal considerations, and pragmatic recommendations for clinics beginning or scaling XR services (Casson, 2019). Two brief closing vignettes are included earlier to demonstrate real-world contingencies and the protective value of clear policies and measurement-driven care.

Extended Reality (XR), including virtual reality (VR), augmented reality (AR), and mixed reality (MR), has matured from a technical novelty into a practical suite of tools that clinicians can integrate into mental health care to create controlled, repeatable, and context-rich experiences (Spytska, 2025). These technologies permit therapists to reconstruct feared situations, rehearse adaptive behavior, and deliver guided cognitive and emotional processing inside environments whose features can be adjusted with precision. In clinical terms, XR supplies therapists with reproducible experiential "laboratories" that can be titrated to a patient's tolerance and therapeutic goals, thereby extending the reach of traditional interventions without sacrificing clinical control (Obermeyer et al., 2019). A concise clinical translation: use XR to simulate important, hard-to-reach experiences safely and deliberately so patients can practice adaptive responses under a clinician's guidance (Obermeyer et al., 2019).

At a perceptual level, XR alters sensory input to redirect attention, elicit emotion, and shape action tendencies; VR typically occludes the surrounding physical world to deliver full immersion, AR overlays digital elements into the patient's actual environment to support in-situ rehearsal, and MR blends virtual and physical objects so they interact in real time. Each modality has distinct affordances that should drive clinical selection: choose VR when maximal stimulus control and immersion are needed; choose AR to support in-the-moment practice within a patient's natural environment; choose MR when the therapeutic aim requires interplay between virtual cues and tangible objects (Mohr et al., 2017). In plain clinical language: modality is a tool choice tied to therapeutic intent, not a technology badge to be used indiscriminately (Mohr et al., 2017).

The central therapeutic mechanisms XR leverages are already familiar to clinicians: emotional engagement, exposure and habituation, expectancy violation, error-based learning, embodiment, and practice in ecologically valid contexts (Methuku et al., 2023). Presence, the subjective experience of "being there", is a key moderator because it determines whether virtual stimuli produce authentic emotional and physiological responses. When presence is sufficient, virtual cues activate the same fear networks and avoidance tendencies seen in vivo, creating opportunities for corrective learning. Clinicians should therefore treat XR as an exposure medium with adjustable dose and repeatability, using it to generate experiences that produce therapeutic learning in ways that can be observed, measured, and integrated (Weiner et al., 2025). To restate clinically: high-presence XR can produce real emotions that patients can learn to tolerate and reinterpret under supervision (Weiner et al., 2025).

Experts such as Thomas Insel, Albert Rizzo, Rosalind Picard have advanced concepts like cognitive-systems perspective.

XR's most developed clinical application is exposure-based treatment for anxiety disorders and specific phobias (Tavory, 2024). VR reliably reproduces contexts, such as airplanes, elevated platforms, or public speaking auditoria, so therapists can deliver graded, repeatable exposures without the logistical complications of arranging in vivo situations. For post-traumatic stress disorder (PTSD), VR permits carefully scaffolded revisiting of trauma-related cues with clinician-controlled pacing and contextualization, minimizing uncontrolled retraumatization while facilitating emotional processing. In substance use treatment, XR can recreate cue-rich environments and social pressure scenarios that provoke craving while providing an opportunity to rehearse refusal strategies under a clinician's supervision (Martinez-Martin et al., 2018). Clinically: XR expands the range and repeatability of exposures clinicians can provide while preserving safety and individualized pacing (Martinez-Martin et al., 2018).

Embodiment and perspective-taking are additional therapeutic uses for XR that go beyond classical exposure (Sun et al., 2025). Allowing patients to inhabit avatars with different body characteristics or social roles creates sensorimotor experiences that can alter self-representation, empathy, and interpersonal behavior. These embodied interventions have been applied to body image disturbance, aggression reduction, and social cognition training; they are particularly useful when corrective, embodiment-based evidence is likely to shift entrenched beliefs. Plainly: avatar-based XR gives patients sensory evidence to challenge distorted self- and other-representations, which therapists can then integrate with cognitive restructuring and behavioral experiments.

The coupling of XR with biometric sensing and analytical algorithms strengthens personalization (Martinez-Martin et al., 2018). Physiological signals, heart rate variability, skin conductance, respiration dynamics, and eye-tracking, provide objective markers of momentary arousal and attention. Machine learning methods can detect patterns and suggest adaptive adjustments, such as pausing an exposure or presenting a calming cue when signs of overload appear (Martinez-Martin et al., 2018). Crucially, the clinician must remain in control: automated suggestions should support, not replace, clinical judgment and the therapeutic alliance (Martinez-Martin et al., 2018). Translation for practice: use biometrics and analytics to inform dosing and to provide objective indices of engagement, but treat them as adjuncts to clinical observation rather than definitive verdicts (Martinez-Martin et al., 2018).

Despite clear promise, XR presents practical and ethical challenges that clinicians must address before adopting it into routine care (Vaidyam et al., 2019). Technical barriers, hardware costs, maintenance requirements, and the need for reliable computing infrastructure, can limit access, particularly in low-resource contexts. Clinically, some patients experience cybersickness, dizziness, or dissociation during immersion; others may lack the cognitive capacity or sensory tolerance to benefit from VR. Ethical complexities include informed consent for immersive experiences, the collection and handling of sensitive biometric data, and maintaining patient autonomy when adaptive algorithms are involved (Ienca et al., 2017). Clinicians must therefore implement standardized screening, robust consent processes that explicitly describe immersion-related risks and data uses, and contingency plans for adverse responses. In summary: adopt XR with explicit policies for screening, consent, and data governance to safeguard patient welfare.

Implementation requires more than buying headsets; it demands attention to space design, workflow integration, staffing, and device lifecycle management. A safe XR suite includes unobstructed movement areas, adjustable lighting, comfortable seating for pre- and post-session processing, and secure storage for devices (Freeman et al., 2017). Operational protocols should cover device sanitation, firmware updates, routine maintenance, and replacement-part planning; predictable upkeep preserves session continuity and patient trust. Clinically relevant workflow elements include pre-session technical checks, a structured patient orientation and tolerance test, integration of XR session notes into the health record, and time allocated for debriefing and between-session assignments (Freeman et al., 2017). Translation: treat XR sessions like any specialized clinical intervention with standardized procedures and documentation (Freeman et al., 2017).

Workforce development is central to successful adoption. Clinicians need competency-based training that blends technical operation with therapeutic integration: hardware setup, sensor calibration, scenario selection, adaptive algorithm oversight, crisis management, and the skills to weave XR experiences into broader formulations and therapeutic plans (Carl et al., 2019). Training should include supervised practice with standardized patients, observed competency assessments, and ongoing supervision that reviews both clinical decisions and technical performance (Pedram & Piatkowski, 2025). Supervisors must be fluent enough in the technology to evaluate fidelity and to guide clinicians on when to escalate or adapt. Clinically: certify clinicians in XR use only after they demonstrate both technical competence and effective therapeutic integration (Pedram & Piatkowski, 2025).

Safety protocols should be explicit and rehearsed. Pre-session screening should identify contraindicating medical or psychiatric conditions, such as uncontrolled epilepsy, severe dissociation, or unstable cardiovascular disease, while relative contraindications require individualized risk-benefit analyses. Sessions should use a patient-led stop-signal, incorporate grounding and stabilization techniques, and include brief post-session integration focused on cognitive processing and behavioral tasks to encourage generalization. Written decision pathways for common contingencies, for example, dissociation, severe cybersickness, or unexpected medical alarms, support consistent, rapid clinician response. Put plainly: establish and rehearse safety checklists so reactions are managed swiftly and predictably.

Informed consent for XR must go beyond standard therapy explanations (Xing et al., 2025). Patients need clear information about the immersive nature of sessions, potential emotional intensity, the collection and storage of biometric data, who will access recordings or logs, and circumstances under which data may be used for supervision or research (Kargarandehkordi et al., 2025). Offering a brief orientation that lets patients sample low-intensity immersion before committing to therapeutic dosing enhances informed choice. Clinically: ensure patients understand experiential and data-related aspects of XR and consent after experiencing a tolerance test when possible (Kargarandehkordi et al., 2025).

Ethical stewardship is particularly important when XR systems employ adaptive algorithms (Mone & Fayazullaeva, 2023). Transparency about algorithmic roles, limits, and the clinician's authority to override automated adjustments should be standard practice. Patients should be informed about potential misclassifications or errors in biometric interpretations and about their right to decline algorithmic features. Data governance must prioritize patient control: encrypted storage, role-based access, retention limits, documented breach response plans, and clear policies on secondary data uses for research or quality improvement. Plain guidance: protect patient data as you would any other health record, and ensure algorithmic assistance remains subordinate to human clinical judgment.

Equity and cultural competence must be embedded in design and deployment. Scenarios must be configurable to reflect diverse cultural, linguistic, and body representations; accessibility features, captioning, alternative input methods, seated-only scenarios, should be default options. Financing models that reduce cost barriers, loaner devices, subsidized programs, grant-supported pilots, help prevent the creation of XR-enabled care deserts (Friend et al., 2024). Clinically: design XR services so they work for patients across demographic and socioeconomic groups, not just those in well-resourced centers (Ricciardi & Zomaya, 2025).

Measurement and quality assurance convert XR from experimental novelty into dependable clinical practice (Walter et al., 2023). Programs should select a compact set of feasible measures that include symptom reduction, functional indicators (work attendance, social participation), process variables (session completion, within-session distress slopes), and safety metrics (rates of cybersickness, dissociation, unplanned terminations). Use brief pre/post session ratings, occasional ecological momentary assessments to track real-world generalization, and biometric indices interpreted in clinical context (De Kock et al., 2021). Create quality improvement cycles, regular data reviews, root-cause analyses when adverse signals appear, and patient interviews to illuminate usability issues, and iterate content and workflows accordingly (De Kock et al., 2021). In brief: measure what matters and use those data to refine care continuously (De Kock et al., 2021).

Research priorities that will accelerate the field's maturity include controlled trials comparing XR modalities to evidence-based comparators, dismantling studies that isolate active features such as embodiment or closed-loop adaptation, trials that examine moderators of treatment response, longitudinal studies on durability and relapse prevention, and implementation research that addresses real-world barriers in diverse care settings (Lorke & Stefanou, 2025). Embedding equity metrics and diverse populations into research designs is essential to avoid a narrow evidence base (Ienca et al., 2017). Clinically: contribute to pragmatic research when possible and collect local outcome data to inform continuous improvement.

Operational governance includes vendor selection and contract negotiation that treat vendors as clinical partners rather than mere suppliers (Pedram & Piatkowski, 2025). Contracts should specify data protections, update processes, algorithmic transparency, and service-level agreements for maintenance and incident response. Avoid lock-in clauses that prevent data portability or require opaque cloud storage without local control. Clinicians and administrators must involve legal and compliance teams early to clarify device classification, data residency requirements, and reimbursement pathways. Practical guidance: secure contracts that prioritize clinical needs and patient protections from the outset (Radanliev, 2025).

Scaling XR beyond specialty centers benefits from hub-and-spoke designs and tele-supervised models. Centralized content libraries and training hubs can support satellite clinics through remote supervision, while mobile kits can bring XR to underserved communities with proper logistical planning for sanitation and technical support. When home-based XR exposures are considered, restrict unsupervised protocols to patients who have demonstrated clinic tolerance, provide remote technical and clinical check-ins, and ensure robust emergency contact procedures. Clinically: expand access thoughtfully, pairing local availability with centralized quality oversight.

Clinician well-being requires deliberate attention. XR sessions demand simultaneous monitoring of affect, device state, and biometric streams, which raises cognitive load and potential emotional fatigue (Engel, 1977). Schedule XR sessions with setup and debrief buffers, rotate high-intensity caseloads, and provide technical support so clinicians are not burdened with device troubleshooting during clinical contact (Weiner et al., 2025). Create forums for peer debrief and supervision to process challenging cases. Plainly: protect clinicians' capacity to deliver safe, empathic care.

Practical implementation tools include short checklists and operational playbooks: pre-session screening and consent; orientation and tolerance test; scenario parameters and stop-signal agreed in writing; biometric calibration where used; structured in-session monitoring; immediate debrief with cognitive integration tasks; documentation of scenario settings and patient responses; scheduled supervision review; and routine device maintenance logs (Martinez-Martin et al., 2018). These tools standardize care and make XR interventions reproducible and auditable (Tsai et al., 2025). Clinically: adopt simple protocols that embed safety, documentation, and iterative learning.

Illustrative vignettes concretize how these principles play out in routine care. A middle-aged woman with severe aviophobia progresses through a VR flight program that sequences boarding, taxiing, turbulence, and landing; biometric monitoring and in-session cognitive reappraisal guide pacing, and after several graded exposures she completes a short real-world flight for work. A young adult with profound body image disturbance uses avatar embodiment to experience different body representations while engaging in cognitive restructuring during debrief; the experiential evidence reduces preoccupations during real-world dressing and improves social participation. A veteran with PTSD who initially dissociates in immersion is managed through shorter, carefully paced exposures, grounding protocols, and iterative clinician-led adjustments that reintroduce trauma cues without overwhelm. These vignettes show

how XR's experiential strength can be harnessed safely when clinicians prepare, monitor, and integrate sessions thoughtfully.

Ethical and legal pitfalls must be anticipated. Obtain explicit consent for recordings, biometric collection, and possible research use; separate clinical care from investigational activities with distinct consent and governance; and maintain transparency when algorithmic adjustments are applied (Freeman et al., 2017). Document clinical rationale for XR use in the record and involve compliance teams regarding device classification and billing codes (Freeman et al., 2017). When adverse events occur, follow pre-specified escalation pathways and report incidents in the clinic's quality system. Plain clinical summary: anticipate the ethical, legal, and clinical contingencies and codify responses before they occur (Freeman et al., 2017).

Financial sustainability depends on realistic accounting that includes device and software costs, training, maintenance, data management, supervision time, and the administrative burden of documentation and measurement (Tizzard, 2025). Funding strategies can combine fee-for-service billing where permitted, grants for innovation and access, partnerships with academic centers, and value-based arrangements that tie reimbursement to functional outcomes. Investment decisions should prioritize applications where XR provides clear added value, such as safe simulation of high-risk exposures or embodiment work that cannot be achieved in vivo (Kim & Backonja, 2025). Clinically: budget for the full operational footprint, not just initial hardware purchases.

Finally, XR's future will be shaped by technological advances, lighter displays, richer haptic feedback, better biometric sensors, and more efficient algorithms, and by human choices about how to integrate these tools into care (Leivaditis & Sepetis, 2025). The clinician's role remains central: to translate immersive experience into psychological change through meaning-making, reflection, and applied behavior change. XR should extend, not replace, the therapeutic relationship; it should generate corrective experiences that therapists use as raw material for formulation and intervention. A final clinical restatement: let XR be a precise instrument in your therapeutic toolkit, tested, measured, and governed, so that technological promise becomes demonstrable, equitable, and durable benefit for the people you serve.

The final phase of integrating Extended Reality into clinical practice concerns translation into everyday decision-making: how to choose XR for an individual patient, how to sequence XR within a broader treatment plan, and how to judge when to stop or transition from XR-supported learning to in vivo practice (Reddy, 2025). Clinicians should adopt a decision rubric that begins with clear clinical aims (what specific behavior, belief, or skill is the session designed to change), assesses suitability (medical, cognitive, and psychosocial contraindications), identifies the minimal XR modality and feature set necessary to achieve the aim (VR versus AR; embodiment versus simple exposure), and specifies measurable progression criteria that determine advancement, maintenance, or termination (Pedram & Piatkowski, 2025). A single-sentence clinical translation: choose XR because it uniquely supports a defined therapeutic aim, not because it is technically novel (Pedram & Piatkowski, 2025). In practice, this means documenting a short treatment plan that states the XR target behavior (for example, entering a crowded bus), the dosing schedule (number and length of exposures), objective metrics for progress (in-session distress slope, between-session behavior), and explicit exit criteria (successful real-world trial or plateau despite adaptations; Pedram & Piatkowski, 2025).

Sequencing XR with other therapeutic elements increases the likelihood that gains will generalize (Singh & Chandra, 2025). XR should rarely function as a standalone "fix"; instead, it should be embedded within a formulation-driven sequence that includes preparation (psychoeducation, coping skills rehearsal), XR practice (graded exposures or embodiment tasks), guided integration (debriefing, cognitive restructuring), and between-session generalization assignments supported by prompts or coach contacts (Rajpal, 2025). A plain clinical clarification follows: experiential gains are consolidated through reflection and real-world practice, not by the XR session alone (Rajpal, 2025). A common sequencing error is to rely on XR exposure without investing time in consolidation; to avoid this, allocate at least one-third of total contact time to pre- and post-exposure therapeutic processes rather than pure in-scenario minutes (Rajpal, 2025).

Transitioning from XR to in vivo exposure or independent functioning should be explicit and data-driven (Johnson et al., 2021). Use staged transfer tasks that mirror the XR exposures in the real world but start at a slightly lower intensity, and couple them with brief "bridge" sessions, either in person or via telehealth, where clinicians review the XR learning points, coach problem-solving for anticipated obstacles, and reinforce coping skills (Fanarioti & Karpouzis, 2025). Objective markers that support transition include sustained reductions in anticipatory anxiety, evidence of coping skill use in naturalistic EMA data, and patient-reported increases in confidence or self-efficacy (Fanarioti & Karpouzis, 2025). To summarize clinically: make transitions explicit, scaffolded, and empirically justified so that XR gains become durable real-world change (Fanarioti & Karpouzis, 2025).

Sustained program quality requires cyclical review and an expectation of iteration. Establish quarterly governance meetings that review aggregated outcomes, safety incidents, patient feedback, and vendor performance; use these meetings to prioritize incremental improvements, whether technical (adjusting motion parameters to reduce cybersickness), clinical (modifying exposure hierarchies), or operational (changing scheduling templates to allow for setup and debrief time; Glass et al., 2022). Embed a lightweight Plan-Do-Study-Act cycle into program management so that changes are implemented with a clear hypothesis and evaluated against short-term metrics

(Li et al., 2025). Clinically stated: treat XR programs as living systems that require deliberate, measurable refinement rather than one-off investments (Li et al., 2025).

A mature XR program contributes to the broader knowledge base through responsible data sharing and collaborative inquiry (Mulukuntla, 2025). When sharing de-identified outcome data, annotate datasets with clear metadata, definitions of scenario parameters, sensor calibration settings, and sample characteristics, so other sites can interpret results accurately (Martinez-Martin et al., 2018). Prioritize contribution to registries that collect common data elements and that incorporate equity metrics to reveal who benefits and who does not (Martinez-Martin et al., 2018). This stewardship approach accelerates learning while minimizing proprietary siloing that impedes cumulative science. A brief clinical guidance: share what you can with safeguards so the field learns faster and more equitably (Martinez-Martin et al., 2018).

Ethical stewardship also extends to the psychosocial meaning of XR experiences (Kumar, 2025). Therapists should anticipate and address existential or identity-related reactions that may arise from deep immersion or embodiment work, changes in self-concept, altered social expectations, or shifts in how patients interpret their past experiences. Integration conversations should explicitly explore meaning, values, and implications for identity and relationships, and clinicians should be ready to link XR work to broader psychotherapeutic aims such as rebuilding trust, repairing relationships, or reframing life goals. Plainly: use XR experiences as a bridge to deeper psychotherapeutic work, not as an end in themselves (Ienca et al., 2017).

Training the next generation of clinicians will require curricular innovations that blend didactic, simulation, and supervised clinical practice (Elfouly & Alouani, 2025). Graduate programs, residency tracks, and continuing education should incorporate case-based XR modules, competency assessments with standardized patients, and supervised clinics where trainees deliver XR-assisted care under experienced mentors (Kim & Backonja, 2025). Certification pathways could formalize competencies across clinical, technical, and ethical domains, making it easier for employers and payers to assess readiness (Kim & Backonja, 2025). A single-sentence clinical takeaway: build XR competency like any other clinical skill, with staged learning, observed practice, and supervised application (Kim & Backonja, 2025).

In closing, Extended Reality is a potent extension of psychotherapy's repertoire: it can make elusive situations tangible, accelerate experiential learning, and provide objective data that enrich clinical judgment (Huang et al., 2024). Yet its value depends entirely on how clinicians use it, selecting the right modality for the right patient, maintaining rigorous safety and ethical standards, embedding XR within a broader therapeutic plan, and measuring outcomes that matter to patients (De Kock et al., 2021). A final clinical summation: let XR serve your formulation and patient goals, protect patients through clear policies and measurement, and contribute your findings to collective learning so that the technology's promise becomes realized and widely beneficent (De Kock et al., 2021).

A brief composite closing vignette illustrates these final principles. A community clinic adopts a VR-assisted exposure pathway for veterans with social reintegration difficulties. The team trains clinicians, sets up a governance cadence, and establishes a transfer protocol linking XR practice to community outings with peer coaches (Hickey et al., 2021). One veteran progress from brief seated VR interactions to full standing simulations with controlled audience reactions; biometric monitoring and EMA confirm reduced anticipatory anxiety and increased social outings (Mohr et al., 2017). The clinician sequences debriefing, values-based goal setting, and real-world coaching until the veteran independently attends a community event. Outcome data are de-identified and contributed to a regional registry that informs subsequent content tailoring (Mohr et al., 2017). This vignette shows the arc from training and safety to measurable real-world gains and shared learning.

The responsibility now rests with clinicians, researchers, institutions, and communities to steward XR's development in ways that maximize benefit and minimize harm (Crameri et al., 2021). That stewardship requires curiosity and skepticism in equal measure: curiosity to explore new therapeutic possibilities and skepticism to demand evidence, to protect patients' rights, and to insist on equitable access. If the field embraces these dual commitments, XR can broaden the reach and effectiveness of mental health care while preserving the therapeutic relationship that remains the heart of healing. A concise closing directive: proceed with thoughtful innovation, measure diligently, and center the humanity of the people you serve.

Organizational culture shapes whether XR becomes a responsible tool or a source of friction (Clemens-Meyer et al., 2021). Programs that treat XR as a flashy add-on rather than a clinical method integrated with supervision, measurement, and ethics tend to produce variable outcomes and staff dissatisfaction (Kim & Backonja, 2025). Clinics that succeed create explicit roles and routines, XR champions who coordinate training and maintenance, data stewards who manage governance, and regular multidisciplinary forums that review cases and metrics (Kim & Backonja, 2025). In simpler clinical terms: build XR into your clinic's routines and responsibilities so it is sustained rather than episodic (Kim & Backonja, 2025).

Intellectual property and proprietary content raise practical and ethical questions about reproducibility and equity. When therapeutic scenarios are locked behind vendor paywalls with opaque update cycles, clinics may face rising costs and limited flexibility to adapt content for cultural relevance. Conversely, open-source or consortium-developed scenario libraries can accelerate equitable access and foster collaborative improvement but require governance to ensure quality and safety. Clinically: balance vendor partnerships with commitments to interoperability and options for local content adaptation.

The pace of technological change invites both opportunity and strategic caution. Emerging hardware, lighter headsets, improved field-of-view, eye- and face-tracking, and better haptic feedback, will increase realism and broaden therapeutic possibilities. Yet each advance brings new testing needs: more sensors means more data to secure; richer immersion may increase cybersickness risk for some patients; and novel interaction paradigms require updated training and consent (Kim & Backonja, 2025). A clear clinical statement: adopt new technologies when they demonstrably improve clinical outcomes or operational safety, not merely when they are novel (Kim & Backonja, 2025).

A responsible innovation pathway reduces risk while enabling progress. Begin with problem-driven pilots that answer a narrowly defined clinical question, use robust measurement to evaluate outcomes and tolerability, and iterate before scaling, Combine pilots with stakeholder engagement that includes patients, family members, frontline clinicians, and technical staff to surface practical and ethical concerns early. When pilots show benefit, expand using hub-and-spoke models with centralized training and quality oversight to maintain fidelity. Clinically: pilot, measure, iterate, and scale thoughtfully rather than leaping to widespread deployment.

Workforce implications extend beyond clinicians to include IT support, biomedical engineers, and data governance specialists (Immanuel et al., 2023). Smaller clinics may partner with regional centers or academic institutions to access these capabilities; larger systems should create roles that blend technical and clinical oversight. Training pathways should also recognize that XR competence is transdisciplinary, clinicians need fluency in device limitations and data interpretation, while engineers benefit from structured exposure to clinical workflows and ethical constraints. A straightforward clinical recommendation: assemble multidisciplinary teams early so operational gaps do not undermine clinical goals.

Patient narratives and qualitative data are invaluable complements to quantitative measures (Mackey et al., 2025). Patients' descriptions of what VR "felt like," how it changed their sense of self, and whether it helped them do things they care about often reveal mechanisms and barriers that numeric scores miss. Routine collection of short narrative responses alongside standardized measures supports richer program evaluation and content refinement. Clinically: ask patients to tell you, in their words, what changed and what remains difficult; those narratives guide better tailoring than numbers alone.

Public communication matters for trust and uptake. Clear, honest messaging about what XR can and cannot do reduces unrealistic expectations and prevents disillusionment. Marketing that overpromises rapid cures risks harm to individuals and erodes professional credibility. Instead, communicate XR as an adjunctive, evidence-informed method that requires clinician oversight and measurement to ensure benefit. Translation for practice: be precise and candid when discussing XR with patients, funders, and the public.

Ethical reflection should be ongoing, not a one-time checkbox at program launch. Establish an ethics review cadence, quarterly or biannual, where new content, algorithm updates, and data-sharing proposals are evaluated by a panel that includes patient representatives and independent ethicists (Ghanim et al., 2023). This practice helps anticipate downstream harms and fosters public confidence. Practically: review ethics repeatedly as your XR program evolves (Robinson et al., 2024).

Long-term impact assessment should include social and systemic effects, not only individual symptom change. Does XR deployment reduce barriers to care across populations, or does it widen existing disparities (Mitsea et al., 2024)? Does it reshape therapeutic norms in ways that privilege technological interventions over human-centered relational work? Evaluations should therefore include equity audits, workforce impact studies, and assessments of how XR changes care pathways over time (Kim & Backonja, 2025). Clinically: look beyond symptom scores to the broader ways XR reshapes care access and clinical culture (Kim & Backonja, 2025).

A final synthesis of immediate, actionable steps distills the chapter into implementable practice. First, define a narrow clinical objective for XR adoption and the minimal feature set required to meet it (Shah et al., 2021). Second, develop a safety and consent protocol that includes orientation, tolerance testing, biometric governance, and stop-signal procedures (Mohr et al., 2017). Third, implement a short measurement bundle, pre/post session symptom ratings, one functional indicator, and a safety log, and review these weekly during initial pilots. Fourth, create multidisciplinary governance with named roles for training, data stewardship, and device maintenance (Mohr et al., 2017). Fifth, pilot with a small, well-screened patient cohort, iterate based on both quantitative and narrative feedback, and only then scale with hub-and-spoke supports. Sixth, document protocols, supervision notes, and outcome data to support replicability and to contribute to collective learning (Mohr et al., 2017). Clinically: take concrete, measurable steps that prioritize safety, measurement, and equity in every XR initiative (Mohr et al., 2017).

In closing, Extended Reality holds great promise as a tool that amplifies clinicians' capacity to deliver controlled experiential learning and personalized dosing. Its benefits will be realized when technological sophistication is married to clinical wisdom, rigorous measurement, ethical governance, and a commitment to equitable access (Moriarty et al., 2022). The invitation to clinicians and leaders is to proceed with purposeful humility, experiment intentionally, measure relentlessly, and center the lived experience of patients so that XR becomes not a technology spectacle but a durable, human-centered extension of effective mental health care, A concise clinical directive: adopt XR deliberately, govern it rigorously, and always translate immersive experience into meaningful change through human clinical work,

Adoption of XR in clinical settings should be governed by simple decision rules that link therapeutic aim to the minimal necessary technology: if the clinical target is best served by controlled immersion and stimulus isolation, select VR; if the target requires practice within the patient's actual environment, select AR; if the intervention needs real-time interaction between virtual and physical objects, select MR, Choose features, embodiment, closed-loop biofeedback, multi-user social simulation, only when they directly serve a clear clinical objective, and document that rationale in the treatment plan (Tsai et al., 2025). A plain clinical rule: use the least complex tool that accomplishes the therapeutic goal and escalate technological complexity only when it demonstrably improves outcomes (Tsai et al., 2025).

Safety must be operationalized through layered protections: systematic pre-session screening that flags absolute and relative contraindications; a concise orientation and tolerance test that includes demonstration immersion and a patient-identified stop-signal; in-session monitoring of subjective distress plus targeted biometric indices when clinically warranted; immediate debrief with cognitive integration tasks; and explicit escalation pathways for medical or psychiatric emergencies that are rehearsed regularly (Freeman et al., 2017). Place a short clarifying sentence here: safety procedures should be standardized, practiced, and reviewed as routinely as any clinical emergency protocol (Freeman et al., 2017).

Training pathways should be competency-based and staged. Early training emphasizes safe device handling, basic scenario control, and procedural checklists; intermediate training focuses on clinical integration, formulation-driven scenario design, adaptive titration, and debrief techniques; advanced training includes supervision of others, interpretation of multimodal biometric data, and participation in program governance (Pruden, 2025). Certification requires observed demonstration of technical fluency and clinical decision-making during simulated and real sessions (Ienca et al., 2017). To restate plainly: clinicians need to prove they can manage both the hardware and the therapy before practicing independently.

Ethical stewardship requires transparency about data and algorithms (Lazarou & Exarchos, 2024). Informed consent documents should clearly state what biometric and behavioral data will be collected, how long it will be stored, who may access it, and under what conditions data might be used for research or supervision (Casson, 2019). When adaptive algorithms are employed, clinicians must be able to explain their role and retain authority to override automated adjustments. Keep this clinical translation in mind: patients must understand both the experience you will create and the data traces it will leave (Casson, 2019).

Practical governance includes vendor contracting that secures clinical rights to data, requires transparent update logs for software and algorithmic changes, and specifies service-level agreements for maintenance and incident response (Ghadi et al., 2025). Prefer vendors who permit local data control or who support auditable, documented cloud architectures that meet healthcare security standards (Li et al., 2025). A short clinical reminder: vendor contracts are clinical governance documents and should be reviewed by compliance and clinical leaders together (Li et al., 2025). Measurement and quality improvement convert XR adoption from an experiment into accountable care (Li et al., 2025). Select a compact measurement bundle, pre/post session symptom rating, a single functional indicator tied to the patient's values, a session tolerability metric, and a safety log, and review these routinely. Use EMA to confirm real-world transfer when that is an explicit treatment aim. Pair quantitative flags with brief qualitative interviews to identify usability or cultural problems that numbers alone miss. To be clear clinically: measure deliberately, act on signals quickly, and prioritize measures that reflect patient-valued change. Research and implementation priorities to accelerate field maturation include dismantling studies that isolate active XR components, pragmatic trials comparing XR to evidence-based comparators, longitudinal designs that assess durability and relapse, and implementation research that focuses on equity, workforce readiness, and cost-effectiveness (Li et al., 2025). Engage in multisite registries where feasible and ensure datasets include demographic and contextual variables that permit analyses of who benefits. A concise clinical exhortation: contribute to the evidence base while protecting patients through careful governance (Li et al., 2025).

Equity and cultural competence must be built into content, procurement, and access strategies. Co-design content with representative patient groups, budget for accessible hardware options or loaner programs, and standardize default accessibility features. Monitor uptake across demographic groups and remediate disparities through targeted outreach and subsidized access. Clinically: make equity an operational goal with measurable targets, not an aspirational aside.

Workforce wellbeing is part of program quality. Structure XR clinical schedules to include setup and debrief time, provide technical support so clinicians are not device troubleshooters in-session, rotate high-intensity caseloads, and create routine forums for case debriefing and emotional processing (Jiao, 2024). Clinician resilience protects patients; an overstretched workforce undermines both care and safety. In practical terms: staff the program to preserve clinician focus on therapeutic work.

Operational playbook for immediate implementation: (Chennupati, 2025) define a narrow clinical use-case and success metrics; (Freeman et al., 2017) select the minimal XR modality and content aligned to that use-case; (Ikwuanusi et al., 2023) draft safety screening and enhanced consent materials; (Godfrey et al., 2021) run a short clinician training and two supervised pilot cases; (Layode et al., 2024) collect the measurement bundle for every session and meet weekly during the pilot to review signals; (Canali et al., 2022) iterate content or procedures based on data and patient narratives; (Ferrar et al., 2021) codify vendor contracts and data governance before scaling; (Hughes & Kalra, 2023) create a supervision cadence and an ethics review schedule; and (Basystiuk et al., 2024) plan for scale with hub-and-spoke or shared-service models (Smuck et al., 2021). A final clarifying sentence: start small, measure faithfully, and scale only when evidence and operations support expansion (Kim & Backonja, 2025).

To close, Extended Reality offers therapists a powerful, generative set of tools for producing controlled experiential learning, but its promise depends on disciplined clinical application. XR should be used to enable experiences that are otherwise difficult to access safely, to provide repeated practice under graded conditions, and to generate objective markers that enrich rather than replace clinical judgment. The clinician's enduring responsibility is to translate immersive experience into durable, meaningful change through careful formulation, ethical governance, measurement, and humane integration. A final clinical summation: introduce XR deliberately, guard patient welfare vigilantly, measure what matters, and let human clinical wisdom guide technological use so that XR becomes a responsible and effective extension of mental health care (Radanliev, 2025).

Ultimately, Extended Reality is a set of clinical instruments whose value will be judged by their ability to produce durable, meaningful change in people's lives (Back et al., 2022). When used thoughtfully, XR can create experiences that are otherwise inaccessible, provide precise titration of challenge, reveal objective markers of engagement, and accelerate therapeutic learning. Yet technology alone does not cure; the therapeutic relationship, clinical formulation, and interpretive work that follow immersion remain the mechanisms by which change generalizes into daily functioning. The practical imperative for clinicians and leaders is therefore clear: adopt XR deliberately, govern it rigorously, measure what matters, and center the humanity of those you serve so that the promise of immersive care translates into equitable, reliable, and lasting benefit. Wearable sensors provide continuous physiological monitoring, supporting adaptive and personalized interventions.

REFERENCES

Adegoke, K., Adegoke, A., Dawodu, D., Bayowa, A., & Adekoya, A (2025). Interoperability in digital healthcare: Enhancing consumer health and transforming care systems.

Agarwal, S., Jalan, M., Hill, R., Pantalone, E., Thrul, J., Sharma, R., Wilcox, H. C., & Robinson, K. A. (2025). Framework to Assist Stakeholders in Technology Evaluation for Recovery (Freeman et al., 2017) to Mental Health and Wellness. *BMC Health Services Research*, *25*, 623. Advance online publication. DOI: 10.1186/s12913-025-12418-0 PMID: 40307807

Aiken, L. H., Lasater, K. B., Sloane, D. M., Pogue, C. A., Rosenbaum, K. E. F., & Muir, K. J.US Clinician Wellbeing Study Consortium. (2023, July). Physician and nurse well-being and preferred interventions to address burnout in hospital practice: Factors associated with turnover, outcomes, and patient safety. [). American Medical Association.]. *JAMA Health Forum*, *4*(7), e231809–e231809. DOI: 10.1001/jamahealthforum.2023.1809 PMID: 37418269

Akhtar, Z. B., & Rawol, A. T. (2024). Artificial intelligence (Tizzard, 2025) and extended reality (XR): A biomedical engineering perspective investigation analysis. *Indonesian Journal of Electronics, Electromedical Engineering, and Medical Informatics*, *6*(3). Advance online publication. DOI: 10.35882/ijeeemi.v6i3.5

Akhtar, Z. B., & Rawol, A. T. (2025). Artificial Intelligence (Leivaditis & Sepetis, 2025) & Extended Reality (Reddy, 2025) within Healthcare: A Multidimensional Biomedical Engineering (Rajpal, 2025) Investigative Exploration. *Biomed. Clin. Res. J*, *1*, 1–22.

Akinode, A. O., Ayadi, O. E., Ezerioha, C. C., & Chika, P (2025). Machine Learning Approaches for Early Detection of Mental Health Disorders Using Wearable Devices and Big Data Analytics. environments, 4, 5.

Allgaier, J., Mulansky, L., Draelos, R. L., & Pryss, R. (2023). How does the model make predictions? A systematic literature review on the explainability power of machine learning in healthcare. *Artificial Intelligence in Medicine*, *143*, 102616. DOI: 10.1016/j.artmed.2023.102616 PMID: 37673561

Almadani, B., Kaisar, H., Thoker, I. R., & Aliyu, F. (2025). A systematic survey of distributed decision support systems in healthcare. *Systems*, *13*(3), 157. DOI: 10.3390/systems13030157

American Psychiatric Association. (2023). Digital [Resource Document. APA.]. *Mental Health (Detroit, Mich.)*, •••, 101.

Anklam, E., Bahl, M. I., Ball, R., Beger, R. D., Cohen, J., Fitzpatrick, S., Girard, P., Halamoda-Kenzaoui, B., Hinton, D., Hirose, A., Hoeveler, A., Honma, M., Hugas, M., Ishida, S., Kass, G. E. N., Kojima, H., Krefting, I., Liachenko, S., Liu, Y., & Slikker, W.Jr. (2022). Emerging technologies and their impact on regulatory science. *Experimental Biology and Medicine (Maywood, N.J.)*, *247*(1), 1–75. DOI: 10.1177/15353702211052280 PMID: 34783606

Babu, A., & Joseph, A. P. (2025). Digital wellness or digital dependency? A critical examination of mental health apps and their implications. *Frontiers in Psychiatry*, *16*, 1581779. DOI: 10.3389/fpsyt.2025.1581779 PMID: 40248604

Back, S. E., Acierno, R., Saraiya, T. C., Harley, B., Wangelin, B., Jarnecke, A. M., McTeague, L. M., Brown, D. G., Santa Ana, E., & Rothbaum, A. O. (2022). Enhancing Prolonged Exposure therapy for PTSD using physiological biomarker-driven technology. *Contemporary Clinical Trials Communications*, *28*, 100940. DOI: 10.1016/j.conctc.2022.100940 PMID: 35664505

Baka, E., Tan, Y.-R., Wong, B. L. H., Xing, Z., & Yap, P. (2025). A scoping review of digital interventions for the promotion of mental health and prevention of mental health conditions for young people. *Oxford Open Digital Health*, *3*, oqaf005. DOI: 10.1093/oodh/oqaf005 PMID: 40230873

Ball, H., Eisner, E., Nicholas, J., Wilson, P., & Bucci, S. (2025). How theories, models, and frameworks have been used to implement digital health interventions in services for people with severe mental health problems: A scoping review. *BMC Public Health*, *25*(1), 1023. DOI: 10.1186/s12889-025-22189-2 PMID: 40098003

Basystiuk, O., Rybchak, Z., Zavushchak, I., & Marikutsa, U. (2024). Evaluation of multimodal data synchronization tools. *Comput. Des. Syst. Theory Pract*, *6*(3), 104–111. DOI: 10.23939/cds2024.03.104

Baumann, S., Stone, R. T., & Abdelall, E. (2024). Introducing a remote patient monitoring usability impact model to overcome challenges. *Sensors (Basel)*, *24*(12), 3977. DOI: 10.3390/s24123977 PMID: 38931760

Bayor, A. A., Li, J., Yang, I. A., & Varnfield, M. (2025). Designing Clinical Decision Support Systems (CDSS)—A User-Centered Lens of the Design Characteristics, Challenges, and Implications: Systematic Review. *Journal of Medical Internet Research*, *27*, e63733. DOI: 10.2196/63733 PMID: 40540451

Bibi, P (2024). Establishing Transparency and Accountability in AI: Ethical Standards for Data Governance and Automated Systems. In.

Boda, V. V. R., & Allam, H. (2022). Ready for Anything: Disaster Recovery Strategies Every Healthcare IT Team Should Know. *International Journal of Emerging Trends in Computer Science and Information Technology*, *3*(1), 38–46. DOI: 10.63282/3050-9246.IJETCSIT-V3I1P105

Boffet, A., Arsac, L. M., Ibanez, V., Sauvet, F., & Deschodt-Arsac, V. (2025). Detection of Cognitive Load Modulation by EDA and HRV. *Sensors (Basel)*, *25*(8), 2343. DOI: 10.3390/s25082343 PMID: 40285033

Bond, R. R., Mulvenna, M. D., Potts, C., O'Neill, S., Ennis, E., & Torous, J. (2023). Digital transformation of mental health services. *Npj Mental Health Research*, *2*(1), 13. DOI: 10.1038/s44184-023-00033-y PMID: 38609479

Canali, S., Schiaffonati, V., & Aliverti, A. (2022). Challenges and recommendations for wearable devices in digital health: Data quality, interoperability, health equity, fairness. *PLOS Digital Health*, *1*(10), e0000104. DOI: 10.1371/journal.pdig.0000104 PMID: 36812619

Carl, E., Stein, A. T., Levihn-Coon, A., Pogue, J. R., Rothbaum, B., Emmelkamp, P., Asmundson, G. J. G., Carlbring, P., & Powers, M. B. (2019). Virtual reality exposure therapy for anxiety and related disorders: A meta-analysis of randomized controlled trials. *Journal of Anxiety Disorders*, *61*, 27–36. DOI: 10.1016/j.janxdis.2018.08.003 PMID: 30287083

Casson, A. J. (2019). Wearable EEG and beyond. *Biomedical Engineering Letters*, *9*(1), 53–71. DOI: 10.1007/s13534-018-00093-6 PMID: 30956880

Chaabene, S., Boudaya, A., Bouaziz, B., & Chaari, L. (2025). An overview of methods and techniques in multimodal data fusion with application to healthcare. *International Journal of Data Science and Analytics*, *20*(4), 1–25. DOI: 10.1007/s41060-025-00715-0

Chen, Z. S., Galatzer-Levy, I. R., Bigio, B., Nasca, C., & Zhang, Y. (2022). Modern views of machine learning for precision psychiatry. *Patterns (New York, N.Y.)*, *3*(11), 100602. DOI: 10.1016/j.patter.2022.100602 PMID: 36419447

Chennupati, N. (2025). Securing the Automated Enterprise: A Framework for Mitigating Security and Privacy Risks in AI-Driven Workflow Automation. *Journal of Computer Science and Technology Studies*, *7*(3), 624–632. DOI: 10.32996/jcsts.2025.7.3.71

Chithra, N., & Bhambri, P. (2024). Ethics in sustainable technology. In *Handbook of Technological Sustainability* (pp. 245–256). CRC Press. DOI: 10.1201/9781003475989-21

Clemens-Meyer, F. H., Lepot, M., Blumensaat, F., Leutnant, D., & Gruber, G. (2021). In Bertrand-Krajewski, J.-L., Clemens-Meyer, F., Lepot, M., & Publishing, I. W. A. (Eds.), *Data validation and data quality assessment. Metrology in Urban Drainage and Stormwater Management: Plug and Pray* (pp. 327–390).

Correa, T., Pavez, I., & Contreras, J. (2021). Digital inequality and mobiles: opportunities and challenges of relying on smartphones for digital inclusion in disadvantaged contexts. Handbook of digital inequality, 62-74.

Crameri, L., Hettiarachchi, I. T., & Hanoun, S. (2021). Effects of dynamic resilience on the reactivity of vagally mediated heart rate variability. *Frontiers in Psychology, 11*, 579210. DOI: 10.3389/fpsyg.2020.579210 PMID: 33551903

Cristofaro, M., & Giardino, P. L. (2025). Surfing the AI waves: The historical evolution of artificial intelligence in management and organizational studies and practices. *Journal of Management History*. Advance online publication. DOI: 10.1108/JMH-01-2025-0002

De Kock, J. H., Latham, H. A., Leslie, S. J., Grindle, M., Munoz, S. A., Ellis, L., Polson, R., & O'Malley, C. M. (2021). A rapid review of the impact of COVID-19 on the mental health of healthcare workers: Implications for supporting psychological well-being. *BMC Public Health, 21*(1), 104. DOI: 10.1186/s12889-020-10070-3 PMID: 33422039

Elfouly, T., & Alouani, A. (2025). A comprehensive survey on wearable computing for mental and physical health monitoring. *Electronics (Basel), 14*(17), 3443. DOI: 10.3390/electronics14173443

Engel, G. L. (1977). The need for a new medical model: A challenge for biomedicine. *Science, 196*(4286), 129–136. DOI: 10.1126/science.847460 PMID: 847460

Fanarioti, A. K., & Karpouzis, K. (2025). Artificial Intelligence and the Future of Mental Health in a Digitally Transformed World. *Computers, 14*(7), 259. DOI: 10.3390/computers14070259

Ferrar, J., Griffith, G. J., Skirrow, C., Cashdollar, N., Taptiklis, N., Dobson, J., Cree, F., Cormack, F. K., Barnett, J. H., & Munafò, M. R. (2021). Developing digital tools for remote clinical research: How to evaluate the validity and practicality of active assessments in field settings. *Journal of Medical Internet Research, 23*(6), e26004. DOI: 10.2196/26004 PMID: 34142972

Ferrara, E. (2024). Large language models for wearable sensor-based human activity recognition, health monitoring, and behavioral modeling: A survey of early trends, datasets, and challenges. *Sensors (Basel), 24*(15), 5045. DOI: 10.3390/s24155045 PMID: 39124092

Fleming, L. E., Maycock, B., White, M. P., & Depledge, M. H. (2019). Fostering human health through ocean sustainability in the 21st century. *People and Nature, 1*(3), 276–283. DOI: 10.1002/pan3.10038

Friend, S. H., Ginsburg, G. S., Picard, R. W., & Drazen, J. M. (2024). Key issues as wearable digital health technologies enter clinical care. *The New England Journal of Medicine, 390*(12), 1118–1127. DOI: 10.1056/NEJMra2307160 PMID: 38507754

Ghadi, Y. Y., Shah, S. F. A., Waheed, W., Mazhar, T., Ahmad, W., Saeed, M. M., & Hamam, H. (2025). Integration of wearable technology and artificial intelligence in digital health for remote patient care. *Journal of Cloud Computing (Heidelberg, Germany), 14*(1), 39. DOI: 10.1186/s13677-025-00759-4

Ghanim, R., Kaushik, A., Park, J., & Abramson, A. (2023). Communication protocols integrating wearables, ingestibles, and implantables for closed-loop therapies. *Device, 1*(3), 100092. DOI: 10.1016/j.device.2023.100092

Gkintoni, E., Vassilopoulos, S. P., & Nikolaou, G. (2025). Next-generation cognitive-behavioral therapy for depression: Integrating digital tools, teletherapy, and personalization for enhanced mental health outcomes. *Medicina (Kaunas, Lithuania), 61*(3), 431. DOI: 10.3390/medicina61030431 PMID: 40142242

Glass, J. E., Tiffany, B., Matson, T. E., Lim, C., Gundersen, G., Kimbel, K., Hartzler, A. L., Curran, G. M., McWethy, A. G., Caldeiro, R. M., & Bradley, K. A. (2022). Approaches for implementing digital interventions for alcohol use disorders in primary care: A qualitative, user-centered design study. *Implementation Research and Practice, 3*, 26334895221135264. DOI: 10.1177/26334895221135264 PMID: 37091101

Godfrey, A., Vandendriessche, B., Bakker, J. P., Fitzer-Attas, C., Gujar, N., Hobbs, M., Liu, Q., Northcott, C. A., Parks, V., Wood, W. A., Zipunnikov, V., Wagner, J. A., & Izmailova, E. S. (2021). Fit-for-purpose biometric monitoring technologies: Leveraging the laboratory biomarker experience. *Clinical and Translational Science, 14*(1), 62–74. DOI: 10.1111/cts.12865 PMID: 32770726

Goktas, P., & Grzybowski, A. (2025). Shaping the future of healthcare: Ethical clinical challenges and pathways to trustworthy AI. *Journal of Clinical Medicine, 14*(5), 1605. DOI: 10.3390/jcm14051605 PMID: 40095575

Hall, C. L., Gómez Bergin, A. D., & Rennick-Egglestone, S. (2024). Research into digital health intervention for mental health: 25-year retrospective on the ethical and legal challenges. *Journal of Medical Internet Research, 26*, e58939. DOI: 10.2196/58939 PMID: 39250796

Hickey, B. A., Chalmers, T., Newton, P., Lin, C.-T., Sibbritt, D., McLachlan, C. S., Clifton-Bligh, R., Morley, J., & Lal, S. (2021). Smart devices and wearable technologies to detect and monitor mental health conditions and stress: A systematic review. *Sensors (Basel), 21*(10), 3461. DOI: 10.3390/s21103461 PMID: 34065620

Hiland, E. B. (2021). *Therapy tech: The digital transformation of mental healthcare*. U of Minnesota Press. DOI: 10.5749/j.ctv1xp9q3t

Hilty, D. M., Armstrong, C. M., Luxton, D. D., Gentry, M. T., & Krupinski, E. A. (2021). A scoping review of sensors, wearables, and remote monitoring for behavioral health: Uses, outcomes, clinical competencies, and research directions. *Journal of Technology in Behavioral Science, 6*(2), 278–313. DOI: 10.1007/s41347-021-00199-2 PMID: 33501372

Holly, L., Thom, S., Elzemety, M., Murage, B., Mathieson, K., & Iñigo Petralanda, M. I. (2023). Strengthening health data governance: New equity and rights-based principles. *International Journal of Health Governance, 28*(3), 225–237. DOI: 10.1108/IJHG-11-2022-0104

Huang, J., Wang, H., Wu, Q., Yin, J., Zhou, H., & He, Y. (2024). Clinical research on neurological and psychiatric diagnosis and monitoring using wearable devices: A literature review. *Interdisciplinary Medicine, 2*(4), e20230037. DOI: 10.1002/INMD.20230037

Hughes, N., & Kalra, D. (2023). Data standards and platform interoperability. In *Real-World Evidence in Medical Product Development* (pp. 79–107). Springer. DOI: 10.1007/978-3-031-26328-6_6

Ienca, M., Fabrice, J., Elger, B., Caon, M., Scoccia Pappagallo, A., Kressig, R. W., & Wangmo, T. (2017). Intelligent assistive technology for Alzheimer's disease and other dementias: A systematic review. *Journal of Alzheimer's Disease, 56*(4), 1301–1340. DOI: 10.3233/JAD-161037 PMID: 28222516

Ikwuanusi, U. F., Adepoju, P. A., & Odionu, C. S (2023). Advancing ethical AI practices to solve data privacy issues in library systems. International journal of multidisciplinary research updates, 6(1), 033-044.

Immanuel, S., Teferra, M. N., Baumert, M., & Bidargaddi, N. (2023). Heart rate variability for evaluating psychological stress changes in healthy adults: A scoping review. *Neuropsychobiology*, *82*(4), 187–202. DOI: 10.1159/000530376 PMID: 37290411

Inkster, B., Knibbs, C., & Bada, M. (2023). Cybersecurity: A critical priority for digital mental health. *Frontiers in Digital Health*, *5*, 1242264. DOI: 10.3389/fdgth.2023.1242264 PMID: 37781452

Islam, R., & Bae, S. W. (2024). Revolutionizing mental health support: An innovative affective mobile framework for dynamic, proactive, and context-adaptive conversational agents. arXiv preprint arXiv:2406.15942.

Iwaya, L. H., Babar, M. A., Rashid, A., & Wijayarathna, C. (2023). On the privacy of mental health apps: An empirical investigation and its implications for app development. *Empirical Software Engineering*, *28*(1), 2. DOI: 10.1007/s10664-022-10236-0 PMID: 36407814

Jain, A., & Jain, A (2025). AI-Based Emotion Detection System in Healthcare for Patient. Generative Artificial Intelligence for Biomedical and Smart Health Informatics, 455-470.

Jiao, C. (2024). A mental health monitoring system based on intelligent algorithms and biosensors: Algorithm behaviour analysis and intervention strategies. *Molecular & Cellular Biomechanics*, *21*(1), 357–357. DOI: 10.62617/mcb.v21i1.357

Johnson, K. B., Wei, W. Q., Weeraratne, D., Frisse, M. E., Misulis, K., Rhee, K., Zhao, J., & Snowdon, J. L. (2021). Precision medicine, AI, and the future of personalized health care. *Clinical and Translational Science*, *14*(1), 86–93. DOI: 10.1111/cts.12884 PMID: 32961010

Kang, H. S., & Exworthy, M. (2022). Wearing the future—wearables to empower users to take greater responsibility for their health and care: Scoping review. *JMIR mHealth and uHealth*, *10*(7), e35684. DOI: 10.2196/35684 PMID: 35830222

Kargarandehkordi, A., Li, S., Lin, K., Phillips, K. T., Benzo, R. M., & Washington, P. (2025). Fusing wearable biosensors with artificial intelligence for mental health monitoring: A systematic review. *Biosensors (Basel)*, *15*(4), 202. DOI: 10.3390/bios15040202 PMID: 40277515

Khoo, Y. X., Kang, R. M., Reynolds, T. L., & Mentis, H. M. (2024). The comprehensiveness of mental health application users' privacy and security concerns. *CHI Conference on Human Factors in Computing Systems*, 16 pages.

Kim, J., & Backonja, U. (2025). Digital health equity frameworks and key concepts: A scoping review. *Journal of the American Medical Informatics Association : JAMIA*, *32*(1), 45–59. DOI: 10.1093/jamia/ocaf017 PMID: 39936843

Kostadimas, D., Kasapakis, V., & Kotis, K. (2025). A systematic review on the combination of VR, IoT and AI technologies, and their integration in applications. *Future Internet*, *17*(4), 163. DOI: 10.3390/fi17040163

Kourtesis, P. (2024). A comprehensive review of multimodal XR applications, risks, and ethical challenges in the metaverse. *Multimodal Technologies and Interaction*, *8*(11), 98. DOI: 10.3390/mti8110098

Kumar, P. (2025). Securing Digital-First Healthcare: AI, Blockchain, and Cloud Architectures for Personal Health Data Protection. *International Journal of Applied Mathematics*, *38*(7s).

Kumar, T., Arora, M., Verma, V., Bhushan, S., & Lalar, S. (2024). Biometric System Integration in Public Health: Challenges and Solutions. In Computational Intelligence and Mathematical Applications (pp. 168-173). CRC Press.

Lamb, R., Choi, I., & Owens, T (2025). Convergence of Extended Reality, Artificial Intelligence, Machine Leaning, and Wearable Sensors in the Field of Education. Mental Health Virtual Reality: The Power of Immersive Worlds, 113-128.

Lay, W., Gasparini, L., Siero, W., & Hughes, E. K. (2025). A rapid review of the benefits and challenges of dynamic consent. *Research Ethics*, *21*(1), 180–202. DOI: 10.1177/17470161241278064

Layode, O., Naiho, H. N. N., Adeleke, G. S., Udeh, E. O., & Labake, T. T. (2024). Data privacy and security challenges in environmental research: Approaches to safeguarding sensitive information. *International Journal of Applied Research in Social Sciences*, *6*(6), 1193–1214. DOI: 10.51594/ijarss.v6i6.1210

Lazarou, E., & Exarchos, T. P. (2024). Predicting stress levels using physiological data: Real-time stress prediction models utilizing wearable devices. *AIMS Neuroscience*, *11*(2), 76–102. DOI: 10.3934/Neuroscience.2024006 PMID: 38988886

Leivaditis, V., & Sepetis, A (2025). Digital Transformation As A Catalyst For Sustainable Health Care Systems: A Narrative Review Of Current Evidence. International Journal of Innovation Management, 29(05n06), 2540009.

Li, M., Patel, J., & Katapally, T. R. (2025). The impact of extended reality cognitive behavioral therapy on mental disorders among children and youth: A systematic review and meta-analysis protocol. *PLoS One*, *20*(3), e0315313. DOI: 10.1371/journal.pone.0315313 PMID: 40048453

Li, M., Patel, J., & Katapally, T. R. (2025). The impact of extended reality cognitive behavioral therapy on mental disorders among children and youth: A systematic review and meta-analysis protocol. *PLoS One*, *20*(3), e0315313. DOI: 10.1371/journal.pone.0315313 PMID: 40048453

Li, M., Patel, J., & Katapally, T. R. (2025). The impact of extended reality cognitive behavioral therapy on mental disorders among children and youth: A systematic review and meta-analysis protocol. *PLoS One*, *20*(3), e0315313. DOI: 10.1371/journal.pone.0315313 PMID: 40048453

Li, M., Patel, J., & Katapally, T. R. (2025). The impact of extended reality cognitive behavioral therapy on mental disorders among children and youth: A systematic review and meta-analysis protocol. *PLoS One*, *20*(3), e0315313. DOI: 10.1371/journal.pone.0315313 PMID: 40048453

Lindner, P., Miloff, A., & Carlbring, P. (2024). The future of virtual reality therapy: Applications, challenges, and research directions. *Frontiers in Virtual Reality*, *5*, 112345.

Liu, M., & Schueller, S. M. (2023). Moving evidence-based mental health interventions into practice: Implementation of digital mental health interventions. *Current Treatment Options in Psychiatry*, *10*(4), 333–345. DOI: 10.1007/s40501-023-00298-2

Livieri, G., Mangina, E., Protopapadakis, E. D., & Panayiotou, A. G. (2025). The gaps and challenges in digital health technology use as perceived by patients: A scoping review and narrative meta-synthesis. *Frontiers in Digital Health*, *7*, 1474956. DOI: 10.3389/fdgth.2025.1474956 PMID: 40212901

Lorke, M., & Stefanou, T. (2025). Improving research and development of wearable assistive and rehabilitation technologies: A systematic review on diversity factors. *Journal of Neuroengineering and Rehabilitation*, *22*(1), 31. DOI: 10.1186/s12984-025-01562-7 PMID: 39985039

Ma, C.-B., Shang, X., Sun, M., Bo, X., Bai, J., Du, Y., & Zhou, M. (2025). Emerging Multifunctional Wearable Sensors: Integrating Multimodal Sweat Analysis and Advanced Material Technologies for Next-Generation Health Monitoring. *ACS Sensors*, *10*(4), 2388–2408. DOI: 10.1021/acssensors.4c03396 PMID: 40162570

Mackey, S., Aghaeepour, N., Gaudilliere, B., Kao, M.-C., Kaptan, M., Lannon, E., Pfyffer, D., & Weber, K. (2025). Innovations in acute and chronic pain biomarkers: Enhancing diagnosis and personalized therapy. *Regional Anesthesia and Pain Medicine*, *50*(2), 110–120. DOI: 10.1136/rapm-2024-106030 PMID: 39909549

Mahon, D. (2023). Empirically Supported Treatments: A Brief History. In Evidence Based Counselling & Psychotherapy for the 21st Century Practitioner (pp. 3-14). Emerald Publishing Limited. DOI: 10.1108/978-1-80455-732-720231001

Martinez-Martin, N., Marcandalli, J., Huang, C. S., Arthur, C. P., Perotti, M., Foglierini, M., Ho, H., Dosey, A. M., Shriver, S., Payandeh, J., Leitner, A., Lanzavecchia, A., Perez, L., & Ciferri, C. (2018). An unbiased screen for human cytomegalovirus identifies neuropilin-2 as a central viral receptor. *Cell*, *174*(5), 1158–1171. DOI: 10.1016/j.cell.2018.06.028 PMID: 30057110

Mitsea, E., Drigas, A., & Skianis, C. (2024). Artificial intelligence, immersive technologies, and neurotechnologies in breathing interventions for mental and emotional health: A systematic review. *Electronics (Basel)*, *13*(12), 2253. DOI: 10.3390/electronics13122253

Mohammad, N. (2021). Enhancing security and privacy in multi-cloud environments: A comprehensive study on encryption techniques and access control mechanisms. [IJCET]. *International Journal of Computer Engineering and Technology*, *12*(2), 51–63.

Mohr, D. C., Zhang, M., & Schueller, S. M. (2017). Personal sensing: Understanding mental health using ubiquitous sensors and machine learning. *Annual Review of Clinical Psychology*, *13*(1), 23–47. DOI: 10.1146/annurev-clinpsy-032816-044949 PMID: 28375728

Mone, V., & Fayazullaeva, S. (2023). Health data on the go: Navigating privacy concerns with wearable technologies. *Legal Information Management*, *23*(3), 179–188. DOI: 10.1017/S1472669623000427

Morey, D. A., Rayo, M. F., & Woods, D. D. (2025). Empirically derived evaluation requirements for responsible deployments of AI in safety-critical settings. *NPJ Digital Medicine*, *8*(1), 374. DOI: 10.1038/s41746-025-01784-y PMID: 40533485

Morgan, J. W., Patel, R. A., & Campbell, S. (2025). Practical considerations of clinical XR (Singh & Chandra, 2025) deployments. *Frontiers in Virtual Reality*, *6*, 1517402. DOI: 10.3389/frvir.2025.1517402

Moriarty, A. S., Meader, N., Snell, K. I., Riley, R. D., Paton, L. W., Dawson, S., Hendon, J., Chew-Graham, C. A., Gilbody, S., Churchill, R., Phillips, R. S., Ali, S., & McMillan, D. (2022). Predicting relapse or recurrence of depression: Systematic review of prognostic models. *The British Journal of Psychiatry : The Journal of Mental Science*, *221*(2), 448–458. DOI: 10.1192/bjp.2021.218 PMID: 35048843

Mulukuntla, S. (2025). Monitoring and Remote Patient Management with Immersive Technologies. In Augmented Wellness: Exploring the Power of VR and AR in Healthcare (pp. 197-218). Springer. DOI: 10.1007/978-981-96-2952-7_9

Obermeyer, Z., Powers, B., Vogeli, C., & Mullainathan, S. (2019). Dissecting racial bias in an algorithm used to manage the health of populations. *Science*, *366*(6464), 447–453. DOI: 10.1126/science.aax2342 PMID: 31649194

Omiyefa, S. (2025). Artificial intelligence and machine learning in precision mental health diagnostics and predictive treatment models. *Int J Res Publ Rev*, *6*(3), 85–99. DOI: 10.55248/gengpi.6.0325.1107

Ong, T., Ivanova, J., Soni, H., Barrera, J., Cummins, M., Welch, B. M., & Bunnell, B. E. (2025). Mental health clients' perspectives on telehealth-based virtual reality therapy. *Frontiers in Virtual Reality*, *6*, 1595326. DOI: 10.3389/frvir.2025.1595326

Panarese, P., Grasso, M. M., & Solinas, C. (2025). Algorithmic bias, fairness, and inclusivity: A multilevel framework for justice-oriented AI. *AI & Society*, •••, 1–23. DOI: 10.1007/s00146-025-02451-2

Pedram, S., & Piatkowski, T. (2025). Exploring the potential of virtual reality (Johnson et al., 2021) in mental healthcare: A systematic literature review. *Virtual Reality (Waltham Cross)*, *29*(3), 135. DOI: 10.1007/s10055-025-01181-6

Pruden, S (2025). Implementing Depression Screening and Treatment Algorithms to Reduce Post-Operative Complications for Patients Undergoing Cardiac Surgery The University of North Carolina at Chapel Hill].

Radanliev, P. (2025). Privacy, ethics, transparency, and accountability in AI systems for wearable devices. *Frontiers in Digital Health*, *7*, 1431246. DOI: 10.3389/fdgth.2025.1431246 PMID: 40599875

Rajpal, S. (2025). Exploring the Role of Virtual Reality and Metaverse in Treating Mental Health: Operating Models and Challenges in Adoption. *Journal of Computer and Communications*, *13*(10), 1–22. DOI: 10.4236/jcc.2025.1310001

Reddy, K. J. (2025). Integrating Technology into Clinical Practice. In Innovations in Neurocognitive Rehabilitation: Harnessing Technology for Effective Therapy (pp. 329-350). Springer. DOI: 10.1007/978-3-031-88117-6_15

Renuka, O., RadhaKrishnan, N., Priya, B. S., Jhansy, A., & Ezekiel, S (2025). Data privacy and protection: Legal and ethical challenges. Emerging Threats and Countermeasures in Cybersecurity, 433-465.

Ricciardi, F., & Zomaya, A. (2025). Perspectives on Managing AI Ethics in the Digital Age. *Information (Basel), 16*(2), 89. DOI: 10.3390/info16040318

Robinson, A., Flom, M., Forman-Hoffman, V. L., Histon, T., Levy, M., Darcy, A., Ajayi, T., Mohr, D. C., Wicks, P., Greene, C., & Montgomery, R. M. (2024). Equity in digital mental health interventions in the United States: Where to next? *Journal of Medical Internet Research, 26*, e59939. DOI: 10.2196/59939 PMID: 39316436

Ross, G., Zhao, Y., Bosman, A., Geballa-Koukoula, A., Zhou, H., Elliott, C., Nielen, M., Rafferty, K., & Salentijn, G (2022). Data handling and ethics of emerging smartphone-based (Glass et al., 2022) sensors–Part 1: best practices and current implementation.

Saganowski, S., Perz, B., Polak, A. G., & Kazienko, P (2022). Emotion recognition for everyday life using physiological signals from wearables: A systematic literature review. IEEE Transactions on Affective Computing, 14(3), 1876-1897. Pinel, P (1793). Traité médico-philosophique sur l'aliénation mentale.

Saksena, N., Matthan, R., Bhan, A., & Balsari, S. (2021). Rebooting consent in the digital age: A governance framework for health data exchange. *BMJ Global Health, 6*(Suppl 5), e005057. DOI: 10.1136/bmjgh-2021-005057 PMID: 34301754

Shah, R. V., Grennan, G., Zafar-Khan, M., Alim, F., Dey, S., Ramanathan, D., & Mishra, J. (2021). Personalized machine learning of depressed mood using wearables. *Translational Psychiatry, 11*(1), 338. DOI: 10.1038/s41398-021-01445-0 PMID: 34103481

Shatte, A. B., Hutchinson, D. M., & Teague, S. J. (2019). Machine learning in mental health: A scoping review of methods and applications. *Psychological Medicine, 49*(9), 1426–1448. DOI: 10.1017/S0033291719000151 PMID: 30744717

Sheikh, M., Qassem, M., & Kyriacou, P. A. (2021). Wearable, environmental, and smartphone-based passive sensing for mental health monitoring. *Frontiers in Digital Health, 3*, 662811. DOI: 10.3389/fdgth.2021.662811 PMID: 34713137

Smith, K. A., Blease, C., Faurholt-Jepsen, M., Firth, J., Van Daele, T., Moreno, C., Carlbring, P., Ebner-Priemer, U. W., Koutsouleris, N., Riper, H., Mouchabac, S., Torous, J., & Cipriani, A. (2023). Digital mental health: Challenges and next steps. *BMJ Mental Health, 26*(1), e300670. DOI: 10.1136/bmjment-2023-300670 PMID: 37197797

Smuck, M., Odonkor, C. A., Wilt, J. K., Schmidt, N., & Swiernik, M. A. (2021). The emerging clinical role of wearables: Factors for successful implementation in healthcare. *NPJ Digital Medicine*, *4*(1), 45. DOI: 10.1038/s41746-021-00418-3 PMID: 33692479

Spytska, L. (2025). The use of artificial intelligence in psychotherapy: Development of intelligent therapeutic systems. *BMC Psychology*, *13*(1), 175. DOI: 10.1186/s40359-025-02491-9 PMID: 40022267

Subu, M. A., Holmes, D., Arumugam, A., Al-Yateem, N., Maria Dias, J., Rahman, S. A., Waluyo, I., Ahmed, F. R., & Abraham, M. S. (2022). Traditional, religious, and cultural perspectives on mental illness: A qualitative study on causal beliefs and treatment use. *International Journal of Qualitative Studies on Health and Well-being*, *17*(1), 2123090. DOI: 10.1080/17482631.2022.2123090 PMID: 36097886

Sun, J., Lu, T., Shao, X., Han, Y., Xia, Y., Zheng, Y., Wang, Y., Li, X., Ravindran, A., Fan, L., Fang, Y., Zhang, X., Ravindran, N., Wang, Y., Liu, X., & Lu, L. (2025). Practical AI application in psychiatry: Historical review and future directions. *Molecular Psychiatry*, *30*(9), 4399–4408. DOI: 10.1038/s41380-025-03072-3 PMID: 40456953

Tavory, T. (2024). Regulating AI in mental health: Ethics of care perspective. *JMIR Mental Health*, *11*, e58493. DOI: 10.2196/58493 PMID: 39298759

Tizzard, C. L. (2025). Re-imagining Care for Aging Disabled Adults.

Tsai, Y. Y., Chen, Y. J., Lin, Y. F., Hsiao, F. C., Hsu, C. H., & Liao, L. D. (2025). Photoplethysmography-based HRV analysis and machine learning for real-time stress quantification in mental health applications. *APL Bioengineering*, *9*(2), 026103. DOI: 10.1063/5.0256590 PMID: 40191605

Vaidyam, A. N., Wisniewski, H., Halamka, J. D., Kashavan, M. S., & Torous, J. B. (2019). Chatbots and conversational agents in mental health: A review of the psychiatric landscape. *Canadian Journal of Psychiatry. Revue Canadienne de Psychiatrie*, *64*(7), 456–464. DOI: 10.1177/0706743719828977 PMID: 30897957

Vaidyam, A. N., Wisniewski, H., Halamka, J. D., Kashavan, M. S., & Torous, J. B. (2019). Chatbots and conversational agents in mental health: A review of the psychiatric landscape. *Canadian Journal of Psychiatry. Revue Canadienne de Psychiatrie*, *64*(7), 456–464. DOI: 10.1177/0706743719828977 PMID: 30897957

Verma, H., Mlynar, J., Schaer, R., Reichenbach, J., Jreige, M., Prior, J., Evéquoz, F., & Depeursinge, A. (2023). Rethinking the role of AI with physicians in oncology: revealing perspectives from clinical and research workflows. *Proceedings of the 2023 CHI conference on human factors in computing systems* DOI: 10.1145/3544548.3581506

Volckens, J., Haynes, E. N., Croisant, S. P., Cui, Y., Errett, N. A., Henry, H. F., Horney, J. A., Kwok, R. K., Magzamen, S., Rappold, A. G., Ravichandran, L., Reinlib, L., Ryan, P. H., & Shaughnessy, D. T. (2023). Health research in the wake of disasters: Challenges and opportunities for sensor science. *Environmental Health Perspectives*, *131*(6), 065002. DOI: 10.1289/EHP12270 PMID: 37389972

Walter, J. R., Xu, S., & Rogers, J. A. (2023). From lab to life: How wearable devices can improve health equity. *Nature Communications*, *14*, 44634. PMID: 38167483

Wang, Z., Xiong, H., Zhang, J., Yang, S., Boukhechba, M., Zhang, D., Barnes, L. E., & Dou, D. (2022). From personalized medicine to population health: A survey of mHealth sensing techniques. *IEEE Internet of Things Journal*, *9*(17), 15413–15434. DOI: 10.1109/JIOT.2022.3161046

Watson, D (2025). The dark side of mental health apps: Privacy concerns and therapeutic limitations. MentalHealthSigns.com.

Weiner, E. B., Dankwa-Mullan, I., Nelson, W. A., & Hassanpour, S. (2025). Ethical challenges and evolving strategies in the integration of artificial intelligence into clinical practice. *PLOS Digital Health*, *4*(4), e0000810. DOI: 10.1371/journal.pdig.0000810 PMID: 40198594

Wibberly, K. H. (2024). Preparing mental health providers for the future: The case for moving beyond the elective telehealth course to integrating telehealth training throughout the curriculum. *Frontiers in Psychology*, *14*, 1301569. DOI: 10.3389/fpsyg.2023.1301569 PMID: 38235285

Xing, Y., Yang, Y., Yang, K., Lu, A., Xing, L., Mackie, K., & Guo, F. (2025). Intelligent sensing devices and systems for personalized mental health. *Med-X*, *3*(1), 10. DOI: 10.1007/s44258-025-00057-3 PMID: 40837134

Zenker, S., Strech, D., Ihrig, K., Jahns, R., Müller, G., Schickhardt, C., Schmidt, G., Speer, R., Winkler, E., von Kielmansegg, S. G., & Drepper, J. (2022). Data protection-compliant broad consent for secondary use of health care data and human biosamples for (Mulukuntla, 2025) medical research: Towards a new German national standard. *Journal of Biomedical Informatics*, *131*, 104096. DOI: 10.1016/j.jbi.2022.104096 PMID: 35643273

Chapter 6
Psychophysiological Measurement in Digital Mental Health

ABSTRACT

Wearable sensors provide continuous, real-time physiological data—such as HRV, EEG, and EDA—offering insights into stress, cognitive load, and emotional regulation (Hilty et al., 2021). These measures enhance assessment accuracy and enable adaptive interventions through closed-loop systems. Clinical integration requires rigorous calibration, artifact rejection, and contextual interpretation to avoid misclassification (Ricciardi & Zomaya, 2025). When combined with behavioral and self-report data, wearables support precision care and proactive monitoring, detecting early signs of relapse or crisis (Ricciardi & Zomaya, 2025). Ethical considerations include consent, privacy, and equity in access. Governance frameworks must enforce encryption, retention limits, and transparency. Properly implemented, wearables bridge subjective experience and objective metrics, empowering both clinicians and patients.

INTRODUCTION

This chapter provides a practical and theoretical overview of psychophysiological measurement as a cornerstone of neuroadaptive mental health systems. It introduces key modalities, including EEG, heart rate variability, galvanic skin response, and functional near-infrared spectroscopy, and explains how these signals index cognitive load, emotional regulation, and stress. Emphasis is placed on multimodal integration, baseline calibration, and artifact management to ensure interpretability and reliability in applied settings. The chapter situates psychophysiological data within

DOI: 10.4018/979-8-3373-4997-8.ch006

the biopsychosocial model, cautioning against simplistic one-to-one mappings between signals and mental states. Clinical examples illustrate how physiological markers can complement self-report and observation in assessment, treatment monitoring, and biofeedback interventions. Limitations such as motion artifacts, contextual confounds, and interpretive ambiguity are discussed alongside advances in AI-enabled signal processing. Ethical considerations, including data sensitivity, consent, and clinical accountability, are woven throughout. By translating technical measurement concepts into clinician-relevant guidance, this chapter establishes psychophysiological sensing as a supportive, not determinative, source of evidence in mental health care.

PSCYHOPHYSIOLOGICAL MEASUREMENT

Psychophysiological measurement refers to the assessment of physiological responses that are associated with psychological processes. This interdisciplinary field combines principles from psychology, physiology, neuroscience, and biomedical engineering to understand how the mind and body interact. Psychophysiological measurements are crucial for exploring the underlying mechanisms of mental health, cognitive functions, and human-computer interactions. By capturing real-time data on physiological changes, researchers and clinicians can gain insights into emotional states, cognitive workload, stress levels, and overall mental well-being (Almadani et al., 2025). To be useful in applied contexts, measurements must be reliable, temporally precise, and interpreted within a pre-specified behavioral or situational frame, so design decisions should specify these criteria up front. For clinical teams, clear protocols for sensor placement, baseline recording, and artifact rejection are essential to produce reproducible signals for decision-making. For researchers, psychophysiological measures offer mechanistic anchors that can validate self-report and behavioral outcomes in experiments. Practitioners should treat physiological readouts as one component in a multimodal assessment strategy that includes observation and patient narrative.

The theoretical foundations of psychophysiological measurement are rooted in the biopsychosocial model, which posits that biological, psychological, and social factors all play a significant role in human health and behavior (Akinode et al., 2025). This model emphasizes the interconnectedness of the mind and body, suggesting that physiological responses can provide valuable information about psychological states (Martinez-Martin et al., 2018). For example, changes in heart rate, skin conductance, and brain activity can reflect emotional arousal, cognitive effort, and stress. When applying this framework, practitioners should operationalize which level (biological, psychological, social) is the primary focus for a given intervention and specify expected physiological correlates. Explicitly defining those expectations improves interpretation and helps avoid overgeneralizing single-sensor findings (Martinez-Martin et al., 2018). Researchers can test these mappings empirically by predefining hypotheses about how specific social contexts will modulate physiological markers. Clinicians can then integrate physiologic trends into case formulations and treatment planning without assuming direct one-to-one mappings to subjective states.

Several key methods are used in psychophysiological measurement, each offering unique insights into different aspects of psychological processes. Electroencephalography (Wang et al., 2022) measures electrical activity in the brain through electrodes placed on the scalp (Volckens et al., 2023). EEG is widely used in both clinical and research settings to monitor brain function, detect abnormalities, and study cognitive processes. For instance, EEG can reveal patterns of brain activity associated with attention, memory, and decision-making. It is also used in neurofeedback therapy, where individuals learn to regulate their brainwave patterns to improve mental health outcomes. To choose the appropriate modality, teams should match the temporal and spatial demands of their questions to the strengths of each sensor. Practical study protocols often combine methods to triangulate findings and increase confidence in inferences about psychological states (Casson, 2019).

Figure 1. Concept map of neuroadaptive systems.

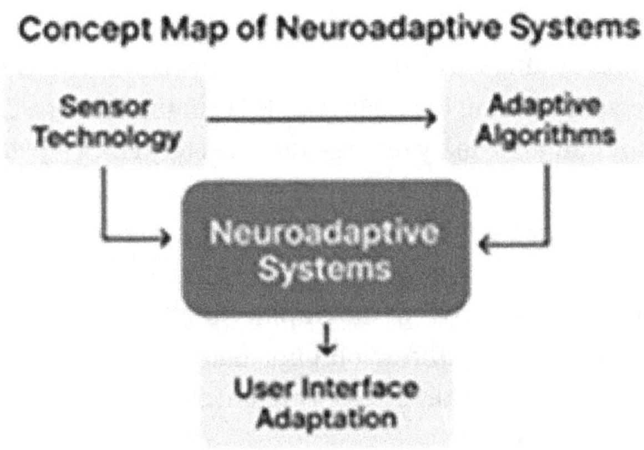

Electroencephalography measures electrical activity in the brain. It involves placing electrodes on the scalp to detect the tiny electrical impulses produced by brain cells, known as neurons. These impulses are recorded as waveforms, which can be analyzed to understand brain function and diagnose neurological conditions. EEG is widely used in both clinical and research settings due to its ability to provide real-time data on brain activity (Holly et al., 2023). For applied work, specify electrode montage, sampling rate, and filtering strategies in advance to ensure interpretability across sessions. Practitioners should expect and plan for common artifacts from muscle activity and eye movements, and include task-based baselines to aid comparison. When combined with behavioral markers or other physiological channels, EEG enhances temporal precision in mapping cognitive events (Obermeyer et al., 2019).

Experts such as Thomas Insel, Albert Rizzo, Rosalind Picard have advanced concepts like neuroadaptive systems.

However, EEG also has limitations (Shah et al., 2022). One major limitation is its sensitivity to motion artifacts, which can distort the recorded signals. This is particularly challenging in real-world settings where individuals may move or speak during the recording. Another limitation is the low spatial resolution of EEG, which makes it difficult to pinpoint the exact location of brain activity (Ricciardi & Zomaya, 2025). Unlike imaging techniques such as fMRI, which provide detailed images of brain structures, EEG provides a more general overview of brain function (Ricciardi & Zomaya, 2025). To mitigate these issues, incorporate artifact-reduction protocols and complementary sensors for source inference. Clearly report preprocessing steps and residual artifact rates when presenting findings. When spatial specificity is required, plan combined-modality recordings or task designs that reduce localization ambiguity.

Despite these limitations, advances in AI and ML have improved the viability of EEG in real-world settings (Kumar et al., 2024). AI models can filter out noise and motion artifacts, enhancing the quality of EEG data (Tsai et al., 2025). Machine learning algorithms can also analyze large datasets to identify patterns and predict outcomes, making EEG a powerful tool for personalized mental health interventions (Tsai et al., 2025). Successful application depends on transparent model evaluation using held-out, ecologically valid datasets. Teams must disclose training data characteristics and performance across demographic subgroups to assess generalizability. Clinicians should test algorithmic outputs against simple rule-based baselines before trust calibration (Tsai et al., 2025). Implement monitoring for model drift to maintain reliability over time .

In conclusion, EEG is a valuable tool for measuring brain activity and understanding cognitive and emotional processes (Akhtar & Rawol, 2025). Its applications in neurofeedback therapy, cognitive load assessment, and decision-making highlight its potential to improve mental health and cognitive performance. The integration of EEG with AI and ML further enhances its capabilities, allowing for adaptive and personalized interventions (Robinson et al., 2024). While EEG has limitations, ongoing research and technological advancements continue to expand its potential in both clinical and research settings (Robinson et al., 2024). To translate EEG research into practice, establish clear protocols, consent procedures, and outcome metrics that align with clinical goals (Robinson et al., 2024). Prioritize interdisciplinary collaboration to ensure technical solutions address real-world clinical constraints (Robinson et al., 2024).

Heart Rate Variability reflects the variation in time between heartbeats and is a key indicator of autonomic nervous system function (Renuka et al., 2025). HRV quantifies R-R interval variability and indexes parasympathetic modulation with high sensitivity to emotional state (Ienca et al., 2017). For reliable interpretation, collect multiple baseline epochs and report both time-domain and frequency-domain metrics. Define whether short-term (Saksena et al., 2021) or ultra-short (30–60 second) measures are acceptable for your clinical or research question (Ienca et al., 2017). Use consistent sensor placement and sampling specifications to ensure within-subject comparability across sessions (Ienca et al., 2017). Predefine artifact-rejection rules for ectopic beats and noisy segments to preserve data integrity (Ienca et al., 2017). When communicating results to patients, present HRV changes relative to their baseline rather than population norms (Ienca et al., 2017).

In mental health, HRV is used to monitor stress, anxiety, and emotional regulation. Research has shown that lower HRV is associated with higher levels of stress and anxiety, while higher HRV indicates better emotional resilience and adaptive capacity. For instance, veterans with PTSD have used HRV biofeedback during mindfulness therapy to improve emotional resilience. By learning to control their breathing and heart rate, they can enhance their HRV and reduce symptoms of anxiety and hyper-arousal. Clinicians should embed HRV training within clear behavioral goals and monitor both physiological and symptom change. Specify session length, breathing cadence targets, and progress markers to operationalize HRV biofeedback protocols. Report adherence metrics because dose of practice influences physiological change and clinical outcomes (Tsai et al., 2025).

Experts such as Thomas Insel, Albert Rizzo, Rosalind Picard have advanced concepts like neuroadaptive systems.

HRV is also used in workplace wellness programs to monitor employee stress levels and promote mental health. Wearable HRV sensors can provide real-time feedback on stress and relaxation, enabling employees to take proactive steps to manage their stress. For example, a company might implement HRV-based interventions such as guided breathing exercises or relaxation breaks during high-stress periods. By promoting better autonomic regulation, these interventions can enhance employee well-being and productivity. Ensure workplace programs respect voluntariness and separate health data from employment evaluative processes. Provide aggregated, de-identified summaries for organizational insights rather than individual-level monitoring. Include clear opt-in consent and data-deletion options to maintain employee autonomy and trust (Freeman et al., 2017).

The integration of HRV with machine learning (Fleming et al., 2019) models trained on large datasets can account for confounding factors such as age, fitness, and medication, improving the reliability of HRV-based assessments (Kang & Exworthy, 2022). ML algorithms can analyze HRV data to identify patterns and predict stress responses, enabling personalized interventions. For example, an AI-driven mental health app might use HRV data to tailor mindfulness exercises or cognitive behavioral therapy (Zenker et al., 2022) sessions to the user's current stress level. For responsible use, document which covariates the model adjusts for and report model performance across demographic strata. Implement continuous monitoring for model drift and periodically retrain models using new, representative data. Combine algorithmic outputs with clinician oversight to preserve safety and contextual judgment. Galvanic skin response measures the electrical conductance of the skin, which varies with its moisture level. This physiological response is primarily driven by sweat gland activity, which is controlled by the sympathetic nervous system. As such, GSR is a valuable indicator of emotional and physiological arousal. This chapter delves into the physiological basis of GSR, its applications in mental health and cognitive science, integration with AI and machine learning, real-world case studies, and its limitations. To apply GSR in clinical or research settings, define whether you are measuring tonic (Panarese et al., 2025) or phasic (Morey et al., 2025) conductance and set sampling and smoothing parameters accordingly. Clarify electrode placement and contact quality standards so that data are comparable across sessions and participants. When reporting results, present both raw conductance and standardized change scores relative to baseline to aid clinical interpretation. Finally, plan complementary measures to disambiguate arousal sources because GSR indicates arousal but not its affective valence (Weiner et al., 2025).

GSR has been widely used in mental health and cognitive science to monitor and assess emotional and physiological states (Correa et al., 2021). In exposure therapy for anxiety disorders, GSR sensors help therapists monitor patients' stress levels in real-time, allowing for adjustments to the therapeutic process. For example, individuals with social anxiety may wear GSR-equipped wristbands during virtual public speaking scenarios, enabling therapists to track their physiological responses and provide immediate feedback. In cognitive science, GSR is used to study the relationship between emotional arousal and cognitive processes. Researchers have employed GSR to investigate how stress and anxiety affect decision-making, attention, and memory. To implement GSR-supported interventions, predefine thresholds for in-session modulation to avoid ad hoc adjustments. Use combined behavioral markers, such as speech rate or task performance, to interpret GSR spikes in context. Train clinicians to translate GSR changes into brief, evidence-based in-session strategies like grounding or cognitive reframing (Kargarandehkordi et al., 2025).

The integration of GSR with AI and machine learning has opened new avenues for personalized and adaptive interventions (Morgan et al., 2025). AI algorithms can analyze GSR data in real-time, detecting patterns and trends that may indicate emotional or physiological states (De Kock et al., 2021). For instance, in adaptive learning environments, AI can use GSR data to identify when a student is experiencing stress or frustration, and adjust the instructional content or pacing accordingly (De Kock et al., 2021). In mental health care, AI-driven systems can leverage GSR data to personalize therapeutic interventions (De Kock et al., 2021). For example, an AI system might detect elevated GSR levels during a therapy session and suggest relaxation techniques or modify the therapeutic approach (De Kock et al., 2021). When deploying AI with GSR inputs, explicitly document model inputs, preprocessing steps, and decision rules so clinicians can evaluate recommendations (De Kock et al., 2021). Validate models on held-out, ecologically valid datasets and test performance across demographic subgroups to avoid biased predictions. Provide clinicians with interpretable summaries that link GSR features to proposed actions rather than opaque risk scores (De Kock et al., 2021).

Experts such as Thomas Insel, Albert Rizzo, Rosalind Picard have advanced concepts like neuroadaptive systems.

Functional near-infrared spectroscopy is a non-invasive imaging technique that measures brain activity by detecting changes in blood oxygenation levels. fNIRS leverages the differing absorption spectra of oxygenated and deoxygenated hemoglobin in the near-infrared range to infer regional cortical activation. For applied research, specify emitter–detector spacing, sampling rate, and baseline calibration procedures to ensure reproducible hemodynamic estimates. Include short task blocks and rest periods to separate neural responses from slow systemic fluctuations. Report both oxygenated and deoxygenated hemoglobin traces and describe any short-separation channel corrections used to remove superficial physiological noise. When integrating fNIRS into clinical studies, preregister hypotheses about which cortical regions will change and how those changes will map onto behavioral outcomes (Tsai et al., 2025).

In mental health, fNIRS has been applied to monitor prefrontal cortex activity in patients with depression during therapy (Bibi, 2024). Researchers have used task-based and resting-state fNIRS protocols to identify patterns of prefrontal engagement that change with symptom improvement (Radanliev, 2025). For clinicians, operationalize which prefrontal metrics (for example, task-evoked oxygenation increase or resting asymmetry) will serve as indicators of treatment response. Establish within-subject baselines and repeated measures to track trajectories rather than relying on single-session comparisons. Provide patients with plain-language explanations about what prefrontal activation implies for attention and emotional control. Use fNIRS changes as one element in a composite outcome that includes symptom ratings and functional measures (Radanliev, 2025).

Experts such as Thomas Insel, Albert Rizzo, Rosalind Picard have advanced concepts like neuroadaptive systems.

One of the key advantages of fNIRS is its portability, which allows for brain imaging in naturalistic settings outside of the laboratory (Lamb et al., 2025). Portable fNIRS systems enable assessment during classroom activities, therapy sessions, and real-world social interactions that are difficult to recreate in a scanner. For field deployments, predefine motion-tolerance thresholds and implement artifact detection pipelines that flag epochs for review. Train technicians and clinicians on comfortable and reproducible probe placement to reduce inter-session variability. Combine portable fNIRS with behavioral logging or video coding to triangulate neural signals with observable behavior. Use pilot data to calibrate expected signal-to-noise ratios in the intended deployment environment (Tsai et al., 2025).

Despite its many advantages, fNIRS also has several limitations (Omiyefa, 2025). Its shallow depth penetration restricts measurement primarily to cortical surfaces and limits access to deep subcortical structures relevant to affective circuitry. Explicitly acknowledge this anatomical constraint in study reports and avoid overinterpreting fNIRS findings as indexing whole-brain activity. Account for individual anatomical differences, such as skull thickness and hair characteristics, by using subject-specific calibration or normalization procedures. Implement motion-correction and physiological-regression methods to mitigate artifacts from movement and systemic signals. When combining fNIRS with other sensors, describe how multimodal fusion will resolve ambiguities arising from fNIRS sensitivity limits (Weiner et al., 2025).

Another limitation of fNIRS is its sensitivity to individual anatomical differences, such as variations in skull thickness and skin pigmentation, which can affect the accuracy of measurements (Chen et al., 2022). These anatomical factors systematically alter photon pathlength and attenuation, creating between-subject variability that complicates group comparisons. To address this, implement subject-specific calibration routines and report calibration outcomes alongside primary results (Ong et al., 2025). Use short-separation channels to estimate and remove superficial hemodynamic noise that differs across individuals. When possible, collect anatomical covariates such as head circumference or simplified photogrammetry to include as model covariates (Ong et al., 2025). Report how calibration and anatomical adjustments influenced effect sizes to improve transparency and replicability (Ong et al., 2025). Provide clinicians with guidelines on expected variability ranges so they can contextualize observed changes within individual anatomy.

In addition to its applications in mental health, fNIRS is also being used to study a wide range of cognitive processes, including attention, memory, and decision-making (De Kock et al., 2021). For example, task-based fNIRS studies can reveal prefrontal engagement patterns during working memory manipulation and sustained attention tasks (Li et al., 2025). Plan experiments with repeated measures and counterbalanced conditions to separate task effects from slow drifts in hemodynamics. Combine behavioral accuracy and reaction-time metrics with fNIRS traces to strengthen inferences about cognitive operations (Li et al., 2025). Use within-subject contrasts to improve sensitivity and reduce the influence of stable individual differences. When reporting, provide both raw hemodynamic responses and normalized effect estimates to aid meta-analytic integration across studies.

The integration of fNIRS with AI and machine learning is a particularly exciting development, as it has the potential to greatly enhance the utility of this technology (Kourtesis, 2024). By leveraging supervised and unsupervised models, researchers can uncover latent patterns that relate cortical activation to cognitive and emotional states. Clearly specify feature extraction procedures and temporal windows used for model training to ensure interpretability and reproducibility (Radanliev, 2025). Validate models using nested cross-validation and external hold-out samples drawn from similar real-world contexts. Share performance metrics that include sensitivity, specificity, and calibration curves to allow clinicians to evaluate trade-offs for applied use (Radanliev, 2025). When deploying models clinically, integrate human review steps and explainable outputs that clinicians can reconcile with patient reports.

In the field of neurorehabilitation, fNIRS is being used to monitor brain activity during rehabilitation exercises, providing real-time feedback to patients and therapists (Li et al., 2025). Therapists can use fNIRS to identify when patients recruit compensatory cortical strategies versus target networks thought to support recovery (Li et al., 2025). Design feedback protocols that translate fNIRS signals into simple, actionable cues such as "increase focus" or "rest briefly," and test their usability prior to clinical rollout (Li et al., 2025). Combine fNIRS monitoring with functional outcome measures to determine whether neural changes translate into meaningful improvements (Li et al., 2025). Document training schedules and adherence to correlate dose with both neural and functional outcomes. Provide therapists with decision rules for adjusting exercise intensity based on observed cortical engagement.

The use of fNIRS in combination with other wearable sensors, such as heart rate variability (Ma et al., 2025) and galvanic skin response (GSR), is also an area of active research (Radanliev, 2025). Multimodal designs increase the likelihood that observed patterns reflect genuine psychophysiological states rather than modality-specific artifacts. Predefine synchronization protocols, sampling alignment, and common preprocessing steps so that signals from different devices can be fused reliably. Use principled fusion strategies, such as hierarchical models or late-fusion ensembles, that preserve modality-specific information while leveraging cross-modal redundancy. Report how multimodal integration altered predictive performance relative to single-modality baselines, and describe failure modes where fusion reduced interpretability. Offer clinicians integrated dashboards that highlight convergent markers and explain discordant signals in plain language.

In conclusion, functional near-infrared spectroscopy is a powerful and versatile tool for studying brain activity and its relationship to cognitive and emotional processes. Its non-invasive nature, portability, and ability to provide real-time feedback make it particularly well-suited for use in both research and clinical settings. While there are still challenges to be addressed, such as shallow depth penetration and sensitivity to motion artifacts, ongoing advancements in signal processing and the integration of AI and machine learning are helping to overcome these limitations and unlock the full potential of fNIRS. As our understanding of the brain continues to grow, fNIRS will undoubtedly play a crucial role in advancing the field of cognitive neuroscience and improving mental health care. To translate fNIRS findings into clinical practice, specify reproducible preprocessing workflows and report expected noise levels for typical deployments. Provide clinicians with practical thresholds for meaningful change and guidelines for combining fNIRS with behavioral data. Encourage pilot testing in realistic care settings to establish feasibility and acceptability before scaling implementations. Maintain transparency about limitations so clinicians can weigh fNIRS evidence appropriately in decision-making (Kim & Backonja, 2025).

Wearable sensors have revolutionized the field of psychophysiological monitoring, providing real-time insights into an individual's emotional and cognitive states (Boffet et al., 2025). These sensors, EEG (electroencephalography), HRV (heart rate variability), GSR (galvanic skin response), and fNIRS (functional near-infrared spectroscopy), have found applications in various domains of mental health care. This chapter delves into the principles, applications, limitations, and integration of these sensors in mental health care. The practical advantage of wearables is continuous, contextualized data that can inform both assessment and intervention in everyday environments. Design choices should prioritize user comfort, battery life, and data security to support sustained use. Clinicians and researchers must also plan for data management, including secure storage, annotation, and audit trails. Evaluate devices against predetermined clinical criteria before adoption to reduce wasted effort on poorly suited hardware (Obermeyer et al., 2019).

The true power of wearable sensors lies in their integration. By combining EEG, HRV, GSR, and fNIRS, researchers can build a comprehensive picture of a person's mental state. Dr. Lamb's lab exemplifies this approach, using AI to fuse multimodal data into actionable insights. For instance, in a digital mental health platform, EEG might detect cognitive fatigue, HRV might signal stress, GSR might indicate arousal, and fNIRS might assess emotional engagement. AI algorithms synthesize this data to deliver closed-loop interventions, adjusting therapy content, suggesting breaks, or initiating relaxation protocols (Freeman et al., 2017). When designing fusion systems, preregister fusion logic and performance targets so stakeholders can evaluate validity. Use interpretable models and visual explanations to support clinician trust and patient understanding. Monitor system performance continuously and provide mechanisms for clinicians to override automated recommendations.

Electroencephalography (Jain & Jain, 2025) measures electrical activity in the brain and is widely used in both clinical and research settings (Ross et al., 2022). In mental health, EEG is central to neurofeedback therapy, where individuals learn to modulate their brainwave patterns. For example, children with Attention-Deficit/Hyperactivity Disorder (ADHD) have used wearable EEG headsets in game-based neurofeedback environments, improving attention and reducing impulsivity. In Dr. Lamb's lab, EEG is used to assess cognitive load and decision-making in high-stress environments, such as emergency response simulations. By applying ML algorithms to EEG data, his team can predict when a user is becoming cognitively overloaded and dynamically adjust the task or environment to reduce strain. To operationalize EEG-based interventions, document decision thresholds and specify clinician review intervals for automated adjustments. Conduct usability testing to ensure interventions are acceptable and do not introduce additional cognitive burden. Maintain logs linking EEG features to outcomes for ongoing validation and quality improvement. Heart Rate Variability (Chaabene et al., 2025) reflects the variation in time between heartbeats and is a key indicator of autonomic nervous system function. In mental health, HRV is used to monitor stress, anxiety, and emotional regulation. Veterans with PTSD, for instance, have used HRV biofeedback during mindfulness therapy to improve emotional resilience. Dr. Lamb's research incorporates HRV sensors into adaptive learning environments, where AI analyzes HRV trends to detect stress and adjust instructional pacing or content difficulty accordingly. To implement HRV-informed adaptations responsibly, predefine response rules and acceptable false-alert rates to avoid desensitizing users. Provide clear patient-facing explanations about what HRV changes mean and which actions may follow (Casson, 2019). Track engagement and efficacy metrics so that adaptive rules can be refined based on observed outcomes and user feedback.

Galvanic Skin Response (Kostadimas et al., 2025) measures skin conductance, which increases with sweat gland activity driven by sympathetic arousal (Islam & Bae, 2024). This physiological response accompanies many forms of emotional activation and is therefore useful as a proximal marker of arousal during tasks or therapy. GSR sensors typically use two electrodes placed on the fingers or palms to capture conductance changes that occur with sweat secretion. The signal is simple to acquire but requires careful preprocessing to remove movement and environmental artifacts. Specify whether your study targets tonic conductance or phasic skin conductance responses, and choose smoothing and peak-detection parameters accordingly. Calibrate sensors against brief standardized stimuli to confirm responsiveness before collecting primary data. When reporting, present both absolute conductance values and normalized change scores to aid comparisons across participants and sessions. Clinicians should interpret GSR rises as indicators of arousal that require contextual behavioral data to determine valence or clinical significance (Tsai et al., 2025).

The integration of GSR with AI and machine learning has opened new avenues for personalized and adaptive interventions (Adegoke et al., 2025). AI algorithms can analyze GSR in real time, identifying patterns that signal sustained stress or transient spikes related to specific tasks or social interactions. In adaptive learning platforms, GSR-informed models can recommend pace adjustments or microbreaks when arousal patterns suggest cognitive overload. Document preprocessing pipelines and feature extraction steps so clinicians can evaluate model transparency and traceability. Validate models on ecologically similar hold-out data and examine performance across demographic subgroups to detect bias. Combine GSR with HRV and motion sensors for richer context and improved specificity before triggering in-the-moment interventions (Obermeyer et al., 2019). Provide clinicians with simple decision rules tied to model outputs to support rapid, defensible in-session responses.

GSR's limitations require explicit management to avoid misinterpretation (Ong et al., 2025). Environmental temperature, humidity, and participant hydration can shift baseline conductance independently of psychological state, and motion artifacts commonly contaminate recordings during real-world use. The measure indexes arousal but not emotional valence, so parallel behavioral or self-report data are necessary to disambiguate fear from excitement (Rajpal, 2025). Implement artifact rejection rules and record ambient conditions to support analytic transparency. Use multimodal fusion to reduce false positives, and report residual artifact rates so readers can judge data quality (Rajpal, 2025). Train clinicians in reading GSR traces and in applying brief in-session calibrations to verify signal validity before acting on spikes (Rajpal, 2025). Maintain conservative thresholds for automated alerts to reduce unnecessary interventions.

A practical clinical vignette illustrates GSR's applied value. During virtual exposure therapy for social anxiety, a patient wore a wristband that recorded frequent phasic GSR peaks during impromptu speech tasks, which the therapist used to pace the exposure more gradually. The therapist paused when high-amplitude GSR responses occurred, used a brief cognitive restructuring exercise, and then resumed the exposure at a lower intensity. Over repeated sessions, the GSR peaks decreased in amplitude and frequency as the patient's tolerance improved, accompanied by reduced avoidance on behavioral tests. This example shows how GSR can guide moment-to-moment clinical decisions when paired with structured therapeutic techniques and ongoing measurement of behavioral outcomes (Obermeyer et al., 2019).

When integrating GSR into clinical workflows, governance and training are essential (Hiland, 2021). Define consent language that explains what GSR measures and its limits, and obtain assent for in-session monitoring with clear opt-out options. Ensure data storage follows institutional security standards and that access is limited to authorized clinical staff. Provide clinicians with quick-reference guides that translate common GSR patterns into recommended, evidence-based in-session actions. Collect implementation metrics, such as frequency of sensor failure, number of false alerts, and clinician response times, to inform iterative improvement. Periodically reverify sensor calibration and update preprocessing procedures as firmware and hardware change (Kargarandehkordi et al., 2025).

The integration of these sensors is also used in AI-powered avatars developed by Lamb's team, which respond to users' emotional and cognitive states in real time (Bond et al., 2023). These avatars provide personalized mental health support, such as guiding users through breathing exercises or cognitive restructuring techniques based on sensor feedback (Ong et al., 2025). To implement avatar-led support responsibly, define clear boundaries for automated coaching and require clinician sign-off for higher-risk recommendations. Document the logic linking sensor patterns to avatar responses so clinicians can audit and adjust behavior rules (Ong et al., 2025). Pilot-test avatars with representative users to identify unexpected interactions and to refine conversational prompts for clarity and safety. Ensure avatars surface uncertainty and recommend human referral for complex or high-risk presentations.

As wearable technology becomes more sophisticated, the integration of AI and ML will be essential for scaling digital mental health solutions (Cristofaro & Giardino, 2025). Dr. Lamb's work points toward a future where adaptive, sensor-driven systems can support mental health across diverse populations and settings, from classrooms to clinics to homes (Mohr et al., 2017). For equitable scaling, explicitly test systems across demographic groups and contexts to detect differential performance and usability issues. Establish governance processes for updating algorithms, including stakeholder review and documentation of each retraining cycle. Define minimal clinical oversight levels that must accompany automated interventions and create escalation pathways for clinician intervention (Mohr et al., 2017). Provide users with concise explanations about what changes when the system adapts and how to access human support.

Emerging trends include smart textiles, emotionally intelligent agents, and predictive diagnostics that anticipate mental health crises before they occur. Smart textiles embed sensors into clothing to reduce device burden and increase adherence during daily life. When deploying these technologies, set clear usability and washability standards, and test sensor durability through realistic wear simulations (Chithra & Bhambri, 2024). For predictive diagnostics, require transparent thresholds and multi-source corroboration before issuing crisis alerts to avoid false positives. Build consent processes that explain predictive functions and potential consequences, and ensure users can opt out of predictive analytics independently of other monitoring.

Engage with ethicists and legal counsel early to align product capabilities with regulatory expectations.

Longitudinal monitoring and digital phenotyping represent a transformative approach in mental health care, leveraging continuous data collection to gain insights into an individual's psychological and behavioral patterns over time (Subu et al., 2022). This method utilizes both passive and active data sources, integrating information from everyday activities such as phone usage, typing patterns, and wearable sensors (Poudel et al., 2025). To operationalize digital phenotypes, predefine which behavioral features will be tracked and how changes will trigger clinical review or automated support (Poudel et al., 2025). Implement data minimization principles by collecting only features relevant to specified outcomes and by applying secure, role-based access controls (Poudel et al., 2025). Periodically reassess the clinical utility of tracked features to avoid persistent collection of low-value data (Poudel et al., 2025). Passive data collection involves gathering information without requiring active input from the user (Poudel et al., 2025). This can include data from smartphones, such as call logs, text messages, app usage, and GPS location (Poudel et al., 2025). Typing patterns, social media activity, and even ambient light and sound levels can provide valuable insights into an individual's mental state. When using passive streams, ensure feature engineering preserves privacy by aggregating sensitive signals and by avoiding storage of raw textual or location traces whenever possible. Communicate clearly which passive features are collected and how they map to interventions so users understand the behavior-to-action pathway. Validate passive-feature models against active self-report and clinician-rated outcomes to confirm clinical relevance (Poudel et al., 2025).

Active data collection requires direct input from the user, such as self-reported mood assessments, cognitive tests, and surveys (Mahon, 2023). These active inputs complement passive streams by providing subjective context that raw sensor data cannot supply. Design short, frequent probes that minimize respondent burden and maximize ecological validity. Use validated brief instruments or single-item measures, when possible, to balance precision with adherence. Schedule prompts at behaviorally relevant times rather than at random to increase response rates and contextual relevance. Ensure user-facing language clarifies purpose and expected time commitment for each prompt. Predefine how active responses will be combined with passive data to inform decision rules (Kim & Backonja, 2025).

Combining active and passive data streams can enhance the accuracy and richness of digital phenotyping (Ienca et al., 2017). For example, a study integrating self-reported mood data with smartphone sensor data found that the combined approach improved prediction of mood fluctuations (Shatte et al., 2019). When fusing data, specify fusion windows and temporal alignment rules to avoid mismatched signals (Shatte et al., 2019). Test multimodal models using cross-validation that preserves temporal order to prevent optimistic bias. Report how missing active responses are handled and consider imputation strategies aligned with the clinical question (Shatte et al., 2019). Use active data to validate passively inferred states before trusting automated interventions (Shatte et al., 2019). Keep patients informed about how active reports influence care decisions.

Despite the potential benefits, maintaining user engagement in longitudinal monitoring poses several challenges. Users may experience fatigue or loss of interest over time, leading to decreased data accuracy and completeness. Implement engagement strategies such as personalized feedback, brief summaries of insights, and occasional rewards to sustain participation. Monitor engagement metrics in real time and adapt prompting schedules when adherence declines. Provide transparent options for users to pause or reduce monitoring intensity without losing access to core services. Co-design engagement features with representative users to ensure cultural and contextual fit. Track reasons for dropout to inform iterative improvements.

Experts such as Thomas Insel, Albert Rizzo, Rosalind Picard have advanced concepts like wearable sensors.

As technology advances, the potential for longitudinal monitoring and digital phenotyping in mental health care continues to grow. Emerging trends include smart textiles and wearable devices that seamlessly integrate into daily life, providing continuous data collection without user intervention (Akhtar & Rawol, 2024). Establish criteria for clinical actionability to avoid overreacting to transient signal fluctuations (Martinez-Martin et al., 2018). Require multi-source corroboration before initiating invasive or high-cost interventions based on predictive alerts. Plan for iterative evaluation cycles that update predictive models while preserving interpretability. Engage regulatory and ethical experts early to align innovations with governance requirements.

The integration of wearable sensors in mental health monitoring has the potential to revolutionize the way we understand and treat mental health conditions (Saganowski et al., 2022). These sensors, which include technologies such as EEG, HRV, GSR, and fNIRS, provide real-time, non-invasive insights into an individual's emotional and cognitive states. However, the use of these technologies raises significant ethical, privacy, and consent concerns that must be carefully considered. This chapter explores these implications, focusing on data ownership, informed consent, algorithmic bias, surveillance risks, and the responsibilities of developers and clinicians. Explicit ethical frameworks must inform study design, procurement, and clinical protocols so stakeholders can evaluate trade-offs before deployment (Tsai et al., 2025). Define the unit of analysis, individual, group, or population, and align data practices accordingly to reduce downstream misuse (Tsai et al., 2025). Ensure multidisciplinary oversight with ethicists, legal counsel, and patient representatives to anticipate foreseeable harms and mitigation strategies.

One of the primary ethical concerns surrounding the use of wearable sensors in mental health monitoring is data ownership (Agarwal et al., 2025). The data collected by these sensors can be highly personal and sensitive, revealing intimate details about an individual's mental and emotional state. As such, it is crucial to establish clear guidelines regarding who owns this data and how it can be used. In many cases, the data collected by wearable sensors is owned by the companies that produce the devices. This can create a power imbalance, as individuals may have little control over how their data is used or shared. To address this issue, it is essential to develop policies that prioritize the rights of individuals to own and control their data. These policies should specify retention limits, permissible secondary uses, and mechanisms for data portability at the individual's request. Create transparent data-use agreements that describe algorithmic uses and commercial partnerships in plain language. Implement role-based access controls and logging so that patients can review who accessed their data and why (Obermeyer et al., 2019).

Informed consent is a fundamental ethical principle in the use of wearable sensors for mental health monitoring (APA, 2023). Individuals must be fully informed about the nature of the data being collected, how it will be used, and the potential risks and benefits of using the technology. This includes providing clear and comprehensive information about the capabilities and limitations of the sensors, as well as any potential privacy and security risks. Obtaining informed consent can be challenging, particularly when dealing with vulnerable populations such as individuals with mental health conditions. It is important to ensure that consent is obtained in a manner that is respectful and considerate of the individual's cognitive and emotional state. This may involve using simplified language, visual aids, or other methods to ensure that individuals fully understand the implications of using the technology. Consent processes should be ongoing, with periodic re-consent for new analytic uses or when algorithms are retrained using pooled data. Offer tiered consent options that let individuals select limited sharing for care versus broader research or development use (Kim & Backonja, 2025). Provide accessible summaries and decision aids that clinicians can use to support shared decision-making.

RESPONSIBILITIES OF DEVELOPERS AND CLINICIANS

Conclusion

The use of wearable sensors in mental health monitoring has the potential to revolutionize the way we understand and treat mental health conditions. However, it is essential to carefully consider the ethical, privacy, and consent implications of using these technologies. By prioritizing data ownership, informed consent, algorithmic bias, surveillance risks, and the responsibilities of developers and clinicians, we can ensure that wearable sensors are used in a manner that is ethical, respectful, and beneficial for all individuals (Ricciardi & Zomaya, 2025). To translate these principles into practice, create implementation checklists that map ethical requirements to operational tasks and responsible parties. Require pilot evaluations that measure both clinical effects and user trust before broad rollout (Ricciardi & Zomaya, 2025). Encourage continuous stakeholder engagement so systems evolve with patient norms and legal frameworks. Maintain public-facing summaries of governance decisions to foster transparency and accountability.

REFERENCES

Adegoke, K., Adegoke, A., Dawodu, D., Bayowa, A., & Adekoya, A (2025). Interoperability in digital healthcare: Enhancing consumer health and transforming care systems.

Agarwal, S., Jalan, M., Hill, R., Pantalone, E., Thrul, J., Sharma, R., Wilcox, H. C., & Robinson, K. A. (2025). Framework to Assist Stakeholders in Technology Evaluation for Recovery (Freeman et al., 2017) to Mental Health and Wellness. *BMC Health Services Research*, *25*, 623. Advance online publication. DOI: 10.1186/s12913-025-12418-0 PMID: 40307807

Akhtar, Z. B., & Rawol, A. T. (2024). Artificial intelligence (Tizzard, 2025) and extended reality (XR): A biomedical engineering perspective investigation analysis. *Indonesian Journal of Electronics, Electromedical Engineering, and Medical Informatics*, *6*(3). Advance online publication. DOI: 10.35882/ijeeemi.v6i3.5

Akhtar, Z. B., & Rawol, A. T. (2025). Artificial Intelligence (Leivaditis & Sepetis, 2025) & Extended Reality (Reddy, 2025) within Healthcare: A Multidimensional Biomedical Engineering (Rajpal, 2025) Investigative Exploration. *Biomed. Clin. Res. J*, *1*, 1–22.

Akinode, A. O., Ayadi, O. E., Ezerioha, C. C., & Chika, P (2025). Machine Learning Approaches for Early Detection of Mental Health Disorders Using Wearable Devices and Big Data Analytics. environments, 4, 5.

Almadani, B., Kaisar, H., Thoker, I. R., & Aliyu, F. (2025). A systematic survey of distributed decision support systems in healthcare. *Systems*, *13*(3), 157. DOI: 10.3390/systems13030157

American Psychiatric Association. (2023). Digital [Resource Document. APA.]. *Mental Health (Detroit, Mich.)*, •••, 101.

Bibi, P (2024). Establishing Transparency and Accountability in AI: Ethical Standards for Data Governance and Automated Systems. In.

Boffet, A., Arsac, L. M., Ibanez, V., Sauvet, F., & Deschodt-Arsac, V. (2025). Detection of Cognitive Load Modulation by EDA and HRV. *Sensors (Basel)*, *25*(8), 2343. DOI: 10.3390/s25082343 PMID: 40285033

Bond, R. R., Mulvenna, M. D., Potts, C., O'Neill, S., Ennis, E., & Torous, J. (2023). Digital transformation of mental health services. *Npj Mental Health Research*, *2*(1), 13. DOI: 10.1038/s44184-023-00033-y PMID: 38609479

Casson, A. J. (2019). Wearable EEG and beyond. *Biomedical Engineering Letters*, *9*(1), 53–71. DOI: 10.1007/s13534-018-00093-6 PMID: 30956880

Chaabene, S., Boudaya, A., Bouaziz, B., & Chaari, L. (2025). An overview of methods and techniques in multimodal data fusion with application to healthcare. *International Journal of Data Science and Analytics*, *20*(4), 1–25. DOI: 10.1007/s41060-025-00715-0

Chen, Z. S., Galatzer-Levy, I. R., Bigio, B., Nasca, C., & Zhang, Y. (2022). Modern views of machine learning for precision psychiatry. *Patterns (New York, N.Y.)*, *3*(11), 100602. DOI: 10.1016/j.patter.2022.100602 PMID: 36419447

Chithra, N., & Bhambri, P. (2024). Ethics in sustainable technology. In *Handbook of Technological Sustainability* (pp. 245–256). CRC Press. DOI: 10.1201/9781003475989-21

Correa, T., Pavez, I., & Contreras, J. (2021). Digital inequality and mobiles: opportunities and challenges of relying on smartphones for digital inclusion in disadvantaged contexts. Handbook of digital inequality, 62-74.

Cristofaro, M., & Giardino, P. L. (2025). Surfing the AI waves: The historical evolution of artificial intelligence in management and organizational studies and practices. *Journal of Management History*. Advance online publication. DOI: 10.1108/JMH-01-2025-0002

De Kock, J. H., Latham, H. A., Leslie, S. J., Grindle, M., Munoz, S. A., Ellis, L., Polson, R., & O'Malley, C. M. (2021). A rapid review of the impact of COVID-19 on the mental health of healthcare workers: Implications for supporting psychological well-being. *BMC Public Health*, *21*(1), 104. DOI: 10.1186/s12889-020-10070-3 PMID: 33422039

Fleming, L. E., Maycock, B., White, M. P., & Depledge, M. H. (2019). Fostering human health through ocean sustainability in the 21st century. *People and Nature*, *1*(3), 276–283. DOI: 10.1002/pan3.10038

Hiland, E. B. (2021). *Therapy tech: The digital transformation of mental healthcare*. U of Minnesota Press. DOI: 10.5749/j.ctv1xp9q3t

Holly, L., Thom, S., Elzemety, M., Murage, B., Mathieson, K., & Iñigo Petralanda, M. I. (2023). Strengthening health data governance: New equity and rights-based principles. *International Journal of Health Governance*, *28*(3), 225–237. DOI: 10.1108/IJHG-11-2022-0104

Ienca, M., Fabrice, J., Elger, B., Caon, M., Scoccia Pappagallo, A., Kressig, R. W., & Wangmo, T. (2017). Intelligent assistive technology for Alzheimer's disease and other dementias: A systematic review. *Journal of Alzheimer's Disease*, *56*(4), 1301–1340. DOI: 10.3233/JAD-161037 PMID: 28222516

Islam, R., & Bae, S. W. (2024). Revolutionizing mental health support: An innovative affective mobile framework for dynamic, proactive, and context-adaptive conversational agents. arXiv preprint arXiv:2406.15942.

Jain, A., & Jain, A (2025). AI-Based Emotion Detection System in Healthcare for Patient. Generative Artificial Intelligence for Biomedical and Smart Health Informatics, 455-470.

Kang, H. S., & Exworthy, M. (2022). Wearing the future—wearables to empower users to take greater responsibility for their health and care: Scoping review. *JMIR mHealth and uHealth*, *10*(7), e35684. DOI: 10.2196/35684 PMID: 35830222

Kargarandehkordi, A., Li, S., Lin, K., Phillips, K. T., Benzo, R. M., & Washington, P. (2025). Fusing wearable biosensors with artificial intelligence for mental health monitoring: A systematic review. *Biosensors (Basel)*, *15*(4), 202. DOI: 10.3390/bios15040202 PMID: 40277515

Kim, J., & Backonja, U. (2025). Digital health equity frameworks and key concepts: A scoping review. *Journal of the American Medical Informatics Association : JAMIA*, *32*(1), 45–59. DOI: 10.1093/jamia/ocaf017 PMID: 39936843

Kostadimas, D., Kasapakis, V., & Kotis, K. (2025). A systematic review on the combination of VR, IoT and AI technologies, and their integration in applications. *Future Internet*, *17*(4), 163. DOI: 10.3390/fi17040163

Kourtesis, P. (2024). A comprehensive review of multimodal XR applications, risks, and ethical challenges in the metaverse. *Multimodal Technologies and Interaction*, *8*(11), 98. DOI: 10.3390/mti8110098

Kumar, T., Arora, M., Verma, V., Bhushan, S., & Lalar, S. (2024). Biometric System Integration in Public Health: Challenges and Solutions. In Computational Intelligence and Mathematical Applications (pp. 168-173). CRC Press.

Lamb, R., Choi, I., & Owens, T (2025). Convergence of Extended Reality, Artificial Intelligence, Machine Leaning, and Wearable Sensors in the Field of Education. Mental Health Virtual Reality: The Power of Immersive Worlds, 113-128.

Li, M., Patel, J., & Katapally, T. R. (2025). The impact of extended reality cognitive behavioral therapy on mental disorders among children and youth: A systematic review and meta-analysis protocol. *PLoS One*, *20*(3), e0315313. DOI: 10.1371/journal.pone.0315313 PMID: 40048453

Ma, C.-B., Shang, X., Sun, M., Bo, X., Bai, J., Du, Y., & Zhou, M. (2025). Emerging Multifunctional Wearable Sensors: Integrating Multimodal Sweat Analysis and Advanced Material Technologies for Next-Generation Health Monitoring. *ACS Sensors*, *10*(4), 2388–2408. DOI: 10.1021/acssensors.4c03396 PMID: 40162570

Mahon, D. (2023). Empirically Supported Treatments: A Brief History. In Evidence Based Counselling & Psychotherapy for the 21st Century Practitioner (pp. 3-14). Emerald Publishing Limited. DOI: 10.1108/978-1-80455-732-720231001

Martinez-Martin, N., Marcandalli, J., Huang, C. S., Arthur, C. P., Perotti, M., Foglierini, M., Ho, H., Dosey, A. M., Shriver, S., Payandeh, J., Leitner, A., Lanzavecchia, A., Perez, L., & Ciferri, C. (2018). An unbiased screen for human cytomegalovirus identifies neuropilin-2 as a central viral receptor. *Cell*, *174*(5), 1158–1171. DOI: 10.1016/j.cell.2018.06.028 PMID: 30057110

Mohr, D. C., Zhang, M., & Schueller, S. M. (2017). Personal sensing: Understanding mental health using ubiquitous sensors and machine learning. *Annual Review of Clinical Psychology*, *13*(1), 23–47. DOI: 10.1146/annurev-clinpsy-032816-044949 PMID: 28375728

Morey, D. A., Rayo, M. F., & Woods, D. D. (2025). Empirically derived evaluation requirements for responsible deployments of AI in safety-critical settings. *NPJ Digital Medicine*, *8*(1), 374. DOI: 10.1038/s41746-025-01784-y PMID: 40533485

Morgan, J. W., Patel, R. A., & Campbell, S. (2025). Practical considerations of clinical XR (Singh & Chandra, 2025) deployments. *Frontiers in Virtual Reality*, *6*, 1517402. DOI: 10.3389/frvir.2025.1517402

Obermeyer, Z., Powers, B., Vogeli, C., & Mullainathan, S. (2019). Dissecting racial bias in an algorithm used to manage the health of populations. *Science*, *366*(6464), 447–453. DOI: 10.1126/science.aax2342 PMID: 31649194

Omiyefa, S. (2025). Artificial intelligence and machine learning in precision mental health diagnostics and predictive treatment models. *Int J Res Publ Rev*, *6*(3), 85–99. DOI: 10.55248/gengpi.6.0325.1107

Ong, T., Ivanova, J., Soni, H., Barrera, J., Cummins, M., Welch, B. M., & Bunnell, B. E. (2025). Mental health clients' perspectives on telehealth-based virtual reality therapy. *Frontiers in Virtual Reality*, *6*, 1595326. DOI: 10.3389/frvir.2025.1595326

Panarese, P., Grasso, M. M., & Solinas, C. (2025). Algorithmic bias, fairness, and inclusivity: A multilevel framework for justice-oriented AI. *AI & Society*, •••, 1–23. DOI: 10.1007/s00146-025-02451-2

Poudel, U., Jakhar, S., Mohan, P., & Nepal, A. (2025). AI in mental health: A review of technological advancements and ethical issues in psychiatry. *Issues in Mental Health Nursing*, *46*(7), 693–701. DOI: 10.1080/01612840.2025.2502943 PMID: 40378075

Radanliev, P. (2025). Privacy, ethics, transparency, and accountability in AI systems for wearable devices. *Frontiers in Digital Health*, *7*, 1431246. DOI: 10.3389/fdgth.2025.1431246 PMID: 40599875

Rajpal, S. (2025). Exploring the Role of Virtual Reality and Metaverse in Treating Mental Health: Operating Models and Challenges in Adoption. *Journal of Computer and Communications*, *13*(10), 1–22. DOI: 10.4236/jcc.2025.1310001

Ricciardi, F., & Zomaya, A. (2025). Perspectives on Managing AI Ethics in the Digital Age. *Information (Basel)*, *16*(2), 89. DOI: 10.3390/info16040318

Robinson, A., Flom, M., Forman-Hoffman, V. L., Histon, T., Levy, M., Darcy, A., Ajayi, T., Mohr, D. C., Wicks, P., Greene, C., & Montgomery, R. M. (2024). Equity in digital mental health interventions in the United States: Where to next? *Journal of Medical Internet Research*, *26*, e59939. DOI: 10.2196/59939 PMID: 39316436

Ross, G., Zhao, Y., Bosman, A., Geballa-Koukoula, A., Zhou, H., Elliott, C., Nielen, M., Rafferty, K., & Salentijn, G (2022). Data handling and ethics of emerging smartphone-based (Glass et al., 2022) sensors–Part 1: best practices and current implementation.

Saganowski, S., Perz, B., Polak, A. G., & Kazienko, P (2022). Emotion recognition for everyday life using physiological signals from wearables: A systematic literature review. IEEE Transactions on Affective Computing, 14(3), 1876-1897. Pinel, P (1793). Traité médico-philosophique sur l'aliénation mentale.

Saksena, N., Matthan, R., Bhan, A., & Balsari, S. (2021). Rebooting consent in the digital age: A governance framework for health data exchange. *BMJ Global Health*, *6*(Suppl 5), e005057. DOI: 10.1136/bmjgh-2021-005057 PMID: 34301754

Shah, B., Allen, J. L. Y., Chaudhury, H., O'Shaughnessy, J., & Tyrrell, C. S. (2022). The role of digital health in the future of integrated care. *Clinics in Integrated Care*, *15*, 100131. DOI: 10.1016/j.intcar.2022.100131

Shatte, A. B., Hutchinson, D. M., & Teague, S. J. (2019). Machine learning in mental health: A scoping review of methods and applications. *Psychological Medicine, 49*(9), 1426–1448. DOI: 10.1017/S0033291719000151 PMID: 30744717

Subu, M. A., Holmes, D., Arumugam, A., Al-Yateem, N., Maria Dias, J., Rahman, S. A., Waluyo, I., Ahmed, F. R., & Abraham, M. S. (2022). Traditional, religious, and cultural perspectives on mental illness: A qualitative study on causal beliefs and treatment use. *International Journal of Qualitative Studies on Health and Well-being, 17*(1), 2123090. DOI: 10.1080/17482631.2022.2123090 PMID: 36097886

Tsai, Y. Y., Chen, Y. J., Lin, Y. F., Hsiao, F. C., Hsu, C. H., & Liao, L. D. (2025). Photoplethysmography-based HRV analysis and machine learning for real-time stress quantification in mental health applications. *APL Bioengineering, 9*(2), 026103. DOI: 10.1063/5.0256590 PMID: 40191605

Volckens, J., Haynes, E. N., Croisant, S. P., Cui, Y., Errett, N. A., Henry, H. F., Horney, J. A., Kwok, R. K., Magzamen, S., Rappold, A. G., Ravichandran, L., Reinlib, L., Ryan, P. H., & Shaughnessy, D. T. (2023). Health research in the wake of disasters: Challenges and opportunities for sensor science. *Environmental Health Perspectives, 131*(6), 065002. DOI: 10.1289/EHP12270 PMID: 37389972

Wang, Z., Xiong, H., Zhang, J., Yang, S., Boukhechba, M., Zhang, D., Barnes, L. E., & Dou, D. (2022). From personalized medicine to population health: A survey of mHealth sensing techniques. *IEEE Internet of Things Journal, 9*(17), 15413–15434. DOI: 10.1109/JIOT.2022.3161046

Weiner, E. B., Dankwa-Mullan, I., Nelson, W. A., & Hassanpour, S. (2025). Ethical challenges and evolving strategies in the integration of artificial intelligence into clinical practice. *PLOS Digital Health, 4*(4), e0000810. DOI: 10.1371/journal.pdig.0000810 PMID: 40198594

Zenker, S., Strech, D., Ihrig, K., Jahns, R., Müller, G., Schickhardt, C., Schmidt, G., Speer, R., Winkler, E., von Kielmansegg, S. G., & Drepper, J. (2022). Data protection-compliant broad consent for secondary use of health care data and human biosamples for (Mulukuntla, 2025) medical research: Towards a new German national standard. *Journal of Biomedical Informatics, 131*, 104096. DOI: 10.1016/j.jbi.2022.104096 PMID: 35643273

Chapter 7
Closed Loop Systems and Multimodal Integration

ABSTRACT

This chapter explores the convergence of AI, XR, and wearable sensors into neuroadaptive ecosystems that personalize care in real time (Hatef et al., 2025). Multimodal integration synthesizes physiological, behavioral, and contextual data to dynamically adjust interventions—such as modifying XR exposure intensity based on HRV or triggering coping prompts during stress spikes (Engel, 1977). Closed-loop systems promise precision and scalability but require interoperability standards, timestamp synchronization, and clinician oversight to prevent harm. Ethical safeguards—layered consent, equity audits, and override protocols—are essential. Implementation science frameworks guide pilot testing, workflow integration, and evaluation across usability, cultural relevance, and cost-effectiveness. The vision: adaptive, context-aware systems that enhance—not replace—human care.

INTRODUCTION

This chapter introduces closed-loop therapeutic systems that integrate sensing, interpretation, and adaptive intervention into continuous cycles of care. It explains how wearable sensors, AI analytics, and XR environments can be combined to provide moment-to-moment responsiveness while preserving clinician oversight. The chapter emphasizes multimodal fusion, integrating physiology, behavior, voice, and context, to improve sensitivity and reduce reliance on single data streams. Baseline personalization, adaptive thresholds, and revalidation are presented as critical design features to prevent drift and misclassification at scale. Through an extended clinical vignette, the chapter illustrates how closed-loop systems can transform between-session practice into measurable, actionable treatment components. Ethical safeguards, including transparency, consent, and override authority, are embedded as

DOI: 10.4018/979-8-3373-4997-8.ch007

design requirements. The chapter cautions against overautomation and highlights the importance of workflow alignment to avoid increasing clinician burden. By framing closed-loop systems as collaborative tools for co-regulation rather than surveillance, the chapter offers a clinically grounded model for adaptive care.

JORDAN'S EXPERIENCE

As Jordan stepped into the counseling center in 2035, the room subtly shifted to meet them: lights dimmed to a warm, calming hue and a soft ambient tone smoothed the air (Babu & Joseph, 2025). This adaptation was guided by preconfigured clinical protocols that aim to standardize low-arousal entry for most clients (Poudel et al., 2025). The system used a short, consented profile to select non-triggering colors and sounds proven to reduce immediate physiological reactivity. Clinicians should document the environmental settings used so subsequent sessions can replicate effective configurations. This procedure reduces initial session time spent on stabilization and allows earlier therapeutic engagement. These operational details support reproducibility across clinicians and sites while preserving individual customization.

The clinic's wearable onboarding system had already synchronized with Jordan's wrist patch and the patient profile indicated a week of disrupted sleep and elevated sympathetic arousal (Hall et al., 2024). The synchronization followed a defined, audited handshake protocol that ensures device identity and data integrity at intake. Staff verified device fit and battery function during onboarding to maximize adherence and data quality over the monitoring period. The profile combined passive sensor streams with brief self-reports to generate a prioritized list of clinical flags for review (Ienca et al., 2017). These flags guided pre-session triage and helped clinicians focus limited session time on the most salient issues.

The environment's immediate adaptation was not theatrical; it was the clinic's standard pre-session coordination designed to reduce the time needed for stabilization and to preserve session minutes for therapeutic work. The coordination protocol included a brief automated consent check and a summary of recent physiological trends presented to clinicians (Iwaya et al., 2023). This standardized approach minimizes variability between sessions and supports consistent measurement of intervention effects. Teams should record both environmental settings and client responses to evaluate which configurations yield the best regulatory outcomes. Implementing this coordination reduces wasted therapeutic time and enhances session efficiency.

Jordan next entered a private XR pod where an AI-driven assistant guided a brief ten-minute mindful-breathing exercise inside a virtual forest (Inkster et al., 2023). The AI delivered the exercise using a scripted but adaptive protocol that adjusted imagery intensity and pacing based on incoming biometric signals (Tsai et al., 2025). Clinicians retained oversight and the ability to abort or modify the exercise at any time to match therapeutic goals. The pod recorded physiological responses to the exercise to provide a baseline regulation metric for the session. These baseline metrics were then used as reference points for in-session exposures and post-session progress tracking.

The exercise was tailored to Jordan's current physiology,breathing cadence and visual contrast adjusted in real time according to heart rate variability (Khoo et al., 2024) and skin conductance. Adaptive tailoring followed prespecified thresholds and smoothing windows to avoid abrupt changes that might confuse the participant. The system prioritized slow, predictable adjustments to support learning of regulatory skills through repeated, gentle feedback. Clinicians should review the recorded adaptation log to understand which adjustments produced the largest shifts in homeostasis. Using HRV and skin conductance together improves sensitivity to both parasympathetic recovery and sympathetic activation (Casson, 2019).

After the warm-up, Jordan met with Dr. Rivera, who had reviewed a dynamic dashboard that synthesized biometric trends, voice-journal sentiment, and behavioral patterns detected by passive sensing (Freeman et al., 2017). The dashboard presented time-aligned widgets so clinicians could rapidly correlate physiology with reported events and speech markers. The summary view prioritized clinically actionable anomalies and suggested focused assessment questions to guide the session. Clinicians should verify automated labels before making diagnostic inferences to maintain clinical responsibility (Freeman et al., 2017). The dashboard included brief confidence scores and timestamps to help clinicians interpret the provenance of each signal.

The dashboard presented a concise timeline that highlighted a midweek spike in stress,an empirical anchor that made what might otherwise be vague subjective reports actionable in session. The timeline allowed clinicians to zoom into specific episodes and listen to time-synced voice excerpts with participant permission. Presenting objective spikes alongside subjective recall helps in collaboratively reconstructing antecedents and consequences. Clinicians should ask targeted questions about context around flagged spikes to confirm internal versus external drivers. This process supports joint formulation and targeted intervention planning.

Together they reviewed an anonymized XR replay of Jordan's week: short vignettes generated from aggregated, consented data that illustrated key moments of escalation and relative calm (Lay et al., 2025). The replay used deidentified avatars and context cues to preserve privacy while conveying sequence and intensity of events. Therapists used the replay to elicit client reflection, explore coping responses, and validate the client's lived experience with concrete, observable patterns. Clients retained control over which vignettes to view and could request deletions or redaction at any time. This process reinforced collaborative transparency and fostered a shared understanding of triggers and regulatory successes.

Jordan recognized a recurring trigger in a particular work meeting; in response, Dr. Rivera deployed a brief cognitive-behavioral rehearsal inside XR in which Jordan practiced assertive language with a virtual coworker while the system provided real-time biofeedback (Baka et al., 2025). The rehearsal environment allowed graded exposure by incrementally increasing conversational difficulty while tracking physiological response. The clinician paused between trials to process thoughts and beliefs that emerged and to reinforce coping strategies. Immediate biofeedback informed pacing and helped the client link cognitive shifts to bodily regulation. Rehearsal sessions were saved as progress markers for future review and reinforcement.

This rehearsal was not experiential novelty but a technique with clear therapeutic logic: it allowed the client to practice cognitive and behavioral strategies in an ecologically valid but safe environment, while physiological markers guided pacing and exposure intensity. The procedure formalized steps for skill acquisition: modeling, guided practice, independent rehearsal, and consolidation with measurable physiological endpoints. Clinicians should document targeted behaviors, success criteria, and planned homework that aligns with in-session gains. This documentation supports reproducibility and allows objective tracking of treatment mechanisms over time. At session close, Dr. Rivera prescribed a 10-minute daily XR resilience module that the system would adapt based on Jordan's ongoing sensor data, and set an alert threshold for clinically concerning patterns (Livieri et al., 2025). The prescription included clear usage instructions and expected goals for the next two weeks to support adherence. The system logged module completion and linked physiological responses to module instances for therapist review. Clinicians should schedule brief check-ins to review module data and troubleshoot barriers to use (De Kock et al., 2021). This arrangement positioned between-session practice as measurable homework that informs subsequent session focus.

The prescription created a continuous, personalized loop of practice and monitoring rather than relying solely on weekly talk therapy to produce change. This loop specified mechanisms of action,practice frequency, targeted skills, and physiological recovery metrics,to make treatment targets explicit. Clinicians should co-define acceptable progress markers with clients to preserve agency and align expectations. Monitoring emphasized small, repeated behavior changes rather than large, episodic shifts. The design thus reorients therapy toward distributed learning and iterative optimization. This vignette is illustrative but also instructive about the working model I describe here: AI, wearable sensors, and Extended Reality (Liu & Schueller, 2023) can be combined into closed-loop therapeutic systems that provide continuous assessment, adaptive intervention, and measurable feedback (Smith et al., 2023). The model foregrounds interoperability, explicit consent, and clinician oversight as prerequisites for ethical use (Fanarioti & Karpouzis, 2025). Implementers should document data lineage and decision logic so clinicians can trace recommendations back to raw signals (Fanarioti & Karpouzis, 2025). This traceability supports both clinical audit and client explanations when needed (Fanarioti & Karpouzis, 2025). The approach reframes assessment and intervention as an integrated, measurable process.

Closed-loop means that data flow is bidirectional and operational: sensors feed data to analysis engines; the analysis informs an intervention; the intervention generates new sensor data; and the system adapts (Shatte et al., 2019). Operational clarity requires specifying latency tolerances and acceptable error rates for each loop component. Teams should map expected data flows and failure modes during implementation planning to reduce downtime. Regular testing of each loop component under realistic conditions prevents silent degradation in performance. These engineering practices translate directly into safer clinical operations (Ienca et al., 2017).

In plainer clinical terms, closed-loop systems automate parts of the assessment-intervention cycle so care can be more responsive to momentary states rather than dependent only on retrospective accounts (Obermeyer et al., 2019). Automation reduces time spent on routine monitoring and frees clinician attention for interpretation and relational work. Clinicians must retain veto authority over automated recommendations to safeguard therapeutic judgment. Training programs should include scenarios where automation is overridden to maintain clinician proficiency. This balance preserves human oversight while leveraging automated responsiveness.

The foundational technologies each contribute a distinct capability. Wearable sensors provide continuous, objective physiological signals, HRV, actigraphy, electrodermal activity (EDA), sleep metrics, and sometimes EEG proxies, that capture momentary states and patterns across contexts (Ball et al., 2025). AI systems ingest these signals and fuse them with behavioral and linguistic inputs to detect patterns, generate predictions, and recommend interventions (Tsai et al., 2025). XR offers an immersive, controllable environment in which rehearsals, exposures, and skills training occur with ecological fidelity (Tsai et al., 2025). For clinicians, this division clarifies that each technology augments a specific clinical function and together they form a complementary toolkit supporting assessment, formulation, and intervention strategies (Tsai et al., 2025). Implementers should map which clinical decisions each modality informs to avoid redundancy and ensure efficient use of clinician time (Tsai et al., 2025). The combined system requires clear interfaces so clinicians can access each modality's outputs without cognitive overload.

A clarifying sentence: think of each technology as a clinical assistant, sensors gather evidence, AI summarizes and suggests, XR provides the practice space, and the clinician remains the integrative decision maker (Fanarioti & Karpouzis, 2025). This framing preserves clinician primacy and assigns bounded roles to automated systems, which reduces role confusion and legal ambiguity. Teams should formalize clinician responsibilities in relation to automated outputs, clarifying who reviews alerts and who communicates changes to clients. Such role definitions reduce missed alerts and ensure consistent therapeutic responsibility across providers.

Multimodal integration is the technical heart of closed-loop therapeutics. Multimodal fusion means combining signals of different kinds, physiology, voice, movement, self-report, contextual markers, so the system produces a more nuanced estimate of mental state than any single input could. For example, a modest HRV drop combined with a flat affect in voice and reduced step count over days provides stronger evidence for a depressive episode than any single indicator alone (Gkintoni et al., 2025). Practically, clinicians should view multimodal outputs as probabilistic indicators that assist, not replace, clinical judgement (Casson, 2019). Implementers should report multimodal confidence scores and example scenarios where combinations improved detection to support clinician trust and comprehension. Transparency about what multimodal fusion can and cannot infer will prevent overreliance on opaque composite metrics.

To clarify: multimodal outputs are best used as supplementary evidence that narrows hypotheses and suggests focused assessment questions rather than as definitive diagnoses (Ricciardi & Zomaya, 2025). Clinicians should train to translate multimodal signals into testable clinical questions that can be validated in session (Rajpal, 2025). This practice preserves hypothesis-testing rigor and integrates quantitative signals into established clinical formulations (Rajpal, 2025). It also reduces risk of confirmation bias by prompting targeted, falsifiable inquiries.

Designing robust closed-loop systems requires careful attention to baseline personalization and adaptive thresholds. Because physiological signals vary widely across individuals and contexts, systems must establish personalized baselines and detect deviation from that baseline rather than rely on fixed population cut points. Personalized baselines reduce false positives and improve specificity for clinically meaningful changes. In clinical language, this means initial onboarding must include sufficiently long baseline sampling, typically several days to a week, so the predictive models calibrate to the individual's normal range (Rajpal, 2025). Operationally, this baseline period should be scheduled and documented during intake, and clinicians should withhold major decisions until adequate baseline data exist (Rajpal, 2025). Systems should also flag low-confidence predictions when baselines are incomplete to prevent premature automated actions.

A clarifying sentence follows: ensure baseline collection is built into intake protocols so the system's alerts reflect meaningful intraindividual change rather than expected variability. Training materials should instruct clinicians how to explain baseline logic to clients and to set appropriate expectations for when adaptive features will become active. Clear client-facing language about timing and data sufficiency promotes adherence during the initial calibration window (Lindner et al., 2024).

Ethical design must be a central, non-negotiable element of any implementation. Consent procedures should specify what data are collected, how they are processed, where they are stored, and how long they are retained; patients must have clear options to opt out of particular data streams without losing access to necessary care (Casson, 2019). Moreover, equity concerns require that models be audited for bias and that alternative care pathways exist for those unwilling or unable to use the technology. Clinicians should treat disclosure and transparency as part of therapeutic alliance rather than administrative overlay. Implementers must create accessible, plain-language consent materials and periodic consent-refresh checkpoints to respect evolving client preferences and understanding. Regular ethics reviews should accompany deployments, with client representatives included to ground decisions in lived experience.

To state this plainly: informed consent in technology-augmented care must be an ongoing, dialogic process, not a one-time signature on a form. Documenting consent dialogues in the clinical record supports accountability and helps resolve future disputes about data use (Spytska, 2025). Several practical challenges shape real-world deployment: device adherence, data integration, clinician burden, and regulatory compliance (Martinez-Martin et al., 2018). Device adherence requires attention to ergonomics, battery life, and clear user instructions to maintain continuous data streams (Martinez-Martin et al., 2018). Data integration depends on interoperable standards and thoughtful dashboard design so clinicians see concise, actionable summaries rather than raw signal dumps (Martinez-Martin et al., 2018). Clinician burden increases if systems generate frequent low-value alerts; design must favor high-specificity notifications and clinician-configurable thresholds. Regulatory compliance demands encrypted transmission, role-based access, and auditable logs to meet legal and institutional requirements. Implementation teams should plan for routine maintenance, user support, and a process for decommissioning devices to manage lifecycle risks.

Device adherence depends on comfort, battery life, and perceived usefulness; if the device is cumbersome, clients stop wearing it and the system loses its utility. Usability testing with representative clients early in procurement helps identify failure points in wearability and interface design. Clear onboarding instructions and quick troubleshooting guides increase sustained use and reduce dropout. Clinicians should monitor wear-time metrics and address adherence barriers collaboratively rather than assuming non-wear indicates noncompliance. Simple technical adjustments, such as alternate attachment methods, often yield large gains in continuous monitoring quality. Collecting qualitative feedback about daily experiences informs iterative device selection and support strategies.

Data integration requires interoperable standards and dashboards that present actionable summaries rather than raw streams (Freeman et al., 2017). Implementers should adopt common data schemas and APIs to reduce brittle point-to-point integrations that break with software updates (Freeman et al., 2017). Dashboards must prioritize a limited number of high-value metrics and allow clinicians to drill down to raw data when needed for verification (Freeman et al., 2017). User-centered design sessions with clinicians produce dashboards aligned with workflow and reduce cognitive load. Regular validation checks should compare dashboard summaries to raw traces to detect transformation errors. Well-designed integration reduces time to insight and increases clinician trust in automated outputs.

Clinician burden is real-systems that produce frequent low-value alerts increase workload and erode trust; alerting logic must prioritize specificity and clinician control. Implement teams should co-design escalation rules with frontline clinicians to ensure alerts are actionable and time-sensitive. Providing clinicians with the ability to mute, Snooze, or batch alerts empowers triage and reduces interruption. Training should include scenarios that simulate false positives and teach appropriate responses to maintain confidence. Monitoring clinician engagement metrics helps identify when alert tuning or additional training is required. Sustained adoption depends on minimizing administrative overhead and preserving time for therapeutic tasks.

Compliance demands secure transmission, encrypted storage, and role-based access that satisfy regulations such as HIPAA while remaining usable in daily practice. Legal teams must be involved early to map data flows and identify jurisdictional constraints for cross-border data (Freeman et al., 2017). Access controls should be fine-grained so only authorized roles see identifiable data, and audit trails must capture who accessed what and when (Freeman et al., 2017). Policies should specify retention periods, deletion procedures, and protocols for data breaches that include client notification templates (Freeman et al., 2017). Regular penetration testing and third-party security reviews provide external validation of safeguards. Balancing high security with seamless clinical usability is essential to maintain trust and legal compliance (Freeman et al., 2017).

A brief vignette illustrates these constraints: a community clinic piloted wrist sensors with a group of university students. The pilot revealed frequent, context-insensitive alerts during late-night social activity that overwhelmed clinicians and reduced trust in the system. Project teams must anticipate common behavioral patterns in target populations and simulate them during testing to reduce false alarms. Collect and analyze pilot logs to identify high-frequency nonactionable events and adjust thresholds accordingly. Engage users in rapid feedback cycles to surface unanticipated use patterns and address usability issues. Document adjustments and rationale so future deployments benefit from lessons learned.

Safety and escalation protocols require explicit mapping. Define which alerts trigger immediate clinician contact, which prompt automated supportive messages, and which require no action. Establish clear on-call roles and expected response timeframes, and rehearse protocols in tabletop exercises to reveal gaps. Include scripted clinician communications and consented automated messages to maintain consistent, trauma-informed responses. Review escalation outcomes regularly and refine thresholds based on real-world alert performance and resource capacity.

To clarify: a technology without an agreed and tested escalation plan is an ethical hazard, not a safety feature. Treat escalation planning as a clinical competency and include it in supervision and performance reviews (Fleming et al., 2019). Require formal sign-off on escalation protocols by clinical leadership before systems go live. Maintain versioned protocol documents and ensure all staff access the latest iteration through a centralized knowledge repository (Ienca et al., 2017). Audit adherence to escalation procedures and remediate identified deviations promptly.

Training clinicians to interpret and integrate AI-derived outputs is a nontrivial competency. Build curricula that combine didactic sessions, hands-on dashboard practice, and case-based role plays that require human judgment in moments of automated suggestion. Require clinicians to demonstrate competency in interpreting confidence scores and tracing recommendations to raw data during supervised practice (Kim & Backonja, 2025). Offer refresher modules and peer-review forums where clinicians discuss challenging cases and share interpretation strategies. Measure training effectiveness through pre/post assessments and incorporate findings into continuous professional development plans.

Measuring outcomes requires both proximal and distal indicators. Define proximal process metrics, module completion rates, immediate physiological changes during tasks, and between-session engagement, to assess mechanism fidelity. Select distal clinical outcomes including symptom reduction and functional improvements to evaluate longer-term effectiveness (Baydili et al., 2025). Use mixed-methods evaluation that combines sensor-derived quantitative trends with qualitative client narratives to capture subjective experience (Robinson et al., 2024). Specify timelines for measurement and interim decision points to decide whether to continue, adapt, or escalate interventions. There are several implementation pathways that fit common clinical contexts (Robinson et al., 2024). Private practices can adopt incremental approaches, beginning with off-the-shelf wearables and subscription XR modules adapted to clinical goals (Robinson et al., 2024). Community clinics may pursue partnerships with academic centers to gain access to pilot funding, shared infrastructure, and training resources that reduce up-front costs. Tertiary care systems can embed closed-loop therapeutics into stepped-care pathways to allocate resources based on clinical risk stratification (Robinson et al., 2024). Each pathway requires tailoring procurement, staffing, and evaluation plans to the local service model and client population (Robinson et al., 2024). Implementers should document decision criteria and expected timelines for each pathway to aid transparency and iterative planning.

To make this practical: start small, evaluate, and scale with clear metrics and staff buy-in. Begin with a limited pilot cohort to establish feasibility and to measure both clinical and operational indicators (Tavory, 2024). Define success criteria up front, including adherence thresholds, alert accuracy, and client satisfaction benchmarks. Use iterative Plan-Do-Study-Act cycles to refine technology configurations and workflow integrations (Tsai et al., 2025). Ensure frontline clinicians participate in decision making to secure their investment in sustainable adoption. Equity concerns must inform procurement and delivery decisions. Devices and access models that require high-end smartphones or persistent broadband will exclude many populations unless mitigations are enacted. Offer clinic-based XR pods, loaner devices, and subsidized connectivity as practical accommodations for those lacking resources (Tsai et al., 2025). Adapt XR content and AI models linguistically and culturally to reflect the diversity of your client population (Tsai et al., 2025). Regularly evaluate differential engagement and outcomes across demographic groups and adjust outreach, training, or device provisioning accordingly.

Plainly: accessibility planning is an implementation priority, not an optional add-on. Embed equity checkpoints into procurement decisions and project milestones so access concerns are considered from day one. Include community representatives in planning bodies to surface local constraints and preferences. Track metrics on access, dropout, and outcome disparities to inform resource reallocation and content localization. Commit to transparent reporting of equity-related outcomes within organizational governance structures.

Experts such as Thomas Insel, Albert Rizzo, Rosalind Picard have advanced concepts like neuroadaptive systems.

Several brief clinical vignettes highlight common therapeutic applications (Sun et al., 2025). First, an anxiety client used wearable-informed XR exposure to practice public speaking. The clinician tracked HRV during graded exposures and used the curve of recovery as a marker of progress; the client reported increased confidence that matched the physiological recordings. Use these vignettes to connect measurement to functional goals and to model clinician interpretation strategies. Second, a client with major depressive disorder received AI-triaged behavioral activation prompts tied to step count. The clinician and client reviewed weekly patterns to co-design incremental activity goals and to set realistic, measurable targets. Third, a veteran with PTSD engaged in XR exposure paired with real-time EDA monitoring; exposure intensity was titrated to maintain an optimal blend of challenge and safety. Collect and archive representative anonymized sessions to build clinical exemplars and training materials for future clinicians. Fourth, a college student used daily 10-

minute XR mindfulness modules after midterms; the system detected disrupted sleep trends and suggested brief sleep-focused modules, prompting a targeted sleep plan in therapy. Routinely translate vignette logic into one-page clinical templates that standardize assessment, intervention, and homework across cases (Ienca et al., 2017).

Risk mitigation includes ongoing audit of algorithmic performance, transparent documentation of model limitations, and accessible routes for client questions and complaints (Vaidyam et al., 2019). Establish a schedule for periodic algorithmic audits and define remediation steps for identified biases or performance degradations. Maintain an accessible policy explaining model scope, known limitations, and expected false positive and false negative rates (Ricciardi & Zomaya, 2025). Provide clients with a clear avenue to request data corrections, deletions, or human review of automated decisions (Ricciardi & Zomaya, 2025). Require vendors to supply explainability documentation that clinical teams can interpret and share with clients (Ricciardi & Zomaya, 2025). Incorporate client-facing FAQs into intake materials to preempt common concerns and to maintain trust.

Audits should examine both technical performance and disparate impact across demographic groups. Include demographic stratification in audit reports and review outcomes for differential performance by age, race, gender, language, and socioeconomic indicators. Engage independent auditors or community advisory boards to validate audit findings and to recommend mitigations when disparities are found. Document remediation actions and monitor their effects in subsequent audit cycles to ensure improvements are realized. Share summary audit outcomes with stakeholders in accessible language to promote transparency and accountability.

Documentation must be written in accessible language that clients can understand. Draft short, plain-English explanations for each major data stream, its intended use, and its known limits (Carl et al., 2019). Integrate these explanations into informed consent conversations and attach them to session notes when relevant. Train clinicians to use standard metaphors and analogies that make technical concepts comprehensible without being patronizing. Regularly solicit client feedback on clarity and revise materials based on their input. Clear documentation reduces misunderstandings and supports sustained engagement. For clinicians, this means maintaining a repository of brief patient-facing explanatory materials and integrating periodic consent refreshers into treatment planning. Store these materials in a shared clinical library with version control and easy search functionality. Schedule consent refreshers at clinically meaningful milestones, such as treatment phase changes or when new data streams are added. Use brief scripted language during refreshers to ensure consistency across clinicians while allowing personalization for individual contexts. Record the outcome of consent refreshers in the clinical record, noting questions and any modifications to client preferences (Ienca et al., 2017).

Looking ahead, the capabilities of these technologies will continue to expand. Expect integrations of environmental sensors, passive behavioral markers, and richer contextual signals to enhance situational awareness. Plan pilot studies that test incremental additions and measure marginal clinical value before full integration.(Xing et al., 2025). Prioritize client consent for each new data stream and document opt-in procedures explicitly in records (Kargarandehkordi et al., 2025). Engage ethics review boards early to evaluate privacy implications and community stakeholders to assess perceived benefits. Budget for additional data storage, annotation, and analyst time as more complex signals arrive (Kargarandehkordi et al., 2025). Establish criteria for retiring sensors that demonstrate low incremental utility or excessive privacy risk.

More sophisticated XR scenarios will be developed to address a broader range of therapeutic goals, and ongoing research will validate and refine these approaches (Friend et al., 2024). Collaborate with content developers to ensure scenarios map directly onto therapeutic targets and measurable learning objectives. Include representative end-users in co-design to improve cultural relevance and accessibility of virtual environments. Predefine metrics for scenario success, such as skill transfer to real-world situations and changes in physiological reactivity. Design randomized or stepped-wedge evaluations to build an evidence base without disrupting ongoing clinical care (Weiner et al., 2025). Share de-identified outcome summaries with the clinical community to accelerate best-practice dissemination (Weiner et al., 2025). Monitor adverse experiences and iterate content to minimize simulator sickness and distress.

However, each added data stream increases privacy complexity and interpretive burden; therefore, additions should follow demonstrable clinical utility and client consent (Walter et al., 2023). Implement a formal review gate where new sensors must meet predefined utility, equity, and privacy criteria before deployment. Require technical documentation that describes data provenance, retention, and de-identification methods for each sensor type .. Limit data access to roles with clear clinical need and record all secondary uses in a governance log .. Offer clients simple dashboards that show which streams are active and allow easy toggling of participation. Conduct periodic privacy impact assessments and publish aggregated results to maintain transparency. Treat removal of non-useful streams as part of ethical stewardship of client data .. Clinicians should adopt a conservative, needs-driven approach to new sensors rather than a maximalist data-collection stance (Pedram & Piatkowski, 2025). Prioritize devices that clearly answer clinical questions and demonstrate measurable impact on outcomes or workflow efficiency .. Integrate decision rules that require clinician confirmation before automated interventions act on novel data types .. Provide training modules that emphasize interpretation limits and common confounds for each sensor .. Encourage clinicians to document rationale when accepting or rejecting sensor-derived recommendations in the clinical record .. Foster a culture of critical appraisal where teams regularly question whether added complexity improves patient care. Reserve broad data collection only for research contexts with explicit participant consent and oversight (Pedram & Piatkowski, 2025).

For practicing clinicians and researchers, the imperative is operational: pilot thoughtfully, center client autonomy, and iteratively refine systems to serve core therapeutic aims rather than technological possibility alone. Start with narrowly defined clinical problems where measurable gains are plausible and scale only after demonstrated benefit (Poudel et al., 2025). Co-design interventions with end users to improve relevance and uptake. Embed evaluation metrics into clinical workflows so decisions to continue, adapt, or discontinue technologies are evidence-driven (Rajpal, 2025). Preserve the therapeutic relationship by making data and decisions interpretable and by involving clients in meaning-making around sensor-derived information (Rajpal, 2025). Adopt technologies that demonstrably improve assessment, augment therapeutic practice, and preserve the therapeutic relationship; everything else follows from rigorous, iterative implementation. Require clear documentation of how each technology affects clinical decision making and client outcomes (Rajpal, 2025). Use mixed-methods evaluation to capture both measurable changes and lived experience. Establish cross-site learning collaboratives to share lessons, avoid repeated errors, and accelerate best practices. Commit to transparent reporting of both successes and failures to build a realistic evidence base (Rajpal, 2025).

REFERENCES

Babu, A., & Joseph, A. P. (2025). Digital wellness or digital dependency? A critical examination of mental health apps and their implications. *Frontiers in Psychiatry*, *16*, 1581779. DOI: 10.3389/fpsyt.2025.1581779 PMID: 40248604

Baka, E., Tan, Y.-R., Wong, B. L. H., Xing, Z., & Yap, P. (2025). A scoping review of digital interventions for the promotion of mental health and prevention of mental health conditions for young people. *Oxford Open Digital Health*, *3*, oqaf005. DOI: 10.1093/oodh/oqaf005 PMID: 40230873

Ball, H., Eisner, E., Nicholas, J., Wilson, P., & Bucci, S. (2025). How theories, models, and frameworks have been used to implement digital health interventions in services for people with severe mental health problems: A scoping review. *BMC Public Health*, *25*(1), 1023. DOI: 10.1186/s12889-025-22189-2 PMID: 40098003

Baydili, İ., Tasci, B., & Tasci, G. (2025). Artificial intelligence in psychiatry: A review of biological and behavioral data analyses. *Diagnostics (Basel)*, *15*(4), 434. DOI: 10.3390/diagnostics15040434 PMID: 40002587

Carl, E., Stein, A. T., Levihn-Coon, A., Pogue, J. R., Rothbaum, B., Emmelkamp, P., Asmundson, G. J. G., Carlbring, P., & Powers, M. B. (2019). Virtual reality exposure therapy for anxiety and related disorders: A meta-analysis of randomized controlled trials. *Journal of Anxiety Disorders*, *61*, 27–36. DOI: 10.1016/j.janxdis.2018.08.003 PMID: 30287083

Casson, A. J. (2019). Wearable EEG and beyond. *Biomedical Engineering Letters*, *9*(1), 53–71. DOI: 10.1007/s13534-018-00093-6 PMID: 30956880

De Kock, J. H., Latham, H. A., Leslie, S. J., Grindle, M., Munoz, S. A., Ellis, L., Polson, R., & O'Malley, C. M. (2021). A rapid review of the impact of COVID-19 on the mental health of healthcare workers: Implications for supporting psychological well-being. *BMC Public Health*, *21*(1), 104. DOI: 10.1186/s12889-020-10070-3 PMID: 33422039

Fanarioti, A. K., & Karpouzis, K. (2025). Artificial Intelligence and the Future of Mental Health in a Digitally Transformed World. *Computers*, *14*(7), 259. DOI: 10.3390/computers14070259

Fleming, L. E., Maycock, B., White, M. P., & Depledge, M. H. (2019). Fostering human health through ocean sustainability in the 21st century. *People and Nature*, *1*(3), 276–283. DOI: 10.1002/pan3.10038

Freeman, D., Reeve, S., Robinson, A., Ehlers, A., Clark, D., Spanlang, B., & Slater, M. (2017). Virtual reality in the assessment, understanding, and treatment of mental health disorders. *Psychological Medicine*, *47*(14), 2393–2400. DOI: 10.1017/S003329171700040X PMID: 28325167

Friend, S. H., Ginsburg, G. S., Picard, R. W., & Drazen, J. M. (2024). Key issues as wearable digital health technologies enter clinical care. *The New England Journal of Medicine*, *390*(12), 1118–1127. DOI: 10.1056/NEJMra2307160 PMID: 38507754

Gkintoni, E., Vassilopoulos, S. P., & Nikolaou, G. (2025). Next-generation cognitive-behavioral therapy for depression: Integrating digital tools, teletherapy, and personalization for enhanced mental health outcomes. *Medicina (Kaunas, Lithuania)*, *61*(3), 431. DOI: 10.3390/medicina61030431 PMID: 40142242

Hall, C. L., Gómez Bergin, A. D., & Rennick-Egglestone, S. (2024). Research into digital health intervention for mental health: 25-year retrospective on the ethical and legal challenges. *Journal of Medical Internet Research*, *26*, e58939. DOI: 10.2196/58939 PMID: 39250796

Ienca, M., Fabrice, J., Elger, B., Caon, M., Scoccia Pappagallo, A., Kressig, R. W., & Wangmo, T. (2017). Intelligent assistive technology for Alzheimer's disease and other dementias: A systematic review. *Journal of Alzheimer's Disease*, *56*(4), 1301–1340. DOI: 10.3233/JAD-161037 PMID: 28222516

Inkster, B., Knibbs, C., & Bada, M. (2023). Cybersecurity: A critical priority for digital mental health. *Frontiers in Digital Health*, *5*, 1242264. DOI: 10.3389/fdgth.2023.1242264 PMID: 37781452

Iwaya, L. H., Babar, M. A., Rashid, A., & Wijayarathna, C. (2023). On the privacy of mental health apps: An empirical investigation and its implications for app development. *Empirical Software Engineering*, *28*(1), 2. DOI: 10.1007/s10664-022-10236-0 PMID: 36407814

Kargarandehkordi, A., Li, S., Lin, K., Phillips, K. T., Benzo, R. M., & Washington, P. (2025). Fusing wearable biosensors with artificial intelligence for mental health monitoring: A systematic review. *Biosensors (Basel)*, *15*(4), 202. DOI: 10.3390/bios15040202 PMID: 40277515

Khoo, Y. X., Kang, R. M., Reynolds, T. L., & Mentis, H. M. (2024). The comprehensiveness of mental health application users' privacy and security concerns. *CHI Conference on Human Factors in Computing Systems*, 16 pages.

Kim, J., & Backonja, U. (2025). Digital health equity frameworks and key concepts: A scoping review. *Journal of the American Medical Informatics Association : JAMIA, 32*(1), 45–59. DOI: 10.1093/jamia/ocaf017 PMID: 39936843

Lay, W., Gasparini, L., Siero, W., & Hughes, E. K. (2025). A rapid review of the benefits and challenges of dynamic consent. *Research Ethics, 21*(1), 180–202. DOI: 10.1177/17470161241278064

Lindner, P., Miloff, A., & Carlbring, P. (2024). The future of virtual reality therapy: Applications, challenges, and research directions. *Frontiers in Virtual Reality, 5*, 112345.

Liu, M., & Schueller, S. M. (2023). Moving evidence-based mental health interventions into practice: Implementation of digital mental health interventions. *Current Treatment Options in Psychiatry, 10*(4), 333–345. DOI: 10.1007/s40501-023-00298-2

Livieri, G., Mangina, E., Protopapadakis, E. D., & Panayiotou, A. G. (2025). The gaps and challenges in digital health technology use as perceived by patients: A scoping review and narrative meta-synthesis. *Frontiers in Digital Health, 7*, 1474956. DOI: 10.3389/fdgth.2025.1474956 PMID: 40212901

Martinez-Martin, N., Marcandalli, J., Huang, C. S., Arthur, C. P., Perotti, M., Foglierini, M., Ho, H., Dosey, A. M., Shriver, S., Payandeh, J., Leitner, A., Lanzavecchia, A., Perez, L., & Ciferri, C. (2018). An unbiased screen for human cytomegalovirus identifies neuropilin-2 as a central viral receptor. *Cell, 174*(5), 1158–1171. DOI: 10.1016/j.cell.2018.06.028 PMID: 30057110

Obermeyer, Z., Powers, B., Vogeli, C., & Mullainathan, S. (2019). Dissecting racial bias in an algorithm used to manage the health of populations. *Science, 366*(6464), 447–453. DOI: 10.1126/science.aax2342 PMID: 31649194

Pedram, S., & Piatkowski, T. (2025). Exploring the potential of virtual reality (Johnson et al., 2021) in mental healthcare: A systematic literature review. *Virtual Reality (Waltham Cross), 29*(3), 135. DOI: 10.1007/s10055-025-01181-6

Poudel, U., Jakhar, S., Mohan, P., & Nepal, A. (2025). AI in mental health: A review of technological advancements and ethical issues in psychiatry. *Issues in Mental Health Nursing, 46*(7), 693–701. DOI: 10.1080/01612840.2025.2502943 PMID: 40378075

Rajpal, S. (2025). Exploring the Role of Virtual Reality and Metaverse in Treating Mental Health: Operating Models and Challenges in Adoption. *Journal of Computer and Communications, 13*(10), 1–22. DOI: 10.4236/jcc.2025.1310001

Ricciardi, F., & Zomaya, A. (2025). Perspectives on Managing AI Ethics in the Digital Age. *Information (Basel), 16*(2), 89. DOI: 10.3390/info16040318

Robinson, A., Flom, M., Forman-Hoffman, V. L., Histon, T., Levy, M., Darcy, A., Ajayi, T., Mohr, D. C., Wicks, P., Greene, C., & Montgomery, R. M. (2024). Equity in digital mental health interventions in the United States: Where to next? *Journal of Medical Internet Research, 26*, e59939. DOI: 10.2196/59939 PMID: 39316436

Shatte, A. B., Hutchinson, D. M., & Teague, S. J. (2019). Machine learning in mental health: A scoping review of methods and applications. *Psychological Medicine, 49*(9), 1426–1448. DOI: 10.1017/S0033291719000151 PMID: 30744717

Smith, K. A., Blease, C., Faurholt-Jepsen, M., Firth, J., Van Daele, T., Moreno, C., Carlbring, P., Ebner-Priemer, U. W., Koutsouleris, N., Riper, H., Mouchabac, S., Torous, J., & Cipriani, A. (2023). Digital mental health: Challenges and next steps. *BMJ Mental Health, 26*(1), e300670. DOI: 10.1136/bmjment-2023-300670 PMID: 37197797

Spytska, L. (2025). The use of artificial intelligence in psychotherapy: Development of intelligent therapeutic systems. *BMC Psychology, 13*(1), 175. DOI: 10.1186/s40359-025-02491-9 PMID: 40022267

Sun, J., Lu, T., Shao, X., Han, Y., Xia, Y., Zheng, Y., Wang, Y., Li, X., Ravindran, A., Fan, L., Fang, Y., Zhang, X., Ravindran, N., Wang, Y., Liu, X., & Lu, L. (2025). Practical AI application in psychiatry: Historical review and future directions. *Molecular Psychiatry, 30*(9), 4399–4408. DOI: 10.1038/s41380-025-03072-3 PMID: 40456953

Tavory, T. (2024). Regulating AI in mental health: Ethics of care perspective. *JMIR Mental Health, 11*, e58493. DOI: 10.2196/58493 PMID: 39298759

Tsai, Y. Y., Chen, Y. J., Lin, Y. F., Hsiao, F. C., Hsu, C. H., & Liao, L. D. (2025). Photoplethysmography-based HRV analysis and machine learning for real-time stress quantification in mental health applications. *APL Bioengineering, 9*(2), 026103. DOI: 10.1063/5.0256590 PMID: 40191605

Vaidyam, A. N., Wisniewski, H., Halamka, J. D., Kashavan, M. S., & Torous, J. B. (2019). Chatbots and conversational agents in mental health: A review of the psychiatric landscape. *Canadian Journal of Psychiatry. Revue Canadienne de Psychiatrie, 64*(7), 456–464. DOI: 10.1177/0706743719828977 PMID: 30897957

Walter, J. R., Xu, S., & Rogers, J. A. (2023). From lab to life: How wearable devices can improve health equity. *Nature Communications, 14*, 44634. PMID: 38167483

Weiner, E. B., Dankwa-Mullan, I., Nelson, W. A., & Hassanpour, S. (2025). Ethical challenges and evolving strategies in the integration of artificial intelligence into clinical practice. *PLOS Digital Health*, *4*(4), e0000810. DOI: 10.1371/journal.pdig.0000810 PMID: 40198594

Xing, Y., Yang, Y., Yang, K., Lu, A., Xing, L., Mackie, K., & Guo, F. (2025). Intelligent sensing devices and systems for personalized mental health. *Med-X*, *3*(1), 10. DOI: 10.1007/s44258-025-00057-3 PMID: 40837134

Section 3
Applications Across the Lifespan

Chapter 8
Digital Mental Health Across the Lifespan

ABSTRACT

Mental health across childhood and adolescence is shaped by developmental trajectories, social environments, and neurobiological changes. This chapter emphasizes age-sensitive assessment and intervention strategies, integrating digital tools like XR and wearables to support engagement and early detection (Engel, 1977). It addresses unique challenges—such as consent complexity, cultural adaptation, and safeguarding privacy for minors—while highlighting opportunities for gamified interventions and family-centered care. Ethical frameworks must prioritize autonomy, parental involvement, and equity. Clinical protocols should embed developmental benchmarks and monitor long-term outcomes beyond symptom reduction, focusing on resilience, functional gains, and socioemotional growth (Rajpal, 2025). Technology must complement—not overshadow—human relationships in pediatric care.

INTRODUCTION

This chapter examines how digital therapeutics can be tailored to developmental stages across the lifespan, from early childhood through older adulthood. It emphasizes that mental health is dynamic and developmentally situated, requiring age-appropriate assessment, consent, and intervention strategies. The chapter explores applications such as gamified XR for children, AI-supported screening in adolescents, workplace interventions for adults, and cognitive support technologies for older adults. Caregiver involvement, autonomy, and ethical safeguards are addressed at each stage. Particular attention is given to neurodevelopmental conditions, including autism and learning differences, highlighting how adaptive systems can support individualized learning and regulation. The chapter stresses equity, accessibility, and cultural fit as essential to lifespan deployment. By integrating developmental science with digital

DOI: 10.4018/979-8-3373-4997-8.ch008

innovation, it demonstrates how technology can support continuity of care while respecting changing capacities and needs over time.

MENTAL HEALTH ACROSS THE LIFESPAN

Mental health is not a static condition but a dynamic continuum that evolves across the human lifespan, shaped by developmental milestones, environmental exposures, social contexts, and biological changes. This definition emphasizes that assessment and intervention must account for temporal change and developmental context in treatment planning. In clinical practice, this means routinely updating formulations as new information emerges and as patients progress through life stages (Martinez-Martin et al., 2018). Researchers should operationalize "continuum" as measurable change over time using longitudinal methods and repeated assessments. Policy and service design must therefore support flexible, stage-appropriate pathways rather than one-size-fits-all programs. From the first stirrings of emotional awareness in childhood to the cognitive complexities of adulthood and the vulnerabilities of aging, mental health care must adapt to the shifting needs of individuals at every stage of life. In this era of digital transformation, the integration of artificial intelligence (AI), extended reality (XR), and wearable sensors offers a revolutionary opportunity to reimagine mental health interventions as not only age-appropriate but also deeply personalized, context-aware, and neuroadaptive (Pedram & Piatkowski, 2025). This paragraph situates the chapter within a lifespan framework and underscores those technological solutions must be evaluated for developmental fit and ethical acceptability.

The journey begins in childhood, a period marked by rapid neurodevelopment, emotional learning, and socialization. Early childhood interventions should therefore prioritize developmental appropriateness and caregiver involvement to maximize learning transfer. Clinically, screening in this period benefits from multimodal data combining observation, caregiver report, and brief objective measures. Researchers should sample across contexts, home, school, clinical settings, to capture representative behavior and avoid false negatives. Practically, educational and pediatric systems need protocols to act on early warning signals with low-burden supports. Mental health challenges in this stage, such as anxiety, attention-deficit/hyperactivity disorder (ADHD), and early signs of mood disorders, often go undetected or are misinterpreted as behavioral issues. Traditional interventions, while effective for some, are often limited by stigma, accessibility, and a lack of engagement. Here, digital therapeutics offer a compelling alternative. Gamified XR environments can transform therapeutic exercises into immersive, playful experiences that resonate with young minds. AI-driven screening tools embedded in school systems or pediatric care settings can detect subtle behavioral patterns indicative of emerging mental health concerns. Wearable sensors, such as wristbands that monitor heart rate variability (Tizzard, 2025) or galvanic skin response (GSR), can provide real-time feedback on emotional regulation, enabling early intervention and fostering emotional literacy. These tools not only enhance clinical insight but also empower children and caregivers with actionable data, creating a feedback loop that supports resilience and self-awareness from an early age (Obermeyer et al., 2019).

As individuals transition into adolescence and young adulthood, the complexity of mental health challenges often intensifies. This developmental window requires interventions that respect growing autonomy while ensuring safety and caregiver collaboration. Clinicians should calibrate consent processes and disclosure protocols to honor adolescent privacy within legal and ethical boundaries. Researchers must design adolescent-focused validation studies that test engagement, safety, and efficacy in real-world settings. Practically, service systems should provide low-threshold access to evidence-based supports that adolescents can use privately and flexibly (Leivaditis & Sepetis, 2025). This period is characterized by identity formation, academic and social pressures, and increased vulnerability to mood disorders, substance use, and self-harm. Digital therapeutics can serve as both a safety net and a scaffold during this critical phase. AI-powered chatbots and virtual therapists offer anonymous, stigma-free access to support, while XR-based exposure therapies can help adolescents confront social anxiety or trauma in controlled, customizable environments (Li et al., 2025). Wearables continue to play a vital role, capturing physiological markers of stress and sleep disruption that often precede psychological symptoms. Importantly, these technologies can be integrated into educational settings, where early detection and intervention can have a profound impact on academic performance, peer relationships, and long-term mental health trajectories.

In adulthood, mental health care must contend with a new set of challenges: the pressures of career, relationships, parenting, and, increasingly, the digital overload of modern life. Adult interventions should be designed to fit within daily routines and to support self-management with clinician oversight when needed. Employers and health systems should consider integrating evidence-based digital therapeutics into employee assistance programs with clear privacy safeguards (Reddy, 2025). Research should test micro-interventions for feasibility and effect in real-world adult populations (Engel, 1977). Workplace stress, burnout, and anxiety are pervasive, yet often underreported due to fear of stigma or professional repercussions. Digital therapeutics offer scalable, discreet solutions that can be embedded into daily routines. AI-driven cognitive behavioral therapy (Rajpal, 2025) platforms can deliver personalized interventions on demand, adapting to the user's mood, behavior, and context (Engel, 1977). XR environments can simulate stressful scenarios, such as public speaking or conflict resolution, allowing users to practice coping strategies in a safe space (Engel, 1977). Wearable sensors can monitor physiological stress markers throughout the workday, prompting micro-interventions such as guided breathing or mindfulness exercises when thresholds are exceeded (Engel, 1977). These tools not only support individual well-being but also offer organizations a data-driven approach to fostering a mentally healthy workplace culture (Engel, 1977).

For adults managing chronic mental health conditions, such as depression, bipolar disorder, or PTSD, digital therapeutics can provide continuity of care that bridges the gaps between clinical visits (Singh & Chandra, 2025). Continuity requires systems that aggregate longitudinal data, enable clinician review, and support stepped care responses based on agreed thresholds. Clinically, integrate passive monitoring with scheduled human contact to avoid overreliance on automated signals. Researchers should validate relapse-prediction models against clinical outcomes and describe false-positive rates transparently. Programs must define escalation pathways so alerts trigger timely, proportionate clinical actions. AI algorithms can analyze longitudinal data from wearables and digital interactions to detect early signs of relapse or crisis, enabling proactive intervention. XR can be used to revisit and reframe traumatic memories in a controlled therapeutic context, while wearable biosensors can track the physiological impact of these sessions, ensuring safety and efficacy (Obermeyer et al., 2019). Moreover, digital platforms can facilitate peer support networks, connecting individuals with shared experiences and reducing the isolation that often accompanies chronic mental illness.

As individuals age, the mental health landscape shifts once again. Older adulthood brings new risk profiles and care needs that require proactive planning and age-informed assessment. Clinicians should incorporate functional assessments, social network mapping, and medication reviews into routine evaluations for older adults. Researchers must adapt measurement tools for sensory and cognitive changes common in aging populations. Service designers should ensure technologies support mobility limitations and simpler interfaces for older users. Older adults face unique challenges, including social isolation, grief, cognitive decline, and increased risk of neurodegenerative disorders such as Alzheimer's disease. Traditional mental health services are often underutilized in this population due to mobility issues, stigma, or lack of specialized providers. Digital therapeutics can bridge these gaps by bringing care directly into the home. XR environments can simulate familiar or meaningful settings, supporting memory recall and emotional engagement in individuals with dementia (Johnson et al., 2021). AI companions, designed with empathetic natural language processing, can provide cognitive stimulation, medication reminders, and even companionship (Ong et al., 2025). Wearable sensors can monitor sleep patterns, gait, and physiological stress, offering early warning signs of cognitive or emotional deterioration (Ong et al., 2025). Importantly, these tools can also support caregivers, providing real-time data and alerts that enhance safety and reduce caregiver burden

(Ong et al., 2025). Developers must prioritize privacy and consent processes tailored for older adults and their proxies to protect autonomy and dignity.

Across all life stages, the integration of AI, XR, and wearable sensors enables a shift from reactive to proactive mental health care (Glass et al., 2022). This shift requires clear clinical protocols that translate sensor-derived signals into meaningful clinical actions (Ricciardi & Zomaya, 2025). Healthcare teams should define thresholds for escalation, verify alerts clinically, and document responses in the medical record. Researchers should test these protocols in pragmatic trials that reflect routine care environments. Payers and policymakers must create reimbursement pathways for continuous monitoring and digital intervention services. Rather than waiting for symptoms to escalate to the point of crisis, digital therapeutics can detect subtle changes in behavior, physiology, or cognition and respond with timely, personalized interventions. This closed-loop model, where data informs intervention and intervention generates new data, creates a dynamic system of care that evolves with the individual (Ricciardi & Zomaya, 2025). Clinicians and patients should co-design response plans so interventions align with personal preferences and values. Moreover, by embedding these technologies into everyday environments, homes, schools, workplaces, they become not just tools for treatment, but integral components of a supportive mental health ecosystem.

However, the promise of lifespan-oriented digital therapeutics is not without challenges. Equity concerns can undermine the benefits if access and literacy are not addressed proactively. Teams should conduct equity impact assessments and deploy targeted supports for underserved populations. Data privacy, informed consent, and algorithmic transparency are central ethical requirements that must be operationalized in each implementation (Mulukuntla, 2025). Clinicians, technologists, and ethicists should collaborate to create understandable consent materials and audit algorithms for bias. Issues of accessibility, digital literacy, and cultural relevance must be addressed to ensure equitable impact. Ethical considerations, particularly around data privacy, algorithmic bias, and informed consent, are paramount, especially when working with vulnerable populations such as children or the elderly (Rajpal, 2025). Interdisciplinary collaboration is essential, bringing together clinicians, technologists, designers, and end-users to co-create solutions that are not only effective but also humane and inclusive. Teams should establish governance structures that include patient representatives to oversee ongoing use and evaluation.

In the chapters that follow, we will explore in greater detail how digital therapeutics are being applied across the lifespan. Each subsequent chapter examines specific age bands, real-world applications, and implementation examples to guide clinicians and researchers. Readers can expect practical recommendations for assessment, intervention selection, and workflow integration in each developmental stage. We will highlight common pitfalls, mitigation strategies, and metrics useful for quality improvement. Case examples and vignettes will illustrate translation from research to practice, emphasizing replicable steps for clinical programs (Kumar, 2025). We begin with pediatric and adolescent mental health, examining how gamified XR and AI-driven screening tools are transforming early intervention (Radanliev, 2025). We then turn to adult mental health and workplace stress, highlighting the role of digital CBT, real-time monitoring, and immersive training environments. Finally, we delve into geriatric mental health and cognitive decline, exploring how digital tools can support aging in place, enhance cognitive function, and provide compassionate care for individuals and their families. Together, these chapters illustrate a vision of mental health care that is continuous, adaptive, and deeply attuned to the rhythms of human life.

The mental health of children and adolescents is a critical area of concern, as early intervention can significantly impact their development and future well-being. Early systems should integrate family, school, and primary care data to form a comprehensive picture (Elfouly & Alouani, 2025). Clinicians must use developmentally sensitive screening tools and interpret results in context. Researchers should evaluate engagement and longer-term functional outcomes beyond symptom reduction. Policy makers should support school-clinic partnerships and funding for validated digital interventions (Engel, 1977). With the advent of digital therapeutics, innovative approaches such as gamified extended reality (XR), early detection methods, and school-based interventions are being explored to address mental health issues in this population (Engel, 1977). This chapter delves into these applications, highlighting their potential benefits and challenges.

CHILDREN WITH AUTISM

Children with autism spectrum disorder (ASD) present with marked heterogeneity across cognitive, sensory, behavioral, and socioemotional domains, making one-size-fits-all intervention models both clinically inefficient and ethically misaligned. Effective support for this population requires approaches that are individualized, developmentally grounded, and responsive to within-person variability over time. From a clinical standpoint, this means moving beyond static diagnostic characterizations toward dynamic, data-informed formulations that integrate caregiver report, direct behavioral observation, and objective psychophysiological indicators of regulation, attention, and stress. Digital therapeutics, particularly those integrating extended reality (XR), wearable sensors, and adaptive machine learning algorithms, are well suited to this task because they can embed assessment within intervention, minimizing disruption while maximizing ecological validity. Gamified XR environments can be designed to target specific skill domains such as joint attention, social communication, emotional labeling, and executive functioning, while simultaneously monitoring physiological markers such as heart rate variability or galvanic skin response to infer cognitive load and emotional arousal. For researchers, these systems offer a powerful platform for identifying digital phenotypes and testing mechanistic hypotheses related to learning, regulation, and generalization in autism within controlled yet realistic contexts. Educators, in turn, benefit from actionable outputs, such as dashboards translating in-session performance into classroom strategies, that align therapeutic goals with instructional practice and individualized education plans. At a policy level, the deployment of such technologies raises critical considerations around evidence standards, data governance, reimbursement, and cross-sector coordination between healthcare and educational systems. When implemented with clear clinical oversight, transparent algorithms, and strong privacy protections, neuroadaptive digital interventions hold the potential to support earlier detection, more precise intervention, and continuity of care, while respecting neurodiversity and promoting autonomy, skill acquisition, and long-term functional participation for children with autism.

CHILDREN WITH DYSLEXIA

Wearable sensors, such as smartwatches, fitness trackers, and EEG headbands, play a pivotal role in this ecosystem (Moriarty et al., 2022). First, define the measurement targets clearly: specify which physiological metrics map to which clinical constructs, such as HRV for autonomic regulation and actigraphy for sleep continuity (Rajpal, 2025). Second, insist on baseline calibration periods to establish individual norms before interpreting deviations (Rajpal, 2025). Third, require data quality checks and signal-processing standards to reduce artifact-driven false alerts (Rajpal, 2025). Clinically, integrate wearable outputs with patient-reported outcomes and behavioral observations to form multi-source assessments (Rajpal, 2025). For example, a consistent elevation in HRV during school hours might indicate social stress or academic pressure (Rajpal, 2025). These devices can continuously monitor physiological parameters like heart rate variability (HRV), galvanic skin response (GSR), and brainwave activity (Rajpal, 2025).

In school-based settings, these technologies can be particularly impactful. Start by specifying implementation prerequisites: obtain district-level approvals, secure parental consent, and allocate staff time for training and monitoring. Recommend pilot phases with mixed-methods evaluation to refine workflows before full rollout. Emphasize partnerships with local clinicians to create clear escalation pathways for identified concerns. For example, a student wearing a sensor-equipped wristband might receive subtle haptic feedback when their stress levels rise, prompting them to use a breathing exercise app or seek support from a counselor (Ghadi et al., 2025). Over time, the system can learn to anticipate stress triggers and offer proactive interventions, creating a preventive mental health framework rather than a reactive one.

EXPOSURE THERAPY AND XR

Exposure therapy remains one of the most empirically supported interventions for anxiety disorders, trauma-related conditions, and avoidance-driven psychopathology, yet its clinical uptake is frequently limited by logistical constraints, patient apprehension, and challenges in maintaining treatment fidelity outside of specialized settings. Extended reality (XR) meaningfully expands the reach and precision of exposure-based interventions by enabling clinicians to design immersive, repeatable, and systematically graded scenarios that closely map onto individualized fear or avoidance hierarchies. From a clinical perspective, XR allows for fine-grained control over stimulus intensity, duration, and complexity, supporting titrated exposure that can be adjusted in real time based on patient response rather than fixed session plans. The integration of physiological monitoring, such as heart rate variability, skin conductance, or respiration, further enhances clinical decision-making by providing objective indicators of arousal and regulation that complement subjective distress ratings. For researchers, XR-based exposure offers a rare balance of experimental control and ecological validity, enabling systematic investigation of habituation, inhibitory learning, and generalization processes across standardized yet lifelike conditions. Educators and trainers can leverage XR to improve workforce capacity by allowing trainees to practice exposure planning, pacing, and response to distress signals in simulated environments before working with patients. At a systems and policy level, XR exposure therapy raises important considerations related to clinical training standards, safety protocols, reimbursement models, and documentation requirements, particularly when deployed outside specialty clinics. When embedded within clinician-guided, human-in-the-loop workflows, with clear consent processes, emergency stop mechanisms, and post-exposure debriefing, XR-enhanced exposure therapy has the potential to improve treatment engagement, extend access to evidence-based care, and strengthen fidelity to core behavioral principles while preserving the central role of therapeutic judgment, collaboration, and ethical responsibility.

INTEGRATION OF BIOFEEDBACK

Biofeedback is a therapeutic technique that involves monitoring physiological signals, such as heart rate, skin conductance, and brain activity, and providing real-time feedback to the individual. Specify calibration procedures and baseline epochs to reduce misinterpretation of momentary fluctuations as clinical change (Chennupati, 2025). Require that biofeedback outputs be displayed in clinically meaningful units and paired with brief coaching scripts to teach self-regulation skills. Build audit trails so clinicians can review physiologic trends alongside session notes and homework adherence. Use mixed-methods evaluation to capture both behavioral change and subjective experience of biofeedback interventions. This feedback helps individuals become more aware of their physiological states and learn to regulate them, which is particularly useful in managing anxiety, stress, and emotional dysregulation.

CHILDREN WITH AUTISM

Moreover, Lamb integrates machine learning algorithms to adapt these XR environments in real time based on the child's behavior and physiological responses (Ferrar et al., 2021). Define adaptation criteria clearly so clinicians know which physiological thresholds trigger changes in the environment. Advise periodic review of adaptation logs with caregivers to explain decisions and plan next steps. Suggest that adaptive models be trained on diverse datasets to improve generalizability and reduce bias. Stress that clinician oversight must remain central, with automated adjustments serving as adjunctive supports. In the context of dyslexia, Lamb's work explores how gamified XR combined with AI can support reading and language development. Clarify that interventions target phonological processing, decoding speed, and orthographic mapping through multisensory scaffolds. Recommend regular validity checks by a reading specialist to ensure game tasks align with proved pedagogical progressions. Suggest embedding teacher dashboards that translate in-game metrics into classroom interventions. Urge early implementation to capitalize on neural plasticity during foundational literacy development.

This dual-purpose design, diagnostic and therapeutic, is a hallmark of Lamb's methodology. Explain that combining assessment within play reduces assessment fatigue and preserves engagement while producing actionable learning data (Fanarioti & Karpouzis, 2025). Recommend clinicians review diagnostic logs weekly and integrate findings into individualized education plans. Encourage researchers to publish transparent feature sets used for diagnostic classifications to aid replication. Reinforce that integrating diagnostics and therapy shortens the feedback loop between detection and tailored intervention.

Lamb's approach aligns with broader findings in the field, such as those from the DysLexML project, which uses machine learning to analyze eye-tracking data for early dyslexia screening (Hughes & Kalra, 2023). Clarify that cross-study alignment improves confidence in candidate digital markers and supports shared measurement standards (Tsai et al., 2025). Advise practitioners to prefer tools that report sensitivity and specificity across age bands comparable to their patient populations. Recommend collaborative networks to pool anonymized data for better model calibration across contexts (Tsai et al., 2025). Highlight that standardized reporting formats facilitate pragmatic adoption in schools and clinics.

These tools can be integrated into XR platforms to provide personalized learning paths, helping children overcome specific challenges in phonemic awareness, decoding, and fluency (Basystiuk et al., 2024). Implement simple decision rules that map in-game performance to instructional adjustments so teachers and clinicians can act on results. Validate the mapping rules against standardized reading assessments before relying on them for formal remediation planning. Include periodic clinician review points to confirm that algorithmic adjustments align with observed classroom progress. Provide teacher training modules that translate game metrics into concrete instructional moves to reinforce learning in multiple contexts.

Moreover, the gamified nature of these XR environments helps reduce the stigma and frustration often associated with traditional reading interventions (Smuck et al., 2021). Frame activities as skill-building quests with clear, measurable objectives to maintain focus on learning rather than deficit. Monitor affective engagement alongside skill metrics to ensure improvements are not driven solely by extrinsic rewards. Encourage teachers and parents to celebrate small mastery milestones to build sustained motivation and self-efficacy in learners. Pair game sessions with brief reflective prompts that help children link in-game successes to real-world reading tasks.

Early detection of mental health issues in children and adolescents is essential for timely intervention and the prevention of long-term psychological and developmental consequences. Specify which outcomes count as meaningful change to avoid overreacting to transient variability in young people's behavior. Use stepped-care pathways that link low-intensity supports to more intensive interventions based on validated thresholds (Ferrara, 2024). Maintain transparent communication with families about what early-detection signals mean and how the care team will respond. Prioritize equitable deployment so that early detection advantages do not concentrate in already well-served populations. Machine learning algorithms can analyze data from a variety of sources, such as mobile app usage, social media activity, and wearable devices, to detect subtle changes in behavior that may signal emerging mental health concerns (Mohr et al., 2017). Require that any algorithm used in practice include readily interpretable outputs and recommended clinician actions to bridge the gap between flagging and care (Mohr et al., 2017). Test algorithms in the specific populations where they will be deployed to ensure local validity and reduce misclassification. Build simple clinician dashboards that highlight actionable trends rather than raw sensor streams to prevent alert fatigue (Mohr et al., 2017).

Wearable sensors, such as smartwatches, fitness trackers, and EEG headbands, play a pivotal role in this ecosystem (Mohr et al., 2017). Clarify measurement intent by mapping each sensor to a specific clinical construct, for example, actigraphy for sleep continuity and HRV for autonomic regulation (Mohr et al., 2017). Require initial baseline monitoring periods to establish normative values for each individual before interpreting deviations. Insist on routine data quality checks and artifact rejection protocols so clinical decisions are not driven by noise (Mohr et al., 2017). Recommend integrating sensor outputs with self-report and collateral observations to improve interpretability and reduce false alarms (Mohr et al., 2017).

Lamb's systems are designed to detect early signs of emotional distress and adjust the digital environment accordingly, whether by reducing sensory input, offering calming stimuli, or alerting a caregiver. Define the operational decision rules that link specific sensor thresholds to system actions so clinicians can audit and override automated responses (Hilty et al., 2021). Recommend documentation of adaptation events and clinical rationales in the patient record to preserve continuity of care (Ricciardi & Zomaya, 2025). Emphasize co-design with families to set acceptable notification preferences and escalation steps. This neuroadaptive feedback loop not only supports early detection but also provides immediate, personalized support (Ricciardi & Zomaya, 2025).

In school-based settings, these technologies can be particularly impactful. Start by outlining governance requirements: district approval, clear data-use agreements, and defined responsibilities for monitoring and response (Almadani et al., 2025). Specify training modules for school staff that cover device use, basic data interpretation, and escalation protocols to clinical services (Tsai et al., 2025). Pilot implementations should measure both student-level outcomes and classroom workflow impacts to ensure feasibility. For example, a student wearing a sensor-equipped wristband might receive subtle haptic feedback when their stress levels rise, prompting them to use a breathing exercise app or seek support from a counselor (Tsai et al., 2025).

EXPOSURE THERAPY AND XR

One of the key advantages of gamified XR is its ability to provide a safe and controlled environment for exposure therapy (Akinode et al., 2025). State explicit session safety procedures including baseline vitals, clinician presence for moderate-to-high intensity exposures, and emergency stop mechanisms. Require pre-session goal-setting and post-session debriefs to translate in-VR learning into in vivo behavior. Recommend collecting both subjective distress ratings and objective physiological markers during exposures to triangulate progress. For instance, children with social anxiety can practice social interactions in a virtual setting, gradually building their confidence and coping skills.

INTEGRATION OF BIOFEEDBACK

Biofeedback is a therapeutic technique that involves monitoring physiological signals, such as heart rate, skin conductance, and brain activity, and providing real-time feedback to the individual. Clarify the instructional aim: teach patients to notice somatic cues and apply learned regulatory strategies when alerted by biofeedback signals. Require standardized coaching scripts that pair each physiological cue with a specific behavioral exercise to build reproducible skills. Implement pre-session baseline epochs to distinguish trait from state variability and set individualized targets. Use visual and auditory feedback modalities that match developmental stage and sensory preferences to maximize learning. Ensure clinicians document biofeedback-guided interventions and progress in the medical record for continuity. This feedback helps individuals become more aware of their physiological states and learn to regulate them, which is particularly useful in managing anxiety, stress, and emotional dysregulation.

These findings collectively underscore the potential of gamified XR as a scalable, engaging, and evidence-based tool for pediatric and adolescent mental health care (Sheikh et al., 2021). Include a systems-level recommendation: pair technology deployment with policy levers such as reimbursement codes, procurement standards, and equity-focused deployment plans. Require that implementers estimate total cost of ownership, including devices, training, and maintenance, before committing to scale. Recommend establishing local advisory groups including parents, educators, and youth to guide culturally responsive content adaptation and deployment decisions.

Lamb's systems are designed to detect early signs of emotional distress and adjust the digital environment accordingly, whether by reducing sensory input, offering calming stimuli, or alerting a caregiver. Define operational decision rules that map sensor thresholds to specific system responses, and require that these rules be documented and reviewable by clinicians and guardians (Mohammad, 2021). Insist on human-in-the-loop architectures where automated adaptations are subject to clinician audit and override to preserve professional responsibility. Log all automated adjustments and clinician interventions to support quality review and ongoing model refinement (Radanliev, 2025). Balance sensitivity and specificity through iterative tuning during pilot phases to reduce both missed events and false alarms. This neuroadaptive feedback loop not only supports early detection but also provides immediate, personalized support (Radanliev, 2025).

In school-based settings, these technologies can be particularly impactful. Start implementation by securing district approvals, clear data-use agreements, and tiered consent processes that differentiate passive monitoring from active interventions (Kang & Exworthy, 2022). Provide succinct training for teachers and school staff that focuses on workflow integration and on recognizing when to escalate to clinical teams (Tsai et al., 2025). Pilot interventions in a limited number of classrooms to evaluate classroom flow impacts and to refine scheduling, device charging logistics, and privacy protections. Ensure that outputs presented to educators are aggregate and actionable, avoiding student-level raw data displays that could breach privacy or overburden staff (Tsai et al., 2025). With these safeguards, a student wearing a sensor-equipped wristband might receive subtle haptic feedback when stress rises, prompting brief in-class coping practices or a counselor check-in (Tsai et al., 2025).

Integrated digital ecosystems combine AI, XR, and biosensing to deliver neuroadaptive mental health care.

Exposure therapy benefits from XR's capacity to present repeatable, controllable scenarios that map onto avoidance hierarchies (Zenker et al., 2022). Require clinicians to construct explicit exposure hierarchies and measurable behavioral goals before XR sessions commence, and to record subjective units of distress alongside objective physiological markers (Mohr et al., 2017). Use graduated stepping with predefined criteria for progression and fallback procedures when arousal exceeds safe levels. Implement post-session generalization tasks that practice skills in vivo and document transfer effects across contexts. Maintain session fidelity checks and adverse-event reporting so treatment teams can monitor safety and effectiveness over time. For many patients, this structured XR approach enables intensive, efficient habituation while preserving clinician oversight and patient safety (Mohr et al., 2017). See the checklist in contained in Chapter 8 Appendix.

REFERENCES

Akinode, A. O., Ayadi, O. E., Ezerioha, C. C., & Chika, P (2025). Machine Learning Approaches for Early Detection of Mental Health Disorders Using Wearable Devices and Big Data Analytics. environments, 4, 5.

Almadani, B., Kaisar, H., Thoker, I. R., & Aliyu, F. (2025). A systematic survey of distributed decision support systems in healthcare. *Systems*, *13*(3), 157. DOI: 10.3390/systems13030157

Basystiuk, O., Rybchak, Z., Zavushchak, I., & Marikutsa, U. (2024). Evaluation of multimodal data synchronization tools. *Comput. Des. Syst. Theory Pract*, *6*(3), 104–111. DOI: 10.23939/cds2024.03.104

Chennupati, N. (2025). Securing the Automated Enterprise: A Framework for Mitigating Security and Privacy Risks in AI-Driven Workflow Automation. *Journal of Computer Science and Technology Studies*, *7*(3), 624–632. DOI: 10.32996/jcsts.2025.7.3.71

Elfouly, T., & Alouani, A. (2025). A comprehensive survey on wearable computing for mental and physical health monitoring. *Electronics (Basel)*, *14*(17), 3443. DOI: 10.3390/electronics14173443

Engel, G. L. (1977). The need for a new medical model: A challenge for biomedicine. *Science*, *196*(4286), 129–136. DOI: 10.1126/science.847460 PMID: 847460

Fanarioti, A. K., & Karpouzis, K. (2025). Artificial Intelligence and the Future of Mental Health in a Digitally Transformed World. *Computers*, *14*(7), 259. DOI: 10.3390/computers14070259

Ferrar, J., Griffith, G. J., Skirrow, C., Cashdollar, N., Taptiklis, N., Dobson, J., Cree, F., Cormack, F. K., Barnett, J. H., & Munafò, M. R. (2021). Developing digital tools for remote clinical research: How to evaluate the validity and practicality of active assessments in field settings. *Journal of Medical Internet Research*, *23*(6), e26004. DOI: 10.2196/26004 PMID: 34142972

Ferrara, E. (2024). Large language models for wearable sensor-based human activity recognition, health monitoring, and behavioral modeling: A survey of early trends, datasets, and challenges. *Sensors (Basel)*, *24*(15), 5045. DOI: 10.3390/s24155045 PMID: 39124092

Ghadi, Y. Y., Shah, S. F. A., Waheed, W., Mazhar, T., Ahmad, W., Saeed, M. M., & Hamam, H. (2025). Integration of wearable technology and artificial intelligence in digital health for remote patient care. *Journal of Cloud Computing (Heidelberg, Germany), 14*(1), 39. DOI: 10.1186/s13677-025-00759-4

Glass, J. E., Tiffany, B., Matson, T. E., Lim, C., Gundersen, G., Kimbel, K., Hartzler, A. L., Curran, G. M., McWethy, A. G., Caldeiro, R. M., & Bradley, K. A. (2022). Approaches for implementing digital interventions for alcohol use disorders in primary care: A qualitative, user-centered design study. *Implementation Research and Practice, 3*, 26334895221135264. DOI: 10.1177/26334895221135264 PMID: 37091101

Hilty, D. M., Armstrong, C. M., Luxton, D. D., Gentry, M. T., & Krupinski, E. A. (2021). A scoping review of sensors, wearables, and remote monitoring for behavioral health: Uses, outcomes, clinical competencies, and research directions. *Journal of Technology in Behavioral Science, 6*(2), 278–313. DOI: 10.1007/s41347-021-00199-2 PMID: 33501372

Hughes, N., & Kalra, D. (2023). Data standards and platform interoperability. In *Real-World Evidence in Medical Product Development* (pp. 79–107). Springer. DOI: 10.1007/978-3-031-26328-6_6

Johnson, K. B., Wei, W. Q., Weeraratne, D., Frisse, M. E., Misulis, K., Rhee, K., Zhao, J., & Snowdon, J. L. (2021). Precision medicine, AI, and the future of personalized health care. *Clinical and Translational Science, 14*(1), 86–93. DOI: 10.1111/cts.12884 PMID: 32961010

Kang, H. S., & Exworthy, M. (2022). Wearing the future—wearables to empower users to take greater responsibility for their health and care: Scoping review. *JMIR mHealth and uHealth, 10*(7), e35684. DOI: 10.2196/35684 PMID: 35830222

Kumar, P. (2025). Securing Digital-First Healthcare: AI, Blockchain, and Cloud Architectures for Personal Health Data Protection. *International Journal of Applied Mathematics, 38*(7s).

Leivaditis, V., & Sepetis, A (2025). Digital Transformation As A Catalyst For Sustainable Health Care Systems: A Narrative Review Of Current Evidence. International Journal of Innovation Management, 29(05n06), 2540009.

Li, M., Patel, J., & Katapally, T. R. (2025). The impact of extended reality cognitive behavioral therapy on mental disorders among children and youth: A systematic review and meta-analysis protocol. *PLoS One, 20*(3), e0315313. DOI: 10.1371/journal.pone.0315313 PMID: 40048453

Martinez-Martin, N., Marcandalli, J., Huang, C. S., Arthur, C. P., Perotti, M., Foglierini, M., Ho, H., Dosey, A. M., Shriver, S., Payandeh, J., Leitner, A., Lanzavecchia, A., Perez, L., & Ciferri, C. (2018). An unbiased screen for human cytomegalovirus identifies neuropilin-2 as a central viral receptor. *Cell, 174*(5), 1158–1171. DOI: 10.1016/j.cell.2018.06.028 PMID: 30057110

Mohammad, N. (2021). Enhancing security and privacy in multi-cloud environments: A comprehensive study on encryption techniques and access control mechanisms. [IJCET]. *International Journal of Computer Engineering and Technology, 12*(2), 51–63.

Mohr, D. C., Zhang, M., & Schueller, S. M. (2017). Personal sensing: Understanding mental health using ubiquitous sensors and machine learning. *Annual Review of Clinical Psychology, 13*(1), 23–47. DOI: 10.1146/annurev-clinpsy-032816-044949 PMID: 28375728

Moriarty, A. S., Meader, N., Snell, K. I., Riley, R. D., Paton, L. W., Dawson, S., Hendon, J., Chew-Graham, C. A., Gilbody, S., Churchill, R., Phillips, R. S., Ali, S., & McMillan, D. (2022). Predicting relapse or recurrence of depression: Systematic review of prognostic models. *The British Journal of Psychiatry : The Journal of Mental Science, 221*(2), 448–458. DOI: 10.1192/bjp.2021.218 PMID: 35048843

Mulukuntla, S. (2025). Monitoring and Remote Patient Management with Immersive Technologies. In Augmented Wellness: Exploring the Power of VR and AR in Healthcare (pp. 197-218). Springer. DOI: 10.1007/978-981-96-2952-7_9

Obermeyer, Z., Powers, B., Vogeli, C., & Mullainathan, S. (2019). Dissecting racial bias in an algorithm used to manage the health of populations. *Science, 366*(6464), 447–453. DOI: 10.1126/science.aax2342 PMID: 31649194

Ong, T., Ivanova, J., Soni, H., Barrera, J., Cummins, M., Welch, B. M., & Bunnell, B. E. (2025). Mental health clients' perspectives on telehealth-based virtual reality therapy. *Frontiers in Virtual Reality, 6*, 1595326. DOI: 10.3389/frvir.2025.1595326

Pedram, S., & Piatkowski, T. (2025). Exploring the potential of virtual reality (Johnson et al., 2021) in mental healthcare: A systematic literature review. *Virtual Reality (Waltham Cross), 29*(3), 135. DOI: 10.1007/s10055-025-01181-6

Radanliev, P. (2025). Privacy, ethics, transparency, and accountability in AI systems for wearable devices. *Frontiers in Digital Health, 7*, 1431246. DOI: 10.3389/fdgth.2025.1431246 PMID: 40599875

Rajpal, S. (2025). Exploring the Role of Virtual Reality and Metaverse in Treating Mental Health: Operating Models and Challenges in Adoption. *Journal of Computer and Communications*, *13*(10), 1–22. DOI: 10.4236/jcc.2025.1310001

Reddy, K. J. (2025). Integrating Technology into Clinical Practice. In Innovations in Neurocognitive Rehabilitation: Harnessing Technology for Effective Therapy (pp. 329-350). Springer. DOI: 10.1007/978-3-031-88117-6_15

Ricciardi, F., & Zomaya, A. (2025). Perspectives on Managing AI Ethics in the Digital Age. *Information (Basel)*, *16*(2), 89. DOI: 10.3390/info16040318

Sheikh, M., Qassem, M., & Kyriacou, P. A. (2021). Wearable, environmental, and smartphone-based passive sensing for mental health monitoring. *Frontiers in Digital Health*, *3*, 662811. DOI: 10.3389/fdgth.2021.662811 PMID: 34713137

Singh, B., & Chandra, S. (2025). Strengthening Sensors and Wearable Technologies in Gauging Healthcare Transmuting Digital Health Technologies: Human Augmentation via Innovation and Implementations of AI. In Cases on AI Innovations in Occupational Health and Safety (pp. 289-308). IGI Global Scientific Publishing.

Smuck, M., Odonkor, C. A., Wilt, J. K., Schmidt, N., & Swiernik, M. A. (2021). The emerging clinical role of wearables: Factors for successful implementation in healthcare. *NPJ Digital Medicine*, *4*(1), 45. DOI: 10.1038/s41746-021-00418-3 PMID: 33692479

Tizzard, C. L. (2025). Re-imagining Care for Aging Disabled Adults.

Tsai, Y. Y., Chen, Y. J., Lin, Y. F., Hsiao, F. C., Hsu, C. H., & Liao, L. D. (2025). Photoplethysmography-based HRV analysis and machine learning for real-time stress quantification in mental health applications. *APL Bioengineering*, *9*(2), 026103. DOI: 10.1063/5.0256590 PMID: 40191605

Zenker, S., Strech, D., Ihrig, K., Jahns, R., Müller, G., Schickhardt, C., Schmidt, G., Speer, R., Winkler, E., von Kielmansegg, S. G., & Drepper, J. (2022). Data protection-compliant broad consent for secondary use of health care data and human biosamples for (Mulukuntla, 2025) medical research: Towards a new German national standard. *Journal of Biomedical Informatics*, *131*, 104096. DOI: 10.1016/j.jbi.2022.104096 PMID: 35643273

Chapter 9
Digital Therapeutics and Workplace Mental Health

ABSTRACT

The modern workplace is marked by rapid technological change, remote work models, and blurred boundaries between professional and personal life. These shifts have increased cognitive load, reduced recovery windows, and amplified stress through constant connectivity and asynchronous demands. This chapter examines how evolving work structures impact mental health, highlighting risks such as burnout, anxiety, and depression. It advocates for assessment protocols that capture altered temporal patterns and organizational stressors, alongside interventions that promote resilience, digital hygiene, and flexible scheduling. Employers and clinicians must collaborate to embed mental health safeguards into workflow design, ensuring equity and sustainability in the digital workplace.

INTRODUCTION

This chapter focuses on the application of digital therapeutics to burnout, stress, and mental health challenges in modern workplaces. It reframes burnout as a systemic, occupational phenomenon shaped by workload, autonomy, and digital overexposure. The chapter explores how wearable sensors, AI analytics, and mobile interventions can enable early detection, resilience training, and preventive care. Ethical governance is emphasized to prevent surveillance and misuse of employee data, including strict separation from performance evaluation. Case examples illustrate how aggregate analytics can inform organizational change while preserving individual privacy. The chapter positions digital workplace mental health as a shared responsibility between clinicians, organizations, and workers, requiring cultural, policy, and infrastructural alignment.

DOI: 10.4018/979-8-3373-4997-8.ch009

DIGITAL THERAPEUTICS

The 21st-century workplace is undergoing a profound transformation, shaped by rapid technological innovation, evolving labor dynamics, and shifting cultural expectations. These shifts alter daily tasks, reporting structures, and the rhythms of work that underpin employee routines. Employers now deploy digital platforms that change when, where, and how work is completed, often increasing asynchronous demands. Workers encounter more frequent interruptions and shorter blocks of focused time, which change recovery windows and cognitive load. Practically, clinicians should assess not only symptom reports but also these altered temporal patterns when formulating work-related stress. While these changes have introduced unprecedented levels of connectivity, flexibility, and productivity, they have also contributed to a growing mental health crisis among working adults. The traditional boundaries between work and personal life have eroded, particularly in the wake of remote and hybrid work models that, while offering convenience, have fostered a culture of constant availability and digital overexposure. This always-on environment has led to rising levels of stress, burnout, and psychological distress, making mental health a central concern not only for individuals but also for organizations striving to maintain a healthy, engaged, and resilient workforce. Burnout, now recognized by the World Health Organization as an occupational phenomenon, exemplifies the systemic dysfunctions of modern work, manifesting as emotional exhaustion, cynicism, and diminished personal efficacy, and resulting in significant costs to both human well-being and organizational performance. In response to these challenges, digital therapeutics have emerged as a promising frontier in mental health care. These evidence-based, software-driven interventions leverage technologies such as artificial intelligence (AI), extended reality (XR), mobile platforms, and wearable sensors to deliver scalable, personalized, and proactive mental health support (Panarese et al., 2025). Unlike traditional wellness apps, digital therapeutics are often clinically validated and designed to integrate seamlessly into daily routines, offering accessible solutions for populations that face barriers to conventional care (Fleming et al., 2019). This chapter explores how digital therapeutics are reshaping the landscape of adult mental health in the workplace, focusing on three key areas: the early detection and prevention of burnout, the cultivation of resilience through structured digital training, and the delivery of cognitive behavioral therapy (Morey et al., 2025) via interactive, mobile-based platforms. These innovations represent a shift from reactive to preventive care, aligning with the broader movement toward precision mental health, which emphasizes individualized, context-aware interventions. However, the successful implementation of these tools requires more than technological sophistication, it demands organizational commitment, ethical oversight, and a culture that prioritizes psychological safety and inclusivity. As we examine the potential of digital therapeutics to transform workplace well-being, we must also consider the broader implications for equity, data privacy, and the future of work itself (Fleming et al., 2019). By embracing these innovations with empathy, intentionality, and a commitment to equity, we can begin to reimagine the workplace not just as a site of productivity, but as a space that actively supports and sustains mental health.

Burnout, once considered a niche concern confined to high-stress professions, has emerged as a global epidemic affecting workers across all sectors. The term now applies beyond frontline fields and includes knowledge workers, service employees, and those in precarious roles. Clinicians and organizations increasingly see overlapping presentations of chronic stress that meet burnout criteria, necessitating cross-disciplinary strategies. Practitioners should therefore assess occupational context, workload patterns, and systemic contributors alongside clinical symptoms (Allgaier et al., 2023). It is no longer a fringe issue but a widespread occupational hazard with profound implications for individual well-being, organizational performance, and public health. Defined by the World Health Organization (Engel, 1977) as a syndrome resulting from chronic workplace stress that has not been successfully managed, burnout is characterized by three core dimensions: emotional exhaustion, depersonalization or cynicism, and a reduced sense of personal accomplishment. These symptoms do not arise in isolation; they are the cumulative result of systemic dysfunctions within the workplace environment.

The recognition of burnout as an occupational phenomenon by the WHO in 2019 marked a pivotal moment in the discourse on workplace mental health (Correa et al., 2021). This designation reframes clinical assessment and organizational responsibility, shifting attention to systemic prevention. It invites employers to adopt structural interventions rather than relying solely on individual-level remedies. In practice, this means clinicians should collaborate with occupational health and leadership to address root causes. It signaled a shift away from viewing burnout as a personal failing or a matter of individual resilience, toward understanding it as a structural issue rooted in organizational culture, leadership practices, and the broader socio-economic context of work. This reframing is essential, as it opens the door to systemic interventions and policy-level changes rather than placing the burden solely on individuals to cope or adapt.

Burnout stems from a complex interplay of organizational, interpersonal, and individual factors. These domains interact dynamically over time, producing cumulative strain or resilience depending on their configuration. Clinicians should map these interacting influences during assessment to prioritize intervention targets. Among the most commonly cited contributors are excessive workloads, unrealistic performance expectations, lack of autonomy, poor leadership, inadequate recognition, and a persistent imbalance between work and personal life. These stressors are often exacerbated by digital technologies that blur the boundaries between professional and private spheres, creating an "always-on" culture that leaves little room for recovery or psychological detachment.

Excessive workload is perhaps the most visible and quantifiable driver of burnout. Workload measures correlate with stress markers and predictable declines in cognitive performance under chronic pressure. Practical assessment should include both objective workload metrics and the employee's subjective experience of capacity. Employees who are consistently expected to perform beyond their capacity, without adequate resources or support, are at high risk of emotional exhaustion. This is particularly true in sectors such as healthcare, education, and technology, where high demands are often coupled with emotional labor and moral distress. Unrealistic expectations, whether self-imposed or externally driven, further compound this pressure, leading to chronic stress and eventual disengagement. Lack of autonomy and control over one's work is another critical factor. When employees lack decision-making authority, they often experience reduced motivation and higher stress reactivity. Clinically, diminished control predicts poorer recovery after work-related setbacks and slows return to baseline functioning. Assess decision latitude by asking about scheduling flexibility, task variety, and input into workload distribution. When employees feel micromanaged, undervalued, or excluded from decision-making processes, their sense of agency diminishes. This not only undermines motivation but also contributes to feelings of helplessness and frustration. Similarly, poor organizational culture, marked by toxic leadership, lack of transparency, and insufficient communication, can erode trust and psychological safety, making it difficult for employees to voice concerns or seek support. For clinicians, distinguishing organizational contributors from individual vulnerabilities guides whether to focus therapy, workplace consultation, or both.

The erosion of work-life boundaries has specific physiological and behavioral consequences. Continuous connectivity increases evening cognitive arousal and reduces time available for restorative activities. Clinicians should assess evening routines, device use patterns, and embedded workplace norms that require off-hours responsiveness. This persistent intrusion into personal time undermines sleep quality and diminishes effective leisure, both vital for stress recovery. The erosion of work-life boundaries, intensified by remote work and digital connectivity, prevents adequate rest and recovery, further accelerating the burnout cycle. Interventions that create clear temporal anchors, scheduled offline periods, protected nonwork hours, and leadership-modeled boundaries, support physiological regeneration. For practical treatment planning, combine behavioral boundary-setting with organizational advocacy for supportive policies.

The consequences of burnout are far-reaching. Individuals may present with a complex symptom cluster that spans affective, cognitive, and somatic domains.

Clinicians should screen for comorbid conditions and functional impairment when burnout features are prominent. At the individual level, burnout is associated with a range of mental and physical health issues, including anxiety, depression, insomnia, cardiovascular disease, and substance use disorders. It impairs cognitive functioning, reduces emotional regulation, and diminishes overall quality of life. At the organizational level, burnout leads to decreased productivity, increased absenteeism, higher turnover rates, and lower employee engagement. This dual impact creates opportunities for interventions that align clinical goals with organizational outcomes, such as workplace accommodations, workload redesign, and population-level prevention programs (Morgan et al., 2025).

In recent years, the advent of digital health technologies has opened new avenues for the early detection and monitoring of burnout. These technologies allow continuous, ecologically valid data collection that complements episodic clinical assessments. Clinicians can use longitudinal digital markers to detect gradual declines in functioning that precede acute crises. These tools leverage advances in artificial intelligence (AI), wearable sensors, and machine learning to provide real-time insights into employees' physiological and behavioral states (De Kock et al., 2021). By identifying early warning signs of stress and fatigue, digital systems can enable timely interventions and support a more proactive approach to mental health care. When integrating digital data into practice, ensure patients understand data limits and consent to its clinical use (De Kock et al., 2021).

Wearable sensors are at the forefront of this transformation (Bibi, 2024). These devices capture continuous physiological and behavioral data in real-world settings (Radanliev, 2025). They provide high-frequency measurements that reveal patterns invisible to single-timepoint assessments. Clinicians should treat wearable outputs as complementary to clinical interviews and validated questionnaires (Radanliev, 2025). Devices such as smartwatches, fitness trackers, and biometric patches can continuously monitor physiological indicators associated with stress and burnout (Radanliev, 2025). These include heart rate variability, galvanic skin response, sleep patterns, physical activity levels, and even respiratory rate. Interpreting these signals requires attention to context, baseline variability, and device-specific limitations.

HRV, for example, is a well-established marker of autonomic nervous system function and has been linked to emotional regulation and resilience (Boda & Allam, 2022). Heart rate variability reflects the flexibility of physiological responses to stress and recovery. Lower HRV over prolonged periods can indicate reduced parasympathetic tone and compromised stress resilience (Tsai et al., 2025). Clinicians should combine HRV trends with symptom reports and functional assessments rather than relying on HRV alone (Tsai et al., 2025). A sustained decrease in HRV may indicate chronic stress or burnout, prompting further assessment or intervention (Tsai et al., 2025).

Galvanic skin response, which measures changes in skin conductivity due to sweat gland activity, is another useful biomarker. GSR indexes sympathetic arousal and can detect transient increases in stress during the workday (Verma et al., 2023). When interpreted alongside contextual data, GSR spikes help identify high-stress tasks or interpersonal triggers (Ong et al., 2025). Combining GSR with sleep and movement metrics strengthens the signal for meaningful stress detection (Ong et al., 2025). It reflects sympathetic nervous system arousal and can signal heightened emotional or cognitive stress. When combined with other metrics such as sleep quality and movement patterns, GSR data can provide a comprehensive picture of an individual's stress profile (Ong et al., 2025).

Artificial intelligence and machine learning algorithms enhance the utility of wearable data by identifying patterns and making predictions (Lamb et al., 2025). These algorithms can handle large, multimodal datasets that are otherwise intractable for manual review. Machine learning models can flag atypical trajectories and cluster users into risk strata to prioritize clinical outreach. Importantly, algorithm outputs should be interpretable and presented with uncertainty estimates to inform clinical decision-making. These systems can analyze large volumes of multimodal data, physiological, behavioral, and contextual, to detect anomalies and generate personalized risk assessments. For instance, a machine learning model might integrate HRV data with calendar activity, email usage, and keystroke dynamics to infer cognitive load, emotional state, and engagement levels (Rajpal, 2025).

Beyond individual monitoring, AI can also be used at the organizational level to assess team dynamics and workplace climate (Omiyefa, 2025). Aggregated analytics can highlight systemic stressors such as misaligned deadlines or uneven workload distribution. Organizations can use these insights to design targeted interventions and resource reallocations. However, team-level analytics require transparent governance and employee input to preserve trust and prevent misuse. Natural language processing tools can analyze communication patterns in emails, chat messages, and meeting transcripts to gauge sentiment, tone, and collaboration quality. These insights can help managers identify areas of concern, such as communication breakdowns, social isolation, or conflict, and take corrective action before these issues escalate.

Importantly, the use of AI and digital monitoring tools must be guided by ethical principles and robust data governance frameworks (Chen et al., 2022). Ethical frameworks should specify consent processes, data minimization strategies, and clear limits on secondary uses of data (Radanliev, 2025). Organizations must establish independent oversight mechanisms to monitor fairness and potential harms. Employees should have accessible avenues to opt out without adverse consequences for their employment. Privacy, consent, and transparency are paramount. Employees must be fully informed about what data is being collected, how it will be used, and who will have access to it (Radanliev, 2025). Anonymization, data minimization, and secure storage are essential to protect sensitive information and maintain trust (Radanliev, 2025).

Moreover, digital tools should be used to empower employees, not to surveil or penalize them. Design principles should favor user control, actionable feedback, and voluntary participation. Providing individuals with their own data summaries and personalized recommendations fosters agency and engagement (Li et al., 2025). Employers should separate health-related analytics from performance evaluations through strict technical and policy firewalls. The goal is to create a supportive environment where technology enhances well-being rather than exacerbates stress. Employees must be fully informed about what data is being collected, how it will be used, and who will have access to it (Rajpal, 2025). Moreover, digital tools should be used to empower employees, not to surveil or penalize them.

The integration of digital detection tools into workplace mental health strategies represents a paradigm shift from reactive to preventive care. Preventive strategies focus on reducing exposure to known stressors and enhancing resilience before crises emerge. Early detection enables stepped-care responses that allocate resources efficiently across populations. Organizations should pair detection with accessible interventions and clear escalation pathways. Instead of waiting for burnout to manifest in absenteeism or clinical symptoms, organizations can now identify and address risk factors in real time (De Kock et al., 2021). This not only improves individual outcomes but also fosters a culture of care, accountability, and continuous improvement.

Digital resilience training programs leverage a range of technologies, including mobile applications, web-based platforms, and immersive extended reality (Kourtesis, 2024) environments, to deliver evidence-based interventions that promote emotional regulation, cognitive flexibility, and social connectedness (Ma et al., 2025). Clarify the implementation goal: deploy short, repeatable modules that users can practice during natural breaks in the workday. This scheduling increases adherence and translates practice into real-world behavior. These platforms are grounded in well-established psychological frameworks such as cognitive behavioral therapy (CBT), mindfulness-based stress reduction (MBSR), and positive psychology. By translating these frameworks into interactive, user-friendly formats, digital tools empower individuals to build resilience in ways that are both engaging and sustainable.

Effective digital resilience programs are typically composed of several interrelated components, each targeting a specific domain of psychological functioning. Note how modular design supports personalization: clinicians or platforms can sequence modules based on assessed need and user preference. This modularity improves relevance and reduces cognitive overload for learners. These components are designed to be modular and adaptive, allowing users to engage with the content at their own pace and according to their unique needs.

Social connection and community features play a central role in sustaining mental health interventions. Begin by creating low-risk, moderated spaces for peer support that include clear guidelines and facilitator oversight. These communities should offer optional anonymity and clear escalation protocols for safety, increasing accessibility and trust among users. Human connection buffers stress by providing practical advice, shared validation, and opportunities for collective problem-solving. Many digital resilience programs incorporate features that facilitate peer support, group challenges, or community forums. These elements foster a sense of belonging and shared purpose, which can buffer against isolation and enhance motivation. Some platforms also offer access to virtual coaches or mental health professionals who provide personalized feedback and encouragement.

Psychoeducation and self-reflection form the cognitive scaffolding for sustainable change. Provide concise, actionable lessons that explain stress mechanisms and link symptoms to specific skill modules to improve transfer. Pair brief educational content with reflection prompts that ask users to connect lessons to recent workplace events. Such pairing enhances insight and promotes deliberate practice rather than passive consumption. In addition to interactive exercises, digital platforms often include educational content that helps users understand the science of stress, resilience, and mental health. This content may be delivered through videos, articles, or infographics, and is designed to increase self-awareness and promote informed self-care. Reflection prompts and journaling tools further support introspection and integration of learning.

These components are typically delivered through intuitive, mobile-friendly interfaces that allow users to engage with the material during breaks, commutes, or other moments of downtime. Prioritize microlearning design: short modules with a single learning objective improve retention and encourage repeated practice. Ensure navigation minimizes cognitive load by limiting choices and using progressive disclosure for complexity. Track engagement metrics to identify drop-off points and iterate on content accordingly. The flexibility and convenience of digital delivery make it easier for individuals to incorporate resilience practices into their daily routines, thereby increasing adherence and impact. Design interfaces that respect privacy, provide clear consent flows, and offer easy access to human support when needed.

ADAPTIVE LEARNING PATHS

As users engage with the platform, AI systems continuously monitor their progress and adjust the training path accordingly (Kostadimas et al., 2025). Define concrete adaptation triggers such as missed sessions, declining mood scores, or multiple failed practice attempts to guide content changes. Schedule periodic reassessments to recalibrate recommendations and avoid overfitting to short-term patterns. When a user shows sustained improvement, the system should reduce prompt frequency and introduce consolidation exercises to maintain gains. If a user is consistently completing exercises and reporting improvements, the system may introduce more advanced content or reduce the frequency of prompts. Conversely, if a user is struggling or disengaging, the platform can offer additional support, simplify tasks, or suggest alternative approaches. This dynamic feedback loop enhances engagement and ensures that the intervention remains aligned with the user's evolving needs.

Natural Language Processing and Conversational Agents

Some platforms incorporate AI-powered chatbots or virtual coaches that use natural language processing (Islam & Bae, 2024) to interact with users in a conversational manner (Ienca et al., 2017). Begin with transparent scope statements that clarify the agent's capabilities and limits to set realistic expectations. Train conversational prompts on diverse language samples to reduce cultural and linguistic bias, and include override pathways to human clinicians when needed. These agents can provide real-time encouragement, answer questions, and guide users through exercises. While not a substitute for human therapists, these tools can offer immediate support and help bridge the gap between sessions or in the absence of professional care.

Predictive Analytics and Risk Stratification

AI can also be used to identify users who may be at higher risk of burnout or mental health decline (Freeman et al., 2017). Implement conservative thresholds for escalation and require human review before any outreach to avoid false positives. Use aggregated monitoring to detect trends while preserving individual anonymity and the option to opt into proactive services. By analyzing patterns in engagement, mood tracking, and biometric data, predictive models can flag individuals who may benefit from additional support or referral to clinical services (Freeman et al., 2017). This proactive approach enables early intervention and reduces the likelihood of crisis. When deploying predictive models, maintain documentation of algorithm performance, update models with new data, and provide accessible appeal mechanisms for users who disagree with automated assessments (Freeman et al., 2017).

Adaptive Learning Paths

As users engage with the platform, AI systems continuously monitor their progress and adjust the training path accordingly (Hiland, 2021). Define concrete adaptation triggers such as missed sessions, declining mood scores, or multiple failed practice attempts to guide content changes. Schedule periodic reassessments to recalibrate recommendations and avoid overfitting to short-term patterns. When a user shows sustained improvement, the system should reduce prompt frequency and introduce consolidation exercises to maintain gains. If a user is consistently completing exercises and reporting improvements, the system may introduce more advanced content or reduce the frequency of prompts. Conversely, if a user is struggling or disengaging, the platform can offer additional support, simplify tasks, or suggest alternative approaches. This dynamic feedback loop enhances engagement and ensures that the intervention remains aligned with the user's evolving needs.

Some platforms incorporate AI-powered chatbots or virtual coaches that use natural language processing (Bond et al., 2023) to interact with users in a conversational manner. Begin with transparent scope statements that clarify the agent's capabilities and limits to set realistic expectations. Train conversational prompts on diverse language samples to reduce cultural and linguistic bias, and include override pathways to human clinicians when needed. These agents can provide real-time encouragement, answer questions, and guide users through exercises. While not a substitute for human therapists, these tools can offer immediate support and help bridge the gap between sessions or in the absence of professional care. Predictive Analytics and Risk Stratification: AI can also be used to identify users who may be at higher risk of burnout or mental health decline. Implement conservative thresholds for escalation and require human review before any outreach to avoid false positives. Use aggregated monitoring to detect trends while preserving individual anonymity and the option to opt into proactive services. By analyzing patterns in engagement, mood tracking, and biometric data, predictive models can flag individuals who may benefit from additional support or referral to clinical services. This proactive approach enables early intervention and reduces the likelihood of crisis. When deploying predictive models, maintain documentation of algorithm performance, update models with new data, and provide accessible appeal mechanisms for users who disagree with automated assessments (Rajpal, 2025).

Progress tracking is another key feature of dCBT. Implement clear, time-bound metrics that show incremental change to sustain user motivation and inform clinical review (Cristofaro & Giardino, 2025). Use visual dashboards that display mood, activity, and cognitive pattern trends with annotations for significant events. Integrate automated summaries that flag nonresponse or worsening symptoms for clinician attention and safe escalation. Ensure reports are exportable in secure formats so clinicians can incorporate them into treatment planning and measurement-based care. AI companions and chatbots are increasingly integrated into dCBT platforms to simulate aspects of the therapeutic relationship (Shatte et al., 2019). Define explicit scope and escalation rules so users and clinicians understand when human support is required. Train conversational agents on diverse, clinically informed scripts to reduce bias and improve cultural relevance. Monitor chatbot interactions for safety signals and implement clinician review workflows for flagged conversations. Use transparent labeling so users know when they are speaking with an automated agent rather than a human clinician.

The flexibility and anonymity of dCBT make it particularly appealing for individuals who might otherwise avoid therapy due to stigma, logistical challenges, or financial constraints. Offer opt-in anonymity features while preserving the ability to transition to identified care when clinically indicated. Provide low-bandwidth and offline options to improve access for users with connectivity limitations and promote equitable uptake. Pair anonymity with clear safety plans that explain how crises will be handled and when identity will be disclosed for safety reasons. The asynchronous nature of digital platforms allows users to engage with the material at their own pace and on their own schedule, which is especially valuable in the context of demanding work environments. The integration of digital CBT into workplace settings represents a significant advancement in organizational health strategy. Begin integration with stakeholder mapping and pilot testing to assess cultural fit, privacy implications, and uptake rates. Establish employee-led advisory groups to guide procurement choices and co-design engagement strategies that respect diverse needs. Create clear policy documents that separate wellness data from performance evaluations and describe consent, retention, and access procedures in plain language.As mental health becomes an increasingly prominent concern for employers, dCBT offers a practical and scalable solution that aligns with the goals of employee wellness, productivity, and retention.

Many organizations now include dCBT platforms as part of their Employee Assistance Programs (Chithra & Bhambri, 2024) or broader wellness initiatives. Require vendor transparency about clinical evidence, safety protocols, and data governance before procurement decisions (Subu et al., 2022). Structure rollout plans with manager training, communications that reduce stigma, and measurable engagement targets tied to program evaluation. Provide parallel human supports for employees who need higher-intensity services and ensure referral pathways are simple and timely. These tools can be offered as standalone resources or integrated with other digital health services, such as teletherapy, mindfulness apps, and wearable devices. These tools can be offered as standalone resources or integrated with other digital health services, such as teletherapy, mindfulness apps, and wearable devices. Begin by mapping interoperability requirements and data flows to prevent inadvertent data leakage between systems. Require vendors to provide Application Programming Interface (API) documentation and consented data schemas to support secure integrations. Pilot small integrations before scaling to identify usability problems and privacy trade-offs in real-world workflows. Integration increases value only when technical, clinical, and legal teams coordinate deployment and monitor outcomes (Mohr et al., 2017).

Integration with HR systems allows for personalized outreach and engagement. Define clear, limited use cases for HR-triggered outreach and require dual consent for any contact initiated from HR. Configure integrations to surface only aggregated wellness signals to HR while preserving individual-level clinical data for care teams (Mahon, 2023). Train HR staff on privacy boundaries and on scripted, non-stigmatizing language to use when outreach is approved and necessary. These precautions maintain trust while enabling targeted support for returning employees or those in transition.

Collaboration with wearable technology further enhances the effectiveness of dCBT (Ienca et al., 2017). Establish standards for data quality and acceptable device types before accepting wearable inputs (Kim & Backonja, 2025). Use pilot data to set clinically meaningful thresholds and to determine which metrics will prompt automated suggestions versus clinician review (Kim & Backonja, 2025). Present users with clear options to control which devices feed into their therapeutic profiles and to revoke access at any time. This approach reduces noise and increases the clinical utility of physiological signals (Kim & Backonja, 2025).

Customization and branding are also important for workplace adoption. Align content tone and examples to the organization's culture without compromising clinical integrity or evidence-based practice (Weiner et al., 2025). Offer multilingual options and culturally adapted scenarios to improve relevance across diverse employee populations. Test branded interfaces with representative user groups and iterate based on feedback to reduce drop-off and increase clarity. Customization should enhance engagement, not obscure safety or data use policies (Rajpal, 2025). Training and support for managers is another critical component of successful integration. Provide concise, skills-focused training that teaches managers to recognize distress signals, have supportive conversations, and connect employees to resources. Include role-play scenarios and short reference scripts managers can use to initiate sensitive discussions while maintaining confidentiality. Measure manager competence through brief post-training assessments and follow-up coaching to sustain changes in behavior. Manager training amplifies digital interventions by creating an environment where employees feel safe to use available tools.

valuation and continuous improvement are essential to ensure the effectiveness of dCBT programs. Establish measurable success criteria before deployment and collect both qualitative and quantitative feedback on user experience. Use iterative Plan-Do-Study-Act cycles to refine content, address usability issues, and respond to emerging safety concerns (Kargarandehkordi et al., 2025). Implement routine outcome monitoring and analyze engagement patterns to detect modules that underperform or create confusion. Involve clinicians in interpreting outcome data to link user metrics with clinical significance (Martinez-Martin et al., 2018). Regularly update content to reflect new evidence while preserving version control and documented change logs (Martinez-Martin et al., 2018). Organizations should establish governance committees that include employee representatives to review evaluation findings and recommend changes.

Digital DBT represents a significant innovation for extending skills-based treatment to broader populations who struggle with emotional regulation. Start by defining appropriate inclusion criteria and clear exclusion thresholds for self-guided use to ensure safety. Provide clinician-oversight pathways that allow therapists to review client entries and intervene when escalation criteria are met. Digital DBT platforms typically include interactive modules that mirror the core skills taught in traditional DBT groups. These modules are often delivered through mobile apps or web-based platforms and include video lessons, guided exercises, and digital worksheets. Users can practice mindfulness techniques, track urges and emotions, and receive real-time coaching prompts during moments of distress.

For providers, digital DBT offers a way to extend the therapeutic alliance beyond the therapy room. Establish clear expectations with clients about response times, data review frequency, and boundaries around after-hours communication (Akhtar & Rawol, 2024). Therapists can assign digital homework, review client entries between sessions, and use data to inform treatment planning (Radanliev, 2025). In group settings, digital platforms can facilitate asynchronous learning, allowing clients to review material at their own pace and revisit challenging concepts. This flexibility is especially beneficial for clients with varying learning styles, cognitive capacities, or scheduling constraints. However, the implementation of digital DBT must be approached with care. Create detailed safety protocols that include risk screening, crisis escalation paths, and coordination with local emergency services where needed. Not all clients are appropriate for self-guided DBT, particularly those with high suicide risk or severe dissociation. Providers must assess readiness, provide appropriate scaffolding, and ensure that digital tools are used as a supplement, not a substitute, for clinical judgment and therapeutic presence (Radanliev, 2025). Ethical considerations around data privacy, informed consent, and crisis response protocols are also paramount, especially given the high-risk populations DBT often serves (Radanliev, 2025).

As digital therapeutics become increasingly embedded in workplace mental health strategies, organizations must navigate a complex landscape of ethical, legal, and cultural considerations. Begin with a cross-functional readiness assessment that includes legal, HR, IT, and clinical stakeholders to identify governance gaps and implementation risks (Saganowski et al., 2022). Define clear objectives for any digital mental health initiative and specify success metrics tied to employee well-being rather than productivity alone. Consider pilot programs with representative user groups to surface accessibility issues and cultural fit before broad rollout. While these technologies offer unprecedented opportunities to support employee well-being, their implementation must be guided by principles of transparency, equity, and organizational responsibility. Without careful planning and ethical foresight, digital tools intended to promote mental health could inadvertently reinforce existing disparities, erode trust, or even cause harm.

One of the most pressing concerns in the deployment of digital mental health tools is the issue of data privacy (Agarwal et al., 2025). Conduct a privacy impact assessment early and publish a concise summary for employees that explains risks, mitigations, and retention limits. Limit collection to data that is necessary for the stated clinical purpose and document deletion timelines for personal information (Robinson et al., 2024). Train technical staff on secure coding and data handling practices and require vendors to demonstrate compliance with recognized security standards (Robinson et al., 2024). These platforms often collect sensitive information, including biometric data, mood logs, behavioral patterns, and communication meta-data (Robinson et al., 2024). When integrated with wearable devices or workplace systems, the scope of data collection can expand significantly, raising questions about surveillance, autonomy, and informed consent (Robinson et al., 2024).

Employers must ensure that all data collected through digital therapeutics is handled with the highest standards of security and confidentiality (APA, 2023). Require end-to-end encryption, role-based access controls, and routine third-party security audits as contractual obligations for vendors. Establish a designated data steward within the organization responsible for oversight, breach response, and employee inquiries (Ienca et al., 2017). Create transparent, easily navigable consent flows that allow employees to revoke permissions and export their personal data (Ienca et al., 2017). This includes implementing end-to-end encryption, secure data storage, and strict access controls (Ienca et al., 2017). More importantly, employees must be fully informed about what data is being collected, how it will be used, who will have access to it, and for what purposes (Ienca et al., 2017).

Clear boundaries must also be established between health monitoring and performance evaluation. Document policy that explicitly forbids the use of health-derived metrics for performance appraisal or disciplinary action, and communicate this policy repeatedly through multiple channels. Use technical segregation, separate databases and access controls, to ensure HR systems cannot query clinical datasets without explicit employee consent (Robinson et al., 2024). Include employee representatives in governance committees to review any proposed cross-functional data use and to maintain accountability (Robinson et al., 2024). Employees should never feel that their mental health data could be used to assess productivity, determine promotions, or justify disciplinary actions (Robinson et al., 2024). To maintain trust, organizations should adopt a "firewall" approach, separating health data from human resources and management functions (Robinson et al., 2024).

Transparency is key. Publish clear, plain-language privacy and governance policies and make them easily discoverable to all employees, with summaries for non-technical readers. Offer periodic training sessions and Q&A forums where staff can ask about data practices and consent options before opting in to programs. Conduct regular audits and publish aggregate findings about uptake, engagement, and safety events while preserving individual anonymity. Organizations should publish clear privacy policies, conduct regular audits, and engage employees in the design and evaluation of digital health initiatives. By fostering a culture of openness and accountability, employers can build trust and encourage meaningful engagement with mental health resources. Equity and accessibility are recurring risks that require proactive mitigation. Include a baseline equity audit that maps digital access gaps, language needs, and assistive technology requirements across the workforce. Engage representative employees in co-design workshops to surface barriers and prioritize inclusive features during procurement. Provide multiple access pathways, such as low-bandwidth web versions and SMS-based options, to reduce exclusion. Track engagement by demographic variables to detect disparities and guide targeted outreach. Digital mental health solutions hold great promise for expanding access to care, but they also risk exacerbating existing inequalities if not designed and implemented with inclusivity in mind. Access to technology is not evenly distributed across the workforce. Employees may differ in their access to smartphones, internet connectivity, digital literacy, and comfort with technology. Moreover, cultural, linguistic, and neurodiversity factors can influence how individuals perceive and engage with digital interventions.

To ensure equity, organizations must adopt inclusive design principles from the outset. Create explicit procurement criteria that require multilingual content, plain language, and WCAG-compliant interfaces from vendors. Include budget lines for translation, accessibility testing, and participant compensation during pilots to ensure representative feedback. Offer training sessions that build digital literacy for employees who report low confidence using apps or platforms. This includes offering content in multiple languages, using plain and culturally sensitive language, and providing alternative formats for individuals with visual, auditory, or cognitive impairments. Platforms should be compatible with assistive technologies and designed with accessibility standards such as WCAG in mind.

Special attention should be given to marginalized and underserved groups, including racial and ethnic minorities, LGBTQ+ individuals, people with disabilities, and those in lower-income or rural settings. Commission targeted needs assessments for these groups to inform culturally adapted content and outreach strategies. Partner with community organizations to validate cultural relevance and to extend access beyond typical corporate channels. Provide dedicated support contacts for employees from underrepresented groups to address concerns and improve uptake. These populations often face additional barriers to mental health care and may be more vulnerable to digital exclusion. Engaging diverse stakeholders in the co-design and testing of digital tools can help ensure that interventions are relevant, respectful, and responsive to the needs of all users.

Equity also extends to the organizational level. Ensure that contractors, part-time staff, and frontline workers receive equivalent access to digital therapeutics through non-corporate login options and inclusive benefit design. Monitor utilization rates across employment categories and adjust outreach strategies where gaps appear. Provide offline resources or printed materials for workers in roles where device access is impractical. Employers must ensure that all employees, regardless of role, location, or status, have equal access to mental health resources. This includes frontline workers, part-time staff, and contractors who may be excluded from traditional wellness programs. Providing flexible access options, such as mobile apps that do not require corporate credentials, can help bridge these gaps. Technology alone cannot solve the complex and deeply human challenges of workplace mental health. Start by recognizing technology as an amplifier of organizational intent rather than a replacement for leadership commitment. Invest in parallel processes that strengthen managerial skills, policy clarity, and frontline supports alongside any digital rollout. Evaluate tools for cultural fit and plan for sustained governance beyond initial procurement to prevent feature drift. The success of digital therapeutics depends on the broader organizational culture in which they are embedded. Leadership commitment, supportive policies, and a climate of psychological safety are essential to creating environments where digital tools can thrive.

Leaders play a critical role in shaping attitudes toward mental health. Require visible leader participation in mental health initiatives to model desired norms and reduce stigma (Watson, 2025). Provide leaders with brief, actionable scripts they can use to open conversations and normalize help-seeking without overstepping privacy. Train leaders in trauma-informed supervision and measurement-based feedback to align managerial actions with well-being goals. When executives and managers openly discuss mental well-being, model healthy behaviors, and actively support mental health initiatives, they signal that these issues are valued and legitimate (Ricciardi & Zomaya, 2025). Conversely, a culture of silence, stigma, or overwork can undermine even the most sophisticated digital interventions. Organizations must invest in leadership training that emphasizes emotional intelligence, trauma-informed supervision, and inclusive communication. Design training that is practical, time-limited, and reinforced through coaching and peer learning circles. Include assessment metrics for leaders' supportive behaviors and tie outcomes to performance reviews where appropriate. Offer follow-up booster sessions and micro-coaching to sustain skill acquisition over time. Leaders should be equipped to recognize signs of distress, initiate supportive conversations, and refer employees to appropriate resources. They should also be held accountable for fostering respectful, equitable, and psychologically safe team environments. Policy infrastructure is equally important. Draft clear policies on flexible work, reasonable accommodations, and mental health leave that prioritize employee dignity and operational continuity. Ensure policy language is accessible, and provide templates managers can use to operationalize accommodations while protecting confidentiality. Set expectations for reasonable response times to accommodation requests and monitor policy adherence through regular audits. Flexible work arrangements, reasonable accommodations, and clear anti-discrimination policies create the conditions for mental health to flourish. Digital tools should be integrated into a comprehensive well-being strategy that includes access to clinical care, peer support, and organizational development initiatives (Ricciardi & Zomaya, 2025).

Finally, organizations must cultivate a culture of continuous learning and improvement. Build feedback loops that gather employee experience data, clinical outcomes, and engagement metrics to inform iterative design (Aiken et al., 2023). Establish multidisciplinary review boards to interpret findings and prioritize modifications that enhance safety, equity, and effectiveness. Share evaluation results transparently with employees and incorporate their recommendations into product roadmaps and training plans. This includes soliciting feedback from employees, evaluating the impact of digital interventions, and iterating based on evidence and experience (Fanarioti & Karpouzis, 2025). Mental health is not a one-time initiative but an ongoing commitment that requires adaptability, humility, and shared responsibility.

The integration of digital therapeutics into adult mental health care represents a profound shift in how we understand, prevent, and treat workplace stress. Clarify the practical aim: move services earlier in the stress trajectory to prevent functional decline and crisis. Operationalize prevention by embedding low-burden screening and brief interventions into routine workflows with clear escalation pathways. Ensure implementation plans specify staffing, training, and measurable outcomes tied to well-being rather than productivity alone. By combining early detection of burnout, personalized resilience training, and scalable digital CBT, we are moving from a reactive model of care to one that is proactive, preventive, and empowering (Kim & Backonja, 2025). These innovations offer the potential to democratize access to mental health support, reduce stigma, and embed well-being into the fabric of organizational life.

However, this transformation is not just about technology, it is about reimagining the workplace as a space where mental health is prioritized, supported, and celebrated. Begin by defining organizational values and metrics that explicitly include psychological safety and employee flourishing. Translate those values into concrete policies, manager competencies, and resource allocations that support sustained implementation. Use pilot feedback to align tools with daily workflows and remove friction that reduces uptake. It requires a commitment to ethical implementation, inclusive design, and cultural change. It demands that we center empathy, equity, and evidence in every decision we make. And it challenges us to see mental health not as a private struggle or a productivity issue, but as a collective responsibility and a fundamental human right. As we continue to innovate, we must do so with care and intention. Establish multidisciplinary governance that includes employees, clinicians, legal counsel, and technical experts to oversee development and deployment. Define clear success criteria and safety metrics before scaling any program and publish aggregate outcomes transparently to employees. Build mechanisms for rapid rollback or mitigation when unintended harms or biases appear in algorithmic outputs. We must listen to the voices of those most affected, confront the structural barriers that perpetuate harm, and build systems that are as compassionate as they are intelligent. In doing so, we can create a future of work that is not only more productive and resilient but also more humane.

A future where every working adult has the tools, support, and dignity they need to thrive, mentally, emotionally, and socially, requires sustained investment across domains. Allocate budget lines for long-term maintenance, evaluation, and accessibility improvements rather than one-time procurement spends. Prioritize workforce development so clinicians and managers can use digital tools responsibly and effectively. Embed continuous quality improvement cycles that incorporate user feedback, equity audits, and outcome monitoring to prevent stagnation. As digital therapeutics become increasingly integrated into mental health care, providers face both unprecedented opportunities and complex challenges. The convergence of artificial intelligence (AI), extended reality (XR), mobile health platforms, and wearable sensors is reshaping how care is delivered, monitored, and experienced (Babu & Joseph, 2025). For mental health and behavioral health professionals, this transformation demands not only technological literacy but also a reimagining of clinical roles, ethical responsibilities, and therapeutic relationships (Engel, 1977). Define minimum competencies for clinicians using digital tools, including basic data interpretation, privacy communication, and escalation protocols (Engel, 1977). Create supervision structures where experienced practitioners support colleagues in blended-care delivery and digital risk management. Encourage clinicians to contribute to tool evaluation and to refuse platforms that lack transparent safety procedures. Digital literacy is no longer optional for mental health professionals. As digital tools become embedded in assessment, intervention, and monitoring, providers must develop fluency in the technologies their clients are using. This includes understanding how digital CBT platforms function, how wearable devices collect and interpret data, and how AI-driven tools personalize care (Engel, 1977).

Pursuing continuing education in digital mental health, including certifications in digital therapeutics or telebehavioral health, is essential. Specify learning objectives for these courses: basic data literacy, privacy law fundamentals, and practical integration techniques for clinical workflows (Hall et al., 2024). Seek programs that include hands-on practice with common platforms and case-based problem solving to translate knowledge into clinical skill (Martinez-Martin et al., 2018). Prioritize accredited training that offers measurable competencies and continuing supervision opportunities. Providers should familiarize themselves with the evidence base behind commonly used digital tools and apps and collaborate with digital health developers to ensure clinical relevance and usability of tools (Martinez-Martin et al., 2018). Establish partnerships with vendors that include clinician advisory roles and transparent documentation of algorithmic logic. Rather than viewing digital therapeutics as separate or competing with traditional therapy, providers should explore ways to integrate them into their clinical workflow (Martinez-Martin et al., 2018). Create clear protocols for when to assign digital modules, how to monitor adherence, and when to escalate to higher-intensity care. Digital tools can enhance therapy by providing between-session support, tracking progress, and offering clients additional resources for skill-building. Integrate brief, documented check-ins to review digital homework and link app-based learning to in-session behavioral experiments.

The use of digital tools introduces new ethical considerations around privacy, consent, and data security (Iwaya et al., 2023). Develop standardized consent templates that explain data flows, retention, and rights in plain language for clients at intake. Revisit consent whenever a new integration or data source is added and document client preferences in the record. Providers must ensure that clients understand what data is being collected, how it is stored, and who has access to it. Include specific discussion points about third-party vendors and downstream data sharing. Informed consent must be ongoing and revisited as technologies evolve. Schedule periodic consent reviews during treatment and provide clients with written summaries of any changes. Clearly explaining the risks and benefits of using digital tools, including data sharing policies, choosing platforms that comply with HIPAA, GDPR, and other relevant privacy regulations, and advocating for transparency and ethical standards in the development and deployment of digital mental health technologies are critical steps. Maintain a curated list of vetted platforms to support transparent clinical recommendations and reduce ad hoc tool adoption (Mohr et al., 2017). Not all clients have equal access to digital tools. Assess digital access and literacy as part of the standard intake process and document any barriers that may affect intervention choices. Offer low-tech or analog alternatives such as printed worksheets, phone-based coaching, or mailed resources when necessary to ensure continuity of care. Socioeconomic status, geographic location, disability, and digital literacy can all affect a client's ability to benefit from digital therapeutics. Create flexible care plans that combine digital and analog methods tailored to client resources and preferences. Providers must be proactive in identifying and addressing these barriers. Collaborate with community organizations and employer programs to connect clients to device subsidies, internet access solutions, or workplace accommodations. Assessing clients' access to technology and comfort with digital tools as part of intake, offering low-tech or analog alternatives when needed, such as printed worksheets or phone-based interventions, and advocating for policies and funding that expand broadband access and digital inclusion are essential practices. Track outcomes for clients using analog pathways to ensure equitable effectiveness and adjust care strategies accordingly.

While digital tools can enhance care, they cannot replace the therapeutic relationship. Define blended-care boundaries that specify the roles of automated feedback versus therapist interpretation to preserve relational depth. Use digital summaries as a springboard for empathy-focused discussion rather than as substitutes for clinical judgment (Inkster et al., 2023). Providers must remain attuned to the emotional and relational dimensions of therapy, ensuring that technology serves to support, not supplant, human connection. Document how digital interactions supplement sessions and specify response time expectations for client messages. Using digital tools to extend your presence, not replace it, e.g., sending personalized messages or check-ins through secure platforms, being mindful of how technology affects rapport, especially in telehealth settings, and regularly soliciting client feedback on their experience with digital tools and adjusting accordingly are important considerations. Build routine review points where clients evaluate the helpfulness of digital tools and jointly decide whether to continue, modify, or stop their use.

The future of mental health care is interdisciplinary. Define actionable collaboration structures such as recurring clinical-tech liaison meetings, joint project charters, and shared KPIs to operationalize interdisciplinary work (Khoo et al., 2024). Encourage short cross-training modules so clinicians learn basic data concepts and technologists learn clinical safety priorities (De Kock et al., 2021). Create formal agreements that specify roles, responsibilities, and escalation pathways for safety incidents. Providers must be prepared to work alongside data scientists, software developers, UX designers, and public health professionals to co-create effective digital solutions (De Kock et al., 2021). Joining interdisciplinary teams or advisory boards for digital health projects, contributing clinical insights to the design and evaluation of digital tools, and advocating for the inclusion of behavioral health perspectives in tech development are valuable strategies (De Kock et al., 2021).

Digital therapeutics are enabling new models of care, including stepped care, blended care, and population-level interventions. Pilot these models with clear triage criteria, measurable outcomes, and clinician oversight to prevent inappropriate stepped-down care. Document pathways that specify when automated care suffices and when escalation is mandatory, and share these protocols with all stakeholders. Train staff on the operational workflows that support blended care delivery and ensure reimbursement pathways are aligned. Providers must be flexible and innovative in adapting to these models while maintaining clinical integrity. Exploring blended care models that combine digital self-help with therapist support, using digital screening tools to triage clients and allocate resources efficiently, and participating in pilot programs or research studies evaluating new care models are recommended approaches (Engel, 1977).

As digital tools evolve, so too must our methods for evaluating their effectiveness and safety. Build evaluation plans that combine randomized designs, implementation metrics, and qualitative user feedback to capture real-world performance. Specify safety endpoints, define non-inferiority margins for clinical outcomes, and use iterative testing to refine algorithms (Lay et al., 2025). Providers have a critical role to play in generating real-world evidence and ensuring that digital interventions meet clinical standards (Ienca et al., 2017). Collecting outcome data and client feedback on digital interventions, participating in research or quality improvement initiatives related to digital mental health, and staying current with literature on digital therapeutics and evidence-based practices are essential activities (Ienca et al., 2017).

Mental health providers are uniquely positioned to influence policy and advocate for systems that support ethical, equitable, and effective use of digital therapeutics. Engage with professional associations to shape policy briefs, reimbursement models, and regulatory guidance relevant to digital care delivery. Advocate for standards that require transparent vendor evidence, independent audits, and patient-accessible summaries of algorithmic functioning (Baka et al., 2025). This includes addressing reimbursement, regulation, and workforce development. Engaging with professional associations to shape digital health policy, advocating for reimbursement models that support hybrid and digital care, and supporting training programs that prepare the next generation of providers for digital practice are critical actions.

By embracing these recommendations, mental health and behavioral health providers can lead the way in integrating digital therapeutics into clinical practice, ensuring that technology enhances care while upholding the highest standards of ethics, equity, and human connection (Livieri et al., 2025). Start with small-scale pilots that prioritize safety, equity, and measurable outcomes before broad rollout to build organizational trust. Document lessons learned and share implementation guides with peers to accelerate collective learning and reduce duplicated errors. Foster mentorship and supervision structures that support clinicians new to digital practice and create communities of practice to disseminate best practices. To illustrate how these elements converge in practice, consider a clinical vignette (Tsai et al., 2025). Maria, a 42-year-old nurse, reports increasing fatigue, irritability, and disengagement after two years of pandemic-related overtime. With a layered approach, begin by mapping her symptom timeline and workplace exposures to identify modifiable stressors and protective factors. Her therapist obtained consent to integrate wearable sleep and activity data into assessment, using trends to prioritize behavioral activation targets and sleep hygiene interventions (Tsai et al., 2025). Coordinate with occupational health using a documented, confidential request to review workload and schedule accommodations, ensuring Maria's clinical information remains separate from performance records (Tsai et al., 2025). A combined intervention plan paired individual therapy with dCBT modules for cognitive restructuring and a resilience app for brief in-shift mindfulness practice. Over three months Maria reports improved sleep, fewer catastrophic thoughts, and a modest return of engagement at work. The combined approach, individual therapy, digital support for skills practice, and a targeted organizational adjustment, illustrates how layered interventions produce more durable recovery than any single component alone.

A second vignette shows the limits of technology without culture change. Jamal, a mid-level manager, begins using a resiliency app that prompts short breathing exercises and prompts for boundary-setting. Despite consistent use, assessors noted his workload and supervisor expectations remained unchanged, underscoring the role of systemic constraints. Embed manager-level interventions alongside individual supports to address workload distribution and recognition practices that maintain healthful norms. Jamal experienced modest symptom relief but continued to feel trapped; the app could not alter structural pressures such as unrealistic deadlines or implicit availability expectations. Clinicians should therefore pair individual strategies with organizational consultation, advocating for managerial training and policy shifts where necessary. Clinically, this case underscores the need for managerial training and policy-level adjustments alongside individual interventions.

A third vignette highlights digital DBT in a safety context. Lauren, a 27-year-old with emotion regulation difficulties, uses a digital DBT coach to practice distress tolerance during moments of overwhelming urge. Before recommending the tool, clinicians should confirm that escalation pathways and crisis contacts are embedded and tested within the platform's workflow. The platform's real-time prompts helped Lauren rehearse grounding and urge-surfing techniques precisely when dysregulation occurred, improving skill generalization. Importantly, her therapist set clear expectations about response times and reviewed automatic alerts to coordinate timely outreach when risk indicators appeared. The platform includes an explicit escalation plan: when certain keywords indicating self-harm appear, the system prompts immediate clinician notification and activates crisis protocols. Here, digital tools extend skills practice while preserving human oversight for acute risk, demonstrating the need for integrated safety workflows.

A fourth vignette demonstrates predictive analytics informing preventive outreach. A large organization's aggregated analytics identify a sudden decline in sleep metrics and rising after-hours communications in one regional office. Use pre-agreed, opt-in monitoring protocols and transparent communication to ensure employees understand the scope and limits of aggregated analytics. Leadership organized a voluntary, non-punitive team check-in and redistributed urgent tasks while offering a short resilience workshop to address immediate skills needs. Early outreach included confidential coaching offers and optional workload adjustments, which reduced distress and prevented escalations in absenteeism. This case shows how ethically governed, aggregated digital signals can guide systemic responses that preserve individual anonymity while enabling targeted support. Early outreach prevents escalation, illustrating how ethically governed, aggregated digital signals can guide systemic responses.

In closing, digital therapeutics are powerful tools that expand what is possible in workplace mental health, but they are not a panacea. Frame digital adoption as one element within a broader strategy that includes policy change, leader development, and direct clinical care (Liu & Schueller, 2023). Prioritize pilots that measure safety, equity, and clinical outcomes, and be prepared to iterate based on employee feedback and objective metrics (Ricciardi & Zomaya, 2025). Their real value lies in thoughtful integration: pairing just-in-time, personalized digital supports with human clinical judgment, ethical governance, accessible design, and organizational changes that reduce upstream sources of harm (Ricciardi & Zomaya, 2025). For clinicians and researchers, the challenge is to apply these tools in ways that preserve the therapeutic relationship, protect privacy, and advance equity. For organizations, the task is to embed technology within policies and leadership practices that model psychological safety and respect (Ricciardi & Zomaya, 2025).

As digital therapeutics become increasingly integrated into mental health care, providers face both unprecedented opportunities and complex challenges. Begin by mapping current clinical workflows to identify where digital tools can add value without duplicating existing processes (Smith et al., 2023). Define clear roles for automated interventions versus clinician-led tasks to prevent responsibility drift and ensure continuity of care. Establish pilot criteria that include safety metrics, user experience goals, and equity checks before wider adoption. The convergence of artificial intelligence (AI), extended reality (XR), mobile health platforms, and wearable sensors is reshaping how care is delivered, monitored, and experienced (Mohr et al., 2017).

For mental health and behavioral health professionals, this transformation demands not only technological literacy but also a reimagining of clinical roles, ethical responsibilities, and therapeutic relationships (Shatte et al., 2019). Create competency checklists that include data interpretation, digital consent practices, and escalation procedures to guide clinician training (Robinson et al., 2024). Implement peer supervision groups focused on blended care to surface dilemmas and share best practices across teams. Encourage clinicians to document digital tool use in clinical notes to maintain transparency and continuity (Robinson et al., 2024). Digital literacy is no longer optional for mental health professionals.

Pursuing continuing education in digital mental health, including certifications in digital therapeutics or telebehavioral health, is essential. Prioritize courses that combine didactic learning with hands-on platform experience and case simulations that reflect common workplace scenarios. Negotiate institutional support for protected time to complete training and for access to vetted learning resources. Track competency attainment and integrate digital skill development into professional development plans. Providers should familiarize themselves with the evidence base behind commonly used digital tools and apps and collaborate with digital health developers to ensure clinical relevance and usability of tools (Obermeyer et al., 2019).

Rather than viewing digital therapeutics as separate or competing with traditional therapy, providers should explore ways to integrate them into their clinical workflow (Ball et al., 2025). Draft standardized protocols that specify how to assign digital modules, how to monitor adherence, and what clinical thresholds trigger escalation to higher-intensity care (Shatte et al., 2019). Pilot blended-care pathways with defined measurement points to evaluate efficacy and adjust procedures before scaling. Use client feedback loops to refine integration practices and address usability problems early. Digital tools can enhance therapy by providing between-session support, tracking progress, and offering clients additional resources for skill-building.

The use of digital tools introduces new ethical considerations around privacy, consent, and data security (Fanarioti & Karpouzis, 2025). Create plain-language consent templates that detail data types collected, intended uses, retention periods, and client rights to revoke consent, and review these at regular treatment intervals (Rajpal, 2025). Require vendors to supply clear documentation on data handling and offer clinicians simple scripts to explain risks and protections to clients. Establish clinic-level policies for secure storage, audit trails, and incident response, and rehearse breach scenarios in team training. Maintain a curated list of vetted platforms and update it based on emerging evidence and safety reviews.

REFERENCES

Agarwal, S., Jalan, M., Hill, R., Pantalone, E., Thrul, J., Sharma, R., Wilcox, H. C., & Robinson, K. A. (2025). Framework to Assist Stakeholders in Technology Evaluation for Recovery (Freeman et al., 2017) to Mental Health and Wellness. *BMC Health Services Research, 25*, 623. Advance online publication. DOI: 10.1186/s12913-025-12418-0 PMID: 40307807

Aiken, L. H., Lasater, K. B., Sloane, D. M., Pogue, C. A., Rosenbaum, K. E. F., & Muir, K. J.US Clinician Wellbeing Study Consortium. (2023, July). Physician and nurse well-being and preferred interventions to address burnout in hospital practice: Factors associated with turnover, outcomes, and patient safety. [). American Medical Association.]. *JAMA Health Forum, 4*(7), e231809–e231809. DOI: 10.1001/jamahealthforum.2023.1809 PMID: 37418269

Akhtar, Z. B., & Rawol, A. T. (2024). Artificial intelligence (Tizzard, 2025) and extended reality (XR): A biomedical engineering perspective investigation analysis. *Indonesian Journal of Electronics, Electromedical Engineering, and Medical Informatics, 6*(3). Advance online publication. DOI: 10.35882/ijeeemi.v6i3.5

American Psychiatric Association. (2023). Digital [Resource Document. APA.]. *Mental Health (Detroit, Mich.)*, •••, 101.

Babu, A., & Joseph, A. P. (2025). Digital wellness or digital dependency? A critical examination of mental health apps and their implications. *Frontiers in Psychiatry, 16*, 1581779. DOI: 10.3389/fpsyt.2025.1581779 PMID: 40248604

Baka, E., Tan, Y.-R., Wong, B. L. H., Xing, Z., & Yap, P. (2025). A scoping review of digital interventions for the promotion of mental health and prevention of mental health conditions for young people. *Oxford Open Digital Health, 3*, oqaf005. DOI: 10.1093/oodh/oqaf005 PMID: 40230873

Ball, H., Eisner, E., Nicholas, J., Wilson, P., & Bucci, S. (2025). How theories, models, and frameworks have been used to implement digital health interventions in services for people with severe mental health problems: A scoping review. *BMC Public Health, 25*(1), 1023. DOI: 10.1186/s12889-025-22189-2 PMID: 40098003

Bibi, P (2024). Establishing Transparency and Accountability in AI: Ethical Standards for Data Governance and Automated Systems. In.

Boda, V. V. R., & Allam, H. (2022). Ready for Anything: Disaster Recovery Strategies Every Healthcare IT Team Should Know. *International Journal of Emerging Trends in Computer Science and Information Technology, 3*(1), 38–46. DOI: 10.63282/3050-9246.IJETCSIT-V3I1P105

Bond, R. R., Mulvenna, M. D., Potts, C., O'Neill, S., Ennis, E., & Torous, J. (2023). Digital transformation of mental health services. *Npj Mental Health Research, 2*(1), 13. DOI: 10.1038/s44184-023-00033-y PMID: 38609479

Chen, Z. S., Galatzer-Levy, I. R., Bigio, B., Nasca, C., & Zhang, Y. (2022). Modern views of machine learning for precision psychiatry. *Patterns (New York, N.Y.), 3*(11), 100602. DOI: 10.1016/j.patter.2022.100602 PMID: 36419447

Chithra, N., & Bhambri, P. (2024). Ethics in sustainable technology. In *Handbook of Technological Sustainability* (pp. 245–256). CRC Press. DOI: 10.1201/9781003475989-21

Cristofaro, M., & Giardino, P. L. (2025). Surfing the AI waves: The historical evolution of artificial intelligence in management and organizational studies and practices. *Journal of Management History*. Advance online publication. DOI: 10.1108/JMH-01-2025-0002

De Kock, J. H., Latham, H. A., Leslie, S. J., Grindle, M., Munoz, S. A., Ellis, L., Polson, R., & O'Malley, C. M. (2021). A rapid review of the impact of COVID-19 on the mental health of healthcare workers: Implications for supporting psychological well-being. *BMC Public Health, 21*(1), 104. DOI: 10.1186/s12889-020-10070-3 PMID: 33422039

Engel, G. L. (1977). The need for a new medical model: A challenge for biomedicine. *Science, 196*(4286), 129–136. DOI: 10.1126/science.847460 PMID: 847460

Fanarioti, A. K., & Karpouzis, K. (2025). Artificial Intelligence and the Future of Mental Health in a Digitally Transformed World. *Computers, 14*(7), 259. DOI: 10.3390/computers14070259

Freeman, D., Reeve, S., Robinson, A., Ehlers, A., Clark, D., Spanlang, B., & Slater, M. (2017). Virtual reality in the assessment, understanding, and treatment of mental health disorders. *Psychological Medicine, 47*(14), 2393–2400. DOI: 10.1017/S003329171700040X PMID: 28325167

Hall, C. L., Gómez Bergin, A. D., & Rennick-Egglestone, S. (2024). Research into digital health intervention for mental health: 25-year retrospective on the ethical and legal challenges. *Journal of Medical Internet Research, 26*, e58939. DOI: 10.2196/58939 PMID: 39250796

Hiland, E. B. (2021). *Therapy tech: The digital transformation of mental healthcare.* U of Minnesota Press. DOI: 10.5749/j.ctv1xp9q3t

Ienca, M., Fabrice, J., Elger, B., Caon, M., Scoccia Pappagallo, A., Kressig, R. W., & Wangmo, T. (2017). Intelligent assistive technology for Alzheimer's disease and other dementias: A systematic review. *Journal of Alzheimer's Disease*, *56*(4), 1301–1340. DOI: 10.3233/JAD-161037 PMID: 28222516

Inkster, B., Knibbs, C., & Bada, M. (2023). Cybersecurity: A critical priority for digital mental health. *Frontiers in Digital Health*, *5*, 1242264. DOI: 10.3389/fdgth.2023.1242264 PMID: 37781452

Iwaya, L. H., Babar, M. A., Rashid, A., & Wijayarathna, C. (2023). On the privacy of mental health apps: An empirical investigation and its implications for app development. *Empirical Software Engineering*, *28*(1), 2. DOI: 10.1007/s10664-022-10236-0 PMID: 36407814

Kargarandehkordi, A., Li, S., Lin, K., Phillips, K. T., Benzo, R. M., & Washington, P. (2025). Fusing wearable biosensors with artificial intelligence for mental health monitoring: A systematic review. *Biosensors (Basel)*, *15*(4), 202. DOI: 10.3390/bios15040202 PMID: 40277515

Khoo, Y. X., Kang, R. M., Reynolds, T. L., & Mentis, H. M. (2024). The comprehensiveness of mental health application users' privacy and security concerns. *CHI Conference on Human Factors in Computing Systems*, 16 pages.

Kim, J., & Backonja, U. (2025). Digital health equity frameworks and key concepts: A scoping review. *Journal of the American Medical Informatics Association : JAMIA*, *32*(1), 45–59. DOI: 10.1093/jamia/ocaf017 PMID: 39936843

Kostadimas, D., Kasapakis, V., & Kotis, K. (2025). A systematic review on the combination of VR, IoT and AI technologies, and their integration in applications. *Future Internet*, *17*(4), 163. DOI: 10.3390/fi17040163

Lamb, R., Choi, I., & Owens, T (2025). Convergence of Extended Reality, Artificial Intelligence, Machine Leaning, and Wearable Sensors in the Field of Education. Mental Health Virtual Reality: The Power of Immersive Worlds, 113-128.

Lay, W., Gasparini, L., Siero, W., & Hughes, E. K. (2025). A rapid review of the benefits and challenges of dynamic consent. *Research Ethics*, *21*(1), 180–202. DOI: 10.1177/17470161241278064

Li, M., Patel, J., & Katapally, T. R. (2025). The impact of extended reality cognitive behavioral therapy on mental disorders among children and youth: A systematic review and meta-analysis protocol. *PLoS One*, *20*(3), e0315313. DOI: 10.1371/journal.pone.0315313 PMID: 40048453

Liu, M., & Schueller, S. M. (2023). Moving evidence-based mental health interventions into practice: Implementation of digital mental health interventions. *Current Treatment Options in Psychiatry, 10*(4), 333–345. DOI: 10.1007/s40501-023-00298-2

Livieri, G., Mangina, E., Protopapadakis, E. D., & Panayiotou, A. G. (2025). The gaps and challenges in digital health technology use as perceived by patients: A scoping review and narrative meta-synthesis. *Frontiers in Digital Health, 7*, 1474956. DOI: 10.3389/fdgth.2025.1474956 PMID: 40212901

Ma, C.-B., Shang, X., Sun, M., Bo, X., Bai, J., Du, Y., & Zhou, M. (2025). Emerging Multifunctional Wearable Sensors: Integrating Multimodal Sweat Analysis and Advanced Material Technologies for Next-Generation Health Monitoring. *ACS Sensors, 10*(4), 2388–2408. DOI: 10.1021/acssensors.4c03396 PMID: 40162570

Mahon, D. (2023). Empirically Supported Treatments: A Brief History. In Evidence Based Counselling & Psychotherapy for the 21st Century Practitioner (pp. 3-14). Emerald Publishing Limited. DOI: 10.1108/978-1-80455-732-720231001

Martinez-Martin, N., Marcandalli, J., Huang, C. S., Arthur, C. P., Perotti, M., Foglierini, M., Ho, H., Dosey, A. M., Shriver, S., Payandeh, J., Leitner, A., Lanzavecchia, A., Perez, L., & Ciferri, C. (2018). An unbiased screen for human cytomegalovirus identifies neuropilin-2 as a central viral receptor. *Cell, 174*(5), 1158–1171. DOI: 10.1016/j.cell.2018.06.028 PMID: 30057110

Mohr, D. C., Zhang, M., & Schueller, S. M. (2017). Personal sensing: Understanding mental health using ubiquitous sensors and machine learning. *Annual Review of Clinical Psychology, 13*(1), 23–47. DOI: 10.1146/annurev-clinpsy-032816-044949 PMID: 28375728

Morgan, J. W., Patel, R. A., & Campbell, S. (2025). Practical considerations of clinical XR (Singh & Chandra, 2025) deployments. *Frontiers in Virtual Reality, 6*, 1517402. DOI: 10.3389/frvir.2025.1517402

Obermeyer, Z., Powers, B., Vogeli, C., & Mullainathan, S. (2019). Dissecting racial bias in an algorithm used to manage the health of populations. *Science, 366*(6464), 447–453. DOI: 10.1126/science.aax2342 PMID: 31649194

Ong, T., Ivanova, J., Soni, H., Barrera, J., Cummins, M., Welch, B. M., & Bunnell, B. E. (2025). Mental health clients' perspectives on telehealth-based virtual reality therapy. *Frontiers in Virtual Reality, 6*, 1595326. DOI: 10.3389/frvir.2025.1595326

Radanliev, P. (2025). Privacy, ethics, transparency, and accountability in AI systems for wearable devices. *Frontiers in Digital Health, 7*, 1431246. DOI: 10.3389/fdgth.2025.1431246 PMID: 40599875

Rajpal, S. (2025). Exploring the Role of Virtual Reality and Metaverse in Treating Mental Health: Operating Models and Challenges in Adoption. *Journal of Computer and Communications, 13*(10), 1–22. DOI: 10.4236/jcc.2025.1310001

Ricciardi, F., & Zomaya, A. (2025). Perspectives on Managing AI Ethics in the Digital Age. *Information (Basel), 16*(2), 89. DOI: 10.3390/info16040318

Robinson, A., Flom, M., Forman-Hoffman, V. L., Histon, T., Levy, M., Darcy, A., Ajayi, T., Mohr, D. C., Wicks, P., Greene, C., & Montgomery, R. M. (2024). Equity in digital mental health interventions in the United States: Where to next? *Journal of Medical Internet Research, 26*, e59939. DOI: 10.2196/59939 PMID: 39316436

Saganowski, S., Perz, B., Polak, A. G., & Kazienko, P. (2022). Emotion recognition for everyday life using physiological signals from wearables: A systematic literature review. *IEEE Transactions on Affective Computing, 14*(3), 1876–1897. DOI: 10.1109/TAFFC.2022.3176135

Shatte, A. B., Hutchinson, D. M., & Teague, S. J. (2019). Machine learning in mental health: A scoping review of methods and applications. *Psychological Medicine, 49*(9), 1426–1448. DOI: 10.1017/S0033291719000151 PMID: 30744717

Smith, K. A., Blease, C., Faurholt-Jepsen, M., Firth, J., Van Daele, T., Moreno, C., Carlbring, P., Ebner-Priemer, U. W., Koutsouleris, N., Riper, H., Mouchabac, S., Torous, J., & Cipriani, A. (2023). Digital mental health: Challenges and next steps. *BMJ Mental Health, 26*(1), e300670. DOI: 10.1136/bmjment-2023-300670 PMID: 37197797

Subu, M. A., Holmes, D., Arumugam, A., Al-Yateem, N., Maria Dias, J., Rahman, S. A., Waluyo, I., Ahmed, F. R., & Abraham, M. S. (2022). Traditional, religious, and cultural perspectives on mental illness: A qualitative study on causal beliefs and treatment use. *International Journal of Qualitative Studies on Health and Well-being, 17*(1), 2123090. DOI: 10.1080/17482631.2022.2123090 PMID: 36097886

Tsai, Y. Y., Chen, Y. J., Lin, Y. F., Hsiao, F. C., Hsu, C. H., & Liao, L. D. (2025). Photoplethysmography-based HRV analysis and machine learning for real-time stress quantification in mental health applications. *APL Bioengineering, 9*(2), 026103. DOI: 10.1063/5.0256590 PMID: 40191605

Verma, H., Mlynar, J., Schaer, R., Reichenbach, J., Jreige, M., Prior, J., Evéquoz, F., & Depeursinge, A. (2023). Rethinking the role of AI with physicians in oncology: revealing perspectives from clinical and research workflows. *Proceedings of the 2023 CHI conference on human factors in computing systems* DOI: 10.1145/3544548.3581506

Watson, D (2025). The dark side of mental health apps: Privacy concerns and therapeutic limitations. MentalHealthSigns.com.

Weiner, E. B., Dankwa-Mullan, I., Nelson, W. A., & Hassanpour, S. (2025). Ethical challenges and evolving strategies in the integration of artificial intelligence into clinical practice. *PLOS Digital Health*, *4*(4), e0000810. DOI: 10.1371/journal.pdig.0000810 PMID: 40198594

Chapter 10
Digital Mental Health in Older Adulthood

ABSTRACT

As global aging accelerates, mental health care for older adults demands integrated strategies addressing mood, cognition, and social determinants. This chapter explores late-life depression, anxiety, and neurodegenerative disorders such as Alzheimer's, emphasizing their interplay with isolation, bereavement, and comorbid illness. It calls for person-centered metrics, functional independence, community participation—and scalable interventions suited to low-resource settings. Digital tools, telehealth, and adaptive cognitive training offer promise but require ethical safeguards and usability testing for older populations. Policy frameworks must prioritize continuity, accessibility, and equity to prevent systemic neglect and support aging with dignity and mental well-being.

INTRODUCTION

This chapter addresses the unique mental health needs of older adults, including depression, anxiety, cognitive decline, and social isolation. It explores how digital monitoring, AI-assisted assessment, and adaptive cognitive supports can extend care beyond clinical settings into daily life. Wearable sensors, ambient monitoring, and passive language analysis are presented as tools for early detection and functional preservation. The chapter emphasizes dignity, autonomy, and caregiver collaboration as guiding principles. Implementation challenges such as accessibility, usability, and consent are addressed alongside real-world clinical vignettes. By focusing on person-centered outcomes rather than cognitive normalization, the chapter positions technology as a means to support aging in place and quality of life.

DOI: 10.4018/979-8-3373-4997-8.ch010

MENTAL HEALTH AND OLDER ADULTS

As the global population ages, the mental health needs of older adults are increasingly complex and demand a fundamental rethinking of how care is delivered. This rethinking requires explicit commitments to continuity, accessibility, and person-centered metrics that can guide practical implementation. Define geriatric mental health broadly to include mood, cognitive, functional, and social dimensions that interact over time. For policy and practice, specify measurable goals such as reduced avoidable hospitalizations and improved community participation. Practitioners should prioritize interventions that align with these goals and that are feasible in low-resource settings. Geriatric mental health spans mood disorders, anxiety, late-life depression, and a range of neurodegenerative illnesses including Alzheimer's disease and other dementias; these conditions impair cognition while also reshaping emotional life, social connection, and daily functioning. Social determinants, social isolation, bereavement, comorbid physical illness, and restricted mobility, amplify vulnerability and complicate treatment. Traditional care models, often episodic, clinic-bound, and reactive, struggle to address the persistent, distributed needs of older adults living with cognitive and affective disorders. In response, digital therapeutics and intelligent environments offer a chance to move from fragmented care to a continuous, person-centered system that supports autonomy and dignity. This shift requires translating data and algorithms into interventions that respect older adults' values, preserve agency, and reinforce human caregiving rather than supplant it (Gkintoni et al., 2025). Put plainly: technology must serve relationships and daily life, not merely generate signals in isolation.

Early detection and continuous monitoring are central to preserving functional independence, slowing decline where possible, and tailoring interventions when needed. Clarify detection goals by specifying sensitivity thresholds and acceptable false positive rates for tools used in routine care. Define monitoring intervals and the types of behavior or physiology that warrant escalation to clinical review (Ricciardi & Zomaya, 2025). Establish metrics for success, such as maintained ADLs or delayed institutionalization, to evaluate monitoring programs. Cognitive impairment exists on a spectrum that includes subjective complaints, mild cognitive impairment (MCI), and progressive dementias; the clinical picture is rarely limited to memory loss alone and often includes executive dysfunction, language changes, visuospatial difficulties, mood disturbance, and social withdrawal. These cognitive and behavioral changes unfold over months and years, and meaningful therapeutic action depends on recognizing patterns before crises arise. Artificial intelligence and machine learning techniques can analyze longitudinal data, from electronic health records and neuropsychological testing to passive signals collected in the home, to reveal subtle deviations from an individual's baseline. By focusing on change at the person-level rather than on population thresholds, these systems can support earlier, more tailored responses that reduce the frequency of emergencies and delay institutionalization.

Vignette 1: Mrs. H is a 78-year-old retired schoolteacher who lives alone after her husband died two years earlier. For practical use, describe clearly which data sources contributed to the detected changes and who will act on alerts (Lindner et al., 2024). Clarify the timeline of monitoring and ensure family and clinicians agree on response steps before activation. Include simple, low-burden interventions as first-line responses to avoid unnecessary escalation and to respect patient preferences. Her daughter reports that Mom's short-term memory lapses seem worse than before, but clinic-based testing is within normal limits for her age. A home-monitoring system combined with simple language-usage analytics detects a gradual increase in word-finding pauses and reduced conversational length across three months. The clinician uses this information to schedule a targeted memory clinic visit, updates her medication to remove an anticholinergic, and begins a home-based cognitive engagement plan that includes brief daily word-recall exercises and weekly phone check-ins. Within six months, Mrs. H reports improved confidence and the family notes fewer missed appointments.

Wearable sensors and ambient monitoring technologies extend clinicians' view of health beyond the clinic and into daily life, offering continuous, objective metrics tied to sleep, activity, gait, heart rate variability, and patterns of social engagement (Casson, 2019). Begin deployment planning by assessing connectivity, device maintenance needs, and the minimal data set required for clinical action (Kargarandehkordi et al., 2025). Specify which team member reviews sensor dashboards and how frequently to prevent alert fatigue and to ensure timely responses (Kargarandehkordi et al., 2025). Train caregivers in interpreting high-level indicators rather than raw sensor output to maintain clinical relevance (Kargarandehkordi et al., 2025). These signals are clinically meaningful: disruption of sleep and circadian rhythm often precedes or co-occurs with cognitive and mood symptoms, changes in gait and balance correlate with fall risk and executive dysfunction, and day-to-day reductions in activity can reflect depressive syndromes or emerging apathy. Devices range from consumer-grade smartwatches to purpose-built biosensors and in-home motion detectors; integration matters more than individual device sophistication. When sensors are coupled with pragmatic dashboards and alert rules that clinicians and caregivers can interpret, they create a feedback loop for targeted intervention, adjusting medications, modifying the environment, or arranging social supports, before deterioration becomes irreversible.

Fall detection and prevention exemplify how wearable technologies can translate into concrete clinical benefit (Spytska, 2025). Start by identifying each person's fall-risk profile and matching sensor sensitivity to that risk to minimize false alarms

(Shatte et al., 2019). Use multidisciplinary input, physical therapy, occupational therapy, and nursing, to design individualized prevention plans tied to detected gait changes. Ensure that automation supports, rather than replaces, human assessment by including clinician review steps in the escalation pathway. A sudden fall is a sentinel event that often triggers hospital admission, functional decline, and accelerated cognitive deterioration. Advanced sensor suites can detect subtle shifts in balance, stride variability, and gait speed that precede falls and can be used to trigger preventive strategies: home-visit physical therapy, adaptive footwear, removal of trip hazards, or closer supervision during high-risk activities (Shatte et al., 2019). Some systems integrate with home automation to turn on lighting at night, unlock doors for emergency responders, or notify designated caregivers. Critically, fall-prevention strategies must be individualized: the same alert might lead to increased supervision for one person and to a targeted exercise plan for another. Technology that supports differentiated responses preserves autonomy while reducing harm.

Wearable-derived markers also provide insight into mental health (Fleming et al., 2019). Allocate specific thresholds for meaningful change in activity, sleep, or physiological markers that trigger outreach protocols. Ensure clinicians document baseline variability so deviations are interpreted against individual norms rather than population averages. Train care teams to prioritize low-burden interventions such as brief check-ins or medication reviews before escalating to intensive services. Abrupt reductions in mobility, prolonged daytime napping, or fragmented nocturnal sleep can signal depressive relapse, anxiety escalation, or medication side effects. These signals should prompt low-burden outreach: a brief telehealth check, a medication reconciliation, or an activation of social services. For older adults in rural areas or those whose mobility is limited, remote monitoring combined with telepsychiatry creates access that previously required significant travel and expense. There is, however, a persistent need to design these systems with accessibility in mind: large, high-contrast interfaces; voice interaction for those with limited dexterity; and minimal cognitive overhead for device setup and charging. Confirm connectivity and user support before roll-out to avoid creating gaps in care or increasing caregiver burden.

AI-enhanced memory supports and adaptive cognitive training extend the clinical toolkit from monitoring to active rehabilitation and compensation. Define clear outcome measures, functional independence, medication adherence, or social participation, to evaluate cognitive supports beyond performance scores. Specify acceptable levels of task difficulty progression and automated adjustment parameters to maintain user confidence and prevent frustration. Include caregiver-facing summaries of progress to align expectations and reduce misinterpretation of daily variability. Cognitive training platforms employ exercises aimed at attention, working memory, processing speed, and problem-solving; when adaptive algorithms tailor difficulty and pacing to the individual, engagement and retention improve. Equally practical are compensatory tools, digital calendars, context-aware reminders, and voice assistants, that scaffold everyday functioning and reduce reliance on fragile memory systems. Importantly, these tools can be used in combination: adaptive training that builds confidence paired with reminders that reduce errors yields better day-to-day functioning than either approach alone. The therapeutic aim is not to produce normal cognition but to maximize preserved skills, reduce distress, and support meaningful participation in life. Require real-world functional endpoints when assessing cognitive tools to ensure clinical relevance.

Beyond training, AI is also being leveraged to support compensatory strategies that help individuals manage the practical challenges of memory loss. When deploying compensation tools, outline user preferences for prompt types, escalation rules, and privacy settings to respect autonomy. Provide simple examples of acceptable reminder phrasing and timing to guide configuration and minimize annoyance. Ensure interoperability so reminders and notes update across devices used by caregivers and clinicians for coordinated support. Digital calendars, voice-activated reminders, and smart assistants can assist with scheduling appointments, taking medications, and completing daily tasks. These tools reduce reliance on memory and executive function, allowing individuals to maintain autonomy in their routines. Some advanced platforms even incorporate facial recognition and contextual cues to help users identify people, places, and objects, features that can significantly reduce confusion and anxiety in those with moderate cognitive impairment. For caregivers, these technologies offer a welcome reprieve by automating routine prompts and monitoring, thereby easing the emotional and logistical burden of care. Pilot compensation tools with caregiver oversight to refine settings and confirm acceptability.

Importantly, AI-driven platforms are also transforming how cognitive assessments are conducted. Establish clear protocols for passive data collection that include opt-in procedures, data retention limits, and review intervals to preserve trust. Define clinician responsibilities for responding to flagged changes and integrate these tasks into existing workflows to avoid unmanaged alerts. Validate algorithms against representative older-adult samples to reduce bias and improve generalizability before clinical deployment. Traditional evaluations, typically administered in clinical settings at infrequent intervals, often fail to capture the subtle, day-to-day fluctuations in cognitive function. In contrast, AI systems can passively monitor a user's interaction with digital devices, analyzing speech patterns, typing behavior, navigation habits, and response times, to detect early signs of cognitive decline (Tsai et al., 2025). These continuous assessments provide a more nuanced and timely understanding of cognitive health, enabling earlier interventions and more precise tracking of disease progression. For example, a decline in verbal fluency or increased hesitation in typing may signal emerging cognitive issues long before they become apparent in formal testing. This shift toward passive, ambient assessment not only enhances diagnostic accuracy but also reduces the stigma and stress often associated with traditional cognitive testing. Pair passive assessments with scheduled clinician reviews to contextualize findings and plan interventions.

As the global population ages, the mental health needs of older adults are increasingly complex and demand a fundamental rethinking of how care is delivered. This rethinking requires explicit commitments to continuity, accessibility, and person-centered metrics that can guide practical implementation. Define geriatric mental health broadly to include mood, cognitive, functional, and social dimensions that interact over time. For policy and practice, specify measurable goals such as reduced avoidable hospitalizations and improved community participation. Practitioners should prioritize interventions that align with these goals and that are feasible in low-resource settings. Geriatric mental health spans mood disorders, anxiety, late-life depression, and a range of neurodegenerative illnesses including Alzheimer's disease and other dementias; these conditions impair cognition while also reshaping emotional life, social connection, and daily functioning. Social determinants, social isolation, bereavement, comorbid physical illness, and restricted mobility, amplify vulnerability and complicate treatment. Traditional care models, often episodic, clinic-bound, and reactive, struggle to address the persistent, distributed needs of older adults living with cognitive and affective disorders. In response, digital therapeutics and intelligent environments offer a chance to move from fragmented care to a continuous, person-centered system that supports autonomy and dignity. This shift requires translating data and algorithms into interventions that respect older adults' values, preserve agency, and reinforce human caregiving rather than supplant it (Baydili et al., 2025). Put plainly: technology must serve relationships and daily life, not merely generate signals in isolation.

Early detection and continuous monitoring are central to preserving functional independence, slowing decline where possible, and tailoring interventions when needed. Clarify detection goals by specifying sensitivity thresholds and acceptable false positive rates for tools used in routine care. Define monitoring intervals and the types of behavior or physiology that warrant escalation to clinical review (Tavory, 2024). Establish metrics for success, such as maintained ADLs or delayed institutionalization, to evaluate monitoring programs. Cognitive impairment exists on a spectrum that includes subjective complaints, mild cognitive impairment (MCI), and progressive dementias; the clinical picture is rarely limited to memory loss alone and often includes executive dysfunction, language changes, visuospatial difficulties, mood disturbance, and social withdrawal. These cognitive and behavioral changes unfold over months and years, and meaningful therapeutic action depends on recognizing patterns before crises arise. Artificial intelligence and machine learning techniques can analyze longitudinal data, from electronic health records and neuropsychological testing to passive signals collected in the home, to reveal subtle deviations from an individual's baseline. By focusing on change at the person-level rather than on population thresholds, these systems can support earlier, more tailored responses that reduce the frequency of emergencies and delay institutionalization.

Vignette 1: Mrs. H is a 78-year-old retired schoolteacher who lives alone after her husband died two years earlier. For practical use, describe clearly which data sources contributed to the detected changes and who will act on alerts (Sun et al., 2025). Clarify the timeline of monitoring and ensure family and clinicians agree on response steps before activation. Include simple, low-burden interventions as first-line responses to avoid unnecessary escalation and to respect patient preferences. Her daughter reports that Mom's short-term memory lapses seem worse than before, but clinic-based testing is within normal limits for her age. A home-monitoring system combined with simple language-usage analytics detects a gradual increase in word-finding pauses and reduced conversational length across three months. The clinician uses this information to schedule a targeted memory clinic visit, updates her medication to remove an anticholinergic, and begins a home-based cognitive engagement plan that includes brief daily word-recall exercises and weekly phone check-ins. Within six months, Mrs. H reports improved confidence and the family notes fewer missed appointments.

Wearable sensors and ambient monitoring technologies extend clinicians' view of health beyond the clinic and into daily life, offering continuous, objective metrics tied to sleep, activity, gait, heart rate variability, and patterns of social engagement (Vaidyam et al., 2019). Begin deployment planning by assessing connectivity, device maintenance needs, and the minimal data set required for clinical action (Ong et al., 2025). Specify which team member reviews sensor dashboards and how frequently to prevent alert fatigue and to ensure timely responses (Ong et al., 2025). Train caregivers in interpreting high-level indicators rather than raw sensor output to maintain clinical relevance (Ong et al., 2025). These signals are clinically meaningful: disruption of sleep and circadian rhythm often precedes or co-occurs with cognitive and mood symptoms, changes in gait and balance correlate with fall risk and executive dysfunction, and day-to-day reductions in activity can reflect depressive syndromes or emerging apathy. Devices range from consumer-grade smartwatches to purpose-built biosensors and in-home motion detectors; integration matters more than individual device sophistication. When sensors are coupled with pragmatic dashboards and alert rules that clinicians and caregivers can interpret, they create a feedback loop for targeted intervention, adjusting medications, modifying the environment, or arranging social supports, before deterioration becomes irreversible.

Fall detection and prevention exemplify how wearable technologies can translate into concrete clinical benefit (Carl et al., 2019). Start by identifying each person's fall-risk profile and matching sensor sensitivity to that risk to minimize false alarms. Use multidisciplinary input, physical therapy, occupational therapy, and nursing, to design individualized prevention plans tied to detected gait changes. Ensure that automation supports, rather than replaces, human assessment by including clinician review steps in the escalation pathway. A sudden fall is a sentinel event that often triggers hospital admission, functional decline, and accelerated cognitive deterioration. Advanced sensor suites can detect subtle shifts in balance, stride variability, and gait speed that precede falls and can be used to trigger preventive strategies: home-visit physical therapy, adaptive footwear, removal of trip hazards, or closer supervision during high-risk activities (Mohr et al., 2017). Some systems integrate with home automation to turn on lighting at night, unlock doors for emergency responders, or notify designated caregivers. Critically, fall-prevention strategies must be individualized: the same alert might lead to increased supervision for one person and to a targeted exercise plan for another. Technology that supports differentiated responses preserves autonomy while reducing harm.

Wearable-derived markers also provide insight into mental health (Xing et al., 2025). Allocate specific thresholds for meaningful change in activity, sleep, or physiological markers that trigger outreach protocols. Ensure clinicians document baseline variability so deviations are interpreted against individual norms rather than population averages. Train care teams to prioritize low-burden interventions such as brief check-ins or medication reviews before escalating to intensive services. Abrupt reductions in mobility, prolonged daytime napping, or fragmented nocturnal sleep can signal depressive relapse, anxiety escalation, or medication side effects. These signals should prompt low-burden outreach: a brief telehealth check, a medication reconciliation, or an activation of social services. For older adults in rural areas or those whose mobility is limited, remote monitoring combined with telepsychiatry creates access that previously required significant travel and expense. There is, however, a persistent need to design these systems with accessibility in mind: large, high-contrast interfaces; voice interaction for those with limited dexterity; and minimal cognitive overhead for device setup and charging. Confirm connectivity and user support before roll-out to avoid creating gaps in care or increasing caregiver burden.

AI-enhanced memory supports and adaptive cognitive training extend the clinical toolkit from monitoring to active rehabilitation and compensation (Mone & Fayazullaeva, 2023). Define clear outcome measures, functional independence, medication adherence, or social participation, to evaluate cognitive supports beyond performance scores. Specify acceptable levels of task difficulty progression and automated adjustment parameters to maintain user confidence and prevent frustration. Include caregiver-facing summaries of progress to align expectations and reduce misinterpretation of daily variability. Cognitive training platforms employ exercises aimed at attention, working memory, processing speed, and problem-solving; when adaptive algorithms tailor difficulty and pacing to the individual, engagement and retention improve. Equally practical are compensatory tools, digital calendars, context-aware reminders, and voice assistants, that scaffold everyday functioning and reduce reliance on fragile memory systems. Importantly, these tools can be used in combination: adaptive training that builds confidence paired with reminders that reduce errors yields better day-to-day functioning than either approach alone. The therapeutic aim is not to produce normal cognition but to maximize preserved skills, reduce distress, and support meaningful participation in life. Require real-world functional endpoints when assessing cognitive tools to ensure clinical relevance (Ricciardi & Zomaya, 2025).

Beyond training, AI is also being leveraged to support compensatory strategies that help individuals manage the practical challenges of memory loss (Friend et al., 2024). When deploying compensation tools, outline user preferences for prompt types, escalation rules, and privacy settings to respect autonomy. Provide simple examples of acceptable reminder phrasing and timing to guide configuration and minimize annoyance. Ensure interoperability so reminders and notes update across devices used by caregivers and clinicians for coordinated support. Digital calendars, voice-activated reminders, and smart assistants can assist with scheduling appointments, taking medications, and completing daily tasks. These tools reduce reliance on memory and executive function, allowing individuals to maintain autonomy in their routines. Some advanced platforms even incorporate facial recognition and contextual cues to help users identify people, places, and objects, features that can significantly reduce confusion and anxiety in those with moderate cognitive impairment. For caregivers, these technologies offer a welcome reprieve by automating routine prompts and monitoring, thereby easing the emotional and logistical burden of care. Pilot compensation tools with caregiver oversight to refine settings and confirm acceptability.

Importantly, AI-driven platforms are also transforming how cognitive assessments are conducted (Walter et al., 2023). Establish clear protocols for passive data collection that include opt-in procedures, data retention limits, and review intervals to preserve trust (Rajpal, 2025). Define clinician responsibilities for responding to flagged changes and integrate these tasks into existing workflows to avoid unmanaged alerts. Validate algorithms against representative older-adult samples to reduce bias and improve generalizability before clinical deployment (Rajpal, 2025). Traditional evaluations, typically administered in clinical settings at infrequent intervals, often fail to capture the subtle, day-to-day fluctuations in cognitive function (Rajpal, 2025). In contrast, AI systems can passively monitor a user's interaction with digital devices, analyzing speech patterns, typing behavior, navigation habits, and response times, to detect early signs of cognitive decline (Rajpal, 2025). These continuous assessments provide a more nuanced and timely understanding of cognitive health, enabling earlier interventions and more precise tracking of disease progression. For example, a decline in verbal fluency or increased hesitation in typing may signal emerging cognitive issues long before they become apparent in formal testing. This shift toward passive, ambient assessment not only enhances diagnostic accuracy but also reduces the stigma and stress often associated with traditional cognitive testing. Pair passive assessments with scheduled clinician reviews to contextualize findings and plan interventions.

Wearable-derived markers also provide insight into mental health (Lorke & Stefanou, 2025). Allocate specific thresholds for meaningful change in activity, sleep, or physiological markers that trigger outreach protocols. Ensure clinicians document baseline variability so deviations are interpreted against individual norms rather than population averages. Train care teams to prioritize low-burden interventions such as brief check-ins or medication reviews before escalating to intensive services. Abrupt reductions in mobility, prolonged daytime napping, or fragmented nocturnal sleep can signal depressive relapse, anxiety escalation, or medication side effects. These signals should prompt low-burden outreach: a brief telehealth check, a medication reconciliation, or an activation of social services. For older adults in rural areas or those whose mobility is limited, remote monitoring combined with telepsychiatry creates access that previously required significant travel and expense. There is, however, a persistent need to design these systems with accessibility in mind: large, high-contrast interfaces; voice interaction for those with limited dexterity; and minimal cognitive overhead for device setup and charging. Confirm connectivity and user support before roll-out to avoid creating gaps in care or increasing caregiver burden.

AI-enhanced memory supports and adaptive cognitive training extend the clinical toolkit from monitoring to active rehabilitation and compensation (Pedram & Piatkowski, 2025). Define clear outcome measures, functional independence, medication adherence, or social participation, to evaluate cognitive supports beyond performance scores. Specify acceptable levels of task difficulty progression and automated adjustment parameters to maintain user confidence and prevent frustration. Include caregiver-facing summaries of progress to align expectations and reduce misinterpretation of daily variability. Cognitive training platforms employ exercises aimed at attention, working memory, processing speed, and problem-solving; when adaptive algorithms tailor difficulty and pacing to the individual, engagement and retention improve. Equally practical are compensatory tools, digital calendars, context-aware reminders, and voice assistants, that scaffold everyday functioning and reduce reliance on fragile memory systems. Importantly, these tools can be used in combination: adaptive training that builds confidence paired with reminders that reduce errors yields better day-to-day functioning than either approach alone. The therapeutic aim is not to produce normal cognition but to maximize preserved skills, reduce distress, and support meaningful participation in life. Require real-world functional endpoints when assessing cognitive tools to ensure clinical relevance (Li et al., 2025).

Beyond training, AI is also being leveraged to support compensatory strategies that help individuals manage the practical challenges of memory loss (Poudel et al., 2025). When deploying compensation tools, outline user preferences for prompt types, escalation rules, and privacy settings to respect autonomy. Provide simple examples of acceptable reminder phrasing and timing to guide configuration and minimize annoyance. Ensure interoperability so reminders and notes update across devices used by caregivers and clinicians for coordinated support. Digital calendars, voice-activated reminders, and smart assistants can assist with scheduling appointments, taking medications, and completing daily tasks. These tools reduce reliance on memory and executive function, allowing individuals to maintain autonomy in their routines. Some advanced platforms even incorporate facial recognition and contextual cues to help users identify people, places, and objects, features that can significantly reduce confusion and anxiety in those with moderate cognitive impairment. For caregivers, these technologies offer a welcome reprieve by automating routine prompts and monitoring, thereby easing the emotional and logistical burden of care. Pilot compensation tools with caregiver oversight to refine settings and confirm acceptability.

Importantly, AI-driven platforms are also transforming how cognitive assessments are conducted (Obermeyer et al., 2019). Establish clear protocols for passive data collection that include opt-in procedures, data retention limits, and review intervals to preserve trust (Obermeyer et al., 2019). Define clinician responsibilities for responding to flagged changes and integrate these tasks into existing workflows to avoid unmanaged alerts. Validate algorithms against representative older-adult samples to reduce bias and improve generalizability before clinical deployment (Obermeyer et al., 2019). Traditional evaluations, typically administered in clinical settings at infrequent intervals, often fail to capture the subtle, day-to-day fluctuations in cognitive function (Obermeyer et al., 2019). In contrast, AI systems can passively monitor a user's interaction with digital devices, analyzing speech patterns, typing behavior, navigation habits, and response times, to detect early signs of cognitive decline (Obermeyer et al., 2019). These continuous assessments provide a more nuanced and timely understanding of cognitive health, enabling earlier interventions and more precise tracking of disease progression. For example, a decline in verbal fluency or increased hesitation in typing may signal emerging cognitive issues long before they become apparent in formal testing. This shift toward passive, ambient assessment not only enhances diagnostic accuracy but also reduces the stigma and stress often associated with traditional cognitive testing. Pair passive assessments with scheduled clinician reviews to contextualize findings and plan interventions.

Building on the capabilities of AI and wearable technologies, extended reality (XR), which includes both virtual reality (Engel, 1977) and augmented reality (AR), is emerging as a powerful tool for enhancing social connection, cognitive stimulation, and emotional well-being in older adults (Martinez-Martin et al., 2018). Define selection criteria for XR candidates, including cognitive load tolerance, sensory limitations, and therapeutic goals. Prepare simple checklists for clinicians and caregivers to screen for adverse vestibular effects and to plan for gradual exposure. Ensure XR content aligns with users' life stories to maximize relevance and reduce disorientation. These immersive technologies offer experiences that transcend the physical limitations often associated with aging, opening new avenues for therapeutic engagement, reminiscence, and community building. In particular, XR environments are uniquely suited to address the psychological and social dimensions of geriatric mental health, which are often overlooked in traditional care models. Establish short session durations and supervision protocols to detect and address discomfort promptly. One of the most compelling applications of XR in this context is VR-based reminiscence therapy. Start by collecting brief life-history details to tailor scenes that are emotionally resonant and culturally appropriate. Use short, repeated sessions and caregiver facilitation to reinforce comfort and to link virtual content with real-world meaning. Monitor affect and orientation during sessions and document responses to guide subsequent exposures. By transporting individuals to familiar or meaningful places, such as childhood homes, natural landscapes, or historical events, VR can evoke autobiographical memories that are deeply tied to identity and emotional continuity. For individuals with dementia, these immersive experiences can be profoundly grounding, helping to reduce agitation, enhance mood, and foster a sense of self that may otherwise feel fragmented. Unlike static photographs or verbal prompts, VR engages multiple senses and creates a sense of presence that can make memories feel more vivid and emotionally resonant. Track changes in agitation and social engagement after VR sessions to evaluate benefit.

Beyond reminiscence, XR platforms are also being used to facilitate social interaction and reduce loneliness, a pervasive issue among older adults, particularly those with mobility impairments or living in long-term care facilities. Set clear facilitation roles for virtual gatherings, including moderators, technical-support staff, and content leads, to ensure sessions remain focused and accessible. Provide orientation sessions for new users and include caregivers in early meetings to normalize the technology and build comfort. Offer a range of activities, shared music, storytelling, gentle movement, that accommodate varied cognitive and physical abilities. Social XR environments allow users to participate in virtual gatherings, where they can interact with peers, family members, or therapists in shared digital spaces (De Kock et al., 2021). These environments can host group therapy sessions, recreational activities, or educational workshops, creating opportunities for meaningful engagement and community building. For many older adults, especially those who are geographically isolated or physically limited, XR offers a vital bridge to the outside world and a renewed sense of belonging (De Kock et al., 2021). Plan for bandwidth and device sharing protocols to extend access in low-resource settings.

XR is also proving valuable in therapeutic contexts beyond socialization and memory support (Tizzard, 2025). Define clinical pathways that specify when XR-based exposure or relaxation is indicated and how to measure response. Train facilitators to titrate exposure intensity and to use biometric feedback when available to guide adjustments. Document contraindications and include emergency stop procedures to preserve safety. Immersive environments can be used for guided relaxation, mindfulness training, and exposure therapy for anxiety or phobias. The immersive nature of XR enhances engagement and can be particularly effective for individuals who may struggle with traditional therapeutic formats. For example, a calming virtual forest or beach scene can be used to facilitate deep breathing exercises and reduce stress, while controlled exposure to anxiety-inducing scenarios can help individuals gradually build coping skills in a safe and supportive setting. When combined with biometric feedback from wearable sensors, such as heart rate or galvanic skin response, XR experiences can be dynamically adjusted in real time to optimize emotional and cognitive outcomes. Ensure XR session notes and biometric summaries populate the clinical record for continuity. As XR technologies become more accessible and user-friendly, their integration into geriatric mental health care is likely to expand. Include version-control processes for XR content and device firmware to avoid unexpected updates during sessions. Establish simple maintenance routines and designate staff responsible for hygiene and headset fitting to reduce infection risk and discomfort. Developers are increasingly designing XR applications with older adults in mind, incorporating features such as simplified interfaces, voice navigation, and adjustable visual settings to accommodate sensory and cognitive changes. Moreover, the convergence of XR with AI and remote monitoring systems holds immense potential for creating fully integrated, adaptive care environments that respond to the unique needs of each individual (Mohr et al., 2017). These innovations not only enhance the quality of life for older adults but also offer new tools for clinicians and caregivers to deliver more effective, personalized, and compassionate care. Include lifecycle costs in procurement decisions, not just device prices.

While the potential of AI, ML, wearable sensors, and XR in geriatric care is immense, their implementation must be approached with ethical sensitivity and user-centered design (Leivaditis & Sepetis, 2025). Begin ethical review early in project planning and include patient advocates and family caregivers on advisory panels. Map potential harms and mitigation strategies, such as re-consenting protocols for cognitive decline and fail-safe mechanisms for device failures. Older adults may face barriers related to digital literacy, sensory impairments, or skepticism toward technology. Interventions must be designed with accessibility in mind, featuring intuitive interfaces, large fonts, voice commands, and culturally relevant content. Privacy and consent are also paramount, particularly when cognitive impairment may affect decision-making capacity. Care must be taken to ensure that individuals understand how their data is used and that caregivers are involved appropriately without undermining autonomy (Li et al., 2025). Transparent data governance, secure storage, and clear communication are essential to maintaining trust (Li et al., 2025). Training for clinicians and caregivers is critical to ensure that digital tools are used effectively and ethically. This includes understanding the capabilities and limitations of the technology, recognizing signs of digital fatigue or frustration, and integrating digital interventions into broader care plans. Interdisciplinary collaboration, between clinicians, technologists, designers, and ethicists, is essential to co-create solutions that are not only effective but also dignified and humane. Require public reporting of data practices and routine audits to maintain accountability (Li et al., 2025). The integration of AI, ML, wearable sensors, and XR into geriatric mental health care represents a paradigm shift toward a more holistic, proactive, and person-centered model (Li et al., 2025). State clear, prioritized goals for system deployment, improved safety, preserved autonomy, reduced loneliness, and measurable functional outcomes, to align stakeholders and funding. These technologies enable early detection, continuous support, and meaningful engagement, empowering older adults to maintain autonomy, connection, and purpose. They also offer caregivers and clinicians powerful tools to deliver more responsive, data-informed, and compassionate care (Li et al., 2025). As we look to the future, the challenge is not merely technological but cultural: to ensure that innovation serves

CAREGIVERS IMPLICATIONS

The integration of artificial intelligence (AI), machine learning (ML), wearable sensors, and extended reality (Reddy, 2025) into geriatric mental health care is profoundly reshaping the caregiving experience, offering both relief and new responsibilities for caregivers (Rajpal, 2025). Identify caregiver competencies required for device management, data interpretation, and ethical decision-making, and include these in training curriculums (Fleming et al., 2019). AI and ML technologies enhance decision-making by analyzing vast datasets to detect early signs of cognitive or emotional decline, enabling caregivers to intervene earlier and more effectively (Fleming et al., 2019). These systems can automate routine tasks such as medication reminders and symptom tracking, reducing the cognitive and emotional load on caregivers while allowing them to focus on more meaningful, human-centered aspects of care. Predictive algorithms also offer foresight into potential health events, such as fall risks or the progression of dementia, empowering caregivers to take preventive action. Wearable sensors complement these capabilities by providing real-time, non-invasive monitoring of vital signs, sleep patterns, activity levels, and emotional states (Fleming et al., 2019). This continuous stream of data allows caregivers to respond swiftly to changes in health status, even from a distance, and facilitates more informed conversations with healthcare providers (Fleming et al., 2019). For family caregivers, especially those balancing multiple responsibilities, this remote oversight offers peace of mind and a greater sense of control. Meanwhile, XR technologies are opening new avenues for therapeutic engagement and social connection (Fleming et al., 2019). Caregivers can use VR-based reminiscence therapy to help individuals with dementia reconnect with meaningful memories, or facilitate virtual gatherings that reduce loneliness and foster community. XR also supports guided relaxation and exposure therapy, offering immersive interventions that may be more engaging and effective than traditional formats (Fleming et al., 2019). These tools not only enrich the lives of older adults but also provide caregivers with innovative ways to deliver care that is both compassionate and stimulating. However, the adoption of these technologies also introduces challenges, including the need for digital literacy, ethical considerations around data privacy, and ensuring equitable access (Fleming et al., 2019). Caregivers must be supported with training and resources to navigate these tools effectively. Ultimately, when thoughtfully implemented, these technologies can transform caregiving from a reactive, labor-intensive role into a more proactive, data-informed, and emotionally sustainable practice, enhancing the quality of care while preserving the dignity and autonomy of those they support (Fleming et al., 2019). Embed respite and peer-support programs into technology roll-outs to mitigate burnout.

As digital technologies become increasingly embedded in geriatric mental health care, the roles of clinicians and caregivers are undergoing a profound transformation. Define role boundaries explicitly to avoid task-shifting that increases caregiver burden without appropriate compensation or training. No longer confined to traditional models of care, these professionals are now expected to navigate a rapidly evolving landscape of artificial intelligence (AI), machine learning (ML), wearable sensors, and extended reality (XR; Weiner et al., 2025). While these tools offer unprecedented opportunities for early detection, personalized intervention, and continuous support, they also demand a new set of competencies and a reimagining of how care is delivered. To ensure that these innovations translate into meaningful improvements in the lives of older adults, it is essential to invest in comprehensive training and support systems for those on the front lines of care. Incorporate digital competency milestones into professional licensing and certification. At the most fundamental level, clinicians and caregivers must develop digital literacy, the ability to confidently and critically engage with digital tools and platforms. Create modular learning pathways that allow busy clinicians and family caregivers to build skills incrementally. This includes understanding how to operate devices, interpret data outputs, and troubleshoot common technical issues. For clinicians, digital literacy extends to navigating electronic health records (Singh & Chandra, 2025) integrated with AI analytics, interpreting predictive models, and incorporating algorithmic insights into clinical decision-making. For caregivers, particularly those without formal medical training, it involves learning how to use wearable devices, respond to alerts, and engage with AI-powered applications that support daily routines and monitor well-being (Weiner et al., 2025). In both cases, digital literacy is not a static skill but a dynamic competency that must evolve alongside technological advancements. Prefer short microlearning modules with practical exercises over lengthy didactic sessions.

Beyond basic literacy, clinicians and caregivers must also cultivate data interpretation and critical thinking skills (Johnson et al., 2021). Offer case-based exercises that demonstrate algorithmic limitations and bias to build healthy skepticism and appropriate reliance. AI and ML systems generate vast amounts of information, ranging from biometric data to behavioral trends, that must be contextualized within the broader picture of an individual's health (Casson, 2019). Clinicians need to understand the limitations and biases of algorithmic models, recognize when to trust automated recommendations, and know when human judgment should override machine-generated insights. This requires a foundational understanding of how algorithms are trained, what data they rely on, and how to assess their accuracy and relevance in real-world settings (Casson, 2019). For caregivers, the challenge lies in translating complex data into actionable steps, such as adjusting a daily schedule based on sleep patterns or recognizing signs of emotional distress from changes in activity levels (Casson, 2019). Include simulated scenarios where caregivers must decide on escalation using device data (Casson, 2019). Another critical area of training involves ethical and privacy considerations. Standardize informed-consent language and procedures for cognitive impairment that permit staged consent and proxy involvement. As digital tools collect and process sensitive health information, clinicians and caregivers must be well-versed in data protection regulations such as HIPAA (in the U. S.) or GDPR (in Europe; Casson, 2019). They must understand how to obtain informed consent, ensure data security, and navigate the ethical dilemmas that arise when balancing autonomy with safety (Casson, 2019). For example, should a caregiver intervene if a wearable sensor detects a fall risk, even if the older adult prefers to maintain independence (Casson, 2019)? These are not merely technical questions but deeply human ones that require empathy, cultural sensitivity, and ethical reasoning. Require documentation of consent discussions and periodic reassessment as cognition changes.

To address these multifaceted training needs, a variety of educational models and programs are emerging. Pilot blended curricula that combine online modules, hands-on device practice, and peer mentoring to accommodate diverse learner needs. Many healthcare institutions are now offering continuing education courses focused on digital health, often in partnership with universities, technology companies, or professional associations. These courses may cover topics such as AI in clinical practice, digital therapeutics, telehealth delivery, and cybersecurity (Glass et al., 2022). Some programs are delivered online to accommodate the demanding schedules of healthcare workers, while others include in-person workshops or simulation labs. For example, XR-based training environments allow clinicians and caregivers to practice responding to real-life scenarios, such as managing a behavioral crisis in a person with dementia, within a safe, controlled, and immersive setting. These simulations not only build technical skills but also enhance emotional intelligence and situational awareness. Plan for ongoing refresher courses and competency checks rather than one-time training. In addition to formal training, peer learning and mentorship play a vital role in building digital competencies. Establish local champions and mentorship pairings to provide just-in-time support and to model best practices. Interdisciplinary learning communities, where clinicians, caregivers, technologists, and researchers come together to share experiences and insights, can foster a culture of innovation and continuous improvement. These communities may take the form of online forums, professional networks, or collaborative workshops. By learning from one another, participants can gain a more holistic understanding of how digital tools function in diverse care settings and how they can be adapted to meet the unique needs of older adults. Fund community-of-practice activities as part of implementation budgets.

The importance of interdisciplinary collaboration cannot be overstated in the context of digital geriatric care. Create formal governance structures that include clinician, design, technical, and ethical representation to guide project decisions. The successful implementation of AI, ML, XR, and wearable technologies requires input from a wide range of stakeholders, including physicians, nurses, occupational therapists, social workers, engineers, designers, and ethicists (Mulukuntla, 2025). Each brings a unique perspective and set of skills that enrich the development and deployment of digital solutions. For instance, while a data scientist may design an algorithm to detect early signs of cognitive decline, a clinician can provide insights into how those signs manifest in daily life, and a caregiver can offer feedback on how the tool fits into the rhythm of home care (Kim & Backonja, 2025). This collaborative approach ensures that technologies are not only scientifically sound but also practical, user-friendly, and aligned with the values of dignity and person-centered care. Schedule regular interdisciplinary reviews to assess performance and address emergent issues. Moreover, interdisciplinary teams are essential for integrating digital tools into existing care pathways. Map decision points where digital inputs influence clinical choices and make these explicit in care protocols (Kim & Backonja, 2025).

Rather than viewing technology as a separate or supplementary component, these teams work to embed digital solutions into the fabric of care delivery. This might involve redesigning workflows to incorporate real-time data from wearable sensors, developing protocols for responding to AI-generated alerts, or creating shared care plans that leverage insights from multiple sources (Kim & Backonja, 2025). In doing so, they help bridge the gap between innovation and implementation, ensuring that digital tools enhance rather than disrupt the continuity of care. Include templated notes and order sets that reflect digital-derived findings.

For caregivers, especially those providing informal or unpaid care, access to training and support is equally important. Offer flexible, nontechnical resources, short videos, pictorial guides, and phone-based coaching, to reach caregivers with varying literacy and time constraints. Many family caregivers find themselves suddenly thrust into complex care roles without adequate preparation or resources. Digital tools can be both a lifeline and a source of stress, depending on how well they are understood and supported. Community organizations, healthcare providers, and advocacy groups can play a crucial role in offering accessible, culturally sensitive training for caregivers. This might include instructional videos, helplines, mobile apps with step-by-step guidance, or in-person support groups where caregivers can learn from one another. Empowering caregivers with knowledge and confidence not only improves care outcomes but also reduces burnout and enhances well-being. Integrate caregiver needs assessment into pre-deployment planning. In addition to technical training, it is essential to address the emotional and psychological dimensions of caregiving in a digital age. Include brief modules on moral distress and boundary-setting to help caregivers navigate tension between surveillance and autonomy. The introduction of monitoring technologies, for example, can raise concerns about surveillance, loss of privacy, or the depersonalization of care. Caregivers may struggle with feelings of guilt or inadequacy if they rely too heavily on technology, or they may feel overwhelmed by the constant stream of data and alerts (Kumar, 2025). Training programs should therefore include components on emotional resilience, ethical reflection, and self-care, helping caregivers navigate the complex interplay between technology and human connection. Provide referral pathways to counseling or respite when caregiver stress is identified.

Looking ahead, the future of training in digital geriatric care will likely involve hybrid models that combine online learning, hands-on practice, and interdisciplinary collaboration. Pilot modular credentialing systems that certify practical competencies and that are portable across care settings. Micro-credentialing and modular learning pathways can allow professionals to build skills incrementally and at their own pace. AI itself may play a role in personalizing training, offering adaptive learning platforms that tailor content to the learner's background, goals, and progress (Elfouly & Alouani, 2025). For example, a nurse might receive targeted modules on interpreting biometric data, while a family caregiver might focus on using voice assistants for medication reminders (Robinson et al., 2024). These personalized learning experiences can make training more relevant, engaging, and effective. Validate training programs by measuring skill retention and impact on care quality.

Ultimately, the goal of training and support is not merely to teach people how to use technology, but to cultivate a mindset of curiosity, adaptability, and empathy. Design curricula that emphasize clinical judgment, ethical decision-making, and communication as much as device operation (Huang et al., 2024). In a field as dynamic and human-centered as geriatric mental health, technology should be seen as a tool to enhance, not replace, the relational aspects of care. By equipping clinicians and caregivers with the skills, knowledge, and confidence to engage with digital tools thoughtfully and ethically, we can create a care environment that is both technologically advanced and deeply compassionate. Align training outcomes with patient-reported measures of dignity and connectedness. As digital therapeutics continue to evolve, the future of geriatric mental health care is poised to be shaped by a new generation of technologies that push the boundaries of what is currently possible. Prioritize translational pathways that move innovations from lab to clinic through staged pilots, regulatory engagement, and clinician involvement. Among the most promising innovations are brain-computer interfaces (BCIs), digital twins, and emotion AI, tools that have the potential to radically transform how we understand, monitor, and support the aging mind (Li et al., 2025). Brain-computer interfaces represent a frontier in neurotechnology, enabling direct communication between the brain and external devices. In the context of geriatric care, BCIs could one day assist individuals with advanced neurodegenerative conditions in expressing needs, navigating digital environments, or even controlling assistive technologies through thought alone. While still largely experimental, early research suggests that BCIs may offer new pathways for restoring agency and communication in individuals with severe cognitive or motor impairments (Li et al., 2025). Require ethical review and staged feasibility studies before clinical use of BCIs (Li et al., 2025).

Digital twins, another emerging innovation, involve creating real-time, virtual replicas of individuals that integrate data from wearable sensors, medical records, and behavioral inputs. Define the minimal data elements required to build a clinically useful digital twin and establish governance for model updates and error-checking. These dynamic models can simulate how a person might respond to different treatments, environmental changes, or lifestyle interventions. For older adults, digital twins could enable highly personalized care planning, allowing clinicians to test and refine interventions in a virtual space before applying them in real life. This approach not only enhances precision but also reduces the risks and costs associated with trial-and-error treatment strategies. Require prospective evaluation comparing digital-twin-guided care to usual care. Emotion AI, or affective computing, is also gaining traction as a tool for enhancing emotional awareness and responsiveness in digital systems. Set clear performance thresholds for emotion-detection models and validate them in diverse older-adult populations to avoid cultural or age-related bias. By analyzing facial expressions, voice tone, and physiological signals, emotion AI can detect subtle shifts in mood or stress levels. In geriatric mental health, this technology could be used to monitor emotional well-being continuously, trigger supportive interventions during periods of distress, or adapt therapeutic content in real time to match the user's emotional state. When integrated with XR environments or AI-driven companions, emotion AI has the potential to create more empathetic and responsive digital experiences. Ensure human oversight for all emotion-based interventions to prevent misclassification harms.

Looking ahead, the future of care will likely be defined by hybrid models that blend human expertise with digital intelligence. Specify governance models that maintain clinician accountability while leveraging algorithmic efficiency for routine monitoring tasks. These models will not replace human caregivers or clinicians but will augment their capabilities, enabling more proactive, personalized, and scalable care. For example, a hybrid system might use AI to flag early signs of depression based on speech patterns, wearable data, and social engagement metrics, prompting a clinician to initiate a check-in or adjust a treatment plan. Similarly, XR platforms could be used to deliver group therapy sessions facilitated by a human therapist but enhanced with immersive, interactive content tailored to each participant's cognitive profile (Ienca et al., 2017). Document decision thresholds where clinician review is mandatory.

To realize the full potential of these innovations, public-private partnerships will play a crucial role. Define shared objectives and accountability mechanisms in partnership agreements to ensure public interest is prioritized. Collaboration between governments, healthcare providers, academic institutions, and technology companies is essential for funding research, developing ethical frameworks, and ensuring equitable access. These partnerships can also help bridge the gap between innovation and implementation by supporting pilot programs, scaling successful interventions, and creating regulatory pathways that encourage responsible adoption. By aligning incentives and pooling expertise, public-private collaborations can accelerate the development of technologies that are not only cutting-edge but also grounded in the real-world needs of older adults and their caregivers. Include commitments to subsidize access for underserved populations in partnership agreements. While the promise of digital therapeutics is vast, it is in real-world applications that their true impact becomes visible. Design pilots with clear success criteria, equity metrics, and realistic timelines to support meaningful evaluation. Across the globe, a growing number of pilot programs and case studies are demonstrating how AI, wearable sensors, XR, and other technologies can be effectively deployed to support geriatric mental health. One notable example is the "VR Reminiscence Therapy" pilot conducted in the UK, where older adults with dementia were immersed in virtual environments replicating familiar places from their past, such as seaside towns, childhood neighborhoods, or historical events. Participants reported improved mood, reduced agitation, and a stronger sense of identity. Caregivers also noted that the therapy sessions sparked meaningful conversations and emotional engagement that had previously been difficult to achieve. The program's success has led to broader adoption in care homes and memory clinics, with ongoing research exploring its long-term cognitive and emotional benefits. Publish operational details from pilots to support adoption and reproducibility. In the United States, the "AI Companion" project at the University of Georgia has piloted the use of voice-activated assistants equipped with natural language processing to monitor speech patterns and detect early signs of cognitive decline and other mental health concerns. When replicating such pilots, ensure linguistic diversity in training data to avoid exclusion of dialects and nonstandard speech patterns. These systems engage users in daily conversations, provide reminders, and offer cognitive games tailored to the individual's abilities. Over time, the AI learns the user's speech habits and can flag deviations that may indicate emerging issues. Preliminary results suggest that this approach not only supports early detection but also enhances user engagement and adherence to care routines. Require transparency with users about model learning and retention practices (Freeman et al., 2017).

Another compelling case comes from Japan, where wearable sensors have been integrated into community-based elder care programs (Hickey et al., 2021). Document the technical and human resources required to maintain sensor networks to inform scalability planning (Kargarandehkordi et al., 2025). These devices track mobility, sleep, heart rate, and social activity, transmitting data to a centralized platform monitored by healthcare professionals (Kargarandehkordi et al., 2025). When anomalies are detected, such as a sudden drop-in activity or irregular sleep patterns, care coordinators are alerted and can initiate follow-up. This system has been credited with reducing hospitalizations, improving medication adherence, and enabling older adults to remain in their homes longer. Importantly, the program includes training for both professional and family caregivers, ensuring that the technology is used effectively and ethically. Adapt protocols to local workforce capacity and connectivity constraints. In Canada, a telehealth initiative using XR for group therapy has shown promise in addressing social isolation and depression among older adults in rural areas (Kargarandehkordi et al., 2025). Include measures for participant engagement and technology usability in program evaluation to guide iterative improvement. Participants join virtual support groups facilitated by mental health professionals, where they can interact in immersive environments designed to foster connection and engagement. The program has been particularly effective for individuals with mobility limitations or those living in geographically isolated communities. Feedback from participants highlights the importance of social presence and the therapeutic value of shared experiences, even in virtual form. Provide low-bandwidth alternatives and device loan programs for remote areas.

Despite these successes, pilot programs also reveal important challenges and lessons learned. Require early equity assessments and community consultations to surface barriers before large investments are made. One recurring issue is the digital divide, many older adults lack access to high-speed internet, modern devices, or the digital literacy needed to engage with new technologies. Programs that have succeeded in overcoming this barrier often include robust onboarding processes, personalized training, and ongoing technical support. Another challenge is interoperability, ensuring that data from different devices and platforms can be integrated into a cohesive care plan (Kargarandehkordi et al., 2025). This requires collaboration between technology providers and healthcare systems, as well as adherence to common data standards (Kargarandehkordi et al., 2025). Scalability is another key consideration. While pilot programs often benefit from dedicated funding and close oversight, expanding these models to larger populations requires sustainable business models, policy support, and infrastructure investment. Public-private partnerships have proven instrumental in this regard, providing the resources and coordination needed to move from proof-of-concept to widespread adoption. For example, government grants have supported the deployment of AI-powered monitoring systems in public elder care facilities, while private companies have contributed technical expertise and product development (Kargarandehkordi et al., 2025). Include maintenance budgets and local capacity-building in scale plans. Ultimately, these case studies underscore the transformative potential of digital therapeutics when implemented thoughtfully and collaboratively. Require routine outcome monitoring and feedback loops to inform continuous improvement. They highlight the importance of user-centered design, interdisciplinary teamwork, and continuous evaluation. Most importantly, they remind us that technology is not a panacea but a powerful tool, one that, when guided by empathy and evidence, can help older adults live with greater dignity, connection, and purpose (Kargarandehkordi et al., 2025). Prioritize patient-reported outcomes alongside clinical metrics (Kargarandehkordi et al., 2025).

As the global population ages, the mental health needs of older adults are becoming increasingly complex and urgent, demanding a fundamental rethinking of how care is delivered. Geriatric mental health encompasses a broad spectrum of conditions, from mood and anxiety disorders to neurodegenerative diseases such as Alzheimer's and other forms of dementia, each of which not only impairs cognitive functioning but also deeply affects emotional well-being, social connectivity, and overall quality of life. These challenges are compounded by social determinants such as isolation, bereavement, declining physical health, and limited mobility, all of which contribute to a heightened vulnerability among older adults. Traditional models of care, often reactive, fragmented, and institutionally bound, are proving inadequate in addressing these multifaceted needs. In this context, the integration of digital therapeutics represents a transformative opportunity to reimagine geriatric mental health care. Technologies such as artificial intelligence (AI), machine learning (ML), wearable sensors, and extended reality (Crameri et al., 2021) are not only reshaping the landscape of diagnosis and treatment but also enabling more personalized, proactive, and dignified approaches to care (Sharma & Meena, 2024). Specify system-level metrics that define success across quality, equity, and cost domains. Understanding cognitive decline in older adults is central to this transformation. Cognitive impairment can range from mild cognitive impairment (Clemens-Meyer et al., 2021) to more severe forms of dementia, including Alzheimer's disease. These conditions are characterized by progressive deterioration in memory, executive function, language, and spatial awareness. Yet the impact extends far beyond cognitive symptoms. Many individuals also experience depression, anxiety, irritability, and social withdrawal, symptoms that are frequently underdiagnosed or misattributed to the natural aging process. The burden of dementia is not only clinical but also deeply social and economic, affecting caregivers, families, and healthcare systems alike (Ong et al., 2025). As the prevalence of cognitive disorders rises, so too does the urgency for innovative approaches that can detect, monitor, and manage these conditions more effectively. Fund longitudinal studies that link sensor-derived markers to functional outcomes (Ong et al., 2025).

Early detection and continuous monitoring are critical to improving outcomes and preserving autonomy. This is where AI and ML technologies are beginning to play a pivotal role. By analyzing large datasets from electronic health records, wearable devices, and behavioral assessments, AI algorithms can identify subtle patterns that may indicate early cognitive decline, often before symptoms become clinically apparent (Shatte et al., 2019). These predictive models enable timely intervention, personalized care planning, and more efficient allocation of healthcare resources. For example, natural language processing (Ong et al., 2025) tools can analyze speech patterns during routine conversations or telehealth visits to detect linguistic markers of cognitive deterioration. Similarly, ML models trained on longitudinal data can forecast the progression of MCI to dementia, allowing clinicians to tailor interventions and support systems accordingly (Shatte et al., 2019). These tools not only enhance diagnostic precision but also reduce the burden on overextended healthcare providers by automating routine assessments and flagging high-risk individuals for further evaluation. Ensure models provide explainable outputs that clinicians can interpret and act upon. In parallel with AI-driven analytics, wearable sensors are emerging as a cornerstone of proactive and personalized mental health care for older adults (Shatte et al., 2019). These devices, ranging from smartwatches and fitness trackers to more specialized biosensors, offer continuous, non-invasive monitoring of physiological and behavioral indicators that are closely linked to cognitive and emotional well-being. For instance, changes in sleep patterns, heart rate variability, gait stability, and physical activity levels can serve as early warning signs of cognitive decline, depression, or anxiety. By capturing these metrics in real time, wearable sensors provide a dynamic picture of an individual's health trajectory, enabling clinicians to detect deviations from baseline functioning that might otherwise go unnoticed in periodic clinical visits (Shatte et al., 2019). Choose devices with open APIs and documented validation studies where possible.

One of the most promising applications of wearable technology lies in fall detection and prevention (Immanuel et al., 2023). Falls are not only a leading cause of injury among older adults but also a significant predictor of cognitive and functional decline. Advanced sensors embedded in wearable devices can monitor balance, posture, and movement patterns, issuing alerts when irregularities suggest an increased risk of falling. Some systems even integrate with home automation technologies to trigger emergency responses or adjust environmental conditions, such as lighting or temperature, to enhance safety and comfort. Beyond physical health, these devices can also track indicators of psychological distress. For example, a sudden drop in activity levels or disrupted sleep may signal the onset of depressive symptoms, prompting timely outreach from caregivers or mental health professionals. Include low-cost device options and device-lending programs in deployment plans.

Moreover, wearable sensors are increasingly being used to support remote patient monitoring and telehealth services, bridging the gap between clinical care and everyday life (Mackey et al., 2025). Data collected from these devices can be transmitted securely to healthcare providers, who can then analyze trends, adjust treatment plans, and engage in more informed, meaningful conversations with patients and their families. This continuous feedback loop not only enhances clinical decision-making but also empowers older adults to take a more active role in managing their health. Importantly, many of these technologies are being designed with user-friendly interfaces and adaptive features to accommodate the sensory, cognitive, and motor limitations that may accompany aging. Document end-to-end data pathways and fallback plans for connectivity loss. Complementing the capabilities of wearable sensors, AI-enhanced memory support tools and cognitive training platforms are redefining how older adults engage with their cognitive health. These digital interventions are designed not only to slow cognitive decline but also to empower individuals with tools that enhance daily functioning and preserve independence. Cognitive training platforms, often gamified to boost motivation and adherence, use exercises that target core domains such as attention, memory, and problem-solving. What sets these platforms apart is their ability to adapt in real time: AI algorithms analyze user performance and dynamically adjust the difficulty, pacing, and content of exercises to ensure that the experience remains both challenging and achievable (Tsai et al., 2025). This level of personalization fosters sustained engagement and may contribute to neuroplasticity, the brain's ability to reorganize and form new neural connections, thereby enhancing cognitive resilience over time. Require trials that include functional and quality-of-life endpoints, not only task performance.

Some advanced platforms even incorporate facial recognition and contextual cues to help users identify people, places, and objects, features that can significantly reduce confusion and anxiety in those with moderate cognitive impairment. Specify consent options for facial-recognition features and allow users or proxies to disable them at any time. Test recognition algorithms with diverse faces and lighting conditions to reduce misidentification and distress. Provide simple onboarding that demonstrates how contextual cues appear and how to interpret them in daily use. For caregivers, these technologies offer a welcome reprieve by automating routine prompts and monitoring, thereby easing the emotional and logistical burden of care.

Importantly, AI-driven platforms are also transforming how cognitive assessments are conducted (Ghanim et al., 2023). Provide clinicians with practical checklists that map passive metrics to clinical interpretations to reduce ambiguity. Require validation studies that compare passive measures with standard neuropsychological tests within representative samples before clinical reliance. Build clinician-facing summaries that highlight clinically actionable changes and suggested next steps rather than raw algorithm outputs. Traditional evaluations, typically administered in clinical settings at infrequent intervals, often fail to capture the subtle, day-to-day fluctuations in cognitive function (Robinson et al., 2024). In contrast, AI systems can passively monitor a user's interaction with digital devices, analyzing speech patterns, typing behavior, navigation habits, and response times, to detect early signs of cognitive decline. These continuous assessments provide a more nuanced and timely understanding of cognitive health, enabling earlier interventions and more precise tracking of disease progression. For example, a decline in verbal fluency or increased hesitation in typing may signal emerging cognitive issues long before they become apparent in formal testing. This shift toward passive, ambient assessment not only enhances diagnostic accuracy but also reduces the stigma and stress often associated with traditional cognitive testing.

Building on the capabilities of AI and wearable technologies, extended reality (XR), which includes both virtual reality (Mitsea et al., 2024) and augmented reality (AR), is emerging as a powerful tool for enhancing social connection, cognitive stimulation, and emotional well-being in older adults (Shah et al., 2021). Draft inclusion criteria that consider sensory impairments, seizure risk, and ability to follow simple instructions to guide safe XR use (Martinez-Martin et al., 2018). Create brief pre-session orientation materials that explain expected sensations and how to signal discomfort. Establish monitoring procedures for disorientation and post-session debriefs to capture subjective experiences and guide future sessions. These immersive technologies offer experiences that transcend the physical limitations often associated with aging, opening new avenues for therapeutic engagement, reminiscence, and community building. In particular, XR environments are uniquely suited to address the psychological and social dimensions of geriatric mental health, which are often overlooked in traditional care models (Martinez-Martin et al., 2018).

One of the most compelling applications of XR in this context is VR-based reminiscence therapy (Pruden, 2025). Create short life-history templates that clinicians can use to select culturally and personally relevant scenes efficiently. Pilot-test scenes with small groups to identify contexts that reliably elicit positive engagement and avoid distressing content. Use simple scales to rate affect before and after sessions so that benefits can be measured and compared across participants. By transporting individuals to familiar or meaningful places, such as childhood homes, natural landscapes, or historical events, VR can evoke autobiographical memories that are deeply tied to identity and emotional continuity. For individuals with dementia, these immersive experiences can be profoundly grounding, helping to reduce agitation, enhance mood, and foster a sense of self that may otherwise feel fragmented. Unlike static photographs or verbal prompts, VR engages multiple senses and creates a sense of presence that can make memories feel more vivid and emotionally resonant.

Beyond reminiscence, XR platforms are also being used to facilitate social interaction and reduce loneliness, a pervasive issue among older adults, particularly those with mobility impairments or living in long-term care facilities. Document facilitation scripts and accessibility adjustments that staff can follow to make gatherings predictable and welcoming. Offer optional caregiver participation in early sessions to model interaction and build confidence for participants. Provide fallback activities for users who experience sensory overload or fatigue to maintain inclusion and dignity. Social XR environments allow users to participate in virtual gatherings, where they can interact with peers, family members, or therapists in shared digital spaces. These environments can host group therapy sessions, recreational activities, or educational workshops, creating opportunities for meaningful engagement and community building. For many older adults, especially those who are geographically isolated or physically limited, XR offers a vital bridge to the outside world and a renewed sense of belonging (Robinson et al., 2024).

XR is also proving valuable in therapeutic contexts beyond socialization and memory support (Lazarou & Exarchos, 2024). Define clear clinical indications and contraindications for XR interventions to guide appropriate referrals (Ricciardi & Zomaya, 2025). Develop short, therapist-led protocols that outline session goals, duration, and expected outcomes for each intervention type. Train staff to monitor biometric and behavioral responses during exposure and to intervene when signs of distress appear (Ricciardi & Zomaya, 2025). Immersive environments can be used for guided relaxation, mindfulness training, and exposure therapy for anxiety or phobias. The immersive nature of XR enhances engagement and can be particularly effective for individuals who may struggle with traditional therapeutic formats (Ricciardi & Zomaya, 2025). For example, a calming virtual forest or beach scene can be used to facilitate deep breathing exercises and reduce stress, while controlled exposure to anxiety-inducing scenarios can help individuals gradually build coping skills in a safe and supportive setting. When combined with biometric feedback from wearable sensors, such as heart rate or galvanic skin response, XR experiences can be dynamically adjusted in real time to optimize emotional and cognitive outcomes (Ricciardi & Zomaya, 2025).

As XR technologies become more accessible and user-friendly, their integration into geriatric mental health care is likely to expand. Assess organizational readiness, including staff bandwidth, technical support capacity, and space for safe VR sessions. Create procurement checklists that include accessibility features, warranty terms, and vendor support for clinical deployments. Engage older adult users in iterative design and testing to ensure interfaces remain simple and intuitive. Developers are increasingly designing XR applications with older adults in mind, incorporating features such as simplified interfaces, voice navigation, and adjustable visual settings to accommodate sensory and cognitive changes. Moreover, the convergence of XR with AI and remote monitoring systems holds immense potential for creating fully integrated, adaptive care environments that respond to the unique needs of each individual (Freeman et al., 2017). These innovations not only enhance the quality of life for older adults but also offer new tools for clinicians and caregivers to deliver more effective, personalized, and compassionate care.

While the potential of AI, ML, wearable sensors, and XR in geriatric care is immense, their implementation must be approached with ethical sensitivity and user-centered design (Jiao, 2024). Convene stakeholder panels, including older adults, caregivers, clinicians, and ethicists, early to shape project aims and acceptable trade-offs. Map consent pathways that accommodate declining capacity and include trigger points for re-consent or proxy involvement. Older adults may face barriers related to digital literacy, sensory impairments, or skepticism toward technology. Interventions must be designed with accessibility in mind, featuring intuitive interfaces, large fonts, voice commands, and culturally relevant content. Privacy and consent are also paramount, particularly when cognitive impairment may affect decision-making capacity. Care must be taken to ensure that individuals understand how their data is used and that caregivers are involved appropriately without undermining autonomy (Martinez-Martin et al., 2018). Transparent data governance, secure storage, and clear communication are essential to maintaining trust (Martinez-Martin et al., 2018). Training for clinicians and caregivers is critical to ensure that digital tools are used effectively and ethically. This includes understanding the capabilities and limitations of the technology, recognizing signs of digital fatigue or frustration, and integrating digital interventions into broader care plans. Interdisciplinary collaboration, between clinicians, technologists, designers, and ethicists, is essential to co-create solutions that are not only effective but also dignified and humane.

The integration of AI, ML, wearable sensors, and XR into geriatric mental health care represents a paradigm shift toward a more holistic, proactive, and person-centered model (Ikwuanusi et al., 2023). Translate this paradigm shift into measurable program goals and implementation milestones to guide evaluation. State clear priorities, safety, autonomy, social connection, and functional outcomes, and report progress against these domains regularly. These technologies enable early detection, continuous support, and meaningful engagement, empowering older adults to maintain autonomy, connection, and purpose. They also offer caregivers and clinicians powerful tools to deliver more responsive, data-informed, and compassionate care. As we look to the future, the challenge is not merely technological but cultural: to ensure that innovation serves human needs rather than organizational convenience.

The integration of artificial intelligence (AI), machine learning (ML), wearable sensors, and extended reality (Godfrey et al., 2021) into geriatric mental health care is profoundly reshaping the caregiving experience, offering both relief and new responsibilities for caregivers (Layode et al., 2024). Begin by mapping specific tasks that technology changes, such as medication reminders, fall alerts, and remote monitoring triage, so training can target real-world duties. Define clear handoffs between automated notifications and human judgment to avoid ambiguity about decision authority. Provide caregivers with simple escalation scripts that guide when to call a clinician, when to perform a home check, and when to activate emergency services. AI and ML technologies enhance decision-making by analyzing vast datasets to detect early signs of cognitive or emotional decline, enabling caregivers to intervene earlier and more effectively. These systems can automate routine tasks such as medication reminders and symptom tracking, reducing the cognitive and emotional load on caregivers while allowing them to focus on more meaningful, human-centered aspects of care. Predictive algorithms also offer foresight into potential health events, such as fall risks or the progression of dementia, empowering caregivers to take preventive action. Wearable sensors complement these capabilities by providing real-time, non-invasive monitoring of vital signs, sleep patterns, activity levels, and emotional states. This continuous stream of data allows caregivers to respond swiftly to changes in health status, even from a distance, and facilitates more informed conversations with healthcare providers. For family caregivers, especially those balancing multiple responsibilities, this remote oversight offers peace of mind and a greater sense of control. Meanwhile,

XR technologies are opening new avenues for therapeutic engagement and social connection. Caregivers can use VR-based reminiscence therapy to help individuals with dementia reconnect with meaningful memories, or facilitate virtual gatherings that reduce loneliness and foster community. XR also supports guided relaxation and exposure therapy, offering immersive interventions that may be more engaging and effective than traditional formats. These tools not only enrich the lives of older adults but also provide caregivers with innovative ways to deliver care that is both compassionate and stimulating. However, the adoption of these technologies also introduces challenges, including the need for digital literacy, ethical considerations around data privacy, and ensuring equitable access. Caregivers must be supported with training and resources to navigate these tools effectively. Ultimately, when thoughtfully implemented, these technologies can transform caregiving from a reactive, labor-intensive role into a more proactive, data-informed, and emotionally sustainable practice, enhancing the quality of care while preserving the dignity and autonomy of those they support (Robinson et al., 2024).

Caregiver preparation must include practical, accessible training that balances technical skills with emotional support and ethical reflection. Structure training into short modules that pair device operation with case scenarios to reinforce decision-making under realistic conditions. Offer on-demand technical support and quick-reference materials caregivers can consult during emergencies or when uncertain about device signals. Integrate discussions about privacy, surveillance, and autonomy so caregivers can honor the older adult's preferences while maintaining safety. The rapid introduction of digital tools can overwhelm caregivers without staged onboarding and clear role definitions; plan deployments that allow acclimation and iterative adjustment. Provide simulations or role-plays that let caregivers practice responding to alerts and interpreting data without risk to a real person (Canali et al., 2022). Ensure training includes guidance on setting reasonable boundaries and on accessing respite services when caregiving demands intensify.

At the most fundamental level, clinicians and caregivers must develop digital literacy, the ability to confidently and critically engage with digital tools and platforms. Begin by defining a concise competency framework that highlights essential skills: device setup, data interpretation, privacy practices, and escalation protocols (Obermeyer et al., 2019). Use blended learning, short videos, hands-on practice, and peer coaching, to accommodate variable schedules and learning styles. Emphasize interpretive skills so clinicians learn when to trust algorithmic outputs and when to investigate discrepancies. Digital literacy should be framed as an ongoing professional development requirement, with periodic refreshers aligned to technological updates and new device introductions. Build simple checklists clinicians can use during visits to reconcile sensor data with patient report and to document decision rationales (Obermeyer et al., 2019).

Beyond basic literacy, clinicians and caregivers must also cultivate data interpretation and critical thinking skills (Ferrar et al., 2021). Provide structured case reviews where teams examine algorithmic recommendations, discuss possible biases, and decide on patient-centered courses of action. Encourage clinicians to demand transparency from vendors about model training data and to prioritize tools validated in older-adult populations (Radanliev, 2025). Train caregivers to recognize common false positives and negatives in device outputs and to use simple heuristics, such as cross-checking multiple signals, before escalating. Develop brief, clinician-facing summaries that translate sensor trends into probable clinical scenarios and recommended first steps (Radanliev, 2025). Promote a culture of skepticism balanced with pragmatic use of technology, ensuring human judgment remains central.

Another critical area of training involves ethical and privacy considerations. Standardize consent processes that allow staged and revisitable agreements, and include explicit documentation of proxy decision-maker roles. Teach clinicians to discuss data-sharing boundaries with patients and families, including who receives which alerts and how long data are retained (Hughes & Kalra, 2023). Build routines for periodic reassessment of consent as cognitive status evolves, and create templates for documenting these reassessments in the medical record. Provide caregivers and clinicians with simple scripts to explain data use in plain language and to address queries about surveillance and autonomy (Ong et al., 2025). Include scenario-based reflection on dilemmas, such as balancing privacy with fall-prevention, to build practical ethical reasoning skills.

To address these multifaceted training needs, a variety of educational models and programs are emerging. Develop modular curricula that map to role-specific competencies and allow incremental credentialing. Partner with local community organizations to deliver culturally tailored training and to support caregivers with limited internet access. Incorporate hands-on device practice sessions and scenario-based assessments that reinforce ethical and practical decision-making. Include follow-up coaching and performance feedback to sustain skill development beyond initial workshops. Many healthcare institutions are now offering continuing education courses focused on digital health, often in partnership with universities, technology companies, or professional associations. These courses may cover topics such as AI in clinical practice, digital therapeutics, telehealth delivery, and cybersecurity (Basystiuk et al., 2024). Some programs are delivered online to accommodate the demanding schedules of healthcare workers, while others include in-person workshops or simulation labs. For example, XR-based training environments allow clinicians and caregivers to practice responding to real-life scenarios, such as managing a behavioral crisis in a person with dementia, within a safe, controlled, and immersive setting (Robinson et al., 2024). These simulations not only build technical skills but also enhance emotional intelligence and situational awareness.

In addition to formal training, peer learning and mentorship play a vital role in building digital competencies. Establish mentorship pairings that match experienced digital-care clinicians with frontline staff and caregivers to facilitate knowledge transfer. Create moderated online forums and regular case-review meetings where practitioners can share implementation challenges and practical solutions. Recognize peer mentors formally through small incentives or continuing education credits to sustain participation. Interdisciplinary learning communities, where clinicians, caregivers, technologists, and researchers come together to share experiences and insights, can foster a culture of innovation and continuous improvement. These communities may take the form of online forums, professional networks, or collaborative workshops. By learning from one another, participants can gain a more holistic understanding of how digital tools function in diverse care settings and how they can be adapted to meet the unique needs of older adults.

The importance of interdisciplinary collaboration cannot be overstated in the context of digital geriatric care. Convene standing advisory committees that include clinicians, designers, engineers, ethicists, and patient representatives to guide development and deployment. Define decision-making processes and feedback loops so that technical changes incorporate clinical realities and user preferences (Smuck et al., 2021). Allocate protected time within clinical schedules for interdisciplinary meetings to ensure sustained engagement and timely problem-solving. The successful implementation of AI, ML, XR, and wearable technologies requires input from a wide range of stakeholders, including physicians, nurses, occupational therapists, social workers, engineers, designers, and ethicists. Each brings a unique perspective and set of skills that enrich the development and deployment of digital solutions. For instance, while a data scientist may design an algorithm to detect early signs of cognitive decline, a clinician can provide insights into how those signs manifest in daily life, and a caregiver can offer feedback on how the tool fits into the rhythm of home care. This collaborative approach ensures that technologies are not only scientifically sound but also practical, user-friendly, and aligned with the values of dignity and person-centered care.

Moreover, interdisciplinary teams are essential for integrating digital tools into existing care pathways. Map workflow integration points explicitly and create standardized protocols that define roles, responsibilities, and escalation criteria. Pilot test workflow changes in small settings and iterate based on user feedback before broader rollout to minimize disruption. Implement simple documentation templates that capture digital-derived findings and follow-up actions to maintain clarity across shifts and providers. Rather than viewing technology as a separate or supplementary component, these teams work to embed digital solutions into the fabric of care delivery. This might involve redesigning workflows to incorporate real-time data from wearable sensors, developing protocols for responding to AI-generated alerts, or creating shared care plans that leverage insights from multiple sources (Baumann et al., 2024). In doing so, they help bridge the gap between innovation and implementation, ensuring that digital tools enhance rather than disrupt the continuity of care.

For caregivers, especially those providing informal or unpaid care, access to training and support is equally important. Design brief, accessible modules that accommodate irregular schedules and varying literacy levels, using multimedia and offline materials. Provide community-based drop-in sessions where caregivers can practice device setup with staff assistance and peer support. Offer multilingual resources and culturally adapted examples to increase relevance and uptake across diverse communities. Many family caregivers find themselves suddenly thrust into complex care roles without adequate preparation or resources. Digital tools can be both a lifeline and a source of stress, depending on how well they are understood and supported. Community organizations, healthcare providers, and advocacy groups can play a crucial role in offering accessible, culturally sensitive training for caregivers. This might include instructional videos, helplines, mobile apps with step-by-step guidance, or in-person support groups where caregivers can learn from one another. Empowering caregivers with knowledge and confidence not only improves care outcomes but also reduces burnout and enhances well-being.

In addition to technical training, it is essential to address the emotional and psychological dimensions of caregiving in a digital age. Incorporate short resilience-building modules that teach stress recognition, practical coping strategies, and quick self-care routines usable between caregiving tasks. Include facilitated reflection sessions where caregivers can discuss ethical tensions and emotional burdens that arise from surveillance technologies and role changes. Provide clear referral pathways to mental health services and respite resources for caregivers who require additional support. The introduction of monitoring technologies, for example, can raise concerns about surveillance, loss of privacy, or the depersonalization of care. Caregivers may struggle with feelings of guilt or inadequacy if they rely too heavily on technology, or they may feel overwhelmed by the constant stream of data and alerts (Ferrara, 2024). Training programs should therefore include components on emotional resilience, ethical reflection, and self-care, helping caregivers navigate the complex interplay between technology and human connection.

Looking ahead, the future of training in digital geriatric care will likely involve hybrid models that combine online learning, hands-on practice, and interdisciplinary collaboration. Pilot competency frameworks that allow incremental credentialing tied to demonstrated skills rather than time-based requirements. Use adaptive learning platforms to tailor content to the learner's role, prior experience, and immediate needs, improving relevance and retention. Plan for ongoing mentorship and periodic reassessment to maintain competencies as devices and algorithms evolve. Micro-credentialing and modular learning pathways can allow professionals to build skills incrementally and at their own pace. AI itself may play a role in personalizing training, offering adaptive learning platforms that tailor content to the learner's background, goals, and progress (Back et al., 2022). For example, a nurse might receive targeted modules on interpreting biometric data, while a family caregiver might focus on using voice assistants for medication reminders (Fanarioti & Karpouzis, 2025). These personalized learning experiences can make training more relevant, engaging, and effective.

Ultimately, the goal of training and support is not merely to teach people how to use technology, but to cultivate a mindset of curiosity, adaptability, and empathy. Embed ethical decision-making exercises and patient-centered communication practice into curricula to reinforce relational care principles. Encourage reflective practice by having trainees document cases where technology aided or complicated care, then discuss these in peer-review sessions. Align training outcomes with measurable patient-reported indicators to ensure that technology adoption translates into better lived experiences for older adults. In a field as dynamic and human-centered as geriatric mental health, technology should be seen as a tool to enhance, not replace, the relational aspects of care. By equipping clinicians and caregivers with the skills, knowledge, and confidence to engage with digital tools thoughtfully and ethically, we can create a care environment that is both technologically advanced and deeply compassionate.

As digital therapeutics continue to evolve, the future of geriatric mental health care is poised to be shaped by a new generation of technologies that push the boundaries of what is currently possible. Establish translational pathways that require early stakeholder engagement, iterative prototyping, and feasibility milestones before broader deployment. Prioritize technologies with clear potential to improve functional outcomes and quality of life rather than novelty alone. Among the most promising innovations are brain-computer interfaces (BCIs), digital twins, and emotion AI, tools that have the potential to radically transform how we understand, monitor, and support the aging mind (Hilty et al., 2021). Brain-computer interfaces represent a frontier in neurotechnology, enabling direct communication between the brain and external devices. In the context of geriatric care, BCIs could one day assist individuals with advanced neurodegenerative conditions in expressing needs, navigating digital environments, or even controlling assistive technologies through thought alone. While still largely experimental, early research suggests that BCIs may offer new pathways for restoring agency and communication in individuals with severe cognitive or motor impairments (Weiner et al., 2025).

The burden of dementia is not only clinical but also deeply social and economic, affecting caregivers, families, and healthcare systems alike (Akinode et al., 2025). Quantify expected resource impacts, care hours, care transitions, and projected costs, to guide service planning and policy advocacy. Encourage health systems to model long-term savings from delayed institutionalization when evaluating investments in digital supports (Radanliev, 2025). Advocate for metrics that capture caregiver time and quality-of-life changes as part of economic assessments. As the prevalence of cognitive disorders rises, so too does the urgency for innovative approaches that can detect, monitor, and manage these conditions more effectively.

Early detection and continuous monitoring are critical to improving outcomes and preserving autonomy. Specify minimum monitoring bundles, for example, sleep, mobility, and social interaction, that balance clinical value with user burden (Wang et al., 2022). Set clear escalation thresholds and response times that integrate with local clinical capacity to ensure timely follow-up. Train teams to interpret multi-signal concordance rather than single-parameter alerts to reduce false positives and unnecessary interventions. This is where AI and ML technologies are beginning to play a pivotal role. By analyzing large datasets from electronic health records, wearable devices, and behavioral assessments, AI algorithms can identify subtle patterns that may indicate early cognitive decline, often before symptoms become clinically apparent. These predictive models enable timely intervention, personalized care planning, and more efficient allocation of healthcare resources. For example, natural language processing (Volckens et al., 2023) tools can analyze speech patterns during routine conversations or telehealth visits to detect linguistic markers of cognitive deterioration. Similarly, ML models trained on longitudinal data can forecast the progression of MCI to dementia, allowing clinicians to tailor interventions and support systems accordingly (Tsai et al., 2025). These tools not only enhance diagnostic precision but also reduce the burden on overextended healthcare providers by automating routine assessments and flagging high-risk individuals for further evaluation.

In parallel with AI-driven analytics, wearable sensors are emerging as a cornerstone of proactive and personalized mental health care for older adults (Holly et al., 2023). Define minimum device feature sets needed for clinical use, reliable time-stamping, battery life, validated sensors, and require vendor evidence of device performance in older populations (Engel, 1977). Create simple consent scripts that explain expected benefits and limitations in plain language and include withdrawal procedures. Plan for periodic device audits and recalibration schedules to maintain data quality over time (Engel, 1977). These devices, ranging from smartwatches and fitness trackers to more specialized biosensors, offer continuous, non-invasive monitoring of physiological and behavioral indicators that are closely linked to cognitive and emotional well-being. For instance, changes in sleep patterns, heart rate variability, gait stability, and physical activity levels can serve as early warning signs of cognitive decline, depression, or anxiety. By capturing these metrics in real time, wearable sensors provide a dynamic picture of an individual's health trajectory, enabling clinicians to detect deviations from baseline functioning that might otherwise go unnoticed in periodic clinical visits (Engel, 1977).

One of the most promising applications of wearable technology lies in fall detection and prevention (Wibberly, 2024). Establish standardized fall-risk assessment templates that incorporate sensor-derived metrics alongside clinical exam findings (Radanliev, 2025). Coordinate with local emergency services to define response expectations for false positives and true events to avoid unnecessary hospital transports. Invest in home-safety assessments triggered by sensor alerts to target environmental modifications where they are most needed (Radanliev, 2025). Falls are not only a leading cause of injury among older adults but also a significant predictor of cognitive and functional decline. Advanced sensors embedded in wearable devices can monitor balance, posture, and movement patterns, issuing alerts when irregularities suggest an increased risk of falling (Radanliev, 2025). Some systems even integrate with home automation technologies to trigger emergency responses or adjust environmental conditions, such as lighting or temperature, to enhance safety and comfort. Beyond physical health, these devices can also track indicators of psychological distress. For example, a sudden drop in activity levels or disrupted sleep may signal the onset of depressive symptoms, prompting timely outreach from caregivers or mental health professionals.

Moreover, wearable sensors are increasingly being used to support remote patient monitoring and telehealth services, bridging the gap between clinical care and everyday life (Bayor et al., 2025). Define secure transmission standards and contingency plans for connectivity loss so that clinical teams can rely on continuous monitoring without gaps. Ensure that data streams include timestamps and simple summary metrics for rapid clinician review rather than raw high-frequency signals. Train clinicians to integrate remote-monitoring summaries into telehealth encounters and to document findings in the medical record for continuity. Data collected from these devices can be transmitted securely to healthcare providers, who can then analyze trends, adjust treatment plans, and engage in more informed, meaningful conversations with patients and their families. This continuous feedback loop not only enhances clinical decision-making but also empowers older adults to take a more active role in managing their health (Weiner et al., 2025). Importantly, many of these technologies are being designed with user-friendly interfaces and adaptive features to accommodate the sensory, cognitive, and motor limitations that may accompany aging.

Complementing the capabilities of wearable sensors, AI-enhanced memory support tools and cognitive training platforms are redefining how older adults engage with their cognitive health (Shah et al., 2022). Specify minimal validation requirements for cognitive-training claims, including real-world functional endpoints and retention assessments. Provide clear user manuals that translate algorithmic adaptation into understandable progress milestones for patients and caregivers. Include caregiver dashboards that summarize progress and recommended practice schedules to coordinate home-based activities with clinician guidance. These digital interventions are designed not only to slow cognitive decline but also to empower individuals with tools that enhance daily functioning and preserve independence. Cognitive training platforms, often gamified to boost motivation and adherence, use exercises that target core domains such as attention, memory, and problem-solving. What sets these platforms apart is their ability to adapt in real time: AI algorithms analyze user performance and dynamically adjust the difficulty, pacing, and content of exercises to ensure that the experience remains both challenging and achievable (Fanarioti & Karpouzis, 2025).

What sets these platforms apart is their ability to adapt in real time: AI algorithms analyze user performance and dynamically adjust the difficulty, pacing, and content of exercises to ensure that the experience remains both challenging and achievable (Akhtar & Rawol, 2025). Provide transparent descriptions of adaptation rules so clinicians can understand how difficulty levels change with performance. Require safety limits on task escalation to prevent frustration and disengagement in vulnerable users. Offer periodic human-led sessions to supplement automated training and to contextualize performance trends for meaningful interpretation. This level of personalization fosters sustained engagement and may contribute to neuroplasticity, the brain's ability to reorganize and form new neural connections, thereby enhancing cognitive resilience over time.

Beyond training, AI is also being leveraged to support compensatory strategies that help individuals manage the practical challenges of memory loss (Renuka et al., 2025). Create clear default settings for reminder frequency, escalation thresholds, and caregiver notifications that can be personalized based on user preference. Offer simple consent flows that explain how contextual cues are gathered and used so users retain control over privacy-sensitive features. Provide examples of common configurations for typical care scenarios, independent living, assisted living, and high-supervision contexts, to guide setup. Digital calendars, voice-activated reminders, and smart assistants can assist with scheduling appointments, taking medications, and completing daily tasks. These tools reduce reliance on memory and executive function, allowing individuals to maintain autonomy in their routines. Some advanced platforms even incorporate facial recognition and contextual cues to help users identify people, places, and objects, features that can significantly reduce confusion and anxiety in those with moderate cognitive impairment.

For caregivers, these technologies offer a welcome reprieve by automating routine prompts and monitoring, thereby easing the emotional and logistical burden of care. Create caregiver-focused interfaces that prioritize urgent alerts and summarize trends rather than overwhelming detail. Include brief coaching tips with each alert suggesting the most appropriate immediate action to reduce decision paralysis. Provide scheduled summary reports that caregivers can review with clinicians to align on care adjustments and to prevent fragmentation. By automating routine tasks, these tools free caregivers to focus on relational care and psychosocial support, improving both provider efficiency and patient well-being.

REFERENCES

Akhtar, Z. B., & Rawol, A. T. (2025). Artificial Intelligence (Leivaditis & Sepetis, 2025) & Extended Reality (Reddy, 2025) within Healthcare: A Multidimensional Biomedical Engineering (Rajpal, 2025) Investigative Exploration. *Biomed. Clin. Res. J*, *1*, 1–22.

Akinode, A. O., Ayadi, O. E., Ezerioha, C. C., & Chika, P (2025). Machine Learning Approaches for Early Detection of Mental Health Disorders Using Wearable Devices and Big Data Analytics. environments, 4, 5.

Back, S. E., Acierno, R., Saraiya, T. C., Harley, B., Wangelin, B., Jarnecke, A. M., McTeague, L. M., Brown, D. G., Santa Ana, E., & Rothbaum, A. O. (2022). Enhancing Prolonged Exposure therapy for PTSD using physiological biomarker-driven technology. *Contemporary Clinical Trials Communications*, *28*, 100940. DOI: 10.1016/j.conctc.2022.100940 PMID: 35664505

Basystiuk, O., Rybchak, Z., Zavushchak, I., & Marikutsa, U. (2024). Evaluation of multimodal data synchronization tools. *Comput. Des. Syst. Theory Pract*, *6*(3), 104–111. DOI: 10.23939/cds2024.03.104

Baumann, S., Stone, R. T., & Abdelall, E. (2024). Introducing a remote patient monitoring usability impact model to overcome challenges. *Sensors (Basel)*, *24*(12), 3977. DOI: 10.3390/s24123977 PMID: 38931760

Baydili, İ., Tasci, B., & Tasci, G. (2025). Artificial intelligence in psychiatry: A review of biological and behavioral data analyses. *Diagnostics (Basel)*, *15*(4), 434. DOI: 10.3390/diagnostics15040434 PMID: 40002587

Bayor, A. A., Li, J., Yang, I. A., & Varnfield, M. (2025). Designing Clinical Decision Support Systems (CDSS)—A User-Centered Lens of the Design Characteristics, Challenges, and Implications: Systematic Review. *Journal of Medical Internet Research*, *27*, e63733. DOI: 10.2196/63733 PMID: 40540451

Canali, S., Schiaffonati, V., & Aliverti, A. (2022). Challenges and recommendations for wearable devices in digital health: Data quality, interoperability, health equity, fairness. *PLOS Digital Health*, *1*(10), e0000104. DOI: 10.1371/journal.pdig.0000104 PMID: 36812619

Carl, E., Stein, A. T., Levihn-Coon, A., Pogue, J. R., Rothbaum, B., Emmelkamp, P., Asmundson, G. J. G., Carlbring, P., & Powers, M. B. (2019). Virtual reality exposure therapy for anxiety and related disorders: A meta-analysis of randomized controlled trials. *Journal of Anxiety Disorders*, *61*, 27–36. DOI: 10.1016/j.janxdis.2018.08.003 PMID: 30287083

Casson, A. J. (2019). Wearable EEG and beyond. *Biomedical Engineering Letters*, *9*(1), 53–71. DOI: 10.1007/s13534-018-00093-6 PMID: 30956880

Clemens-Meyer, F. H., Lepot, M., Blumensaat, F., Leutnant, D., & Gruber, G. (2021). In Bertrand-Krajewski, J.-L., Clemens-Meyer, F., Lepot, M., & Publishing, I. W. A. (Eds.), *Data validation and data quality assessment. Metrology in Urban Drainage and Stormwater Management: Plug and Pray* (pp. 327–390).

Crameri, L., Hettiarachchi, I. T., & Hanoun, S. (2021). Effects of dynamic resilience on the reactivity of vagally mediated heart rate variability. *Frontiers in Psychology*, *11*, 579210. DOI: 10.3389/fpsyg.2020.579210 PMID: 33551903

De Kock, J. H., Latham, H. A., Leslie, S. J., Grindle, M., Munoz, S. A., Ellis, L., Polson, R., & O'Malley, C. M. (2021). A rapid review of the impact of COVID-19 on the mental health of healthcare workers: Implications for supporting psychological well-being. *BMC Public Health*, *21*(1), 104. DOI: 10.1186/s12889-020-10070-3 PMID: 33422039

Elfouly, T., & Alouani, A. (2025). A comprehensive survey on wearable computing for mental and physical health monitoring. *Electronics (Basel)*, *14*(17), 3443. DOI: 10.3390/electronics14173443

Engel, G. L. (1977). The need for a new medical model: A challenge for biomedicine. *Science*, *196*(4286), 129–136. DOI: 10.1126/science.847460 PMID: 847460

Fanarioti, A. K., & Karpouzis, K. (2025). Artificial Intelligence and the Future of Mental Health in a Digitally Transformed World. *Computers*, *14*(7), 259. DOI: 10.3390/computers14070259

Fleming, L. E., Maycock, B., White, M. P., & Depledge, M. H. (2019). Fostering human health through ocean sustainability in the 21st century. *People and Nature*, *1*(3), 276–283. DOI: 10.1002/pan3.10038

Freeman, D., Reeve, S., Robinson, A., Ehlers, A., Clark, D., Spanlang, B., & Slater, M. (2017). Virtual reality in the assessment, understanding, and treatment of mental health disorders. *Psychological Medicine*, *47*(14), 2393–2400. DOI: 10.1017/S003329171700040X PMID: 28325167

Friend, S. H., Ginsburg, G. S., Picard, R. W., & Drazen, J. M. (2024). Key issues as wearable digital health technologies enter clinical care. *The New England Journal of Medicine*, *390*(12), 1118–1127. DOI: 10.1056/NEJMra2307160 PMID: 38507754

Ghanim, R., Kaushik, A., Park, J., & Abramson, A. (2023). Communication protocols integrating wearables, ingestibles, and implantables for closed-loop therapies. *Device*, *1*(3), 100092. DOI: 10.1016/j.device.2023.100092

Gkintoni, E., Vassilopoulos, S. P., & Nikolaou, G. (2025). Next-generation cognitive-behavioral therapy for depression: Integrating digital tools, teletherapy, and personalization for enhanced mental health outcomes. *Medicina (Kaunas, Lithuania), 61*(3), 431. DOI: 10.3390/medicina61030431 PMID: 40142242

Glass, J. E., Tiffany, B., Matson, T. E., Lim, C., Gundersen, G., Kimbel, K., Hartzler, A. L., Curran, G. M., McWethy, A. G., Caldeiro, R. M., & Bradley, K. A. (2022). Approaches for implementing digital interventions for alcohol use disorders in primary care: A qualitative, user-centered design study. *Implementation Research and Practice, 3*, 26334895221135264. DOI: 10.1177/26334895221135264 PMID: 37091101

Godfrey, A., Vandendriessche, B., Bakker, J. P., Fitzer-Attas, C., Gujar, N., Hobbs, M., Liu, Q., Northcott, C. A., Parks, V., Wood, W. A., Zipunnikov, V., Wagner, J. A., & Izmailova, E. S. (2021). Fit-for-purpose biometric monitoring technologies: Leveraging the laboratory biomarker experience. *Clinical and Translational Science, 14*(1), 62–74. DOI: 10.1111/cts.12865 PMID: 32770726

Hickey, B. A., Chalmers, T., Newton, P., Lin, C.-T., Sibbritt, D., McLachlan, C. S., Clifton-Bligh, R., Morley, J., & Lal, S. (2021). Smart devices and wearable technologies to detect and monitor mental health conditions and stress: A systematic review. *Sensors (Basel), 21*(10), 3461. DOI: 10.3390/s21103461 PMID: 34065620

Hilty, D. M., Armstrong, C. M., Luxton, D. D., Gentry, M. T., & Krupinski, E. A. (2021). A scoping review of sensors, wearables, and remote monitoring for behavioral health: Uses, outcomes, clinical competencies, and research directions. *Journal of Technology in Behavioral Science, 6*(2), 278–313. DOI: 10.1007/s41347-021-00199-2 PMID: 33501372

Holly, L., Thom, S., Elzemety, M., Murage, B., Mathieson, K., & Iñigo Petralanda, M. I. (2023). Strengthening health data governance: New equity and rights-based principles. *International Journal of Health Governance, 28*(3), 225–237. DOI: 10.1108/IJHG-11-2022-0104

Huang, J., Wang, H., Wu, Q., Yin, J., Zhou, H., & He, Y. (2024). Clinical research on neurological and psychiatric diagnosis and monitoring using wearable devices: A literature review. *Interdisciplinary Medicine, 2*(4), e20230037. DOI: 10.1002/INMD.20230037

Hughes, N., & Kalra, D. (2023). Data standards and platform interoperability. In *Real-World Evidence in Medical Product Development* (pp. 79–107). Springer. DOI: 10.1007/978-3-031-26328-6_6

Ienca, M., Fabrice, J., Elger, B., Caon, M., Scoccia Pappagallo, A., Kressig, R. W., & Wangmo, T. (2017). Intelligent assistive technology for Alzheimer's disease and other dementias: A systematic review. *Journal of Alzheimer's Disease*, *56*(4), 1301–1340. DOI: 10.3233/JAD-161037 PMID: 28222516

Ikwuanusi, U. F., Adepoju, P. A., & Odionu, C. S (2023). Advancing ethical AI practices to solve data privacy issues in library systems. International journal of multidisciplinary research updates, 6(1), 033-044.

Immanuel, S., Teferra, M. N., Baumert, M., & Bidargaddi, N. (2023). Heart rate variability for evaluating psychological stress changes in healthy adults: A scoping review. *Neuropsychobiology*, *82*(4), 187–202. DOI: 10.1159/000530376 PMID: 37290411

Johnson, K. B., Wei, W. Q., Weeraratne, D., Frisse, M. E., Misulis, K., Rhee, K., Zhao, J., & Snowdon, J. L. (2021). Precision medicine, AI, and the future of personalized health care. *Clinical and Translational Science*, *14*(1), 86–93. DOI: 10.1111/cts.12884 PMID: 32961010

Kargarandehkordi, A., Li, S., Lin, K., Phillips, K. T., Benzo, R. M., & Washington, P. (2025). Fusing wearable biosensors with artificial intelligence for mental health monitoring: A systematic review. *Biosensors (Basel)*, *15*(4), 202. DOI: 10.3390/bios15040202 PMID: 40277515

Kim, J., & Backonja, U. (2025). Digital health equity frameworks and key concepts: A scoping review. *Journal of the American Medical Informatics Association : JAMIA*, *32*(1), 45–59. DOI: 10.1093/jamia/ocaf017 PMID: 39936843

Kumar, P. (2025). Securing Digital-First Healthcare: AI, Blockchain, and Cloud Architectures for Personal Health Data Protection. *International Journal of Applied Mathematics*, *38*(7s).

Layode, O., Naiho, H. N. N., Adeleke, G. S., Udeh, E. O., & Labake, T. T. (2024). Data privacy and security challenges in environmental research: Approaches to safeguarding sensitive information. *International Journal of Applied Research in Social Sciences*, *6*(6), 1193–1214. DOI: 10.51594/ijarss.v6i6.1210

Lazarou, E., & Exarchos, T. P. (2024). Predicting stress levels using physiological data: Real-time stress prediction models utilizing wearable devices. *AIMS Neuroscience*, *11*(2), 76–102. DOI: 10.3934/Neuroscience.2024006 PMID: 38988886

Li, M., Patel, J., & Katapally, T. R. (2025). The impact of extended reality cognitive behavioral therapy on mental disorders among children and youth: A systematic review and meta-analysis protocol. *PLoS One*, *20*(3), e0315313. DOI: 10.1371/journal.pone.0315313 PMID: 40048453

Li, M., Patel, J., & Katapally, T. R. (2025). The impact of extended reality cognitive behavioral therapy on mental disorders among children and youth: A systematic review and meta-analysis protocol. *PLoS One*, *20*(3), e0315313. DOI: 10.1371/journal.pone.0315313 PMID: 40048453

Lindner, P., Miloff, A., & Carlbring, P. (2024). The future of virtual reality therapy: Applications, challenges, and research directions. *Frontiers in Virtual Reality*, *5*, 112345.

Lorke, M., & Stefanou, T. (2025). Improving research and development of wearable assistive and rehabilitation technologies: A systematic review on diversity factors. *Journal of Neuroengineering and Rehabilitation*, *22*(1), 31. DOI: 10.1186/s12984-025-01562-7 PMID: 39985039

Mackey, S., Aghaeepour, N., Gaudilliere, B., Kao, M.-C., Kaptan, M., Lannon, E., Pfyffer, D., & Weber, K. (2025). Innovations in acute and chronic pain biomarkers: Enhancing diagnosis and personalized therapy. *Regional Anesthesia and Pain Medicine*, *50*(2), 110–120. DOI: 10.1136/rapm-2024-106030 PMID: 39909549

Martinez-Martin, N., Marcandalli, J., Huang, C. S., Arthur, C. P., Perotti, M., Foglierini, M., Ho, H., Dosey, A. M., Shriver, S., Payandeh, J., Leitner, A., Lanzavecchia, A., Perez, L., & Ciferri, C. (2018). An unbiased screen for human cytomegalovirus identifies neuropilin-2 as a central viral receptor. *Cell*, *174*(5), 1158–1171. DOI: 10.1016/j.cell.2018.06.028 PMID: 30057110

Mitsea, E., Drigas, A., & Skianis, C. (2024). Artificial intelligence, immersive technologies, and neurotechnologies in breathing interventions for mental and emotional health: A systematic review. *Electronics (Basel)*, *13*(12), 2253. DOI: 10.3390/electronics13122253

Mohr, D. C., Zhang, M., & Schueller, S. M. (2017). Personal sensing: Understanding mental health using ubiquitous sensors and machine learning. *Annual Review of Clinical Psychology*, *13*(1), 23–47. DOI: 10.1146/annurev-clinpsy-032816-044949 PMID: 28375728

Mone, V., & Fayazullaeva, S. (2023). Health data on the go: Navigating privacy concerns with wearable technologies. *Legal Information Management*, *23*(3), 179–188. DOI: 10.1017/S1472669623000427

Mulukuntla, S. (2025). Monitoring and Remote Patient Management with Immersive Technologies. In Augmented Wellness: Exploring the Power of VR and AR in Healthcare (pp. 197-218). Springer. DOI: 10.1007/978-981-96-2952-7_9

Obermeyer, Z., Powers, B., Vogeli, C., & Mullainathan, S. (2019). Dissecting racial bias in an algorithm used to manage the health of populations. *Science*, *366*(6464), 447–453. DOI: 10.1126/science.aax2342 PMID: 31649194

Ong, T., Ivanova, J., Soni, H., Barrera, J., Cummins, M., Welch, B. M., & Bunnell, B. E. (2025). Mental health clients' perspectives on telehealth-based virtual reality therapy. *Frontiers in Virtual Reality*, *6*, 1595326. DOI: 10.3389/frvir.2025.1595326

Pedram, S., & Piatkowski, T. (2025). Exploring the potential of virtual reality (Johnson et al., 2021) in mental healthcare: A systematic literature review. *Virtual Reality (Waltham Cross)*, *29*(3), 135. DOI: 10.1007/s10055-025-01181-6

Poudel, U., Jakhar, S., Mohan, P., & Nepal, A. (2025). AI in mental health: A review of technological advancements and ethical issues in psychiatry. *Issues in Mental Health Nursing*, *46*(7), 693–701. DOI: 10.1080/01612840.2025.2502943 PMID: 40378075

Pruden, S (2025). Implementing Depression Screening and Treatment Algorithms to Reduce Post-Operative Complications for Patients Undergoing Cardiac Surgery The University of North Carolina at Chapel Hill].

Radanliev, P. (2025). Privacy, ethics, transparency, and accountability in AI systems for wearable devices. *Frontiers in Digital Health*, *7*, 1431246. DOI: 10.3389/fdgth.2025.1431246 PMID: 40599875

Rajpal, S. (2025). Exploring the Role of Virtual Reality and Metaverse in Treating Mental Health: Operating Models and Challenges in Adoption. *Journal of Computer and Communications*, *13*(10), 1–22. DOI: 10.4236/jcc.2025.1310001

Ricciardi, F., & Zomaya, A. (2025). Perspectives on Managing AI Ethics in the Digital Age. *Information (Basel)*, *16*(2), 89. DOI: 10.3390/info16040318

Robinson, A., Flom, M., Forman-Hoffman, V. L., Histon, T., Levy, M., Darcy, A., Ajayi, T., Mohr, D. C., Wicks, P., Greene, C., & Montgomery, R. M. (2024). Equity in digital mental health interventions in the United States: Where to next? *Journal of Medical Internet Research*, *26*, e59939. DOI: 10.2196/59939 PMID: 39316436

Shah, B., Allen, J. L. Y., Chaudhury, H., O'Shaughnessy, J., & Tyrrell, C. S. (2022). The role of digital health in the future of integrated care. *Clinics in Integrated Care*, *15*, 100131. DOI: 10.1016/j.intcar.2022.100131

Shah, R. V., Grennan, G., Zafar-Khan, M., Alim, F., Dey, S., Ramanathan, D., & Mishra, J. (2021). Personalized machine learning of depressed mood using wearables. *Translational Psychiatry*, *11*(1), 338. DOI: 10.1038/s41398-021-01445-0 PMID: 34103481

Sharma, R., & Meena, H. K. (2024). Emerging trends in EEG signal processing: A systematic review. *SN Computer Science*, *5*(4), 415. DOI: 10.1007/s42979-024-02773-w

Shatte, A. B., Hutchinson, D. M., & Teague, S. J. (2019). Machine learning in mental health: A scoping review of methods and applications. *Psychological Medicine*, *49*(9), 1426–1448. DOI: 10.1017/S0033291719000151 PMID: 30744717

Smuck, M., Odonkor, C. A., Wilt, J. K., Schmidt, N., & Swiernik, M. A. (2021). The emerging clinical role of wearables: Factors for successful implementation in healthcare. *NPJ Digital Medicine*, *4*(1), 45. DOI: 10.1038/s41746-021-00418-3 PMID: 33692479

Spytska, L. (2025). The use of artificial intelligence in psychotherapy: Development of intelligent therapeutic systems. *BMC Psychology*, *13*(1), 175. DOI: 10.1186/s40359-025-02491-9 PMID: 40022267

Sun, J., Lu, T., Shao, X., Han, Y., Xia, Y., Zheng, Y., Wang, Y., Li, X., Ravindran, A., Fan, L., Fang, Y., Zhang, X., Ravindran, N., Wang, Y., Liu, X., & Lu, L. (2025). Practical AI application in psychiatry: Historical review and future directions. *Molecular Psychiatry*, *30*(9), 4399–4408. DOI: 10.1038/s41380-025-03072-3 PMID: 40456953

Tavory, T. (2024). Regulating AI in mental health: Ethics of care perspective. *JMIR Mental Health*, *11*, e58493. DOI: 10.2196/58493 PMID: 39298759

Tizzard, C. L. (2025). Re-imagining Care for Aging Disabled Adults.

Tsai, Y. Y., Chen, Y. J., Lin, Y. F., Hsiao, F. C., Hsu, C. H., & Liao, L. D. (2025). Photoplethysmography-based HRV analysis and machine learning for real-time stress quantification in mental health applications. *APL Bioengineering*, *9*(2), 026103. DOI: 10.1063/5.0256590 PMID: 40191605

Vaidyam, A. N., Wisniewski, H., Halamka, J. D., Kashavan, M. S., & Torous, J. B. (2019). Chatbots and conversational agents in mental health: A review of the psychiatric landscape. *Canadian Journal of Psychiatry. Revue Canadienne de Psychiatrie*, *64*(7), 456–464. DOI: 10.1177/0706743719828977 PMID: 30897957

Volckens, J., Haynes, E. N., Croisant, S. P., Cui, Y., Errett, N. A., Henry, H. F., Horney, J. A., Kwok, R. K., Magzamen, S., Rappold, A. G., Ravichandran, L., Reinlib, L., Ryan, P. H., & Shaughnessy, D. T. (2023). Health research in the wake of disasters: Challenges and opportunities for sensor science. *Environmental Health Perspectives*, *131*(6), 065002. DOI: 10.1289/EHP12270 PMID: 37389972

Walter, J. R., Xu, S., & Rogers, J. A. (2023). From lab to life: How wearable devices can improve health equity. *Nature Communications*, *14*, 44634. PMID: 38167483

Wang, Z., Xiong, H., Zhang, J., Yang, S., Boukhechba, M., Zhang, D., Barnes, L. E., & Dou, D. (2022). From personalized medicine to population health: A survey of mHealth sensing techniques. *IEEE Internet of Things Journal*, *9*(17), 15413–15434. DOI: 10.1109/JIOT.2022.3161046

Weiner, E. B., Dankwa-Mullan, I., Nelson, W. A., & Hassanpour, S. (2025). Ethical challenges and evolving strategies in the integration of artificial intelligence into clinical practice. *PLOS Digital Health*, *4*(4), e0000810. DOI: 10.1371/journal.pdig.0000810 PMID: 40198594

Wibberly, K. H. (2024). Preparing mental health providers for the future: The case for moving beyond the elective telehealth course to integrating telehealth training throughout the curriculum. *Frontiers in Psychology*, *14*, 1301569. DOI: 10.3389/fpsyg.2023.1301569 PMID: 38235285

Xing, Y., Yang, Y., Yang, K., Lu, A., Xing, L., Mackie, K., & Guo, F. (2025). Intelligent sensing devices and systems for personalized mental health. *Med-X*, *3*(1), 10. DOI: 10.1007/s44258-025-00057-3 PMID: 40837134

Section 4
Clinical and Research Implications

Chapter 11
Clinical Validation and Evidence Standards

ABSTRACT

This chapter provides a roadmap for translating digital mental health innovations into practice through rigorous evidence generation (Kang & Exworthy, 2022). It outlines sequential steps: defining clinical need, co-designing prototypes, validating efficacy via randomized trials, and embedding implementation science to monitor fidelity, reach, and sustainability (Pedram & Piatkowski, 2025). Emphasis is placed on pragmatic trials, equity audits, and post-market surveillance to detect performance drift and subgroup disparities. The chapter underscores the necessity of transparent reporting, independent replication, and participatory governance to ensure accountability. By linking design principles to measurable outcomes, it positions evidence-based validation as the cornerstone of ethical and effective digital mental health care (Pedram & Piatkowski, 2025).

INTRODUCTION

This chapter examines the methodological challenges of validating digital mental health interventions. It contrasts traditional randomized controlled trials with adaptive, hybrid, and implementation-focused designs better suited to evolving technologies. The chapter outlines evidence standards required by regulators, payers, and clinicians, emphasizing transparency, reproducibility, and representativeness. Implementation outcomes, such as acceptability, feasibility, and maintenance, are presented as essential complements to efficacy metrics. By bridging research and practice, the chapter provides guidance on generating evidence that supports safe and scalable deployment.

DOI: 10.4018/979-8-3373-4997-8.ch011

VALIDATION OF MODELS

Collaborative models such as co-design, translational research teams, and public-private partnerships can facilitate the integration of diverse perspectives and skill sets (Correa et al., 2021). Give an example of a translational team that included frontline clinicians and community advocates, which improved external validity and recruitment success. Recommend establishing memoranda of understanding to clarify roles, data governance, and intellectual property before projects scale (Engel, 1977). Stress that these models enhance relevance, usability, and the likelihood that validated tools will be adopted in real-world care (Engel, 1977). The focus is on practical translation rather than technical exposition. It defines "clinical validation" as evidence demonstrating safety and therapeutic effect in real-world care settings (Morgan et al., 2025). It explains "implementation" as the set of organizational, workflow, and economic steps required for routine use. It clarifies "inclusive design" as practices that ensure access across abilities, languages, and socioeconomic conditions. It emphasizes that the chapters that follow will connect conceptual frameworks to actionable steps for researchers, clinicians, and policy makers.

As digital therapeutics continue to evolve, their integration into mental health care systems demands rigorous clinical validation, thoughtful implementation, and inclusive design. To be actionable, these three aims require distinct but coordinated study designs, training pipelines, and design standards (Rajpal, 2025). Each aim poses methodological questions that shape how we measure outcomes, train clinicians, and evaluate equity. Coordinated planning across these domains reduces the risk that a validated tool cannot be implemented or is inaccessible to vulnerable groups (Rajpal, 2025). Together, they establish the infrastructure needed for durable and equitable clinical impact (Rajpal, 2025).

While the preceding sections of this book have explored the technological foundations and applications of artificial intelligence (AI), extended reality (XR), and wearable sensors, Part IV shifts the focus to the critical infrastructure that supports the responsible and effective deployment of these tools in real-world clinical settings (Bibi, 2024). This shift moves from describing what the technologies can do to answering how they should be tested, adopted, and governed in care systems. It foregrounds practical constraints such as clinician time, reimbursement, and information governance that determine real-world feasibility. It also considers patient-centered factors like digital literacy, device ownership, and privacy preferences that influence uptake. These considerations bridge the prior technical chapters with the implementation challenges clinicians face daily.

This part addresses three interrelated pillars: evidence-based validation, clinician training, and design for engagement and accessibility (Boda & Allam, 2022). Each pillar contributes distinct evidence needs, workforce competencies, and design choices that interact during deployment (Radanliev, 2025). For example, validation studies inform what clinicians should learn, while training affects fidelity and therefore trial outcomes (Radanliev, 2025). Design choices influence both engagement metrics and the kinds of evidence necessary to demonstrate effectiveness across populations (Radanliev, 2025). Explicitly treating these domains as linked reduces fragmentation between research and practice and improves the chances of successful scale-up (Radanliev, 2025).

These domains are essential not only for ensuring the safety and efficacy of digital interventions but also for fostering trust, adoption, and sustained use among diverse populations and practitioners. Trust depends on transparent evidence, clear clinician guidance, and understandable user interfaces (Verma et al., 2023). Adoption requires fit with clinical workflows, billing structures, and staff capacity (Shatte et al., 2019). Sustained use hinges on ongoing support, iterative updates, and demonstrated value for patients and systems. In short, success demands more than technical performance; it requires coordinated attention to evidence, people, and context (Shatte et al., 2019).

The Imperative of Evidence-Based Validation (Lamb et al., 2025). The promise of digital mental health tools is vast, but without robust clinical trials and empirical validation, their potential remains speculative (Mohr et al., 2017). This statement underscores that technical feasibility does not equal clinical effectiveness, and that empirical evidence is necessary for responsible adoption (Mohr et al., 2017). It clarifies that "robust" evidence should include reproducible outcomes, representative samples, and transparent analytic plans (Mohr et al., 2017). It provides an example where initial pilot success did not generalize in pragmatic trials due to sample differences. It connects these needs to regulatory expectations and payer demands for measurable benefit. It reiterates that rigorous validation protects patients, guides clinicians, and supports sustainable implementation.

Figure 1. Panel A: Trial Outcome Comparison Panel B: Radar Chart RE-AIM framework dashboard

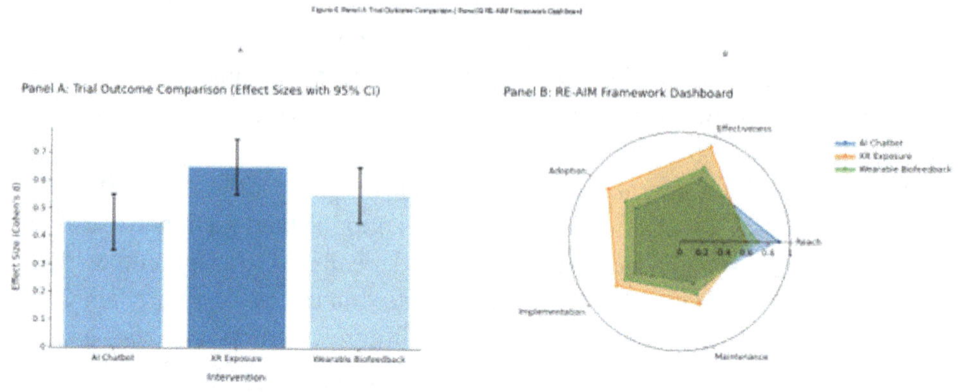

Effect sizes (Cohen's d) for three digital mental health interventions, AI Chatbot, XR Exposure Therapy, and Wearable Biofeedback, are shown with 95% confidence intervals. XR Exposure demonstrates the largest effect size (d ≈ 0.65), followed by Wearable Biofeedback (d ≈ 0.55) and AI Chatbot (d ≈ 0.45), indicating differential efficacy across modalities (Omiyefa, 2025). Radar chart comparing AI Chatbot, XR Exposure, and Wearable Biofeedback across five implementation dimensions: Reach, Effectiveness, Adoption, Implementation, and Maintenance. XR Exposure scores highest on Effectiveness and Adoption, while AI Chatbot leads in Reach. Wearable Biofeedback shows moderate performance across all dimensions, highlighting trade-offs between scalability and sustainability.

Unlike traditional pharmaceuticals or psychotherapeutic interventions, digital therapeutics often operate at the intersection of software engineering, behavioral science, and neurotechnology. This interdisciplinary character complicates trial design, outcome selection, and implementation strategies (Mohr et al., 2017). It requires teams with complementary expertise in clinical measurement, data governance, and user-centered design (Mohr et al., 2017). It clarifies that software development lifecycles and clinical research timelines must be synchronized early in a project (Mohr et al., 2017). It offers a brief example where engineers and clinicians co-planned release schedules to avoid mid-trial software changes (Mohr et al., 2017). It emphasizes that deliberate coordination reduces costly protocol amendments and preserves trial validity (Mohr et al., 2017).

This complexity necessitates novel approaches to clinical research that can accommodate rapid iteration, adaptive algorithms, and multimodal data streams (Chen et al., 2022). Traditional fixed-protocol trials may be insufficient when interventions learn from user interaction or when devices produce continuous physiological data (Ricciardi & Zomaya, 2025). Adaptive, modular, and hybrid trial designs provide flexible structures that preserve inferential integrity while allowing iterative improvements (Ricciardi & Zomaya, 2025). This clarification notes that pre-specifying update procedures and analytic adjustments is essential for interpretability. It gives an example of a trial that used a prespecified algorithm update plan to maintain consistency across sites (Ricciardi & Zomaya, 2025). It links these methodological adaptations back to earlier chapters on AI and sensors to show continuity across the book (Ricciardi & Zomaya, 2025).

Randomized controlled trials (Li et al., 2025) remain the gold standard for establishing efficacy, but they must be adapted to the unique characteristics of digital interventions. For example, how do we account for updates to an AI model mid-trial (De Kock et al., 2021)? How do we measure the therapeutic impact of immersive XR environments or real-time biofeedback from wearable sensors (Robinson et al., 2024)? These practical questions demand preplanned protocols that specify version control, update thresholds, and analytic contingencies. A clarification: define what constitutes a substantive software change that triggers re-randomization or sensitivity analyses. An illustrative example: a trial pre-registered a plan to stratify analyses by software version when model updates exceeded a performance threshold (Robinson et al., 2024). This approach preserves the strengths of RCTs while acknowledging digital intervention realities.

Moreover, regulatory bodies such as the Food and Drug Administration (FDA) and EMA are beginning to develop frameworks for digital therapeutics, but these are still in flux. Researchers and developers must navigate a landscape where the boundaries between medical devices, wellness tools, and clinical interventions are increasingly blurred (Radanliev, 2025). This regulatory uncertainty creates both opportunity and risk for innovators and clinicians. A clarification: engage early with regulators to clarify intended device classification and evidence expectations (Ienca et al., 2017). An example: a development team consulted the regulator's pre-submission process to align trial endpoints with regulatory standards (Ienca et al., 2017). Proactive regulatory engagement reduces the risk of later noncompliance and accelerates potential adoption.

The clinician of the future will need to interpret data from wearable sensors, understand the logic behind AI-driven decision support systems, and facilitate therapeutic experiences in virtual environments (Ma et al., 2025). Educational programs should teach clinicians how to translate raw sensor outputs into clinically meaningful signals (Ricciardi & Zomaya, 2025). Offer a concrete classroom exercise where trainees review anonymized HRV traces and make treatment-relevant interpretations (Ricciardi & Zomaya, 2025). Teach clinicians to evaluate AI outputs for common failure modes and to communicate uncertainty to patients in plain language (Ricciardi & Zomaya, 2025). These competencies are not traditionally taught in medical or psychology programs, necessitating a rethinking of curricula and continuing education. Equip clinicians with checklists and decision aids that integrate digital outputs into routine assessments.

Interdisciplinary collaboration is key. Clinicians must work alongside data scientists, engineers, and designers to co-create tools that are clinically relevant and user-friendly (Boffet et al., 2025). Establish regular co-design sessions where clinicians provide scenario-based feedback and engineers prototype live adjustments. Create governance forums that include clinicians to oversee design trade-offs and prioritize clinical safety (Kim & Backonja, 2025). Certification programs, digital literacy initiatives, and experiential learning opportunities can help bridge the gap between clinical expertise and technological fluency (Kim & Backonja, 2025). Include supervised practicum experiences with digital tools to ensure competence in real-world workflows. These measures promote shared language and mutual accountability across disciplines.

Importantly, the integration of technology should not come at the expense of the therapeutic relationship. Empathy, presence, and trust remain central to effective mental health care. Trainings must emphasize communication skills that preserve empathic attunement when interacting through screens or avatars. Provide an illustrative role-play where clinicians practice reflective listening while guiding a patient through an XR exposure session (Jain & Jain, 2025). Highlight practical strategies such as explicit check-ins about privacy, collaborative review of algorithmic recommendations, and shared decision-making around digital tool use. Training programs must therefore emphasize how to maintain these human elements in digitally mediated contexts. Reinforce that technology should augment, not replace, core therapeutic skills.

Designing for engagement involves understanding the psychological and behavioral drivers of user interaction. Operationalize engagement by defining proximal behaviors, such as daily check-ins or completion of therapeutic exercises. Use behavior-change techniques and validated engagement heuristics to map features to intended mechanisms of action (Kostadimas et al., 2025). Gamification, personalization, and adaptive feedback can enhance motivation and retention. Explain that gamified elements should reinforce therapeutic tasks rather than distract from them. However, these features must be grounded in clinical goals and ethical considerations (Martinez-Martin et al., 2018). Require that any persuasive design be accompanied by safeguards that prevent manipulation or overuse.

Accessibility is equally critical. Define accessibility in practical terms, including readable font sizes, high-contrast color schemes, and alternative input methods. Digital mental health tools must be usable by individuals across a wide range of abilities, languages, cultures, and socioeconomic backgrounds. Include explicit testing with screen readers and simplified navigation for users with low literacy. This includes designing for people with visual, auditory, cognitive, or motor impairments, as well as those with limited digital literacy or internet access. Specify fallback options, such as SMS-based content or offline modes, to accommodate low-connectivity contexts. Ensure that accessibility accommodations are documented and tested as part of trial protocols (Islam & Bae, 2024).

Cultural sensitivity is also paramount. Define cultural adaptation steps, such as language translation, idiom review, and validation of symptom descriptions. Mental health experiences and expressions vary widely across cultures, and digital tools must be adaptable to these differences. Require engagement of community stakeholders to surface local meanings and concerns. Inclusive design practices, such as participatory design, localization, and community engagement, can help ensure that interventions are relevant and respectful. Recommend that pilot studies explicitly evaluate cultural acceptability and that iterative changes respond to stakeholder feedback.

Bridging the Gap Between Innovation and Implementation. Many promising tools are developed in academic or startup settings but fail to reach clinical practice or scale effectively (Adegoke et al., 2025). Identify common failure points early, such as misaligned incentives, fragile business models, and lack of clinician workflow fit. Provide practical criteria for transition readiness, including interoperability, reimbursement strategy, and clinician training plans. Highlight that successful translation requires measurable implementation outcomes alongside efficacy metrics. Emphasize the need for pilot implementations in routine care to reveal operational barriers before wide release.

This "valley of death" is often due to a lack of alignment between technological innovation and the realities of clinical workflows, reimbursement models, and user needs (Ong et al., 2025). Clarify that alignment means matching product capabilities with clinician time constraints, billing codes, and patient access patterns. Offer an example where a digital assessment required 30 minutes of clinician time and failed because workflows allowed only five. Recommend stakeholder mapping early in development to identify decision-makers, payers, and clinical champions who influence adoption (Radanliev, 2025). Stress that economic and human factors are as decisive as technical performance.

Ethical and Policy Considerations. As digital mental health tools become more embedded in care systems, ethical and policy considerations take on increasing importance. Clarify that ethical review must address data governance, consent processes, equity impacts, and algorithmic fairness throughout the product lifecycle (Casson, 2019). Provide an example where a trial's consent materials were co-designed with patient advocates to improve comprehension and trust (Casson, 2019). Explain that policy review should align institutional procurement, privacy, and clinical governance policies with trial and deployment plans (Casson, 2019). Require a documented risk assessment that identifies potential harms and mitigation plans before scaling.

Issues such as data privacy, algorithmic bias, informed consent, and digital equity must be addressed proactively and transparently (Freeman et al., 2017). Define algorithmic bias in clinically relevant terms and list concrete assessment steps, such as subgroup performance checks and audit logging. Offer a research vignette where subgroup analyses revealed differential classifier performance that led to retraining on more representative data (Freeman et al., 2017). Emphasize that informed consent must be iterative and accessible, using layered disclosures and plain-language summaries. Finally, state that equity assessments should be embedded in trial design, not appended after efficacy claims (Freeman et al., 2017).

Clinical validation processes must include safeguards to ensure that digital tools do not exacerbate existing disparities or introduce new forms of harm (Hiland, 2021). Specify safeguards such as stratified enrollment targets, continuous monitoring for differential outcomes, and predefined stopping criteria for harm signals. Provide an example in which an implementation pilot paused enrollment when remote-monitoring alerts disproportionately failed for participants with older devices. Recommend routine equity audits and stakeholder review panels to interpret findings and direct remediation. These practices help ensure interventions serve rather than harm vulnerable groups.

Training programs must include ethical literacy and critical thinking about the implications of technology use. Integrate case-based ethics modules that require clinicians to evaluate scenarios involving privacy breaches, algorithmic errors, and consent complexity. Provide a classroom example in which trainees role-play obtaining consent for passive data collection and discuss boundary issues for remote monitoring (Engel, 1977). Recommend competency assessments that include ethical decision-making and documentation of risk communication. Ethical literacy prepares clinicians to support patient autonomy and to intervene when technology-related risks arise.

Policy frameworks at the institutional, national, and international levels will play a crucial role in shaping the future of digital mental health. Clarify that policy development should be iterative, evidence-informed, and inclusive of clinician and patient voices (Bond et al., 2023). Offer an example where a hospital's procurement policy required demonstration of clinical benefit, equity assessment, and a maintenance plan before approving digital tools (Kim & Backonja, 2025). Recommend engagement with regulators early and documentation of compliance pathways to reduce deployment delays. These policy actions create predictable environments that encourage responsible innovation.

Unlike traditional pharmaceuticals or psychotherapeutic modalities, digital interventions, ranging from AI-driven diagnostic tools to immersive XR therapies and wearable sensor platforms, present unique challenges and opportunities for clinical evaluation (Weiner et al., 2025). Explain that software updates, adaptive algorithms, and multimodal data streams complicate trial fidelity and endpoint definition (Robinson et al., 2024). Offer a concrete example where sensor drift required recalibration and revalidation prior to efficacy analysis (Robinson et al., 2024). Emphasize that reproducible analytic pipelines and version-controlled artifacts are essential for credible results. Stress that interdisciplinary teams must document technical decisions alongside clinical protocols (Robinson et al., 2024).

This chapter explores the evolving landscape of clinical trials for digital mental health tools, examining methodological innovations, regulatory considerations, and best practices for generating robust, generalizable evidence (Kargarandehkordi et al., 2025). Clarify that "generalizable evidence" refers to results that apply across relevant clinical settings and patient subgroups, not only tightly controlled samples (Engel, 1977). Provide a brief example of a multisite pragmatic trial that tested a mobile CBT program across urban and rural clinics to assess external validity (Engel, 1977). State that the chapter emphasizes practical guidance for designing trials that balance internal rigor with real-world relevance. Conclude that readers will find templates and decision rules to operationalize these recommendations.

THE NEED FOR EVIDENCE-BASED VALIDATION IN DIGITAL MENTAL HEALTH INTERVENTIONS

In recent years, digital mental health interventions have emerged as promising tools for addressing various psychological and psychiatric conditions. Explain that promise refers to scalable access, personalized delivery, and continuous monitoring capabilities unique to digital platforms. Provide an example of an app-based intervention that increased access in regions lacking specialty care, demonstrating potential reach advantages. Clarify that promise alone does not substitute for rigorous outcome data and that promising features must be tied to measurable clinical benefit (Saganowski et al., 2022). Emphasize the necessity of balancing enthusiasm with methodological restraint to protect patients and preserve trust.

Current Challenges. Despite the potential benefits of digital mental health interventions, several challenges hinder their widespread adoption and acceptance. One major challenge is the lack of standardized methodologies for evaluating these interventions. Clarify that the field lacks consensus on key outcome definitions, minimal clinically important differences, and standard engagement metrics. Provide an example where two trials used different adherence thresholds, complicating meta-analytic synthesis. State that harmonized measurement frameworks would improve comparability and accelerate cumulative knowledge.

METHODOLOGICAL CONSIDERATIONS

To address these challenges, researchers and developers must adopt innovative methodologies for evidence-based validation of digital mental health interventions (Aiken et al., 2023). Clarify that methodological innovation should aim to preserve causal inference while accommodating iterative software development and user-driven adaptation. Define criteria for when adaptive methods are preferable to fixed protocols, such as when the intervention learns from individual behavior or when rapid iteration is essential for safety. Provide an explicit research example in which an adaptive design allowed midstream tuning of a conversational agent's feedback parameters without compromising primary endpoint integrity (Fanarioti & Karpouzis, 2025). Explain that pre-specifying adaptation rules, decision thresholds, and analysis plans is essential to prevent post hoc bias and to support reproducibility (Fanarioti & Karpouzis, 2025).

Adaptive trial designs, which allow for modifications to the study protocol based on interim results, are particularly useful for digital interventions (Kim & Backonja, 2025). These designs enable researchers to update algorithms, adjust sample sizes, and refine intervention components without compromising the validity of the study (De Kock et al., 2021). Clarify that every adaptive element must be governed by a prespecified statistical plan that controls Type I error and preserves interpretability. Offer an example where a sample size re-estimation protected power after early effect-size estimates differed from projections. State that adaptive designs require close collaboration with statisticians and regulatory liaisons to ensure acceptability for stakeholders and potential approval pathways.

Micro-randomized trials are another promising approach for evaluating digital interventions. MRTs involve randomizing intervention components at multiple time points, allowing researchers to assess the effectiveness of different elements of the intervention. Provide a concrete MRT vignette where a JITAI randomized prompt timing and content across days to determine which context-sensitive cue most effectively reduced momentary craving. Clarify that MRTs estimate proximal, time-varying effects rather than cumulative treatment effects, and that their analytic models must account for temporal dependence and varying exposure histories. Recommend that MRT planning include simulation studies to inform power and sampling schedules.

N-of-1 trials, which focus on individual participants undergoing multiple treatment and control periods, are well-suited for personalized digital interventions.

These trials provide detailed insights into individual variability and can inform the development of tailored treatment plans. Explain that aggregating many N-of-1 trials can also yield population-level inferences about heterogeneity of treatment effect. Provide an applied example in which a series of N-of-1 evaluations informed personalized threshold settings for a wearable-guided panic-prevention algorithm (De Kock et al., 2021). State that careful randomization, washout specification, and adherence monitoring are necessary to preserve internal validity in N-of-1 designs.

Hybrid effectiveness-implementation designs, which simultaneously evaluate clinical outcomes and implementation factors, are valuable for assessing the real-world applicability and scalability of digital interventions (De Kock et al., 2021). These designs are particularly useful when implementation barriers are likely to moderate clinical effectiveness (De Kock et al., 2021). Clarify that hybrid trials should predefine both effectiveness and implementation endpoints, such as reach, fidelity, and cost-effectiveness, and plan integrated analyses that link these domains. Offer an example where a hybrid trial compared centralized versus decentralized deployment strategies while measuring symptom change and clinician time burden (De Kock et al., 2021). Recommend early engagement with health system stakeholders to define pragmatic success criteria that align with operational priorities.

THE CHALLENGE OF BLINDING IN DIGITAL CONTEXTS

Despite the numerous advantages of digital mental health interventions, one of the primary challenges in conducting rigorous clinical trials is mitigating bias (Kim & Backonja, 2025). Bias can significantly impact the validity and reliability of trial outcomes, leading to skewed results and potentially misleading conclusions (Kim & Backonja, 2025). Clarify that bias sources include expectancy, differential dropout, selective engagement, and analyst degrees of freedom. Recommend embedding bias-detection checks, such as baseline imbalance testing and sensitivity analyses for missing-not-at-random patterns. Provide an example where pre-specified sensitivity analyses altered the interpretation of an apparent treatment effect. Emphasize that active bias mitigation plans should be part of the registered protocol (Kim & Backonja, 2025).

USING OBJECTIVE OUTCOME MEASURES

One of the most effective ways to mitigate bias in digital mental health trials is to incorporate objective, quantifiable outcome measures that are less susceptible to subjective interpretation. Clarify that objective measures complement, rather than replace, validated self-report instruments and clinician ratings (Inkster et al., 2023). Specify common objective domains: physiological signals, passive behavior metrics, and application-derived performance indicators. Give a concrete example where heart rate variability tracked via a wrist sensor served as a corroborating endpoint alongside depression scales (Pedram & Piatkowski, 2025). Recommend predefining signal-processing pipelines and quality-control thresholds to avoid post hoc analytic choices that introduce bias.

BLINDED ASSESSMENTS

Blinded assessments play a critical role in preserving internal validity in clinical trials of digital mental health interventions, where traditional forms of blinding are often difficult or impossible to achieve. Unlike pharmacological trials, participants and clinicians interacting with apps, wearable sensors, or XR systems are typically aware of the intervention being delivered, increasing the risk of expectancy effects and observer bias. Blinded outcome assessment offers a pragmatic safeguard by ensuring that individuals responsible for measuring primary and secondary outcomes, such as symptom severity, functional improvement, or diagnostic status, are unaware of treatment allocation, intervention version, or level of participant engagement. In practice, this often involves the use of independent evaluators conducting structured interviews, centralized rating teams reviewing de-identified data, or automated scoring pipelines that separate outcome computation from intervention delivery. Within digital mental health research, blinded assessments help disentangle true therapeutic effects from improvements driven by novelty, motivation, or participant beliefs about technology.

Implementing blinded assessments in digital contexts requires deliberate procedural and technical design. Outcome assessors must be insulated not only from group assignment but also from metadata that could inadvertently reveal exposure, such as app usage frequency, device type, or version identifiers. This often necessitates parallel data streams, one supporting intervention delivery and another supporting outcome evaluation, governed by clear data access controls and documentation. Automated and semi-automated assessment tools, including algorithm-scored questionnaires or sensor-derived metrics processed through pre-specified pipelines, can further reduce assessor bias when appropriately validated. However, blinding does not eliminate all sources of bias; it must be complemented by pre-registered analytic plans, robust handling of missing data, and transparency about where blinding was partial or infeasible. For researchers and clinicians interpreting trial results, the presence of blinded outcome assessment remains a key indicator of methodological rigor and strengthens confidence that observed effects are attributable to the intervention rather than to measurement artifacts or expectancy-driven distortions.

AUTOMATING DATA COLLECTION AND ANALYSIS

Automating data collection and analysis is a defining feature of digital mental health interventions, offering both methodological advantages and new responsibilities for researchers and clinicians. Unlike traditional trials that rely on episodic self-reports or clinician-administered assessments, digital systems can passively and continuously capture high-resolution data streams, including physiological signals, behavioral patterns, and interaction logs. Automated collection reduces recall bias, minimizes clinician burden, and improves ecological validity by capturing experiences as they unfold in real-world contexts. When paired with ecological momentary assessment, wearable sensing, or application-derived metrics, automation enables a more dynamic understanding of symptom trajectories, treatment adherence, and context-sensitive responses. For researchers, this richness expands analytic possibilities, but it also demands careful specification of what constitutes meaningful data versus noise, as continuous collection can easily outpace theoretical clarity if not grounded in prespecified constructs and hypotheses.

Automated analysis pipelines further enhance scalability and reproducibility when they are transparent, version-controlled, and locked prior to outcome evaluation. Predefined signal-processing steps, quality-control thresholds, and analytic decision rules are essential to prevent post hoc flexibility that can undermine causal inference. In clinical contexts, automation can translate raw data into actionable indicators, such as thresholds for clinical alerts or summaries for treatment planning, but these outputs must be interpretable and aligned with clinician workflows. Importantly, automation does not eliminate the need for oversight; continuous data increase privacy risks and amplify the consequences of analytic errors or algorithmic drift. As emphasized in this chapter, effective automation requires governance structures that document data provenance, restrict unnecessary access, and clearly separate intervention delivery from outcome evaluation. When thoughtfully designed, automated data collection and analysis can strengthen both scientific rigor and clinical feasibility, supporting digital mental health tools that are not only innovative but also trustworthy and ready for real-world use.

PLACEBO-LIKE CONTROLS

Incorporating placebo-like controls is essential for reducing expectancy effects and disentangling true therapeutic impact from non-specific engagement benefits in digital mental health trials. Because participants are often aware that they are interacting with an active digital system, traditional inert placebos are rarely feasible. Instead, researchers employ carefully designed comparator conditions that match the intervention on factors such as time, interface complexity, attention, and interaction frequency, while omitting key therapeutic mechanisms. Examples include attention-matched wellness apps, neutral XR environments without exposure hierarchies, or wearable platforms that provide non-contingent feedback. These controls help isolate whether observed improvements are attributable to specific intervention components, such as adaptive feedback, exposure protocols, or algorithmic personalization, rather than to novelty, perceived support, or increased self-monitoring. For both researchers and clinicians, the presence of a credible placebo-like control strengthens confidence that reported effects reflect meaningful clinical change.

Designing effective placebo-like controls requires both methodological rigor and ethical sensitivity. Control conditions must be sufficiently engaging to maintain adherence and minimize differential dropout, yet transparent enough to avoid deception that could undermine trust or informed consent. In digital contexts, this balance is often achieved through partial disclosure, for example, explaining that participants will receive different versions of a digital program without emphasizing presumed superiority. Analytically, placebo-like controls are particularly important when outcomes rely on self-report or subjective clinician ratings, which are more vulnerable to expectancy bias. However, their use also complicates interpretation when controls themselves produce modest benefits, as is common in supportive or self-monitoring conditions. As emphasized in this chapter, the goal is not to eliminate all non-specific effects but to account for them systematically. When thoughtfully implemented, placebo-like controls improve causal inference, clarify mechanisms of action, and provide more reliable guidance for clinical decision-making and policy adoption.

OUTCOME MEASURES AND DATA COLLECTION IN DIGITAL MENTAL HEALTH TRIALS

Ecological Momentary Assessment (Obermeyer et al., 2019) is one such method, involving real-time self-reports collected via mobile devices. EMA allows for the capture of data in the user's natural environment, providing a more accurate and dynamic picture of their mental health status (Ball et al., 2025). Provide a practical example: random prompts four times daily over two weeks can reveal diurnal mood patterns linked to relapse risk. Clarify that EMA designs must balance sampling frequency with participant burden and incorporate strategies to limit reactivity. State that time-stamped EMA linked to passive sensors increases ecological validity and supports causal inference about proximal effects.

Digital interventions have the unique capability to generate continuous, high-resolution data over extended periods (Fanarioti & Karpouzis, 2025). This enables several advanced analytical techniques that can enhance our understanding of intervention effects and user behavior. Define trajectory analyses, personalization algorithms, and predictive modeling as distinct analytic aims that require different sampling densities and preprocessing pipelines. Recommend establishing data quality thresholds and missingness rules before analysis to prevent post hoc decisions (Fleming et al., 2019). Finally, note that continuous data increase privacy obligations and should be governed by strict access and retention policies (Fleming et al., 2019).

MICRO-RANDOMIZED TRIALS (MRTS)

Micro-randomized trials (Ricciardi & Zomaya, 2025) involve randomizing intervention components at multiple time points. Explain that MRTs estimate time-varying, proximal effects rather than cumulative outcomes, which is essential for just-in-time adaptive interventions. Offer a research example: randomize prompt timing and content across hours to determine optimal delivery windows for momentary support (Lindner et al., 2024). Clarify that MRT analytic models must account for serial correlation and differing exposure histories across participants. Recommend iterative simulations during design to set sampling rates and ensure adequate power for detecting proximal effects. Emphasize that MRTs complement, rather than replace, longer-term RCTs when designing adaptive digital therapeutics.

N-OF-1 TRIALS

N-of-1 trials represent a particularly well-suited evaluation strategy for personalized digital mental health interventions, where treatment effects may vary substantially across individuals. Unlike traditional randomized controlled trials that estimate average effects across groups, N-of-1 designs involve repeated within-person comparisons across multiple treatment and control periods. This structure allows each participant to serve as their own control, making it possible to detect individual-level response patterns that would otherwise be obscured by between-subject variability. In digital contexts, such as adaptive CBT platforms, wearable-guided interventions, or just-in-time adaptive systems, N-of-1 trials align closely with the goal of tailoring interventions to an individual's cognitive, behavioral, or physiological profile. For researchers, these designs generate high-resolution evidence about heterogeneity of treatment effects, while for clinicians, they offer a rigorous framework for determining whether a specific digital tool is beneficial for a particular patient rather than relying solely on population-level averages.

Methodologically, N-of-1 trials in digital mental health require careful attention to randomization schedules, washout periods, and adherence monitoring to preserve internal validity. Digital interventions are especially amenable to these designs because software can automate treatment switching, data capture, and outcome measurement with minimal participant burden. However, researchers must clearly define stable outcome measures, ensure that intervention effects are reversible or time-limited, and guard against carryover effects that could confound interpretation. Aggregating results across multiple N-of-1 trials can further support population-level inferences about variability in response and help identify subgroups most likely to benefit. As emphasized in this chapter, N-of-1 trials should not be viewed as a replacement for larger trials, but as a complementary approach that strengthens precision, supports shared clinical decision-making, and advances the broader goal of personalized, evidence-based digital mental health care.

HYBRID EFFECTIVENESS-IMPLEMENTATION DESIGNS

Hybrid designs simultaneously evaluate clinical effectiveness and implementation outcomes (Poudel et al., 2025). Clarify that hybrid Type 1 prioritizes effectiveness while collecting implementation data, Type 2 balances both aims, and Type 3 focuses on implementation with clinical monitoring (Poudel et al., 2025). Provide a concrete illustration: a hybrid trial that measures symptom change while assessing fidelity, reach, and cost across clinic sites (Poudel et al., 2025). Recommend specifying implementation metrics, such as adoption rate, clinician burden, and maintenance, alongside primary clinical endpoints (Poudel et al., 2025). State that hybrid designs shorten the translation pathway by informing both efficacy and real-world scale-up concurrently. Encourage early stakeholder engagement to define pragmatic success criteria aligned with health system needs.

REGULATORY AND ETHICAL CONSIDERATIONS

Regulatory agencies are developing frameworks for digital therapeutics, but the landscape remains complex. Clarify that device classification, evidence expectations, and post-market surveillance requirements vary by jurisdiction and risk level (Spytska, 2025). Provide an example of a pre-submission meeting with regulators that clarified required endpoints and safety monitoring plans. Recommend mapping regulatory touchpoints into the trial timeline and allocating budget for compliance activities (Kim & Backonja, 2025). Emphasize proactive engagement with institutional review boards and privacy officers to align consent processes and data governance with regulatory standards (Kim & Backonja, 2025).

CASE STUDIES IN DIGITAL MENTAL HEALTH

AI-Powered CBT App for Depression

Cognitive Behavioral Therapy is a well-established treatment for depression, focusing on changing negative thought patterns and behaviors. Clarify that AI augmentation typically personalizes content sequencing and adapts feedback based on user inputs and engagement patterns (Baydili et al., 2025). Provide a brief trial example: a randomized trial compared the AI-enhanced app to a matched journaling control over 12 weeks with engagement tracked continuously (Kim & Backonja, 2025). Explain that analysis controlled for baseline severity, platform version, and differential dropout to isolate the app's specific contribution (Kim & Backonja, 2025). Emphasize that implementation considerations included clinician referral workflows and data-sharing agreements for safety alerts (Kim & Backonja, 2025).

VR Exposure Therapy for PTSD

VR Exposure Therapy for PTSD serves as a central case study in this chapter, illustrating how immersive technologies can be rigorously validated and pragmatically implemented within evidence-based mental health care. Building on decades of research supporting exposure-based treatments for PTSD, VR platforms enable clinicians to deliver controlled, repeatable, and graded exposure to trauma-relevant cues that may be difficult to access through imaginal or in vivo approaches alone. In clinical trials discussed in this section, VR environments were designed to align tightly with established exposure hierarchies, allowing clinicians to modulate sensory intensity while maintaining therapeutic intent. Outcome evaluation combined standardized PTSD symptom measures with session-level distress ratings, behavioral avoidance indicators, and engagement metrics, providing a multidimensional view of treatment response. As a case example, VR exposure demonstrated clinically meaningful symptom reduction while improving treatment adherence among individuals who struggled with traditional exposure formats, reinforcing its potential as a translational enhancement rather than a theoretical departure from established care.

From an implementation perspective, the VR exposure case study underscores the interdependence of validation, clinician training, and workflow integration emphasized throughout the chapter. Trial success depended not only on symptom change but also on equipment reliability, software version stability, and clinician competence in managing immersive sessions while maintaining empathic presence. Training protocols emphasized both technical fluency and preservation of the therapeutic relationship, positioning VR as a medium through which core clinical skills are applied rather than replaced. The case also highlights practical barriers encountered during pilot deployment, including scheduling constraints, hardware maintenance, and patient tolerability, all of which informed subsequent implementation refinements. By situating VR exposure therapy within the broader Case Studies section, the chapter demonstrates how methodological rigor, ethical oversight, and real-world feasibility must converge for digital mental health tools to move from promising innovation to sustainable clinical practice, particularly in the treatment of complex conditions such as PTSD.

Wearable Sensor Platform for Anxiety Monitoring

Anxiety disorders are among the most common mental health conditions, characterized by excessive worry and physiological arousal. Clarify that wearable platforms blend continuous physiological sensing with just-in-time interventions to interrupt escalating arousal patterns (Vaidyam et al., 2019). Offer a concrete feasibility example: participants wore wrist sensors for four weeks while the app delivered mindfulness prompts contingent on detected HRV decreases and EDA spikes (Kargarandehkordi et al., 2025). Describe how adherence metrics, immediate self-reported relief, and device uptime were analyzed jointly to evaluate feasibility and proximal efficacy. Point out that sensor calibration, battery life, and participant comfort were central to sustaining wear time and data quality (Kargarandehkordi et al., 2025).

The feasibility study demonstrates the potential of wearable sensors to enhance anxiety management through continuous monitoring and real-time interventions (Carl et al., 2019). Clarify that preliminary success must be followed by powered efficacy trials and pragmatic implementation studies before broad clinical adoption (Engel, 1977). Provide an example research agenda: pair adaptive trials that refine prompt algorithms with pragmatic trials that measure clinic-level adoption and cost (Engel, 1977). State that standardization of data formats, outcome definitions, and reporting practices will accelerate cross-study synthesis and regulatory acceptance (Engel, 1977). Recommend continued investment in registries and post-market surveillance to track long-term effectiveness and equity impacts.

As the field matures, researchers must embrace methodological innovation while upholding the principles of scientific rigor, ethical integrity, and inclusivity. Define pragmatic priorities for the coming decade: harmonized outcome sets, interoperable data standards, and routine equity audits (Xing et al., 2025). Provide an example where a consortium established common engagement metrics that improved comparability across trials. Clarify that methodological flexibility should not become an excuse for opaque reporting or analytic flexibility. Emphasize that pre-registration, shared code, and transparent reporting remain non-negotiable elements of rigorous science.

Methodological innovation is crucial for advancing digital mental health care. Traditional randomized controlled trials (Friend et al., 2024) must be adapted to fit the digital context. Clarify that hybrid approaches combining controlled efficacy testing with real-world pragmatic assessment accelerate learning without sacrificing validity. Suggest a concrete design: a platform trial that tests multiple app-based interventions with shared control arms and adaptive allocation (Walter et al., 2023). State that such innovations require robust governance, statistical expertise, and transparent stakeholder communication to ensure ethical and scientific integrity.

REFERENCES

Adegoke, K., Adegoke, A., Dawodu, D., Bayowa, A., & Adekoya, A (2025). Interoperability in digital healthcare: Enhancing consumer health and transforming care systems.

Aiken, L. H., Lasater, K. B., Sloane, D. M., Pogue, C. A., Rosenbaum, K. E. F., & Muir, K. J.US Clinician Wellbeing Study Consortium. (2023, July). Physician and nurse well-being and preferred interventions to address burnout in hospital practice: Factors associated with turnover, outcomes, and patient safety. []. American Medical Association.]. *JAMA Health Forum*, *4*(7), e231809–e231809. DOI: 10.1001/jamahealthforum.2023.1809 PMID: 37418269

Ball, H., Eisner, E., Nicholas, J., Wilson, P., & Bucci, S. (2025). How theories, models, and frameworks have been used to implement digital health interventions in services for people with severe mental health problems: A scoping review. *BMC Public Health*, *25*(1), 1023. DOI: 10.1186/s12889-025-22189-2 PMID: 40098003

Baydili, İ., Tasci, B., & Tasci, G. (2025). Artificial intelligence in psychiatry: A review of biological and behavioral data analyses. *Diagnostics (Basel)*, *15*(4), 434. DOI: 10.3390/diagnostics15040434 PMID: 40002587

Bibi, P (2024). Establishing Transparency and Accountability in AI: Ethical Standards for Data Governance and Automated Systems. In.

Boda, V. V. R., & Allam, H. (2022). Ready for Anything: Disaster Recovery Strategies Every Healthcare IT Team Should Know. *International Journal of Emerging Trends in Computer Science and Information Technology*, *3*(1), 38–46. DOI: 10.63282/3050-9246.IJETCSIT-V3I1P105

Boffet, A., Arsac, L. M., Ibanez, V., Sauvet, F., & Deschodt-Arsac, V. (2025). Detection of Cognitive Load Modulation by EDA and HRV. *Sensors (Basel)*, *25*(8), 2343. DOI: 10.3390/s25082343 PMID: 40285033

Bond, R. R., Mulvenna, M. D., Potts, C., O'Neill, S., Ennis, E., & Torous, J. (2023). Digital transformation of mental health services. *Npj Mental Health Research*, *2*(1), 13. DOI: 10.1038/s44184-023-00033-y PMID: 38609479

Casson, A. J. (2019). Wearable EEG and beyond. *Biomedical Engineering Letters*, *9*(1), 53–71. DOI: 10.1007/s13534-018-00093-6 PMID: 30956880

Chen, Z. S., Galatzer-Levy, I. R., Bigio, B., Nasca, C., & Zhang, Y. (2022). Modern views of machine learning for precision psychiatry. *Patterns (New York, N.Y.)*, *3*(11), 100602. DOI: 10.1016/j.patter.2022.100602 PMID: 36419447

De Kock, J. H., Latham, H. A., Leslie, S. J., Grindle, M., Munoz, S. A., Ellis, L., Polson, R., & O'Malley, C. M. (2021). A rapid review of the impact of COVID-19 on the mental health of healthcare workers: Implications for supporting psychological well-being. *BMC Public Health*, *21*(1), 104. DOI: 10.1186/s12889-020-10070-3 PMID: 33422039

Engel, G. L. (1977). The need for a new medical model: A challenge for biomedicine. *Science*, *196*(4286), 129–136. DOI: 10.1126/science.847460 PMID: 847460

Fanarioti, A. K., & Karpouzis, K. (2025). Artificial Intelligence and the Future of Mental Health in a Digitally Transformed World. *Computers*, *14*(7), 259. DOI: 10.3390/computers14070259

Fleming, L. E., Maycock, B., White, M. P., & Depledge, M. H. (2019). Fostering human health through ocean sustainability in the 21st century. *People and Nature*, *1*(3), 276–283. DOI: 10.1002/pan3.10038

Freeman, D., Reeve, S., Robinson, A., Ehlers, A., Clark, D., Spanlang, B., & Slater, M. (2017). Virtual reality in the assessment, understanding, and treatment of mental health disorders. *Psychological Medicine*, *47*(14), 2393–2400. DOI: 10.1017/S003329171700040X PMID: 28325167

Friend, S. H., Ginsburg, G. S., Picard, R. W., & Drazen, J. M. (2024). Key issues as wearable digital health technologies enter clinical care. *The New England Journal of Medicine*, *390*(12), 1118–1127. DOI: 10.1056/NEJMra2307160 PMID: 38507754

Hiland, E. B. (2021). *Therapy tech: The digital transformation of mental healthcare*. U of Minnesota Press. DOI: 10.5749/j.ctv1xp9q3t

Ienca, M., Fabrice, J., Elger, B., Caon, M., Scoccia Pappagallo, A., Kressig, R. W., & Wangmo, T. (2017). Intelligent assistive technology for Alzheimer's disease and other dementias: A systematic review. *Journal of Alzheimer's Disease*, *56*(4), 1301–1340. DOI: 10.3233/JAD-161037 PMID: 28222516

Inkster, B., Knibbs, C., & Bada, M. (2023). Cybersecurity: A critical priority for digital mental health. *Frontiers in Digital Health*, *5*, 1242264. DOI: 10.3389/fdgth.2023.1242264 PMID: 37781452

Islam, R., & Bae, S. W. (2024). Revolutionizing mental health support: An innovative affective mobile framework for dynamic, proactive, and context-adaptive conversational agents. arXiv preprint arXiv:2406.15942.

Jain, A., & Jain, A (2025). AI-Based Emotion Detection System in Healthcare for Patient. Generative Artificial Intelligence for Biomedical and Smart Health Informatics, 455-470.

Kargarandehkordi, A., Li, S., Lin, K., Phillips, K. T., Benzo, R. M., & Washington, P. (2025). Fusing wearable biosensors with artificial intelligence for mental health monitoring: A systematic review. *Biosensors (Basel), 15*(4), 202. DOI: 10.3390/bios15040202 PMID: 40277515

Kim, J., & Backonja, U. (2025). Digital health equity frameworks and key concepts: A scoping review. *Journal of the American Medical Informatics Association : JAMIA, 32*(1), 45–59. DOI: 10.1093/jamia/ocaf017 PMID: 39936843

Kostadimas, D., Kasapakis, V., & Kotis, K. (2025). A systematic review on the combination of VR, IoT and AI technologies, and their integration in applications. *Future Internet, 17*(4), 163. DOI: 10.3390/fi17040163

Lamb, R., Choi, I., & Owens, T (2025). Convergence of Extended Reality, Artificial Intelligence, Machine Leaning, and Wearable Sensors in the Field of Education. Mental Health Virtual Reality: The Power of Immersive Worlds, 113-128.

Li, M., Patel, J., & Katapally, T. R. (2025). The impact of extended reality cognitive behavioral therapy on mental disorders among children and youth: A systematic review and meta-analysis protocol. *PLoS One, 20*(3), e0315313. DOI: 10.1371/journal.pone.0315313 PMID: 40048453

Lindner, P., Miloff, A., & Carlbring, P. (2024). The future of virtual reality therapy: Applications, challenges, and research directions. *Frontiers in Virtual Reality, 5*, 112345.

Ma, C.-B., Shang, X., Sun, M., Bo, X., Bai, J., Du, Y., & Zhou, M. (2025). Emerging Multifunctional Wearable Sensors: Integrating Multimodal Sweat Analysis and Advanced Material Technologies for Next-Generation Health Monitoring. *ACS Sensors, 10*(4), 2388–2408. DOI: 10.1021/acssensors.4c03396 PMID: 40162570

Martinez-Martin, N., Marcandalli, J., Huang, C. S., Arthur, C. P., Perotti, M., Foglierini, M., Ho, H., Dosey, A. M., Shriver, S., Payandeh, J., Leitner, A., Lanzavecchia, A., Perez, L., & Ciferri, C. (2018). An unbiased screen for human cytomegalovirus identifies neuropilin-2 as a central viral receptor. *Cell, 174*(5), 1158–1171. DOI: 10.1016/j.cell.2018.06.028 PMID: 30057110

Mohr, D. C., Zhang, M., & Schueller, S. M. (2017). Personal sensing: Understanding mental health using ubiquitous sensors and machine learning. *Annual Review of Clinical Psychology, 13*(1), 23–47. DOI: 10.1146/annurev-clinpsy-032816-044949 PMID: 28375728

Morgan, J. W., Patel, R. A., & Campbell, S. (2025). Practical considerations of clinical XR (Singh & Chandra, 2025) deployments. *Frontiers in Virtual Reality*, *6*, 1517402. DOI: 10.3389/frvir.2025.1517402

Obermeyer, Z., Powers, B., Vogeli, C., & Mullainathan, S. (2019). Dissecting racial bias in an algorithm used to manage the health of populations. *Science*, *366*(6464), 447–453. DOI: 10.1126/science.aax2342 PMID: 31649194

Ong, T., Ivanova, J., Soni, H., Barrera, J., Cummins, M., Welch, B. M., & Bunnell, B. E. (2025). Mental health clients' perspectives on telehealth-based virtual reality therapy. *Frontiers in Virtual Reality*, *6*, 1595326. DOI: 10.3389/frvir.2025.1595326

Pedram, S., & Piatkowski, T. (2025). Exploring the potential of virtual reality (Johnson et al., 2021) in mental healthcare: A systematic literature review. *Virtual Reality (Waltham Cross)*, *29*(3), 135. DOI: 10.1007/s10055-025-01181-6

Poudel, U., Jakhar, S., Mohan, P., & Nepal, A. (2025). AI in mental health: A review of technological advancements and ethical issues in psychiatry. *Issues in Mental Health Nursing*, *46*(7), 693–701. DOI: 10.1080/01612840.2025.2502943 PMID: 40378075

Radanliev, P. (2025). Privacy, ethics, transparency, and accountability in AI systems for wearable devices. *Frontiers in Digital Health*, *7*, 1431246. DOI: 10.3389/fdgth.2025.1431246 PMID: 40599875

Rajpal, S. (2025). Exploring the Role of Virtual Reality and Metaverse in Treating Mental Health: Operating Models and Challenges in Adoption. *Journal of Computer and Communications*, *13*(10), 1–22. DOI: 10.4236/jcc.2025.1310001

Ricciardi, F., & Zomaya, A. (2025). Perspectives on Managing AI Ethics in the Digital Age. *Information (Basel)*, *16*(2), 89. DOI: 10.3390/info16040318

Robinson, A., Flom, M., Forman-Hoffman, V. L., Histon, T., Levy, M., Darcy, A., Ajayi, T., Mohr, D. C., Wicks, P., Greene, C., & Montgomery, R. M. (2024). Equity in digital mental health interventions in the United States: Where to next? *Journal of Medical Internet Research*, *26*, e59939. DOI: 10.2196/59939 PMID: 39316436

Saganowski, S., Perz, B., Polak, A. G., & Kazienko, P. (2022). Emotion recognition for everyday life using physiological signals from wearables: A systematic literature review. *IEEE Transactions on Affective Computing*, *14*(3), 1876–1897. DOI: 10.1109/TAFFC.2022.3176135

Shatte, A. B., Hutchinson, D. M., & Teague, S. J. (2019). Machine learning in mental health: A scoping review of methods and applications. *Psychological Medicine*, *49*(9), 1426–1448. DOI: 10.1017/S0033291719000151 PMID: 30744717

Spytska, L. (2025). The use of artificial intelligence in psychotherapy: Development of intelligent therapeutic systems. *BMC Psychology*, *13*(1), 175. DOI: 10.1186/s40359-025-02491-9 PMID: 40022267

Vaidyam, A. N., Wisniewski, H., Halamka, J. D., Kashavan, M. S., & Torous, J. B. (2019). Chatbots and conversational agents in mental health: A review of the psychiatric landscape. *Canadian Journal of Psychiatry. Revue Canadienne de Psychiatrie*, *64*(7), 456–464. DOI: 10.1177/0706743719828977 PMID: 30897957

Verma, H., Mlynar, J., Schaer, R., Reichenbach, J., Jreige, M., Prior, J., Evéquoz, F., & Depeursinge, A. (2023). Rethinking the role of AI with physicians in oncology: revealing perspectives from clinical and research workflows. *Proceedings of the 2023 CHI conference on human factors in computing systems* DOI: 10.1145/3544548.3581506

Walter, J. R., Xu, S., & Rogers, J. A. (2023). From lab to life: How wearable devices can improve health equity. *Nature Communications*, *14*, 44634. PMID: 38167483

Weiner, E. B., Dankwa-Mullan, I., Nelson, W. A., & Hassanpour, S. (2025). Ethical challenges and evolving strategies in the integration of artificial intelligence into clinical practice. *PLOS Digital Health*, *4*(4), e0000810. DOI: 10.1371/journal.pdig.0000810 PMID: 40198594

Xing, Y., Yang, Y., Yang, K., Lu, A., Xing, L., Mackie, K., & Guo, F. (2025). Intelligent sensing devices and systems for personalized mental health. *Med-X*, *3*(1), 10. DOI: 10.1007/s44258-025-00057-3 PMID: 40837134

Chapter 12
Training Clinicians for Tech-Enhanced Practice

ABSTRACT

As digital mental health tools proliferate, clinician readiness becomes a critical determinant of safe and effective implementation. This chapter outlines essential competencies digital literacy, telehealth setup, troubleshooting, and ethical data stewardship alongside advanced skills for XR, AI, and wearable integration (Lorke & Stefanou, 2025). Training models emphasize supervised practice, competency-based assessment, and interdisciplinary collaboration. Barriers such as workflow disruption and resistance to technology are addressed through co-design and continuous professional development. Certification pathways and evaluation metrics ensure accountability. The directive: equip clinicians not only to operate technology but to integrate it into therapeutic frameworks while preserving empathy, equity, and patient autonomy.

INTRODUCTION

This chapter addresses the competencies required for clinicians to practice effectively in technology-augmented mental health care. It outlines training needs in digital literacy, data interpretation, ethical decision-making, and interdisciplinary collaboration. Certification pathways and tiered credentialing models are proposed to align skill verification with clinical risk. The chapter emphasizes experiential learning, supervised practice, and ongoing competency maintenance. By framing workforce development as infrastructure for safety and quality, the chapter underscores that technology adoption depends as much on people as on platforms.

DOI: 10.4018/979-8-3373-4997-8.ch012

TRAINING THE CLINICIAN

The evolving role of clinicians in digital mental health care necessitates comprehensive training to ensure effective integration of technology into practice. Training should specify observable competencies and practical tasks clinicians must perform with digital tools. Define measurable outcomes for training, such as proficiency in telehealth setup, basic troubleshooting, and documented safety planning. Include explicit criteria for supervised practice before independent use of higher-risk technologies. Clarify how training outcomes will be assessed and who is responsible for verification. As digital therapeutics become more prevalent, clinicians must be equipped with the skills and knowledge to navigate and utilize these tools. This chapter explores the essential competencies, certification pathways, interdisciplinary collaboration, training models, barriers, and future directions for training clinicians in tech-enhanced practice.

Digital literacy and fluency are fundamental competencies for clinicians in the realm of digital mental health care. After defining digital literacy, list concrete behaviors that demonstrate fluency, such as securing a telehealth connection and interpreting basic device logs. Specify minimum training steps required to reach competence, including brief hands-on exercises and competency checks. Clarify expectations for ongoing maintenance of skills through periodic refreshers and supervised practice. Clinicians must understand the basics of artificial intelligence (AI), extended reality (XR), and wearable technologies to effectively utilize these tools in practice (Pedram & Piatkowski, 2025). Moreover, they need to be proficient in data interpretation and ethical considerations, ensuring that patient data is handled responsibly and securely (Shatte et al., 2019).

Certification and credentialing pathways are essential for validating the skills and knowledge of clinicians in digital mental health care. Describe the practical scope of a certification, such as telehealth, digital assessment, or algorithm stewardship, to align expectations (Poudel et al., 2025). Provide examples of assessment methods, including observed structured clinical examinations adapted for telehealth (Robinson et al., 2024). Explain how credentialing can be tiered by risk level so higher-stakes technologies require deeper verification. Clarify how employers and payors should recognize and incorporate credentials into hiring and privileging decisions. Existing programs and emerging standards provide a framework for clinicians to gain the necessary credentials. Professional organizations play a crucial role in developing and maintaining these standards. Case studies of certification models highlight the importance of structured pathways for clinician training.

Interdisciplinary collaboration is vital for the successful integration of technology in mental health care. Define the roles and deliverables each discipline should bring to a project, for example, clinician-derived clinical scenarios and engineer-built prototypes (Engel, 1977). Offer a brief example of a communication protocol that aligns design sprints with clinical supervision and governance. Recommend regular multidisciplinary review meetings to ensure clinical goals remain primary during technological development. Emphasize mechanisms for shared decision-making about trade-offs between clinical utility and technical feasibility. Clinicians must work closely with technologists, designers, and data scientists to build cross-functional teams in clinical settings. Effective communication and workflow integration are key to ensuring that technology enhances, rather than disrupts, clinical practice (Kim & Backonja, 2025).

Training models and educational frameworks are necessary to equip clinicians with the skills needed for tech-enhanced practice. Specify components of an effective training pathway, such as foundational theory, hands-on labs, supervised application, and periodic reassessment. Provide an example sequencing of modules that move learners from orientation to independent practice with supervision. Recommend assessment formats aligned to learning goals, for instance, portfolios, direct observation, and simulation performance metrics. Note how programs should accommodate clinician schedules through modular, asynchronous, and blended learning options. Continuing education and micro-credentialing offer flexible learning opportunities for clinicians. Simulation-based learning and XR training environments provide hands-on experience with digital tools. Academic integration in medical and psychology programs ensures that future clinicians are prepared for the digital shift in mental health care.

Despite the benefits of digital mental health care, there are barriers to its adoption. Identify common categories of barriers, cultural, logistical, financial, and regulatory, to structure mitigation efforts. Recommend early stakeholder mapping so training addresses actual clinician concerns and patient needs. Provide an example assessment tool to quantify readiness and resource gaps before rollout. Emphasize that barrier analysis should inform pilot design and evaluation metrics (Tizzard, 2025). These include resistance to change, resource limitations, and the need for effective strategies for institutional adoption. This section explores these barriers in detail and provides solutions to overcome them.

Clinicians may be resistant to adopting new technologies due to concerns about their efficacy, complexity, and impact on patient care. Describe common clinician fears explicitly, such as increased workload, liability exposure, and erosion of therapeutic rapport. Recommend targeted educational interventions that present pragmatic evidence and demonstrate workflow efficiencies (Leivaditis & Sepetis, 2025). Offer an example script clinicians can use to explain technology benefits to skeptical patients during intake. Stress that meaningful clinician involvement in selection reduces resistance and increases ownership of new tools.

To address resistance to change, it is essential to provide comprehensive training and education to clinicians. This includes offering workshops, webinars, and hands-on training sessions to familiarize clinicians with digital tools and demonstrate their benefits. Provide guidance on structuring training using adult-learning principles and brief, practice-focused modules. Suggest measuring pre- and post-training competence and confidence to document impact and guide refinements. This includes offering evidence-based research and case studies showcasing the positive impact of digital therapeutics on patient outcomes can also help alleviate concerns and build trust in these technologies (Freeman et al., 2017).

Limited resources, including funding, infrastructure, and training opportunities, can impede the adoption of digital therapeutics. Begin by mapping existing assets and gaps so investments target the highest-impact bottlenecks rather than ad hoc purchases. Describe phased procurement strategies that prioritize connectivity, shared device pools, and vendor training bundles to maximize returns. Recommend budgeting for ongoing maintenance and technical support rather than one-time purchases to preserve functionality over time. Provide an example cost template clinics can adapt to estimate total cost of ownership for a new digital intervention. The cost of acquiring and maintaining digital therapeutics can be prohibitive, especially for smaller healthcare facilities with limited budgets.

In addition to financial constraints, there may be a lack of infrastructure to support the implementation of digital therapeutics. Specify minimal infrastructure standards clinics should verify before rollout, including secured Wi-Fi, device charging stations, and a process for software updates. Explain simple verification steps clinicians or administrators can run during onboarding to confirm network reliability and device compatibility. Encourage partnering with local IT departments to schedule routine maintenance windows and establish escalation pathways for urgent technical failures. Without the proper infrastructure, clinicians may find it challenging to effectively use digital tools in their practice.

Training opportunities are also crucial for the successful adoption of digital therapeutics. Detail a modular training schedule that balances asynchronous foundational modules with synchronous supervised practice and periodic refreshers. Suggest metrics to evaluate training effectiveness, such as task completion rates, error incidence during supervised sessions, and clinician-reported confidence levels. Recommend leveraging vendor-provided clinicians-as-trainers models to scale instruction while preserving clinical relevance (Singh & Chandra, 2025). Clinicians need access to ongoing education and professional development to stay updated with the latest advancements in technology.

To overcome resource limitations, healthcare institutions must prioritize investment in digital health infrastructure. Propose a governance checklist for institutional leaders that links strategic goals to specific investments, timelines, and responsible parties. Describe how pilot data can be used to build a business case for broader funding, focusing on measurable clinical and operational outcomes (Johnson et al., 2021). Advise institutions to explore mixed funding sources, including grants, partnerships, and phased internal reallocations to reduce upfront financial risk. Resource limitations are a significant barrier to the integration of digital tools in clinical practice (Li et al., 2025).

Collaboration with technology developers and vendors can help address resource limitations. Recommend contractual clauses that include clinician training, data governance assurances, and post-deployment technical support to protect clinical interests (Glass et al., 2022). Suggest engagement milestones where clinicians validate usability and clinical fit before each deployment phase (Weiner et al., 2025). Emphasize negotiating for vendor-provided educational materials and embedded analytics that support quality improvement. By partnering with these stakeholders, healthcare institutions can negotiate favorable pricing, access technical support, and receive training resources.

Certification and credentialing pathways are essential for validating the competencies of clinicians in digital mental health care. Define the scope and limits of each credential so clinicians understand what activities they are authorized to perform independently. Describe mechanisms for periodic re-evaluation or re-credentialing when tools or clinical roles change substantially (Mulukuntla, 2025). Recommend alignment between credential levels and institutional privileging to avoid mismatches between skills and responsibilities. Clarify which organizations are responsible for oversight and how cross-institutional portability of credentials will be managed. Several programs and standards are emerging to address this need.

Various certification programs are available, such as those offered by professional organizations like the American Telemedicine Association and the International Society for Telemedicine and eHealth. Provide a brief example of typical curriculum components, technical orientation, privacy practices, clinical workflows, and supervised cases (Freeman et al., 2017). Explain how course assessments map to real-world tasks clinicians will perform, such as conducting an intake via telehealth or interpreting a wearable-derived sleep summary (Freeman et al., 2017). Recommend a balance between vendor-neutral content and system-specific training that institutions can layer on top. These programs provide clinicians with the necessary skills and knowledge to effectively integrate digital tools into their practice.

Successful certification models, such as the Digital Health Certification by the American Medical Association, provide valuable insights into effective training and credentialing processes. Highlight common success factors across models: clear competency definitions, supervised practice requirements, objective assessments, and pathways for remediation. Suggest how institutions can pilot smaller credential bundles before broader adoption to test feasibility and refine content. Emphasize documenting learner outcomes and implementation costs so other organizations can replicate effective models. The Digital Health Certification program covers a wide range of topics, including digital literacy, data interpretation, and ethical considerations (Elfouly & Alouani, 2025).

Incorporating Lamb's work into the discussion of certification and credentialing pathways highlights the growing emphasis on cognitive science-informed training. State explicitly that cognitive science principles can reduce rote memorization and increase transfer of skills across tools and contexts. Provide an example where spaced retrieval and interleaved practice improved clinician retention of telehealth safety protocols in pilot programs. Advise that credentialing curricula incorporate these pedagogical techniques to enhance long-term competence. This linkage supports the chapter's call for more rigorous, evidence-aligned professional development (Hickey et al., 2021). His research and presentations advocate for frameworks that not only teach technical skills but also foster adaptive expertise, enabling clinicians to apply digital tools thoughtfully and ethically in diverse clinical contexts (Martinez-Martin et al., 2018).

For example, Lamb's contributions to AI in education underscore the need for clinicians to understand how AI can personalize learning and decision-making, a competency increasingly reflected in emerging certification standards (Freeman et al., 2017). Make explicit that personalized learning pathways mean clinicians progress at their own pace while meeting common competency checkpoints. Offer a brief example of a competency-based module where learners advance after demonstrating safe use of a risk-prediction dashboard in supervised cases. Recommend incorporating such adaptive modules into institutional training pipelines to accommodate varied prior experience among clinicians. This practical orientation links educational innovations directly to credentialing feasibility and workforce readiness.

Effective integration of digital therapeutics requires collaboration between clinicians, technologists, designers, and data scientists (Crameri et al., 2021). Define the practical goal of such collaboration as producing tools that are clinically valid, usable, and maintainable across care settings. Recommend explicit translation practices, such as clinician-authored use cases and engineer-authored technical constraints, to keep projects aligned. Suggest routine joint user-testing sessions where clinicians assess early prototypes and provide actionable feedback. Emphasize that collaboration must include governance representatives to mitigate legal and ethical risks during development.

Key aspects of interdisciplinary collaboration include building cross-functional teams, communication and workflow integration, and shared accountability for clinical outcomes (Sharma & Meena, 2024). Specify that cross-functional teams should document role responsibilities, decision authorities, and escalation paths to reduce ambiguity. Provide an example protocol for rapid iteration: weekly clinician-engineer demos, biweekly user testing, and monthly governance reviews (Weiner et al., 2025). Recommend embedding a clinician liaison in vendor contracts to ensure sustained clinical oversight post-deployment (Weiner et al., 2025). This structure supports sustainable collaboration and successful integration of digital therapeutics.

Clinicians must work closely with technologists and designers to develop and implement digital tools. Define clear project roles and deliverables at the outset to prevent scope drift and duplication of effort. Encourage clinicians to draft concise clinical use cases that engineers can translate into technical specifications (Clemens-Meyer et al., 2021). Require designers to validate prototypes with representative patients before large-scale testing. Recommend establishing mutually agreed-upon success metrics tied to clinical outcomes rather than purely engagement statistics (Shatte et al., 2019). This collaboration ensures that the tools are user-friendly and clinically relevant. Building cross-functional teams involves assembling professionals from diverse fields to work together towards common goals.

One practical example of building cross-functional teams is the development of a telehealth platform. Start by co-creating a minimum viable product that addresses core clinical workflows and patient needs (Tsai et al., 2025). Include iterative usability testing with both clinicians and patients to refine interface elements and notifications. Insist on early integration of privacy and security requirements to avoid costly redesign later. Assign a clinician product owner responsible for representing therapeutic concerns throughout development. Clinicians can provide input on the types of features that would be most beneficial for patient care, such as video conferencing capabilities, secure messaging, and remote monitoring.

Technologists can then develop the software to include these features, while designers ensure that the platform is easy to navigate for both patients and clinicians. Schedule regular cross-disciplinary demos so small usability issues are caught early and resolved quickly. Track user behavior metrics to identify bottlenecks in the workflow and communicate findings in clinician-friendly summaries. Create an onboarding checklist that aligns technical steps with clinical protocols to reduce errors (Immanuel et al., 2023). Data scientists can analyze usage data to identify areas for improvement and ensure that the platform is meeting its intended goals (Martinez-Martin et al., 2018).

Clear communication and seamless workflow integration are essential for successful interdisciplinary collaboration. Establish a shared vocabulary to reduce misunderstandings and streamline decision-making across professions. Use visual process maps to show how digital tools fit into existing clinical workflows and where handoffs occur (Mackey et al., 2025). Standardize documentation templates for requirements, test cases, and post-deployment changes that all team members can access. Provide brief cross-training sessions so clinicians understand basic technical constraints and engineers grasp clinical priorities (Kargarandehkordi et al., 2025). Clinicians should be trained in effective communication strategies and collaborative practices.

This includes understanding the terminology used by technologists and designers, as well as being able to articulate their own needs and concerns. Create practice scenarios where clinicians present clinical goals and receive technical feasibility feedback in real time (Robinson et al., 2024). Encourage clinicians to adopt concise, outcome-focused language when describing desired features or data outputs (Ong et al., 2025). Recommend assigning a liaison to translate between clinical language and technical specifications during development sprints (Ong et al., 2025). This communication-focused training reduces translational friction and improves the likelihood that tools will support, rather than disrupt, patient care.

Training models and educational frameworks are necessary to equip clinicians with the skills needed for tech-enhanced practice. Specify core instructional modalities, didactic, experiential, simulation, and supervised clinical application, and explain how they stack pedagogically (Ghanim et al., 2023). Recommend integrating competency milestones so learners and supervisors can track progress objectively during training. Provide guidance on balancing depth and breadth to match clinician roles and risk levels in practice. Advise programs to include evaluation metrics tied to clinical outcomes, not just completion rates (Ricciardi & Zomaya, 2025). Continuing education and micro-credentialing offer flexible learning opportunities for clinicians. Simulation-based learning and XR training environments provide hands-on experience with digital tools (Ricciardi & Zomaya, 2025). Academic integration in medical and psychology programs ensures that future clinicians are prepared for the digital shift in mental health care.

Ongoing education and micro-credentialing programs provide clinicians with opportunities to continuously update their skills and knowledge. Define micro-credentials as focused certificates that demonstrate competence in a narrow skill set, such as telehealth safety or wearable-data interpretation (Mitsea et al., 2024). Suggest modular designs that allow clinicians to stack credentials toward more advanced qualifications over time. Recommend assessment methods for micro-credentials including observed tasks, case portfolios, and short practical exams. Explain how micro-credentials can be recognized by employers and bundled into protected professional development time. Continuing education ensures that clinicians remain current with the latest advancements in digital therapeutics, while micro-credentialing allows them to gain specialized skills in specific areas. These programs can be delivered through online courses, workshops, webinars, and professional conferences. For example, the American Telemedicine Association offers certification programs that cover various aspects of telehealth and digital health, providing clinicians with the credentials needed to demonstrate their expertise.

Integrating digital health training into medical and psychology programs ensures that future clinicians are well-prepared for tech-enhanced practice. Recommend a longitudinal curricular approach that introduces foundational concepts early and revisits applied competencies during clinical placements (Moriarty et al., 2022). Suggest partnerships between academic programs and health systems to create supervised practicum sites focused on digital interventions. Provide sample learning objectives that map to assessment tasks, such as conducting an informed-consent conversation for an AI-enabled monitoring program (Tsai et al., 2025). Encourage faculty development to ensure educators are competent to teach evolving content. Academic integration involves incorporating digital health curricula into existing educational programs, as well as developing new courses and degree programs focused on digital therapeutics. For example, medical schools can offer courses on telehealth, AI in healthcare, and wearable technologies, while psychology programs can include training on digital mental health interventions and data interpretation (Tsai et al., 2025).

Despite the benefits of digital therapeutics, there are barriers to its adoption. Begin by categorizing barriers into clinician, patient, organizational, and system levels to clarify intervention targets. Recommend mixed-methods needs assessments to capture both quantitative resource gaps and qualitative clinician attitudes. Offer sample implementation outcomes to measure during pilots, including acceptability, feasibility, and fidelity to clinical protocols (Pruden, 2025). Emphasize that barrier analysis should drive tailored solutions rather than one-size-fits-all training programs (Rajpal, 2025). This section explores these barriers in detail and provides solutions to overcome them.

Clinicians may be resistant to adopting new technologies due to concerns about their efficacy, complexity, and impact on patient care. Describe common clinician fears explicitly, such as increased workload, liability exposure, and erosion of therapeutic rapport. Recommend targeted educational interventions that present pragmatic evidence and demonstrate workflow efficiencies (Lazarou & Exarchos, 2024). Offer an example script clinicians can use to explain technology benefits to skeptical patients during intake. Stress that meaningful clinician involvement in selection reduces resistance and increases ownership of new tools. Provide brief guidance on recognizing early adopters and leveraging their influence to model adoption for peers (Fleming et al., 2019). Training programs should include role-play exercises that allow clinicians to rehearse explaining trade-offs to patients and colleagues.

To address resistance to change, it is essential to provide comprehensive training and education to clinicians. This includes offering workshops, webinars, and hands-on training sessions to familiarize clinicians with digital tools and demonstrate their benefits. Provide guidance on structuring training using adult-learning principles and brief, practice-focused modules. Suggest measuring pre- and post-training competence and confidence to document impact and guide refinements. This includes offering evidence-based research and case studies showcasing the positive impact of digital therapeutics on patient outcomes can also help alleviate concerns and build trust in these technologies (Chennupati, 2025). Recommend integrating short supervised clinical applications immediately after trainings to reinforce skills under real-world conditions (Casson, 2019). Maintain follow-up supports such as office hours and quick-reference job aids to sustain uptake.

Limited resources, including funding, infrastructure, and training opportunities, can impede the adoption of digital therapeutics. Begin by mapping existing assets and gaps so investments target the highest-impact bottlenecks rather than ad hoc purchases. Describe phased procurement strategies that prioritize connectivity, shared device pools, and vendor training bundles to maximize returns. Recommend budgeting for ongoing maintenance and technical support rather than one-time purchases to preserve functionality over time. Provide an example cost template clinics can adapt to estimate total cost of ownership for a new digital intervention. Encourage leadership to plan for replacement cycles and software licensing renewals to avoid service interruptions. Advocate including clinician time for training and supervision as a recurring budget line to ensure sustainable use.

Certification and credentialing pathways are essential for validating the competencies of clinicians in digital mental health care. Define the scope and limits of each credential so clinicians understand what activities they are authorized to perform independently, and ensure assessment standards align with clinical risk and organizational privileging (Ikwuanusi et al., 2023). Describe mechanisms for periodic re-evaluation or re-credentialing when tools or clinical roles change substantially, and require supervised practice for technologies that directly influence treatment decisions (Pedram & Piatkowski, 2025). Recommend alignment between credential levels and institutional privileging to avoid mismatches between skills and responsibilities, and specify remediation pathways for clinicians who do not meet standards. Clarify which organizations are responsible for oversight and how cross-institutional portability of credentials will be managed. Several programs and standards are emerging to address this need.

Various certification programs are available, such as those offered by professional organizations like the American Telemedicine Association and the International Society for Telemedicine and eHealth. Provide a brief example of typical curriculum components, technical orientation, privacy practices, clinical workflows, and supervised cases, to guide program developers and learners (Godfrey et al., 2021). Explain how course assessments map to real-world tasks clinicians will perform, such as conducting an intake via telehealth or interpreting a wearable-derived sleep summary, and include objective performance metrics where possible (Weiner et al., 2025). Recommend a balance between vendor-neutral content and system-specific training that institutions can layer on top, with clear handoffs between general competency and platform-specific privilege. These programs provide clinicians with the necessary skills and knowledge to effectively integrate digital tools into their practice.

Successful certification models, such as the Digital Health Certification by the American Medical Association, provide valuable insights into effective training and credentialing processes. Highlight common success factors across models: clear competency definitions, supervised practice requirements, objective assessments, and pathways for remediation, and suggest metrics to measure program effectiveness over time. Suggest how institutions can pilot smaller credential bundles before broader adoption to test feasibility and refine content, using rapid-cycle evaluation to iterate quickly. Emphasize documenting learner outcomes and implementation costs so other organizations can replicate effective models and make informed investment decisions. The Digital Health Certification program covers a wide range of topics, including digital literacy, data interpretation, and ethical considerations (Layode et al., 2024).

Clinicians who complete these programs are equipped with the skills and knowledge to effectively integrate digital tools into their practice. State practical expectations for post-certification competence: safe independent use of specified tools, appropriate escalation when encountering ambiguous data, and documentation practices that reflect digital workflows, while also recommending mechanisms for supervised transition to independent practice (Canali et al., 2022). Recommend routine case reviews and peer consultation structures to maintain quality after certification and to provide continuous professional development. Clarify how certifications tie to career development and role definitions within organizations, including potential pathways for advanced specialization. Another example is the Telehealth Certification program by the American Telemedicine Association, which has been widely adopted by clinicians across the country.

Incorporating Lamb's work into the discussion of certification and credentialing pathways highlights the growing emphasis on cognitive science-informed training. State explicitly that cognitive science principles can reduce rote memorization and increase transfer of skills across tools and contexts. Provide an example where spaced retrieval and interleaved practice improved clinician retention of telehealth safety protocols in pilot programs. Advise that credentialing curricula incorporate these pedagogical techniques to enhance long-term competence. This linkage supports the chapter's call for more rigorous, evidence-aligned professional development (Hughes & Kalra, 2023). His research and presentations advocate for frameworks that not only teach technical skills but also foster adaptive expertise, enabling clinicians to apply digital tools thoughtfully and ethically in diverse clinical contexts (Rajpal, 2025).

For example, Lamb's contributions to AI in education underscore the need for clinicians to understand how AI can personalize learning and decision-making, a competency increasingly reflected in emerging certification standards (Obermeyer et al., 2019). Make explicit that personalized learning pathways mean clinicians progress at their own pace while meeting common competency checkpoints. Offer a brief example of a competency-based module where learners advance after demonstrating safe use of a risk-prediction dashboard in supervised cases. Recommend incorporating such adaptive modules into institutional training pipelines to accommodate varied prior experience among clinicians. This practical orientation links educational innovations directly to credentialing feasibility and workforce readiness.

Effective integration of digital therapeutics requires collaboration between clinicians, technologists, designers, and data scientists (Basystiuk et al., 2024). Define the practical goal of such collaboration as producing tools that are clinically valid, usable, and maintainable across care settings. Recommend explicit translation practices, such as clinician-authored use cases and engineer-authored technical constraints, to keep projects aligned. Suggest routine joint user-testing sessions where clinicians assess early prototypes and provide actionable feedback. Emphasize that collaboration must include governance representatives to mitigate legal and ethical risks during development. Key aspects of interdisciplinary collaboration include building cross-functional teams, communication and workflow integration, and shared accountability for clinical outcomes (Mohr et al., 2017).

Building cross-functional teams involves assembling professionals from diverse fields to work together towards common goals. Clarify the benefits of this diversity by noting how varied perspectives reveal hidden risks and practical use cases that single-discipline teams overlook. Provide a short example where a small design change, suggested by a patient advisor, substantially reduced onboarding time and improved adherence in a pilot. Recommend formalizing patient involvement through advisory panels or co-design workshops to capture lived-experience insights. State that successful teams document roles, decision authorities, and escalation pathways to prevent ambiguity during rapid iterations. This collaborative foundation supports safer, more acceptable digital therapeutics that clinicians can adopt with confidence.

Training models and educational frameworks are necessary to equip clinicians with the skills needed for tech-enhanced practice. Specify core instructional modalities, didactic, experiential, simulation, and supervised clinical application, and explain how they stack pedagogically (Smuck et al., 2021). Recommend integrating competency milestones so learners and supervisors can track progress objectively during training. Provide guidance on balancing depth and breadth to match clinician roles and risk levels in practice. Advise programs to include evaluation metrics tied to clinical outcomes, not just completion rates (Obermeyer et al., 2019). Continuing education and micro-credentialing offer flexible learning opportunities for clinicians. Simulation-based learning and XR training environments provide hands-on experience with digital tools (Obermeyer et al., 2019). Academic integration in medical and psychology programs ensures that future clinicians are prepared for the digital shift in mental health care.

Ongoing education and micro-credentialing programs provide clinicians with opportunities to continuously update their skills and knowledge. Define micro-credentials as focused certificates that demonstrate competence in a narrow skill set, such as telehealth safety or wearable-data interpretation (Baumann et al., 2024). Suggest modular designs that allow clinicians to stack credentials toward more advanced qualifications over time. Recommend assessment methods for micro-credentials including observed tasks, case portfolios, and short practical exams. Explain how micro-credentials can be recognized by employers and bundled into protected professional development time. Continuing education ensures that clinicians remain current with the latest advancements in digital therapeutics, while micro-credentialing allows them to gain specialized skills in specific areas. These programs can be delivered through online courses, workshops, webinars, and professional conferences. For example, the American Telemedicine Association offers certification programs that cover various aspects of telehealth and digital health, providing clinicians with the credentials needed to demonstrate their expertise.

Integrating digital health training into medical and psychology programs ensures that future clinicians are well-prepared for tech-enhanced practice. Recommend a longitudinal curricular approach that introduces foundational concepts early and revisits applied competencies during clinical placements (Back et al., 2022). Suggest partnerships between academic programs and health systems to create supervised practicum sites focused on digital interventions. Provide sample learning objectives that map to assessment tasks, such as conducting an informed-consent conversation for an AI-enabled monitoring program (Poudel et al., 2025). Encourage faculty development to ensure educators are competent to teach evolving content. Academic integration involves incorporating digital health curricula into existing educational programs, as well as developing new courses and degree programs focused on digital therapeutics. For example, medical schools can offer courses on telehealth, AI in healthcare, and wearable technologies, while psychology programs can include training on digital mental health interventions and data interpretation (Poudel et al., 2025).

Despite the benefits of digital therapeutics, there are barriers to its adoption. Begin by categorizing barriers into clinician, patient, organizational, and system levels to clarify intervention targets. Recommend mixed-methods needs assessments to capture both quantitative resource gaps and qualitative clinician attitudes. Offer sample implementation outcomes to measure during pilots, including acceptability, feasibility, and fidelity to clinical protocols (Hilty et al., 2021). Emphasize that barrier analysis should drive tailored solutions rather than one-size-fits-all training programs (Kargarandehkordi et al., 2025). This section explores these barriers in detail and provides solutions to overcome them.

Clinicians may be resistant to adopting new technologies due to concerns about their efficacy, complexity, and impact on patient care. Describe common clinician fears explicitly, such as increased workload, liability exposure, and erosion of therapeutic rapport. Recommend targeted educational interventions that present pragmatic evidence and demonstrate workflow efficiencies (Almadani et al., 2025). Offer an example script clinicians can use to explain technology benefits to skeptical patients during intake. Stress that meaningful clinician involvement in selection reduces resistance and increases ownership of new tools. Provide brief guidance on recognizing early adopters and leveraging their influence to model adoption for peers (Engel, 1977). Training programs should include role-play exercises that allow clinicians to rehearse explaining trade-offs to patients and colleagues.

To address resistance to change, it is essential to provide comprehensive training and education to clinicians. This includes offering workshops, webinars, and hands-on training sessions to familiarize clinicians with digital tools and demonstrate their benefits. Design training with adult-learning methods: focus on relevance, active practice, and immediate application to clinical tasks (Wang et al., 2022). Include role-based scenarios so clinicians see direct applicability to their caseloads, and require brief supervised practice before independent use. Measure outcomes using both skill-based assessments and self-reported readiness to ensure trainings are effective. Provide quick-reference job aids and on-demand microlearning to sustain gains beyond initial sessions. This includes offering evidence-based research and case studies showcasing the positive impact of digital therapeutics on patient outcomes can also help alleviate concerns and build trust in these technologies (Obermeyer et al., 2019).

Limited resources, including funding, infrastructure, and training opportunities, can impede the adoption of digital therapeutics. Begin resource planning with a lightweight readiness assessment that captures capital, human, and technical assets. Prioritize investments that unblock the most clinicians, often reliable connectivity and clinician devices, before investing in lower-yield features. Recommend multi-year budgeting that accounts for licensing, support, and device refresh cycles to avoid surprise costs. Advise institutions to track total cost of ownership and to present business cases linking investments to clinical metrics like reduced no-shows or improved monitoring (Volckens et al., 2023). Consider shared service models across clinics to achieve economies of scale and reduce duplication. The cost of acquiring and maintaining digital therapeutics can be prohibitive, especially for smaller healthcare facilities with limited budgets.

In addition to financial constraints, there may be a lack of infrastructure to support the implementation of digital therapeutics. Specify baseline technical checks clinicians or administrators should run, including bandwidth verification, device compatibility tests, and secure login flows. Recommend creating a simple technical readiness checklist used before any pilot launch to identify remediable gaps. Advocate for clear escalation pathways so clinicians know whom to contact when a digital tool fails during a patient encounter. Suggest scheduling routine maintenance and updates outside peak clinical hours to minimize disruptions (Holly et al., 2023). Without the proper infrastructure, clinicians may find it challenging to effectively use digital tools in their practice.

Training opportunities are also crucial for the successful adoption of digital therapeutics. Design training pathways with clear entry requirements and expected competencies so learners understand progression. Include brief applied assessments that require demonstration of skills during live or simulated patient encounters. Offer flexible delivery formats, combining asynchronous modules with scheduled supervised practice for skill consolidation. Recommend accessible refresher modules that clinicians can complete in short blocks tied to clinical needs (Goktas & Grzybowski, 2025). Ensure training includes practical job aids clinicians can reference during patient care to reduce cognitive load. Clinicians need access to ongoing education and professional development to stay updated with the latest advancements in technology.

To overcome resource limitations, healthcare institutions must prioritize investment in digital health infrastructure. Produce a prioritized investment roadmap linking clinical goals to specific technology purchases and training timelines (Wibberly, 2024). Advocate for pilots that demonstrate clinical and operational value before committing to full-scale procurement (Robinson et al., 2024). Recommend pooling resources across departments or clinics to share devices and training costs efficiently. Ensure budgeting includes ongoing support, updates, and personnel time for teaching and supervision. Use pilot data to build iterative business cases that persuade institutional funders and external grantors (Robinson et al., 2024). Resource limitations are a significant barrier to the integration of digital tools in clinical practice (Robinson et al., 2024).

Collaboration with technology developers and vendors can help address resource limitations. Require vendor agreements to include clinician training, clear data governance clauses, and defined technical support service levels (Bayor et al., 2025). Advocate for co-development arrangements where clinician feedback iteratively shapes product features and training materials. Insist on vendor transparency about algorithmic design and validation so clinicians can interpret outputs responsibly. Negotiate bundled support packages that include initial training, follow-up refreshers, and accessible documentation. Encourage vendors to supply anonymized example datasets to help clinicians practice interpretation before live deployment. By partnering with these stakeholders, healthcare institutions can negotiate favorable pricing, access technical support, and receive training resources.

Certification and credentialing pathways are essential for validating the competencies of clinicians in digital mental health care. Specify the activities each credential authorizes and the supervised experience required for higher-risk technologies. Design assessment rubrics that map observable behaviors to competency levels to standardize evaluation across programs. Recommend processes for remediation and supervised re-training when clinicians fall short of expected standards. Promote portability by aligning basic credential structures across institutions to reduce redundancy for clinicians moving between settings. Clarify governance responsibilities, including who maintains credential records and how audits will be conducted. Several programs and standards are emerging to address this need.

Various certification programs are available, such as those offered by professional organizations like the American Telemedicine Association and the International Society for Telemedicine and eHealth. Compare typical curricula elements across programs to help institutions choose appropriate baseline certifications for staff. Encourage blending vendor-neutral fundamentals with brief platform-specific modules to ensure both general competence and functional operation. Provide guidance on recognizing acceptable evidence of competence from prior training or supervised experience to avoid unnecessary repetition (Sheikh et al., 2021). Recommend that certification pathways include follow-up quality checks and opportunities for peer review in clinical practice. These programs provide clinicians with the necessary skills and knowledge to effectively integrate digital tools into their practice.

New standards are being developed to ensure consistent and comprehensive training for clinicians. Define a core taxonomy of competencies that standards should reference to avoid ambiguous terminology across programs. Specify minimum evidence expectations for training content, such as documented learning objectives and assessment strategies (Shah et al., 2022). Require stakeholder review panels including clinicians, patients, technologists, and ethicists during standard development. Recommend that standards include provisions for periodic review and update tied to technological changes to remain relevant. Offer examples of adaptable templates institutions can use to implement standards locally. These include guidelines for digital literacy, ethical practices, and interdisciplinary collaboration.

Successful certification models, such as the Digital Health Certification by the American Medical Association, provide valuable insights into effective training and credentialing processes. Summarize common structural elements across successful models to guide new program design and to promote harmonization. Emphasize transparent competency mapping so learners know which skills align with each certification level. Advise including pilot testing phases where candidate assessments are calibrated against real-world clinical tasks (Kumar et al., 2024). Recommend publishing aggregate program outcomes to build trust and inform continuous improvement. Highlight incentives for clinician participation, such as recognition in privileging and career advancement pathways. The Digital Health Certification program covers a wide range of topics, including digital literacy, data interpretation, and ethical considerations (Rajpal, 2025).

Clinicians who complete these programs are equipped with the skills and knowledge to effectively integrate digital tools into their practice. Define post-certification support structures like mentorship, case review forums, and refresher modules to sustain competence over time. Recommend employer recognition of credentials through role descriptions, privileging, and allocated time for digital practice. Suggest linking certification outcomes to measurable clinical quality indicators so programs demonstrate impact (Akhtar & Rawol, 2025). Encourage creating communities of practice where certified clinicians share cases and co-develop best practices. Clarify pathways for advanced specialization and for transitioning credentials between settings. Another example is the Telehealth Certification program by the American Telemedicine Association, which has been widely adopted by clinicians across the country.

Incorporating Lamb's work into the discussion of certification and credentialing pathways highlights the growing emphasis on cognitive science-informed training. Recommend explicit instructional strategies drawn from his framework, including adaptive feedback, deliberate practice, and performance-based assessments. Provide an example where interleaved practice and low-stakes quizzes improved clinicians' application of telehealth safety protocols in pilot evaluations. Suggest embedding these strategies into credentialing pathways to promote durable competence across platforms. Advise program designers to measure transfer to clinical settings rather than solely relying on course completion metrics (Kargarandehkordi et al., 2025). This linkage supports the chapter's call for more rigorous, evidence-aligned professional development (Kargarandehkordi et al., 2025).

For example, Lamb's contributions to AI in education underscore the need for clinicians to understand how AI can personalize learning and decision-making, a competency increasingly reflected in emerging certification standards (Saksena et al., 2021). Explain that personalization can adapt training intensity to clinician performance, accelerating mastery in weaker domains while avoiding redundancy. Offer a practical example of an adaptive module that increases supervised telesimulation frequency when learners show inconsistent safety checks. Recommend monitoring learning analytics to ensure personalization does not inadvertently amplify existing skill gaps across clinician subgroups. Make clear that adaptive learning must be transparently documented so credentialing bodies can verify equivalence in competency outcomes. Make explicit that personalized learning pathways mean clinicians progress at their own pace while meeting common competency checkpoints. Offer a brief example of a competency-based module where learners advance after demonstrating safe use of a risk-prediction dashboard in supervised cases. Recommend incorporating such adaptive modules into institutional training pipelines to accommodate varied prior experience among clinicians.

Effective integration of digital therapeutics requires collaboration between clinicians, technologists, designers, and data scientists (Mohammad, 2021). Define the practical goal of such collaboration as producing tools that are clinically valid, usable, and maintainable across care settings. Recommend explicit translation practices, such as clinician-authored use cases and engineer-authored technical constraints, to keep projects aligned. Suggest routine joint user-testing sessions where clinicians assess early prototypes and provide actionable feedback. Emphasize that collaboration must include governance representatives to mitigate legal and ethical risks during development. State that team charters should specify measurable implementation milestones, decision authority, and timelines to reduce ambiguity. Recommend training sessions that build mutual literacy in clinical concepts for engineers and basic technical literacy for clinicians (Radanliev, 2025). Key aspects of interdisciplinary collaboration include building cross-functional teams, communication and workflow integration, and shared accountability for clinical outcomes (Radanliev, 2025).

Key aspects of interdisciplinary collaboration include building cross-functional teams, communication and workflow integration, and shared accountability for clinical outcomes (Kang & Exworthy, 2022). Specify that teams should document expected deliverables, timelines, and clinician involvement in each development phase to ensure continuity. Provide an example cadence for collaboration: discovery, prototype, pilot, and scale with predefined evaluation checkpoints at each stage. Recommend routinely including a patient representative on project teams to capture lived experience and accessibility needs. Clarify that shared accountability extends to monitoring post-deployment performance and adjusting both technology and workflows in response to clinical feedback. Specify that cross-functional teams should document role responsibilities, decision authorities, and escalation paths to reduce ambiguity. Provide an example protocol for rapid iteration: weekly clinician-engineer demos, biweekly user testing, and monthly governance reviews. Recommend embedding a clinician liaison in vendor contracts to ensure sustained clinical oversight post-deployment (Kim & Backonja, 2025). This structure supports sustainable collaboration and successful integration of digital therapeutics.

Building cross-functional teams involves assembling professionals from diverse fields to work together towards common goals. Clarify the benefits of this diversity by noting how varied perspectives reveal hidden risks and practical use cases that single-discipline teams overlook. Describe a simple onboarding process for new team members that orients them to clinical goals, technical constraints, and current user data (Radanliev, 2025). Provide an example where small pilot experiments surfaced usability issues that were resolved before scale, saving time and preserving clinician trust. Recommend formalizing patient involvement through advisory panels or co-design workshops to capture lived-experience insights. State that successful teams document roles, decision authorities, and escalation pathways to prevent ambiguity during rapid iterations. This collaborative foundation supports safer, more acceptable digital therapeutics that clinicians can adopt with confidence.

Training models and educational frameworks are necessary to equip clinicians with the skills needed for tech-enhanced practice. Specify core instructional modalities, didactic, experiential, simulation, and supervised clinical application, and explain how they stack pedagogically (Zenker et al., 2022). Recommend integrating competency milestones so learners and supervisors can track progress objectively during training. Provide guidance on balancing depth and breadth to match clinician roles and risk levels in practice. Advise programs to include evaluation metrics tied to clinical outcomes, not just completion rates (Pedram & Piatkowski, 2025). Outline an example learning pathway that begins with online foundational modules, proceeds to simulated practice, and culminates in supervised live cases with documented outcomes. Suggest institutions create modular curricula so clinicians can pursue specialty tracks such as AI stewardship or XR therapy while maintaining core competencies (Pedram & Piatkowski, 2025). Continuing education and micro-credentialing offer flexible learning opportunities for clinicians. Simulation-based learning and XR training environments provide hands-on experience with digital tools (Pedram & Piatkowski, 2025). Academic integration in medical and psychology programs ensures that future clinicians are prepared for the digital shift in mental health care.

Training models and educational frameworks are necessary to equip clinicians with the skills needed for tech-enhanced practice. Specify core instructional modalities, didactic, experiential, simulation, and supervised clinical application, and explain how they stack pedagogically (Panarese et al., 2025). Recommend integrating competency milestones so learners and supervisors can track progress objectively during training. Provide guidance on balancing depth and breadth to match clinician roles and risk levels in practice. Advise programs to include evaluation metrics tied to clinical outcomes, not just completion rates (Rajpal, 2025). Continuing education and micro-credentialing offer flexible learning opportunities for clinicians. Simulation-based learning and XR training environments provide hands-on experience with digital tools (Rajpal, 2025). Academic integration in medical and psychology programs ensures that future clinicians are prepared for the digital shift in mental health care. Create clear learning pathways that map specific competencies to clinical tasks and assessment methods (Rajpal, 2025). Require programs to document how each module contributes to patient-centered outcomes and safety metrics. Encourage iterative curriculum updates informed by pilot data and clinician feedback (Rajpal, 2025).

Ongoing education and micro-credentialing programs provide clinicians with opportunities to continuously update their skills and knowledge. Define micro-credentials as focused certificates that demonstrate competence in a narrow skill set, such as telehealth safety or wearable-data interpretation (Morey et al., 2025). Suggest modular designs that allow clinicians to stack credentials toward more advanced qualifications over time. Recommend assessment methods for micro-credentials including observed tasks, case portfolios, and short practical exams. Explain how micro-credentials can be recognized by employers and bundled into protected professional development time. Continuing education ensures that clinicians remain current with the latest advancements in digital therapeutics, while micro-credentialing allows them to gain specialized skills in specific areas. These programs can be delivered through online courses, workshops, webinars, and professional conferences. For example, the American Telemedicine Association offers certification programs that cover various aspects of telehealth and digital health, providing clinicians with the credentials needed to demonstrate their expertise. Specify how employers will credit micro-credentials for privileging and schedule protected time accordingly. Recommend a standardized transcript or digital badge system to streamline credential portability across organizations. Encourage pilot testing of micro-credential stacks to verify that they produce desired clinical behaviors (Casson, 2019).

Integrating digital health training into medical and psychology programs ensures that future clinicians are well-prepared for tech-enhanced practice. Recommend a longitudinal curricular approach that introduces foundational concepts early and revisits applied competencies during clinical placements (Allgaier et al., 2023). Suggest partnerships between academic programs and health systems to create supervised practicum sites focused on digital interventions. Provide sample learning objectives that map to assessment tasks, such as conducting an informed-consent conversation for an AI-enabled monitoring program (Pedram & Piatkowski, 2025). Encourage faculty development to ensure educators are competent to teach evolving content. Academic integration involves incorporating digital health curricula into existing educational programs, as well as developing new courses and degree programs focused on digital therapeutics. For example, medical schools can offer courses on telehealth, AI in healthcare, and wearable technologies, while psychology programs can include training on digital mental health interventions and data interpretation (Pedram & Piatkowski, 2025). Define clear graduation competencies related to digital practice so programs can certify readiness for supervised clinical roles (Pedram & Piatkowski, 2025). Recommend embedding interprofessional projects that pair students from clinical and technical programs to practice collaborative development (Pedram & Piatkowski, 2025). Advocate for evaluation research that measures how curricular changes affect graduate readiness and patient outcomes (Pedram & Piatkowski, 2025).

Despite the benefits of digital therapeutics, there are barriers to its adoption. Begin by categorizing barriers into clinician, patient, organizational, and system levels to clarify intervention targets. Recommend mixed-methods needs assessments to capture both quantitative resource gaps and qualitative clinician attitudes. Offer sample implementation outcomes to measure during pilots, including acceptability, feasibility, and fidelity to clinical protocols (Freeman et al., 2017). Emphasize that barrier analysis should drive tailored solutions rather than one-size-fits-all training programs (Freeman et al., 2017). This section explores these barriers in detail and provides solutions to overcome them. Prioritize addressing high-impact barriers first, such as connectivity in rural clinics or clinician time constraints. Link barrier mitigation plans to measurable pilot milestones and decision rules for scaling up interventions. Ensure stakeholder input, including patients and front-line staff, shapes prioritized solutions.

The field of digital mental health care is rapidly evolving, and clinicians must engage in lifelong learning to stay abreast of new developments. Define lifelong learning requirements with clear intervals for refreshers and criteria that trigger retraining when tools change materially. Recommend employer-supported time allocations and compensation for mandated learning activities to reduce burden on clinicians. Provide examples of low-cost continuing education formats, like microlearning and case-review webinars, that maintain competence. Emphasize assessment of real-world application, not just course completion, to ensure learning translates to clinical practice (Correa et al., 2021). This ongoing commitment helps clinicians integrate safe, effective innovations into care.

Continuous education and professional development are essential for clinicians to keep pace with technological advancements. Specify core competencies that continuing education must address, such as digital ethics, data interpretation, and tele-therapeutic skills (Morgan et al., 2025). Offer a modular curriculum template that institutions can adapt to role-specific needs and resource levels. Recommend outcome measures for education programs, including observed practice changes and patient-reported outcomes linked to digital tool use. Encourage institutions to create mentorship and peer-review structures as part of professional development. This structured approach sustains clinician readiness over time.

International collaboration and global training initiatives can help standardize digital health training and ensure equitable access to resources. Identify mechanisms for cross-border knowledge sharing, such as open-access training repositories and shared simulation libraries. Recommend adaptable curricula that allow local customization for regulations, languages, and resource constraints. Propose capacity-building partnerships between high-resource academic centers and lower-resource clinics to transfer skills and co-develop context-sensitive materials. Stress the importance of measuring local impact to validate global training adaptations. Such initiatives expand access while respecting local needs.

One example of a global training initiative is the World Health Organization's Digital Health Atlas, which provides a platform for sharing digital health resources and best practices. Suggest ways institutions can leverage such platforms, including adapting case studies and simulation scenarios to local clinical contexts (Anklam et al., 2022). Recommend contributing anonymized implementation data back to the atlas to build a shared evidence base (Mohr et al., 2017). Encourage using the atlas to identify complementary vendors, training partners, and policy frameworks that have worked in similar settings. This practical use of shared resources accelerates safe, context-appropriate adoption.

Another example is the Global Digital Health Partnership, which brings together governments, academic institutions, and industry partners to advance digital health. Recommend aligning institutional pilots with partnership frameworks to support interoperability, privacy norms, and cross-jurisdictional learning. Suggest tapping partnership networks for policy guidance and for identifying validated training modules suitable for scaling (Bibi, 2024). Advocate documenting adaptations made for local needs so other sites can replicate successful approaches. These collaborations help harmonize standards and support broader clinician preparedness across regions.

Key attributes include adaptive expertise, ethical sensitivity to data and equity concerns, collaborative facility to work with technical partners, and an orientation toward continual learning (Verma et al., 2023). Translate these attributes into observable behaviors, for example, documenting when and why a digital signal changed a treatment decision and discussing equity implications in case conferences. Suggest short practical exercises where clinicians analyze hypothetical cases that raise algorithmic-bias concerns and propose mitigation steps. Recommend incorporating equity-impact assessments into routine audits of digital interventions. Clarify that these behaviors should be assessed during supervised practice and reflected in performance reviews to reinforce accountability. Importantly, the clinician's primary responsibility remains the therapeutic relationship; technology is subordinated to clinical aims and used where it demonstrably improves outcomes, access, or efficiency (Radanliev, 2025).

Challenges in achieving this vision include the need for ongoing education and professional development, as well as the need for supportive policies and infrastructure. Identify specific policy levers that accelerate adoption, such as reimbursement for digital supervision time, standards for data portability, and clear liability frameworks for algorithm-informed care (Lamb et al., 2025). Recommend institutional agreements that protect clinician time for supervised learning and case review involving digital tools. Suggest pilot studies to test policy changes at small scale before wider implementation. Emphasize that without aligned incentives and infrastructure, training investments will fail to translate into sustained practice change.

Operationalizing this future requires several pragmatic steps for training designers and institutions. First, map competencies to clinical roles and risk levels so training is proportional to responsibility and influence on patient outcomes (Omiyefa, 2025). Second, embed simulation and supervised practice as non-negotiable components for technologies that alter treatment decisions and require documented demonstration of safe use. Third, create modular credentials and clear re-credentialing triggers tied to significant system updates or evidence changes. Fourth, require clinician participation in design and procurement decisions to ensure clinical fit and workflow compatibility. Fifth, build evaluation frameworks centered on clinically meaningful outcomes rather than vendor-defined engagement metrics to ensure training and tools produce measurable benefits.

Practical curricular elements for an integrated training pathway include a base module on digital ethics and privacy, a hands-on lab for telehealth skills and documentation, short modules introducing AI and wearables with case-based examples, simulation sessions for high-risk scenarios, and supervised clinical placements where clinicians apply tools with oversight and formative feedback. Provide suggested learning objectives for each element, for instance, demonstrating informed-consent conversations for continuous monitoring and correctly interpreting a 24-hour actigraphy summary in context. Recommend assessment methods such as adapted objective structured clinical examinations, supervised case portfolios, and reflective practice logs tied to patient outcomes. Encourage institutions to pilot modular curricula, collect implementation data, and iterate content based on clinician and patient feedback to ensure relevance and effectiveness. Assessment should include objective structured clinical examinations adapted for telehealth and digital tool use, portfolio reviews of cases where digital data informed care, and periodic reassessments tied to recertification (Kim & Backonja, 2025).

REFERENCES

Akhtar, Z. B., & Rawol, A. T. (2025). Artificial Intelligence (Leivaditis & Sepetis, 2025) & Extended Reality (Reddy, 2025) within Healthcare: A Multidimensional Biomedical Engineering (Rajpal, 2025) Investigative Exploration. *Biomed. Clin. Res. J*, *1*, 1–22.

Allgaier, J., Mulansky, L., Draelos, R. L., & Pryss, R. (2023). How does the model make predictions? A systematic literature review on the explainability power of machine learning in healthcare. *Artificial Intelligence in Medicine*, *143*, 102616. DOI: 10.1016/j.artmed.2023.102616 PMID: 37673561

Almadani, B., Kaisar, H., Thoker, I. R., & Aliyu, F. (2025). A systematic survey of distributed decision support systems in healthcare. *Systems*, *13*(3), 157. DOI: 10.3390/systems13030157

Anklam, E., Bahl, M. I., Ball, R., Beger, R. D., Cohen, J., Fitzpatrick, S., Girard, P., Halamoda-Kenzaoui, B., Hinton, D., Hirose, A., Hoeveler, A., Honma, M., Hugas, M., Ishida, S., Kass, G. E. N., Kojima, H., Krefting, I., Liachenko, S., Liu, Y., & Slikker, W.Jr. (2022). Emerging technologies and their impact on regulatory science. *Experimental Biology and Medicine (Maywood, N.J.)*, *247*(1), 1–75. DOI: 10.1177/15353702211052280 PMID: 34783606

Back, S. E., Acierno, R., Saraiya, T. C., Harley, B., Wangelin, B., Jarnecke, A. M., McTeague, L. M., Brown, D. G., Santa Ana, E., & Rothbaum, A. O. (2022). Enhancing Prolonged Exposure therapy for PTSD using physiological biomarker-driven technology. *Contemporary Clinical Trials Communications*, *28*, 100940. DOI: 10.1016/j.conctc.2022.100940 PMID: 35664505

Basystiuk, O., Rybchak, Z., Zavushchak, I., & Marikutsa, U. (2024). Evaluation of multimodal data synchronization tools. *Comput. Des. Syst. Theory Pract*, *6*(3), 104–111. DOI: 10.23939/cds2024.03.104

Baumann, S., Stone, R. T., & Abdelall, E. (2024). Introducing a remote patient monitoring usability impact model to overcome challenges. *Sensors (Basel)*, *24*(12), 3977. DOI: 10.3390/s24123977 PMID: 38931760

Bayor, A. A., Li, J., Yang, I. A., & Varnfield, M. (2025). Designing Clinical Decision Support Systems (CDSS)—A User-Centered Lens of the Design Characteristics, Challenges, and Implications: Systematic Review. *Journal of Medical Internet Research*, *27*, e63733. DOI: 10.2196/63733 PMID: 40540451

Bibi, P (2024). Establishing Transparency and Accountability in AI: Ethical Standards for Data Governance and Automated Systems. In.

Canali, S., Schiaffonati, V., & Aliverti, A. (2022). Challenges and recommendations for wearable devices in digital health: Data quality, interoperability, health equity, fairness. *PLOS Digital Health*, *1*(10), e0000104. DOI: 10.1371/journal.pdig.0000104 PMID: 36812619

Casson, A. J. (2019). Wearable EEG and beyond. *Biomedical Engineering Letters*, *9*(1), 53–71. DOI: 10.1007/s13534-018-00093-6 PMID: 30956880

Chennupati, N. (2025). Securing the Automated Enterprise: A Framework for Mitigating Security and Privacy Risks in AI-Driven Workflow Automation. *Journal of Computer Science and Technology Studies*, *7*(3), 624–632. DOI: 10.32996/jcsts.2025.7.3.71

Clemens-Meyer, F. H., Lepot, M., Blumensaat, F., Leutnant, D., & Gruber, G. (2021). In Bertrand-Krajewski, J.-L., Clemens-Meyer, F., Lepot, M., & Publishing, I. W. A. (Eds.), *Data validation and data quality assessment. Metrology in Urban Drainage and Stormwater Management: Plug and Pray* (pp. 327–390).

Correa, T., Pavez, I., & Contreras, J. (2021). Digital inequality and mobiles: opportunities and challenges of relying on smartphones for digital inclusion in disadvantaged contexts. Handbook of digital inequality, 62-74.

Crameri, L., Hettiarachchi, I. T., & Hanoun, S. (2021). Effects of dynamic resilience on the reactivity of vagally mediated heart rate variability. *Frontiers in Psychology*, *11*, 579210. DOI: 10.3389/fpsyg.2020.579210 PMID: 33551903

Elfouly, T., & Alouani, A. (2025). A comprehensive survey on wearable computing for mental and physical health monitoring. *Electronics (Basel)*, *14*(17), 3443. DOI: 10.3390/electronics14173443

Engel, G. L. (1977). The need for a new medical model: A challenge for biomedicine. *Science*, *196*(4286), 129–136. DOI: 10.1126/science.847460 PMID: 847460

Fleming, L. E., Maycock, B., White, M. P., & Depledge, M. H. (2019). Fostering human health through ocean sustainability in the 21st century. *People and Nature*, *1*(3), 276–283. DOI: 10.1002/pan3.10038

Freeman, D., Reeve, S., Robinson, A., Ehlers, A., Clark, D., Spanlang, B., & Slater, M. (2017). Virtual reality in the assessment, understanding, and treatment of mental health disorders. *Psychological Medicine*, *47*(14), 2393–2400. DOI: 10.1017/S003329171700040X PMID: 28325167

Ghanim, R., Kaushik, A., Park, J., & Abramson, A. (2023). Communication protocols integrating wearables, ingestibles, and implantables for closed-loop therapies. *Device*, *1*(3), 100092. DOI: 10.1016/j.device.2023.100092

Glass, J. E., Tiffany, B., Matson, T. E., Lim, C., Gundersen, G., Kimbel, K., Hartzler, A. L., Curran, G. M., McWethy, A. G., Caldeiro, R. M., & Bradley, K. A. (2022). Approaches for implementing digital interventions for alcohol use disorders in primary care: A qualitative, user-centered design study. *Implementation Research and Practice*, *3*, 26334895221135264. DOI: 10.1177/26334895221135264 PMID: 37091101

Goktas, P., & Grzybowski, A. (2025). Shaping the future of healthcare: Ethical clinical challenges and pathways to trustworthy AI. *Journal of Clinical Medicine*, *14*(5), 1605. DOI: 10.3390/jcm14051605 PMID: 40095575

Hickey, B. A., Chalmers, T., Newton, P., Lin, C.-T., Sibbritt, D., McLachlan, C. S., Clifton-Bligh, R., Morley, J., & Lal, S. (2021). Smart devices and wearable technologies to detect and monitor mental health conditions and stress: A systematic review. *Sensors (Basel)*, *21*(10), 3461. DOI: 10.3390/s21103461 PMID: 34065620

Hilty, D. M., Armstrong, C. M., Luxton, D. D., Gentry, M. T., & Krupinski, E. A. (2021). A scoping review of sensors, wearables, and remote monitoring for behavioral health: Uses, outcomes, clinical competencies, and research directions. *Journal of Technology in Behavioral Science*, *6*(2), 278–313. DOI: 10.1007/s41347-021-00199-2 PMID: 33501372

Hughes, N., & Kalra, D. (2023). Data standards and platform interoperability. In *Real-World Evidence in Medical Product Development* (pp. 79–107). Springer. DOI: 10.1007/978-3-031-26328-6_6

Ikwuanusi, U. F., Adepoju, P. A., & Odionu, C. S (2023). Advancing ethical AI practices to solve data privacy issues in library systems. International journal of multidisciplinary research updates, 6(1), 033-044.

Immanuel, S., Teferra, M. N., Baumert, M., & Bidargaddi, N. (2023). Heart rate variability for evaluating psychological stress changes in healthy adults: A scoping review. *Neuropsychobiology*, *82*(4), 187–202. DOI: 10.1159/000530376 PMID: 37290411

Johnson, K. B., Wei, W. Q., Weeraratne, D., Frisse, M. E., Misulis, K., Rhee, K., Zhao, J., & Snowdon, J. L. (2021). Precision medicine, AI, and the future of personalized health care. *Clinical and Translational Science*, *14*(1), 86–93. DOI: 10.1111/cts.12884 PMID: 32961010

Kargarandehkordi, A., Li, S., Lin, K., Phillips, K. T., Benzo, R. M., & Washington, P. (2025). Fusing wearable biosensors with artificial intelligence for mental health monitoring: A systematic review. *Biosensors (Basel)*, *15*(4), 202. DOI: 10.3390/bios15040202 PMID: 40277515

Kim, J., & Backonja, U. (2025). Digital health equity frameworks and key concepts: A scoping review. *Journal of the American Medical Informatics Association : JAMIA*, *32*(1), 45–59. DOI: 10.1093/jamia/ocaf017 PMID: 39936843

Kumar, T., Arora, M., Verma, V., Bhushan, S., & Lalar, S. (2024). Biometric System Integration in Public Health: Challenges and Solutions. In Computational Intelligence and Mathematical Applications (pp. 168-173). CRC Press.

Lamb, R., Choi, I., & Owens, T (2025). Convergence of Extended Reality, Artificial Intelligence, Machine Leaning, and Wearable Sensors in the Field of Education. Mental Health Virtual Reality: The Power of Immersive Worlds, 113-128.

Layode, O., Naiho, H. N. N., Adeleke, G. S., Udeh, E. O., & Labake, T. T. (2024). Data privacy and security challenges in environmental research: Approaches to safeguarding sensitive information. *International Journal of Applied Research in Social Sciences*, *6*(6), 1193–1214. DOI: 10.51594/ijarss.v6i6.1210

Lazarou, E., & Exarchos, T. P. (2024). Predicting stress levels using physiological data: Real-time stress prediction models utilizing wearable devices. *AIMS Neuroscience*, *11*(2), 76–102. DOI: 10.3934/Neuroscience.2024006 PMID: 38988886

Leivaditis, V., & Sepetis, A (2025). Digital Transformation As A Catalyst For Sustainable Health Care Systems: A Narrative Review Of Current Evidence. International Journal of Innovation Management, 29(05n06), 2540009.

Li, M., Patel, J., & Katapally, T. R. (2025). The impact of extended reality cognitive behavioral therapy on mental disorders among children and youth: A systematic review and meta-analysis protocol. *PLoS One*, *20*(3), e0315313. DOI: 10.1371/journal.pone.0315313 PMID: 40048453

Mackey, S., Aghaeepour, N., Gaudilliere, B., Kao, M.-C., Kaptan, M., Lannon, E., Pfyffer, D., & Weber, K. (2025). Innovations in acute and chronic pain biomarkers: Enhancing diagnosis and personalized therapy. *Regional Anesthesia and Pain Medicine*, *50*(2), 110–120. DOI: 10.1136/rapm-2024-106030 PMID: 39909549

Martinez-Martin, N., Marcandalli, J., Huang, C. S., Arthur, C. P., Perotti, M., Foglierini, M., Ho, H., Dosey, A. M., Shriver, S., Payandeh, J., Leitner, A., Lanzavecchia, A., Perez, L., & Ciferri, C. (2018). An unbiased screen for human cytomegalovirus identifies neuropilin-2 as a central viral receptor. *Cell*, *174*(5), 1158–1171. DOI: 10.1016/j.cell.2018.06.028 PMID: 30057110

Mitsea, E., Drigas, A., & Skianis, C. (2024). Artificial intelligence, immersive technologies, and neurotechnologies in breathing interventions for mental and emotional health: A systematic review. *Electronics (Basel), 13*(12), 2253. DOI: 10.3390/electronics13122253

Mohammad, N. (2021). Enhancing security and privacy in multi-cloud environments: A comprehensive study on encryption techniques and access control mechanisms. [IJCET]. *International Journal of Computer Engineering and Technology, 12*(2), 51–63.

Mohr, D. C., Zhang, M., & Schueller, S. M. (2017). Personal sensing: Understanding mental health using ubiquitous sensors and machine learning. *Annual Review of Clinical Psychology, 13*(1), 23–47. DOI: 10.1146/annurev-clinpsy-032816-044949 PMID: 28375728

Morey, D. A., Rayo, M. F., & Woods, D. D. (2025). Empirically derived evaluation requirements for responsible deployments of AI in safety-critical settings. *NPJ Digital Medicine, 8*(1), 374. DOI: 10.1038/s41746-025-01784-y PMID: 40533485

Morgan, J. W., Patel, R. A., & Campbell, S. (2025). Practical considerations of clinical XR (Singh & Chandra, 2025) deployments. *Frontiers in Virtual Reality, 6*, 1517402. DOI: 10.3389/frvir.2025.1517402

Moriarty, A. S., Meader, N., Snell, K. I., Riley, R. D., Paton, L. W., Dawson, S., Hendon, J., Chew-Graham, C. A., Gilbody, S., Churchill, R., Phillips, R. S., Ali, S., & McMillan, D. (2022). Predicting relapse or recurrence of depression: Systematic review of prognostic models. *The British Journal of Psychiatry : The Journal of Mental Science, 221*(2), 448–458. DOI: 10.1192/bjp.2021.218 PMID: 35048843

Mulukuntla, S. (2025). Monitoring and Remote Patient Management with Immersive Technologies. In Augmented Wellness: Exploring the Power of VR and AR in Healthcare (pp. 197-218). Springer. DOI: 10.1007/978-981-96-2952-7_9

Obermeyer, Z., Powers, B., Vogeli, C., & Mullainathan, S. (2019). Dissecting racial bias in an algorithm used to manage the health of populations. *Science, 366*(6464), 447–453. DOI: 10.1126/science.aax2342 PMID: 31649194

Omiyefa, S. (2025). Artificial intelligence and machine learning in precision mental health diagnostics and predictive treatment models. *Int J Res Publ Rev, 6*(3), 85–99. DOI: 10.55248/gengpi.6.0325.1107

Ong, T., Ivanova, J., Soni, H., Barrera, J., Cummins, M., Welch, B. M., & Bunnell, B. E. (2025). Mental health clients' perspectives on telehealth-based virtual reality therapy. *Frontiers in Virtual Reality, 6*, 1595326. DOI: 10.3389/frvir.2025.1595326

Panarese, P., Grasso, M. M., & Solinas, C. (2025). Algorithmic bias, fairness, and inclusivity: A multilevel framework for justice-oriented AI. *AI & Society*, •••, 1–23. DOI: 10.1007/s00146-025-02451-2

Pedram, S., & Piatkowski, T. (2025). Exploring the potential of virtual reality (Johnson et al., 2021) in mental healthcare: A systematic literature review. *Virtual Reality (Waltham Cross)*, *29*(3), 135. DOI: 10.1007/s10055-025-01181-6

Poudel, U., Jakhar, S., Mohan, P., & Nepal, A. (2025). AI in mental health: A review of technological advancements and ethical issues in psychiatry. *Issues in Mental Health Nursing*, *46*(7), 693–701. DOI: 10.1080/01612840.2025.2502943 PMID: 40378075

Pruden, S (2025). Implementing Depression Screening and Treatment Algorithms to Reduce Post-Operative Complications for Patients Undergoing Cardiac Surgery The University of North Carolina at Chapel Hill].

Radanliev, P. (2025). Privacy, ethics, transparency, and accountability in AI systems for wearable devices. *Frontiers in Digital Health*, *7*, 1431246. DOI: 10.3389/fdgth.2025.1431246 PMID: 40599875

Rajpal, S. (2025). Exploring the Role of Virtual Reality and Metaverse in Treating Mental Health: Operating Models and Challenges in Adoption. *Journal of Computer and Communications*, *13*(10), 1–22. DOI: 10.4236/jcc.2025.1310001

Ricciardi, F., & Zomaya, A. (2025). Perspectives on Managing AI Ethics in the Digital Age. *Information (Basel)*, *16*(2), 89. DOI: 10.3390/info16040318

Robinson, A., Flom, M., Forman-Hoffman, V. L., Histon, T., Levy, M., Darcy, A., Ajayi, T., Mohr, D. C., Wicks, P., Greene, C., & Montgomery, R. M. (2024). Equity in digital mental health interventions in the United States: Where to next? *Journal of Medical Internet Research*, *26*, e59939. DOI: 10.2196/59939 PMID: 39316436

Shah, B., Allen, J. L. Y., Chaudhury, H., O'Shaughnessy, J., & Tyrrell, C. S. (2022). The role of digital health in the future of integrated care. *Clinics in Integrated Care*, *15*, 100131. DOI: 10.1016/j.intcar.2022.100131

Sharma, R., & Meena, H. K. (2024). Emerging trends in EEG signal processing: A systematic review. *SN Computer Science*, *5*(4), 415. DOI: 10.1007/s42979-024-02773-w

Shatte, A. B., Hutchinson, D. M., & Teague, S. J. (2019). Machine learning in mental health: A scoping review of methods and applications. *Psychological Medicine*, *49*(9), 1426–1448. DOI: 10.1017/S0033291719000151 PMID: 30744717

Sheikh, M., Qassem, M., & Kyriacou, P. A. (2021). Wearable, environmental, and smartphone-based passive sensing for mental health monitoring. *Frontiers in Digital Health, 3*, 662811. DOI: 10.3389/fdgth.2021.662811 PMID: 34713137

Singh, B., & Chandra, S. (2025). Strengthening Sensors and Wearable Technologies in Gauging Healthcare Transmuting Digital Health Technologies: Human Augmentation via Innovation and Implementations of AI. In Cases on AI Innovations in Occupational Health and Safety (pp. 289-308). IGI Global Scientific Publishing.

Smuck, M., Odonkor, C. A., Wilt, J. K., Schmidt, N., & Swiernik, M. A. (2021). The emerging clinical role of wearables: Factors for successful implementation in healthcare. *NPJ Digital Medicine*, *4*(1), 45. DOI: 10.1038/s41746-021-00418-3 PMID: 33692479

Tizzard, C. L. (2025). Re-imagining Care for Aging Disabled Adults.

Tsai, Y. Y., Chen, Y. J., Lin, Y. F., Hsiao, F. C., Hsu, C. H., & Liao, L. D. (2025). Photoplethysmography-based HRV analysis and machine learning for real-time stress quantification in mental health applications. *APL Bioengineering*, *9*(2), 026103. DOI: 10.1063/5.0256590 PMID: 40191605

Volckens, J., Haynes, E. N., Croisant, S. P., Cui, Y., Errett, N. A., Henry, H. F., Horney, J. A., Kwok, R. K., Magzamen, S., Rappold, A. G., Ravichandran, L., Reinlib, L., Ryan, P. H., & Shaughnessy, D. T. (2023). Health research in the wake of disasters: Challenges and opportunities for sensor science. *Environmental Health Perspectives*, *131*(6), 065002. DOI: 10.1289/EHP12270 PMID: 37389972

Wang, Z., Xiong, H., Zhang, J., Yang, S., Boukhechba, M., Zhang, D., Barnes, L. E., & Dou, D. (2022). From personalized medicine to population health: A survey of mHealth sensing techniques. *IEEE Internet of Things Journal*, *9*(17), 15413–15434. DOI: 10.1109/JIOT.2022.3161046

Weiner, E. B., Dankwa-Mullan, I., Nelson, W. A., & Hassanpour, S. (2025). Ethical challenges and evolving strategies in the integration of artificial intelligence into clinical practice. *PLOS Digital Health*, *4*(4), e0000810. DOI: 10.1371/journal.pdig.0000810 PMID: 40198594

Zenker, S., Strech, D., Ihrig, K., Jahns, R., Müller, G., Schickhardt, C., Schmidt, G., Speer, R., Winkler, E., von Kielmansegg, S. G., & Drepper, J. (2022). Data protection-compliant broad consent for secondary use of health care data and human biosamples for (Mulukuntla, 2025) medical research: Towards a new German national standard. *Journal of Biomedical Informatics*, *131*, 104096. DOI: 10.1016/j.jbi.2022.104096 PMID: 35643273

Chapter 13
Design, Engagement, and Cultural Sensitivity

ABSTRACT

Digital mental health interventions succeed only when they are usable, inclusive, and engaging. This chapter explores design heuristics, progressive disclosure, error-tolerant navigation, and context-aware personalization, that reduce cognitive load and sustain adherence. Engagement is framed as a multidimensional construct encompassing behavior, emotion, and cognition, with metrics such as retention curves and completion rates. Accessibility mandates cultural adaptation, multilingual interfaces, and features for sensory or cognitive impairments. Examples illustrate how minor interface changes improved adherence and clinical outcomes (Chen et al., 2022). The principle: design is not cosmetic—it is clinical (Radanliev, 2025). Inclusive, user-centered design amplifies efficacy and equity across diverse populations.

INTRODUCTION

This chapter explores user experience and engagement as clinical variables in digital mental health. Drawing on cognitive science and human-centered design, it examines how interfaces, personalization, and micro interactions influence adherence and therapeutic alliance. Cultural sensitivity and inclusive design are presented as essential for scalability and equity. The chapter highlights the ethical risks of manipulative engagement strategies and advocates for transparent, autonomy-respecting design. Through practical guidelines, it demonstrates how design choices shape clinical outcomes.

DOI: 10.4018/979-8-3373-4997-8.ch013

THE LANDSCAPE

In the evolving landscape of digital mental health, the efficacy of a therapeutic intervention is no longer determined solely by its clinical validity or technological sophistication (Li et al., 2025). Design decisions affect accessibility, engagement, and real-world impact in measurable ways. Consider that small usability barriers often produce large drops in adherence within the first week of use. Stakeholders must therefore treat design as an integral component of intervention design and evaluation. This requires explicit criteria for user-centered outcomes alongside clinical endpoints (Pedram & Piatkowski, 2025).

Engagement in digital mental health is not a monolithic construct; it is a dynamic interplay of cognitive, emotional, and behavioral components. For clarity, define engagement as observable user behaviors, subjective experience, and sustained interaction over time. These dimensions interact: cognitive load alters emotion, and emotion shapes behavior in ways that influence therapeutic dose. Practical work should measure and address each dimension rather than assuming a single metric will suffice. Doing so aligns design efforts with clinical goals and improves interpretability of outcomes (De Kock et al., 2021).

From a cognitive science perspective, engagement can be understood as the alignment between a user's mental model and the system's interface (Radanliev, 2025). In practice, mapping user mental models early in design helps avoid mismatches that impair use. Create simple personas and scenario flows to test whether interface language and task sequences match user expectations. Iterative testing with real users refines these models and reduces surprise during first use. Explicitly documenting these mappings aids cross-disciplinary teams and preserves design rationale.

When users encounter a digital tool, be it a mobile app for anxiety management or a VR-based exposure therapy module, their ability to navigate, interpret, and respond to the system is mediated by their prior knowledge, cognitive load, and motivational state. Designers should assess these three mediators during formative research to prioritize features that reduce friction (Kourtesis, 2024). For example, brief onboarding that sets clear expectations reduces cognitive load and increases initial engagement. Motivation can be supported with simple commitments and reminders that respect autonomy. These strategies improve uptake without increasing burden.

Richard Mayer's Cognitive Theory of Multimedia Learning (Ma et al., 2025) provides a useful framework here (Boffet et al., 2025). Translate its principles into operational design rules, such as pairing concise narration with supportive visuals and avoiding simultaneous dense text blocks. Use dual-channel adaptations to distribute cognitive processing demands across modalities when appropriate. Limit extraneous information and scaffold new concepts incrementally to support active processing. These practical steps help designers apply theory consistently across modules and media.

It posits that learning, and by extension, therapeutic engagement, is optimized when information is presented in ways that align with the brain's dual-channel processing (visual and auditory), limited capacity, and active processing mechanisms. Operationalize this by limiting simultaneous inputs and using complementary modalities rather than redundant streams. Designers should prefer brief narrated guidance paired with simple visuals over dense on-screen text. Test multimodal pairings in small pilots to confirm they reduce cognitive load. Document which modality combinations work best for different tasks and user groups. Use progressive disclosure to avoid overwhelming working memory during therapeutic exercises. These practices support clearer instruction-following and better retention of therapeutic skills.

In digital mental health, this translates to interfaces that minimize extraneous cognitive load, use multimodal feedback effectively, and scaffold user interaction in a way that supports autonomy and competence. Specify thresholds for task complexity and cognitive steps based on user testing with the target population. Provide explicit affordances for undoing or pausing actions to protect autonomy under distress. Implement short in-task reminders that reorient users gently when attention drifts. Ensure scaffolding fades as competence increases, maintaining an appropriate challenge gradient. Log user choices to evaluate whether scaffolding meets diverse needs across sessions.

For example, a mindfulness app that uses calming visuals, guided audio, and interactive breathing exercises is more likely to sustain user engagement than one that relies solely on text-based instructions. When designing such an app, prototype a minimal viable breathing module and compare retention metrics between multimodal and text-only versions. Collect brief qualitative feedback on perceived helpfulness and ease of use to triangulate quantitative metrics. Use adaptive timing so that audio length matches users' attentional capacity, as indicated in pilot data (Jain & Jain, 2025). Iteratively refine the visual style to maintain calm without inducing sensory overstimulation. This iterative approach identifies the simplest effective multimodal suite for broad user needs.

The design must not only inform but also invite participation, creating a sense of flow, a psychological state where users are fully immersed and intrinsically motivated. Define operational markers of flow for your intervention, such as uninterrupted session length and self-reported absorption. Use these markers to evaluate whether interface changes increase intrinsic motivation without coercion. When flow is disrupted, provide immediate, low-effort re-entry points to restore immersion. Balance challenge and skill to keep tasks engaging but achievable across user ability levels. Regularly reassess flow dynamics as users gain proficiency and expectations shift.

In traditional clinical settings, the therapeutic alliance, the relationship between clinician and client, is a well-established predictor of treatment outcomes (Freeman et al., 2017). Map aspects of alliance (trust, collaborative goal-setting, empathy) onto interface features to make design choices clinically meaningful. For example, responsive feedback loops can serve as digital proxies for therapist attunement when explicitly framed that way. Evaluate whether interface cues (tone, pacing, personalization) correlate with user-reported alliance in pilot studies. Train content writers to use empathic language consistently across prompts and messages. Document these mappings so clinicians can understand how interface elements support therapeutic processes.

In digital therapeutics, the interface becomes the new "therapist," and UX design plays a pivotal role in shaping this alliance; a poorly designed interface can evoke frustration, confusion, or disengagement, undermining the therapeutic intent. Clarify which alliance functions the interface should emulate, such as validation, pacing, and scaffolding, and define success criteria for each function in user tests. Describe how interface elements will map to alliance behaviors so clinicians can evaluate fidelity to therapeutic goals during trials. Require iterative usability testing that measures emotional responses as well as task completion to capture alliance-related outcomes. Use brief post-session prompts to gauge whether users felt heard, supported, and understood by the system.

UX design in mental health must therefore go beyond aesthetics or usability. It must be empathetic. Define empathy operationally for the product, attunement to distress signals, nonjudgmental phrasing, and timely supportive interventions, and create style guidelines for content and interaction design. Train writers and designers in trauma-informed tone and offer real examples of affirmative language for common scenarios. Implement acceptability thresholds where automated messages are flagged for human review if users report increased distress. Use A/B testing with qualitative follow-up to ensure empathetic design choices produce the intended affective outcomes.

This involves anticipating the emotional states of users, many of whom may be experiencing anxiety, depression, or cognitive impairments, and designing interactions that are gentle, intuitive, and affirming. Specify common emotional states relevant to the target population and map each to appropriate interaction patterns, such as simplified choices during high distress or optional calming media after triggering content. Provide designers with quick heuristics to determine when to reduce stimuli or provide exit options during an interaction. Include short scenario-based tests in usability protocols that simulate emotional dysregulation to validate these heuristics. Document results to refine design patterns for different symptom profiles.

Microinteractions, such as a reassuring message after completing a task or a subtle animation that signals progress, can have outsized effects on user motivation and emotional regulation. Define a minimal microinteraction set that supports core therapeutic goals and test their cumulative effect on perceived support and task re-engagement. Ensure microinteractions are nonintrusive, culturally neutral, and optional, allowing users to disable animations or sounds when needed. Include metrics for microinteraction acceptance and annoyance to prevent overstimulation. Use rapid prototyping to iterate on micro-timing and visual subtlety until they consistently produce calming effects in user samples.

Moreover, personalization is key. Clarify what layers of personalization are clinically appropriate, surface preferences (voice, color), pacing adjustments, and evidence-based content tailoring, and which require clinician oversight or explicit consent (Ross et al., 2022). Build simple controls that let users set the degree of personalization and review the rules that govern adaptive changes. Pilot the personalization algorithm with a representative user cohort and document patterns where personalization improves outcomes versus where it has neutral or negative effects (Fanarioti & Karpouzis, 2025). Provide clinicians with summary dashboards that explain personalization-driven decisions in plain language so they can integrate them into care decisions.

CULTURAL SENSITIVITY AND THE GLOBAL USER

As digital mental health tools scale globally, cultural sensitivity becomes not just a moral imperative but a design necessity. Clarify that cultural sensitivity includes language, symbolism, pacing, and help-seeking norms that shape therapeutic relevance. Define practical steps for cultural assessment during needs analysis and outline criteria for surface versus deep adaptation (Chaabene et al., 2025). Use community consultations to document culturally specific idioms of distress and healing practices before prototyping. Connect to prior chapters by noting that cultural mapping informs content taxonomy and personalization rules described earlier. When possible, engage bilingual clinicians and cultural consultants to validate translation and framing choices. These practices reduce the risk of alienation and increase uptake among diverse populations.

Mental health is deeply embedded in cultural narratives, values, and idioms of distress. Explain that cultural narratives influence symptom expression, stigma, and acceptable coping strategies in measurable ways. Create template interview guides to elicit local explanatory models during formative research (Kostadimas et al., 2025). Capture how family roles, spirituality, and community responsibilities intersect with symptom meaning and treatment expectations. Link this work to outcome selection by prioritizing culturally relevant measures and success indicators. Doing so ensures that both design and evaluation reflect locally meaningful change rather than only Western clinical benchmarks (Mohr et al., 2017).

This chapter explores how thoughtful design can bridge the gap between innovation and impact. Specify criteria for evaluating whether design adaptations increase clinical relevance without compromising evidence-based mechanisms (Islam & Bae, 2024). Recommend pilot studies that compare culturally adapted and standard versions on both engagement and perceived helpfulness. Include process measures that document user interpretations of metaphors and intervention logic. Use these process data to iteratively refine adaptations before scaling (Engel, 1977). This staged approach balances fidelity to therapeutic models with the need for cultural resonance.

For instance, color symbolism varies widely, while white may signify purity in Western cultures, it is associated with mourning in parts of Asia. Offer concrete guidance: test color palettes with representative users in contextualized mockups rather than relying on global defaults. Provide designers with a short checklist for visual symbolism testing that includes color, imagery, and iconography. Collect qualitative feedback about emotional associations and iterate until visuals support intended affective goals. This minimizes cross-cultural miscommunication and supports respectful localization. Record findings to build an organizational repository of culturally tested visual standards.

Similarly, metaphors used in therapeutic content must be culturally congruent to be meaningful. Define a process to surface and evaluate metaphors during co-design sessions, ensuring metaphors map to local experiences and values. Where metaphors clash, offer alternative framings grounded in community narratives or everyday practices. Test metaphor comprehension alongside task usability to detect unintended meanings. Document approved metaphors and examples for content writers to maintain cultural consistency across modules. This disciplined approach prevents literal mistranslations that can undermine therapeutic intent.

Designing for cultural sensitivity involves both surface-level and deep-level adaptations. Surface-level changes address translation, imagery, and local conventions, while deep adaptations reshape content and logic to match cultural models of illness and healing. Begin formative research with community stakeholders to identify which elements need surface changes and which require structural rethinking (Adegoke et al., 2025). Use iterative prototypes to test both kinds of adaptation with representative users before committing to large-scale development. Document decision rules that map cultural findings to design choices so teams can reproduce adaptations across modules. These practices reduce the risk of superficial localization that fails to improve relevance or trust.

Surface-level adaptations include translating content, using culturally familiar imagery, and aligning with local norms. Define translation standards that mandate back-translation and cultural review by native speakers. Test imagery in-context to avoid unintended associations and collect user ratings on perceived relevance. Create a repository of culturally vetted assets to streamline future localization work. Train content teams in cultural humility so they prioritize consultation over assumption. This structured approach improves initial acceptability and reduces later redesign costs.

Deep-level adaptations require engaging with cultural models of illness, healing, and help-seeking. Explicitly map local explanatory models during co-design sessions, noting causal beliefs, preferred interventions, and family involvement. Use these maps to inform intervention logic, sequencing, and outcome priorities, rather than overlaying Western therapeutic metaphors. Pilot adapted workflows with local clinicians to ensure alignment with practice patterns and referral pathways. Maintain versioned content artifacts so researchers can compare outcomes across cultural adaptations. Such rigor preserves therapeutic mechanisms while enhancing cultural fit.

This may involve co-designing with local stakeholders, incorporating indigenous knowledge systems, or allowing users to customize their experience in culturally relevant ways. Establish community advisory boards early and compensate members fairly for their expertise. Create co-design workshops that prioritize narrative methods to elicit metaphors and rituals relevant to healing. Provide users configurable cultural frames that influence language, imagery, and intervention metaphors. Evaluate whether customization improves engagement or creates fragmentation, and iterate accordingly. These participatory steps build trust and produce interventions that communities accept as legitimate.

One promising approach is the use of culturally adaptive algorithms, machine learning models that adjust content delivery based on cultural data (Ong et al., 2025). Define transparent rules for how cultural signals inform algorithmic choices and require manual oversight for culturally sensitive adaptations. Prioritize training datasets that reflect the target cultural diversity to reduce misclassification and bias. Implement audit logs that show why a recommendation was made and allow users or clinicians to override algorithmic choices. Conduct fairness testing across cultural groups to detect disparate impacts and refine models prior to deployment. These safeguards help harness adaptive personalization while protecting cultural integrity.

This includes designing for users with sensory, motor, cognitive, and emotional differences. Define categories of difference to guide recruitment of participants during co-design, including low-vision, limited dexterity, executive dysfunction, and emotional lability. Require prototype sessions that simulate common situational impairments, such as noisy environments and single-handed device use. Use plain-language summaries after testing to translate findings into design tickets for engineers. Encourage cross-functional participation in testing so product, clinical, and accessibility experts share learning (Hiland, 2021). Such practices ensure that design choices address functional needs rather than stereotypes.

For instance, individuals with autism may benefit from predictable interfaces and reduced sensory input, while those with depression may need interfaces that are forgiving of lapses in engagement. Offer concrete design patterns: reduced animation, linear navigation, and persistent save-states for users needing predictability. Suggest fallback modes that minimize sensory load and allow progressive disclosure of complexity. Recommend that systems provide gentle nudges rather than punitive reminders to re-engage users who miss sessions. Test these patterns with representative users and iterate based on subjective reports of comfort and comprehension. This approach balances structure with autonomy to support diverse symptom presentations.

Inclusive design also considers situational impairments, such as using an app in a noisy environment or with limited connectivity, and designs for resilience. Specify feature priorities for low-resource contexts: offline caching, small payload media, and concise interaction flows. Encourage default settings that optimize for low bandwidth while allowing users to opt into richer experiences when available. Build fast-paths for common tasks that work under connectivity constraints, such as a single-tap grounding exercise. Validate resilience by stress-testing prototypes under simulated poor network conditions. These measures reduce exclusion and improve real-world reliability.

Importantly, inclusive design is not about creating separate versions for different users. It is about creating flexible systems that adapt to user needs. Recommend an architecture pattern that supports modular feature flags and user-level preferences without fragmenting codebases. Provide guidelines for designing universal defaults that work acceptably for most users while exposing accessible customizations. Train content and design teams to think in terms of optional layers rather than separate products. Monitor usage patterns to ensure that customization options are discoverable and actually used. This strategy preserves cohesion while enabling individualized experiences.

THE ETHICS OF ENGAGEMENT

Techniques that increase engagement, such as gamification, persuasive design, or behavioral nudges, can also be manipulative if not used transparently. Define acceptable uses of persuasive techniques in clinical contexts and create a checklist for ethical review (Cristofaro & Giardino, 2025). Require explicit opt-in for gamified elements when users are vulnerable or in crisis. Provide examples of noncoercive nudges that support autonomy, such as respectful reminders and motivational framing.

Mandate monitoring for adverse psychological responses to engagement mechanics and plan mitigation strategies.

Ethical UX design requires transparency, consent, and user control. Specify granular consent mechanisms that allow users to enable or disable personalization and data-driven features (Chithra & Bhambri, 2024). Offer clear, plain-language explanations of how engagement data is used to tailor experiences (Casson, 2019). Provide users with accessible controls to review and revoke permissions at any time. Document consent flows in clinical records when interventions are part of treatment plans (Casson, 2019). These practices preserve trust and respect users' decision-making authority.

Users should understand how their data is used to personalize their experience, have the ability to opt out of certain features, and be empowered to set their own goals and boundaries (Subu et al., 2022). Offer templates for goal-setting dialogs that align with therapeutic objectives and respect user priorities. Include visible settings that let users opt out of social sharing, leaderboards, or reminder nudges. Ensure clinicians can view but not override a patient's personal privacy choices without documented consent. This alignment reduces the risk of coercive clinical workflows (Radanliev, 2025).

Ethical design also involves being honest about the limitations of the tool, what it can and cannot do, and providing pathways to human support when needed. Incorporate clear disclaimers that state the tool's scope in user onboarding and help centers. Provide an always-accessible pathway to escalate concerns to a human clinician or crisis resource. Train support staff to respond to escalations originating from digital tools. Maintain referral lists for local services and update them regularly to ensure reliable handoffs.

In the design of digital mental health tools, user experience (Mahon, 2023) and user interface (Ienca et al., 2017) principles are not peripheral considerations but central pillars that determine the therapeutic potential, emotional resonance, and ethical integrity of the intervention. Clarify that UX/UI choices shape clinical dose, user retention, and perceived safety in measurable ways (Weiner et al., 2025). Define core UX outcomes for teams, ease of use, emotional attunement, accessibility, and clarity of therapeutic intent. Require design teams to link each interface decision to a hypothesized clinical mechanism before development (Kim & Backonja, 2025). Include brief usability benchmarks that align with clinical goals and set target thresholds for pilot testing (Kim & Backonja, 2025).

Unlike traditional therapy, where the clinician's presence provides structure, empathy, and real-time feedback, digital tools must rely entirely on design to fulfill these roles. State that the interface must intentionally reproduce critical functions of clinician contact, including pacing, validation, and contingency planning. Map therapeutic functions to concrete interaction patterns that can be tested with users.

Use clinician-informed heuristics to assess whether the interface supports therapeutic pacing and contingency handling. Ensure workflows include explicit handoffs to human care when interactions exceed predefined risk thresholds.

At the heart of effective UX/UI design lies the imperative to reduce cognitive load, particularly for users who may be navigating psychological distress, cognitive fatigue, or emotional dysregulation. Operationalize cognitive-load reduction by limiting on-screen options, offering progressive disclosure, and standardizing visual affordances. Create a short checklist for designers that includes maximum choice thresholds and recommended chunk sizes for information. Test cognitive load empirically using brief task-based measures during usability sessions. Iterate designs until target populations can complete core tasks within defined cognitive thresholds.

Mental health conditions such as anxiety, depression, PTSD, and ADHD often impair executive function, attention, and working memory, making even simple digital interactions potentially overwhelming. Require formative research to document common functional limitations within the target population and use those findings to set design constraints (Kargarandehkordi et al., 2025). Provide examples of lowered-demand modes, simplified navigation, one-tap coping tools, and optional stepwise exercises, for users with executive challenges. Validate these modes through scenario-based usability testing that simulates symptomatic states. Record outcomes to inform inclusive defaults for all users.

In this context, clarity and simplicity are not just aesthetic preferences, they are therapeutic necessities. Specify minimum clarity standards for content: plain language at an appropriate reading level, consistent iconography, and direct-action labels. Implement content style guides that prioritize short sentences and clear imperatives for therapeutic tasks. Build automated checks into content pipelines to flag jargon and long sentences. Evaluate content clarity during pilot tests with representative users and refine until comprehension metrics meet predefined goals.

Interfaces must be designed to minimize decision fatigue and cognitive friction. Provide explicit design constraints: limit primary choices to three or fewer, present progressive next steps, and prioritize one-tap recovery actions. Use cognitive walk-throughs with representative users to validate that navigation is intuitive under stress. Define measurable success criteria, such as time-to-core-function and error rates, for each release milestone. Require that onboarding teaches the shortest path to a core task in under 60 seconds. These constraints reduce abandonment and support therapeutic continuity for users with limited cognitive bandwidth.

This involves streamlined navigation structures, consistent visual language, and progressive disclosure of information. Specify a modular information architecture that groups tools by therapeutic purpose, not by technical type, to match clinical workflows (Akhtar & Rawol, 2024). Create template screens that enforce visual consistency across modules, including standardized iconography and whitespace rules. Test navigation paths using first-use and return-use scenarios to ensure repeatability and ease. Document any deviations from templates with rationale tied to clinical goals (Ong et al., 2025). This disciplined approach reduces surprises and supports predictable use patterns.

For example, a user should never be more than two or three taps away from a core function, and the interface should avoid presenting too many options at once. Operationalize this rule by mapping tap-depth for every primary workflow and flagging flows that exceed the threshold. Prototype minimal-path designs and measure completion rates against the tap-depth target during usability testing. Include fallback quick-actions on persistent UI chrome to maintain access during high distress. Use analytics to monitor real-world deviations and iterate until pathways meet prescribed limits. These refinements make core support reliably reachable in moments of need.

Visual consistency, through the use of standardized icons, color schemes, and typography, helps users form mental models of the system, reducing the need for constant reorientation. Define a concise visual system guide that specifies type scales, color roles, and icon semantics tied to therapeutic functions. Require accessibility contrast checks and iconography tests with users from varied cultural backgrounds. Keep the visual vocabulary small to reduce learning cost and speed recognition. Maintain a living component library so teams reuse validated patterns across features (Saganowski et al., 2022). This consistency accelerates mastery and lowers cognitive friction during repeated use.

Progressive disclosure ensures that users are not overwhelmed by complexity; instead, advanced features are revealed gradually, as needed, supporting a sense of mastery and control. Establish default beginner modes and optional advanced paths, with clear signals indicating how to access each level. Use onboarding to surface foundational features, then trigger access to advanced tools when users demonstrate readiness. Track transition rates and user feedback to determine whether disclosure pacing supports competence without surprise. Link disclosure stages to clinical milestones so clinicians can align treatment pacing with app complexity (Agarwal et al., 2025). This calibrated exposure enhances retention and supports skill acquisition.

These principles align with Sweller's Cognitive Load Theory, which emphasizes the importance of reducing extraneous load to facilitate learning and engagement. To operationalize this, create concrete rules for information density, such as maximum words per screen and allowable simultaneous inputs. Require designers to document choices that reduce split-attention and extraneous processing. Pilot tasks should measure subjective cognitive effort in addition to performance. Embed cognitive-load checks into acceptance criteria for each feature to ensure continued alignment with therapeutic aims.

In digital mental health, reducing cognitive friction can mean the difference between a user completing a therapeutic exercise or abandoning the app altogether.

Specify measurable engagement thresholds and dropout risk indicators to guide iterative fixes. Use short in-session surveys to detect moments of overload and map them to interface elements. Provide rapid remediation patterns, such as simplified views or one-tap exits, to recover users during overload. Link these remediation tools to clinician alerts when repeated abandonment signals clinical concern (APA, 2023).

Beyond clarity, the organization of information, its visual hierarchy and architecture, plays a critical role in shaping user experience. Define a standard information architecture that prioritizes user goals and therapeutic intentions rather than feature lists. Use card sorting and tree testing with representative users to validate labels and groupings. Require that primary therapeutic actions occupy prime visual real estate and secondary items be de-emphasized. Document architecture decisions so clinicians and researchers can anticipate user pathways during trials.

Visual hierarchy refers to the arrangement of elements in a way that guides the user's attention and supports intuitive interaction. Provide designers with explicit rules for contrast, scale, and grouping that correspond to therapeutic priority. Test whether primary actions attract attention within three seconds during first-use sessions. Include whitespace and grouping metrics in design reviews to prevent clutter. Align labels and icons with clinical language to reduce translation between app and therapy discussions.

In mental health applications, where users may be emotionally dysregulated or cognitively fatigued, a strong visual hierarchy can provide a sense of order and calm. Establish calming design affordances, consistent alignment, muted palettes, and stable layouts, to support regulation. Evaluate whether these affordances reduce reported anxiety during use by collecting brief mood ratings before and after tasks. Train design teams to recognize when aesthetic choices may inadvertently increase arousal. Integrate these checks into iterative usability cycles to preserve emotional safety.

Yet functionality alone is insufficient. Designers must account for affective experience as deliberately as for task completion, and they should treat emotional affordances as testable design variables. Specify which emotional responses the product intends to evoke, calm, confidence, reduced shame, and link those to measurable indicators such as brief in-session mood ratings. Build style guides that align visual and verbal tone to those intended affects and include examples of acceptable language and imagery. Require iterative testing that captures both task success and emotional response to ensure the interface supports healing as well as usability. Incorporate clinician review of emotionally salient content to verify that therapeutic tone is preserved across updates. These steps help translate design intent into reproducible practice without compromising clinical fidelity (Watson, 2025).

Emotional design is the practice of creating interfaces that evoke positive emotional responses and support users' psychological needs. Define a taxonomy of emotional design elements, tone, imagery, motion, and feedback, and document how each element should be used to support therapeutic aims. Provide exemplars that show acceptable and unacceptable uses of motion and metaphor to avoid accidental trigger creation. Require that copy and microcopy be reviewed by clinicians and lived-experience advisors to verify compassionate framing. Include short tests that measure whether specific design choices increase perceived warmth, trust, or safety among representative users. Use these data to refine guidelines and maintain consistent emotional scaffolding across features (Aiken et al., 2023).

In this context, the interface becomes a proxy for the therapeutic relationship. Operationalize which relational functions the interface must provide, validation, pacing, and contingency planning, and create design heuristics to match them. For example, validation can be operationalized through confirming language and visible acknowledgement of user effort; pacing can be supported by adjustable session lengths and easy pause/resume behavior. Provide clinicians with a mapping document that links interface heuristics to therapeutic intents so they can interpret user-reported data clinically (Kim & Backonja, 2025). Test whether users perceive relational presence by including short alliance items in longitudinal assessments. These practices make relational design explicit and auditable within clinical workflows (Fleming et al., 2019).

Personalization deepens this connection by allowing users to tailor their experience to their needs, preferences, and goals. Define clear boundaries for personalization: user-facing preferences, behaviorally driven adjustments, and clinician-mediated adaptations, and describe consent requirements for each. Implement transparent explanations for adaptive changes and provide simple toggles to accept, pause, or revert personalization choices. Pilot personalization features with diverse user cohorts to surface differential effects and unintended consequences. Maintain logs that explain adaptation rationales in clinician-facing summaries so care teams can contextualize automated recommendations. This disciplined approach preserves autonomy while leveraging personalization to increase relevance and adherence.

Feedback is another cornerstone of effective UX/UI design in mental health. Specify the types of feedback, confirmatory, reflective, and progress-oriented, and provide examples of nonjudgmental phrasing that emphasize effort and growth. Set rules for timing and frequency of feedback so it informs without nagging, and allow users to adjust intensity through preferences. Test feedback framing with users who have perfectionistic or depressive tendencies to ensure messages are motivating rather than discouraging. Provide clinicians with aggregated feedback visualizations and guidance on interpreting patterns for treatment planning. These measures ensure feedback supports therapeutic processes while mitigating psychological risk.

Trust is the cornerstone of any therapeutic relationship, and in digital contexts, it must be earned through design. Make explicit trust criteria early in the product lifecycle: data minimization, clear consent, and predictable behavior are nonnegotiable design constraints. Provide users concise, readable summaries of privacy practices and visible controls rather than burying choices in dense policy text. Use incremental consent patterns that allow users to grant permissions gradually as they experience benefit. Validate trust-building features through qualitative interviews that probe perceived safety and willingness to disclose sensitive information. Track trust signals over time to detect erosion and prioritize remediation promptly.

Users must feel confident that their data is secure, their privacy respected, and their autonomy preserved (Freeman et al., 2017). Define measurable privacy experience indicators such as comprehension of privacy summaries, frequency of consent changes, and rates of feature opt-out. Offer transparent audit trails that show when and why data was accessed or shared, and provide simple interfaces for users to manage data retention (Freeman et al., 2017). Integrate privacy training in clinician workflows so care teams understand how patient data flows between app and record systems (Freeman et al., 2017). Use user feedback to refine consent language and to surface common points of confusion for targeted clarification.

UX/UI principles that support trust include clear privacy policies, granular consent flows, and intuitive data management interfaces (Babu & Joseph, 2025). Operationalize these elements into prototype consent dialogs that are tested for comprehension and burden. Provide plain-language explanations next to each toggle and surface the consequences of choices succinctly. Require that consent dialogs include links to short explanatory videos or examples for users who prefer multimedia explanations. Evaluate whether consent flows increase drop-off and iterate to balance ethical transparency with usability.

Visual indicators such as lock icons or secure connection messages can reinforce a sense of safety when paired with plain explanations. Standardize these indicators in the design system and test whether users interpret them correctly across cultures and literacy levels. Avoid overreliance on icons alone; always pair visual cues with short text labels that explain what the indicator means in practice. Monitor whether these trust indicators correlate with increased disclosure of clinically relevant information during use. Use mixed-methods evaluation to ensure that visual reassurance aligns with actual security and governance practices.

Avoiding dark patterns, design tactics that manipulate users into actions they might not otherwise take, is essential. Establish a governance checklist that flags potential dark-pattern patterns during design reviews and requires ethics sign-off for any persuasive element. Train teams to recognize manipulative defaults and reward transparency in design decisions during product retrospectives. Implement an internal dashboard of ethical issues discovered in user feedback and track remediation steps publicly in release notes when appropriate. This accountability reduces the risk of erosion of trust and supports long-term therapeutic engagement.

Finally, digital mental health tools must be designed to accommodate emotional variability and crisis states. Define a crisis design mode that simplifies the interface and prioritizes immediate regulation and connection tools. Ensure crisis mode is discoverable but not intrusive, and provide clear user control for exiting it when safe. Collaborate with clinicians to define clinical thresholds and escalation pathways that the system can surface without making clinical decisions autonomously (Hall et al., 2024). Simulate crisis scenarios in usability testing with appropriate safeguards and measure response times and user perceptions of helpfulness.

Design considerations include simplified "crisis modes," rapid access to grounding tools, and emotionally responsive prompts. Specify the minimum viable crisis feature set, one-tap breathing, distraction choices, and quick contact options, and require performance testing under real-device constraints. Provide configurable escalation settings so clinicians or organizations can tailor response thresholds to local resources and legal requirements. Include a user-facing explanation of what crisis mode does and how it interacts with emergency services or clinician notifications. Track usage and outcomes of crisis interventions to refine content and make evidence-informed adjustments (Iwaya et al., 2023).

A crisis mode might strip the interface down to its most essential elements, offering immediate access to breathing exercises, calming visuals, or emergency contacts. Design the stripped interface to reduce cognitive demand and sensory stimulation while preserving clear exit paths and options to reach human help. Validate that the reduced interface remains legible under stress by testing with users after a brief stress induction and measure whether they can successfully initiate a calming practice within 30 seconds. Provide options for users to pin or favorite specific crisis tools for even faster access in future moments of need. Document the decision logic so clinicians know what users experience during a crisis activation.

Emotional check-ins, regular prompts that allow users to report their mood, can help the system respond appropriately and offer tailored support. Standardize mood scales with simple anchors and offer optional contextual prompts to reduce burden. Allow users to silence check-ins temporarily and to choose the cadence that fits their life, honoring variability in engagement capacity. Use aggregated, anonymized mood trends to inform population-level service planning while ensuring individual privacy choices are respected. Integrate check-ins with clinician dashboards so care teams can contextualize in-session observations with between-session data when consented (Inkster et al., 2023).

Non-linear navigation allows users to jump directly to the tools they need, rather than following a rigid sequence. Design navigation so core regulation tools are accessible from persistent UI elements and minimize nested menus for crisis-relevant functions. Provide clear affordances for discovery of advanced features while preserving a fast path to core supports. Test navigation under conditions of reduced attention and measure successful access rates to critical tools. Use these findings to refine the balance between discoverability and immediacy for emotionally salient features.

UX/UI design in digital mental health is not a one-time task but an ongoing process of iteration, testing, and refinement. Build continuous feedback loops into the product lifecycle that collect usability, emotional response, and clinical outcome data at regular intervals (Khoo et al., 2024). Schedule periodic co-design reviews with lived-experience advisors to ensure evolving relevance and to surface emergent harms quickly. Treat design debt as a clinical risk and prioritize fixes that affect safety and accessibility in sprint planning (Engel, 1977). Document iteration rationales to preserve institutional learning and to support reproducible evaluation across deployments. It must be grounded in continuous feedback from users with lived experience.

Evaluation metrics should go beyond clicks and time-on-task to include emotional responses, therapeutic outcomes, and long-term engagement. Define a balanced metric set that includes behavioral engagement, self-reported safety, symptom-reduction proxies, and equity indicators disaggregated by demographic groups. Use short validated measures and ultra-brief mood scales during pilots to reduce burden while capturing meaningful change signals. Triangulate quantitative metrics with qualitative narratives to interpret anomalies and to generate actionable design hypotheses. Report evaluation findings in clinician-accessible formats that connect interface changes to likely clinical effects (Ong et al., 2025).

In this way, UX/UI design contributes to both scientific validity and ethical deployment of digital therapeutics. Make explicit how interface choices map onto hypothesized mechanisms of change and include those mappings in study protocols and implementation plans (Lay et al., 2025). Require pre-specified process measures that document whether users experienced the intended affordances, such as perceived safety or ease of use. Use these process outcomes to interpret efficacy results and to inform decisions about scaling or adaptation. Framing UX as part of the intervention model elevates design from cosmetic work to core clinical science (Rajpal, 2025).

CULTURAL SENSITIVITY IN DIGITAL MENTAL HEALTH DESIGN

In the rapidly evolving field of digital mental health, the imperative to design for cultural sensitivity is not merely a matter of ethical obligation, it is a foundational requirement for clinical efficacy, user engagement, and global scalability (Rajpal, 2025). Begin cultural planning by defining target populations and specifying culturally relevant success metrics tied to local values. Require cultural gap analyses early in development to identify potential misalignments with therapeutic metaphors or help-seeking norms. Use these analyses to prioritize adaptation activities and to allocate budget for deep cultural work. Treat cultural sensitivity as an ongoing maintenance item that requires re-evaluation when scaling into new communities.

At its core, cultural sensitivity in design begins with the recognition that mental health is not a universal construct but a culturally mediated experience. Clarify that designers must treat cultural models as variables that shape symptom definitions, help-seeking, and recovery expectations. Provide a short protocol for eliciting local explanatory models during formative research phases (Baka et al., 2025). Emphasize that valid adaptation requires both linguistic translation and conceptual translation of therapeutic goals. Connect this requirement to measurement by recommending culturally appropriate outcome indicators. Use local clinical advisors to vet conceptual mappings before piloting interventions (Ricciardi & Zomaya, 2025).

What constitutes "normal" or "pathological" behavior varies across societies, as do the idioms through which distress is expressed. Recommend developing a taxonomy of local idioms of distress to inform both content and natural-language processing models. Require that screening items be validated against community norms rather than imported thresholds (Livieri et al., 2025). Include examples of somatic versus emotional presentations and instruct teams to adjust prompts accordingly. Document mapping decisions so future localization work can reuse validated instruments (Pedram & Piatkowski, 2025). This improves diagnostic sensitivity and cultural relevance in assessment.

This translation of meaning requires a shift from surface-level localization to deep cultural adaptation. Define decision rules that distinguish surface from deep adaptations and link each rule to measurable testing protocols. Use staged adaptation workflows that move from prototype testing to small-scale efficacy pilots before wider deployment. Insist on iterative feedback loops with community members to refine metaphors, narratives, and help-seeking pathways. Archive adaptation artifacts to permit replication and to support cross-cultural comparisons. These steps reduce the risk of superficial fixes that fail to affect engagement.

Surface-level localization involves modifying superficial elements of the interface, such as language, color schemes, or imagery, to align with local norms. Specify acceptance criteria for surface adaptations, including back-translation validation and user-rated cultural fit metrics. Require representative user testing for imagery and iconography to detect unintended, culturally specific meanings. Create a lightweight approval workflow that documents who validated each asset and why (Liu & Schueller, 2023). Encourage reuse of validated assets to reduce duplication while maintaining local authenticity (Weiner et al., 2025). This approach accelerates localization while preserving quality.

Deep cultural adaptation involves rethinking the structure, content, and logic of the intervention to align with culturally specific models of mental health. Provide teams with a templated co-design agenda that surfaces local causal beliefs, treatment norms, and communal healing practices. Require pilot comparators that test adapted versus standard workflows for engagement and perceived helpfulness. Use mixed methods to evaluate whether adapted logic preserves therapeutic mechanisms in context. Report adaptation outcomes transparently so other teams can learn from both successes and failures. This rigor supports ethical, effective scaling across cultural contexts.

One promising approach is the use of culturally adaptive algorithms, machine learning models that adjust content delivery based on cultural data (Smith et al., 2023). Define transparent governance for algorithmic cultural adaptation, specifying which cultural signals are admissible and why. Require representative training sets and documented provenance for cultural labels used in models. Mandate human-in-the-loop review for any adaptation that materially changes therapeutic framing. Include audit procedures to detect differential performance across cultural groups and publish remediation plans when disparities are found.

INCLUSIVE DESIGN IN DIGITAL MENTAL HEALTH

Inclusive design in digital mental health is not simply about compliance with accessibility standards or the accommodation of specific impairments, it is a design philosophy rooted in the recognition of human diversity as a source of strength, innovation, and ethical responsibility. Clarify that inclusive design requires proactive recruitment of diverse users across ability, language, age, and cultural lines during formative work. Specify organizational commitments, budget, timelines, and stakeholder roles, to embed inclusivity as a project deliverable. Require teams to translate inclusive findings into prioritized, testable feature requests with measurable acceptance criteria. Frame inclusivity as both an ethical mandate and an evidence-generating practice (Shatte et al., 2019).

At its foundation, inclusive design begins with the understanding that disability is not a fixed attribute of an individual but a mismatch between a person's abilities and the environment in which they operate. Operationalize this social model by creating task-based scenarios that surface environmental barriers and by measuring task success under varied conditions (Obermeyer et al., 2019). Use scenario matrices that combine device constraints, connectivity, and symptomatic states to identify persistent mismatches. Require that accessibility fixes address environmental sources of difficulty rather than solely individual adaptations. Document environmental assumptions in design specs so future teams can reproduce inclusive decisions.

One of the core principles of inclusive design is flexibility in use. Specify a modular interaction architecture that supports multiple input and output modes without duplicating content maintenance. Define minimal viable modes, voice, text, and gesture, and require parity of critical therapeutic functions across modes. Provide clear defaults that are broadly usable while exposing controls for personalized adjustments. Test equivalence across modes in usability studies to ensure therapeutic fidelity is maintained regardless of interaction pathway.

Another key principle is equitable use, ensuring that the design is useful and marketable to people with diverse abilities without segregating or stigmatizing any group. Require that no accessibility feature be hidden behind a separate product tier and mandate parity testing to confirm features perform equally across demographic groups. Use inclusive language templates and neutral imagery in default experiences to avoid signaling a "special" mode. Track adoption of inclusive features and interview users to confirm that options reduce stigma and improve perception of dignity. Simple and intuitive use is another cornerstone of inclusive design. Specify a target reading level and require plain-language rewriting for all prompts and instructions to meet it. Provide a short checklist for interface clarity that includes single-step directives, explicit affordances, and example-driven prompts. Test comprehension with brief teach-back tasks during usability sessions to confirm that instructions are actionable under distress. Ensure that error recovery paths are explicit and forgiving, allowing users to undo or resume without penalty. These measures reduce cognitive burden and support consistent use across varying literacy and cognitive states.

Interfaces should be easy to understand, regardless of the user's experience, knowledge, language skills, or current emotional state. Require first-use walkthroughs that are optional, skippable, and resumable, and evaluate whether they improve task completion without increasing friction. Create localized content bundles that pair simple language with culturally appropriate examples for nonnative speakers. Include quick help overlays that provide context-sensitive guidance without interrupting the task flow. Use contextual analytics to identify where users hesitate and prioritize those spots for microcopy or design tweaks.

This is particularly important in mental health contexts, where users may be experiencing cognitive fog, emotional dysregulation, or crisis. Define scenario-based acceptance tests that simulate symptomatic states and measure successful access to core tools under those conditions. Provide designers with empathy maps that describe cognitive and emotional constraints common to target users. Require that trauma-informed language alternatives be available on-demand, especially for modules that address sensitive topics. Use brief post-task mood checks to ensure the interface did not increase distress and to capture opportunities for immediate remediation.

Clear navigation, consistent layout, and plain language are essential. Create a modular content grid that enforces consistent placement of primary actions and secondary information across screens. Require that all interactive elements include explicit labels and predictable behavior to reduce surprise under stress. Maintain a short library of validated microcopy that can be reused across features to ensure tonal consistency and reduce content debt (Ball et al., 2025). Measure navigation efficiency with simple metrics such as time-to-primary-action and number-of-taps to completion across representative users.

Visual cues, such as icons, progress bars, and color coding, can support comprehension and reduce cognitive load. Standardize icon semantics and provide hover or tap explanations for ambiguous symbols to aid learning. Use progressive affordances that reveal contextual cues only when needed to prevent clutter and sensory overload. Validate color-coding choices with accessibility contrast checks and cultural review panels to avoid misinterpretation. Track whether visual cues reduce error rates and improve perceived clarity in iterative usability cycles.

Universal design goes beyond accessibility by recognizing that all users benefit from flexible, intuitive systems. Define universal design objectives that improve usability for everyone, such as consistent affordances, multiple input modes, and compact interaction paths. Require that new features pass a universal usability check before release, demonstrating benefit across diverse user scenarios. Provide examples where universal features reduced support requests or improved completion rates in pilots. Link universal design goals to equity outcomes to make impact visible to stakeholders. Maintain a registry of universal patterns that teams can adopt to speed inclusive development.

Captions on videos help not only users with hearing impairments but also those in noisy environments or with limited data plans (Fanarioti & Karpouzis, 2025). Specify captioning standards, accurate speech-to-text, speaker labels, and time-synced display, and require human review for sensitive content. Offer low-bandwidth alternatives such as downloadable transcripts and audio-only modes to accommodate connectivity constraints. Test caption visibility and comprehension on small screens and in motion to ensure real-world usefulness. Track usage of captions and transcripts to inform priorities for media accessibility investment. These practices broaden access and support diverse usage contexts.

Designing for the margins creates systems that are more robust, resilient, and inclusive for everyone. Articulate a margin-first development policy that prioritizes edge-case testing with real users who have significant accessibility needs. Use findings from these tests to inform default behaviors so that edge-case fixes benefit the majority. Require that product roadmaps allocate time for inclusive retrofits rather than deferring them indefinitely. Publish anonymized case studies showing how margin-driven changes improved outcomes at scale. Framing margin-driven design as risk reduction and value creation builds organizational commitment.

Trust is the cornerstone of any therapeutic relationship, and in digital contexts, it must be earned through design. Make explicit trust criteria early in the product lifecycle: data minimization, clear consent, and predictable behavior are nonnegotiable design constraints (Gkintoni et al., 2025). Provide users concise, readable summaries of privacy practices and visible controls rather than burying choices in dense policy text. Use incremental consent patterns that allow users to grant permissions gradually as they experience benefit. Validate trust-building features through qualitative interviews that probe perceived safety and willingness to disclose sensitive information. Track trust signals over time to detect erosion and prioritize remediation promptly.

Users must feel confident that their data is secure, their privacy respected, and their autonomy preserved (Ricciardi & Zomaya, 2025). Define measurable privacy experience indicators such as comprehension of privacy summaries, frequency of consent changes, and rates of feature opt-out. Offer transparent audit trails that show when and why data was accessed or shared, and provide simple interfaces for users to manage data retention (Tsai et al., 2025). Integrate privacy training in clinician workflows so care teams understand how patient data flows between app and record systems (Tsai et al., 2025). Use user feedback to refine consent language and to surface common points of confusion for targeted clarification.

REFERENCES

Adegoke, K., Adegoke, A., Dawodu, D., Bayowa, A., & Adekoya, A (2025). Interoperability in digital healthcare: Enhancing consumer health and transforming care systems.

Agarwal, S., Jalan, M., Hill, R., Pantalone, E., Thrul, J., Sharma, R., Wilcox, H. C., & Robinson, K. A. (2025). Framework to Assist Stakeholders in Technology Evaluation for Recovery (Freeman et al., 2017) to Mental Health and Wellness. *BMC Health Services Research*, *25*, 623. Advance online publication. DOI: 10.1186/s12913-025-12418-0 PMID: 40307807

Aiken, L. H., Lasater, K. B., Sloane, D. M., Pogue, C. A., Rosenbaum, K. E. F., & Muir, K. J.US Clinician Wellbeing Study Consortium. (2023, July). Physician and nurse well-being and preferred interventions to address burnout in hospital practice: Factors associated with turnover, outcomes, and patient safety. [). American Medical Association.]. *JAMA Health Forum*, *4*(7), e231809–e231809. DOI: 10.1001/jamahealthforum.2023.1809 PMID: 37418269

Akhtar, Z. B., & Rawol, A. T. (2024). Artificial intelligence (Tizzard, 2025) and extended reality (XR): A biomedical engineering perspective investigation analysis. *Indonesian Journal of Electronics, Electromedical Engineering, and Medical Informatics*, *6*(3). Advance online publication. DOI: 10.35882/ijeeemi.v6i3.5

American Psychiatric Association. (2023). Digital [Resource Document. APA.]. *Mental Health (Detroit, Mich.)*, •••, 101.

Babu, A., & Joseph, A. P. (2025). Digital wellness or digital dependency? A critical examination of mental health apps and their implications. *Frontiers in Psychiatry*, *16*, 1581779. DOI: 10.3389/fpsyt.2025.1581779 PMID: 40248604

Baka, E., Tan, Y.-R., Wong, B. L. H., Xing, Z., & Yap, P. (2025). A scoping review of digital interventions for the promotion of mental health and prevention of mental health conditions for young people. *Oxford Open Digital Health*, *3*, oqaf005. DOI: 10.1093/oodh/oqaf005 PMID: 40230873

Ball, H., Eisner, E., Nicholas, J., Wilson, P., & Bucci, S. (2025). How theories, models, and frameworks have been used to implement digital health interventions in services for people with severe mental health problems: A scoping review. *BMC Public Health*, *25*(1), 1023. DOI: 10.1186/s12889-025-22189-2 PMID: 40098003

Casson, A. J. (2019). Wearable EEG and beyond. *Biomedical Engineering Letters*, *9*(1), 53–71. DOI: 10.1007/s13534-018-00093-6 PMID: 30956880

Chaabene, S., Boudaya, A., Bouaziz, B., & Chaari, L. (2025). An overview of methods and techniques in multimodal data fusion with application to healthcare. *International Journal of Data Science and Analytics*, *20*(4), 1–25. DOI: 10.1007/s41060-025-00715-0

Chithra, N., & Bhambri, P. (2024). Ethics in sustainable technology. In *Handbook of Technological Sustainability* (pp. 245–256). CRC Press. DOI: 10.1201/9781003475989-21

Cristofaro, M., & Giardino, P. L. (2025). Surfing the AI waves: The historical evolution of artificial intelligence in management and organizational studies and practices. *Journal of Management History*. Advance online publication. DOI: 10.1108/JMH-01-2025-0002

De Kock, J. H., Latham, H. A., Leslie, S. J., Grindle, M., Munoz, S. A., Ellis, L., Polson, R., & O'Malley, C. M. (2021). A rapid review of the impact of COVID-19 on the mental health of healthcare workers: Implications for supporting psychological well-being. *BMC Public Health*, *21*(1), 104. DOI: 10.1186/s12889-020-10070-3 PMID: 33422039

Engel, G. L. (1977). The need for a new medical model: A challenge for biomedicine. *Science*, *196*(4286), 129–136. DOI: 10.1126/science.847460 PMID: 847460

Fanarioti, A. K., & Karpouzis, K. (2025). Artificial Intelligence and the Future of Mental Health in a Digitally Transformed World. *Computers*, *14*(7), 259. DOI: 10.3390/computers14070259

Freeman, D., Reeve, S., Robinson, A., Ehlers, A., Clark, D., Spanlang, B., & Slater, M. (2017). Virtual reality in the assessment, understanding, and treatment of mental health disorders. *Psychological Medicine*, *47*(14), 2393–2400. DOI: 10.1017/S003329171700040X PMID: 28325167

Gkintoni, E., Vassilopoulos, S. P., & Nikolaou, G. (2025). Next-generation cognitive-behavioral therapy for depression: Integrating digital tools, teletherapy, and personalization for enhanced mental health outcomes. *Medicina (Kaunas, Lithuania)*, *61*(3), 431. DOI: 10.3390/medicina61030431 PMID: 40142242

Hall, C. L., Gómez Bergin, A. D., & Rennick-Egglestone, S. (2024). Research into digital health intervention for mental health: 25-year retrospective on the ethical and legal challenges. *Journal of Medical Internet Research*, *26*, e58939. DOI: 10.2196/58939 PMID: 39250796

Hiland, E. B. (2021). *Therapy tech: The digital transformation of mental healthcare*. U of Minnesota Press. DOI: 10.5749/j.ctv1xp9q3t

Ienca, M., Fabrice, J., Elger, B., Caon, M., Scoccia Pappagallo, A., Kressig, R. W., & Wangmo, T. (2017). Intelligent assistive technology for Alzheimer's disease and other dementias: A systematic review. *Journal of Alzheimer's Disease*, *56*(4), 1301–1340. DOI: 10.3233/JAD-161037 PMID: 28222516

Inkster, B., Knibbs, C., & Bada, M. (2023). Cybersecurity: A critical priority for digital mental health. *Frontiers in Digital Health*, *5*, 1242264. DOI: 10.3389/fdgth.2023.1242264 PMID: 37781452

Islam, R., & Bae, S. W. (2024). Revolutionizing mental health support: An innovative affective mobile framework for dynamic, proactive, and context-adaptive conversational agents. arXiv preprint arXiv:2406.15942.

Iwaya, L. H., Babar, M. A., Rashid, A., & Wijayarathna, C. (2023). On the privacy of mental health apps: An empirical investigation and its implications for app development. *Empirical Software Engineering*, *28*(1), 2. DOI: 10.1007/s10664-022-10236-0 PMID: 36407814

Jain, A., & Jain, A (2025). AI-Based Emotion Detection System in Healthcare for Patient. Generative Artificial Intelligence for Biomedical and Smart Health Informatics, 455-470.

Kargarandehkordi, A., Li, S., Lin, K., Phillips, K. T., Benzo, R. M., & Washington, P. (2025). Fusing wearable biosensors with artificial intelligence for mental health monitoring: A systematic review. *Biosensors (Basel)*, *15*(4), 202. DOI: 10.3390/bios15040202 PMID: 40277515

Khoo, Y. X., Kang, R. M., Reynolds, T. L., & Mentis, H. M. (2024). The comprehensiveness of mental health application users' privacy and security concerns. *CHI Conference on Human Factors in Computing Systems*, 16 pages.

Kim, J., & Backonja, U. (2025). Digital health equity frameworks and key concepts: A scoping review. *Journal of the American Medical Informatics Association : JAMIA*, *32*(1), 45–59. DOI: 10.1093/jamia/ocaf017 PMID: 39936843

Kostadimas, D., Kasapakis, V., & Kotis, K. (2025). A systematic review on the combination of VR, IoT and AI technologies, and their integration in applications. *Future Internet*, *17*(4), 163. DOI: 10.3390/fi17040163

Lay, W., Gasparini, L., Siero, W., & Hughes, E. K. (2025). A rapid review of the benefits and challenges of dynamic consent. *Research Ethics*, *21*(1), 180–202. DOI: 10.1177/17470161241278064

Li, M., Patel, J., & Katapally, T. R. (2025). The impact of extended reality cognitive behavioral therapy on mental disorders among children and youth: A systematic review and meta-analysis protocol. *PLoS One*, *20*(3), e0315313. DOI: 10.1371/journal.pone.0315313 PMID: 40048453

Liu, M., & Schueller, S. M. (2023). Moving evidence-based mental health interventions into practice: Implementation of digital mental health interventions. *Current Treatment Options in Psychiatry*, *10*(4), 333–345. DOI: 10.1007/s40501-023-00298-2

Livieri, G., Mangina, E., Protopapadakis, E. D., & Panayiotou, A. G. (2025). The gaps and challenges in digital health technology use as perceived by patients: A scoping review and narrative meta-synthesis. *Frontiers in Digital Health*, *7*, 1474956. DOI: 10.3389/fdgth.2025.1474956 PMID: 40212901

Ma, C.-B., Shang, X., Sun, M., Bo, X., Bai, J., Du, Y., & Zhou, M. (2025). Emerging Multifunctional Wearable Sensors: Integrating Multimodal Sweat Analysis and Advanced Material Technologies for Next-Generation Health Monitoring. *ACS Sensors*, *10*(4), 2388–2408. DOI: 10.1021/acssensors.4c03396 PMID: 40162570

Mohr, D. C., Zhang, M., & Schueller, S. M. (2017). Personal sensing: Understanding mental health using ubiquitous sensors and machine learning. *Annual Review of Clinical Psychology*, *13*(1), 23–47. DOI: 10.1146/annurev-clinpsy-032816-044949 PMID: 28375728

Obermeyer, Z., Powers, B., Vogeli, C., & Mullainathan, S. (2019). Dissecting racial bias in an algorithm used to manage the health of populations. *Science*, *366*(6464), 447–453. DOI: 10.1126/science.aax2342 PMID: 31649194

Ong, T., Ivanova, J., Soni, H., Barrera, J., Cummins, M., Welch, B. M., & Bunnell, B. E. (2025). Mental health clients' perspectives on telehealth-based virtual reality therapy. *Frontiers in Virtual Reality*, *6*, 1595326. DOI: 10.3389/frvir.2025.1595326

Pedram, S., & Piatkowski, T. (2025). Exploring the potential of virtual reality (Johnson et al., 2021) in mental healthcare: A systematic literature review. *Virtual Reality (Waltham Cross)*, *29*(3), 135. DOI: 10.1007/s10055-025-01181-6

Radanliev, P. (2025). Privacy, ethics, transparency, and accountability in AI systems for wearable devices. *Frontiers in Digital Health*, *7*, 1431246. DOI: 10.3389/fdgth.2025.1431246 PMID: 40599875

Rajpal, S. (2025). Exploring the Role of Virtual Reality and Metaverse in Treating Mental Health: Operating Models and Challenges in Adoption. *Journal of Computer and Communications*, *13*(10), 1–22. DOI: 10.4236/jcc.2025.1310001

Ricciardi, F., & Zomaya, A. (2025). Perspectives on Managing AI Ethics in the Digital Age. *Information (Basel)*, *16*(2), 89. DOI: 10.3390/info16040318

Ross, G., Zhao, Y., Bosman, A., Geballa-Koukoula, A., Zhou, H., Elliott, C., Nielen, M., Rafferty, K., & Salentijn, G (2022). Data handling and ethics of emerging smartphone-based (Glass et al., 2022) sensors–Part 1: best practices and current implementation.

Saganowski, S., Perz, B., Polak, A. G., & Kazienko, P. (2022). Emotion recognition for everyday life using physiological signals from wearables: A systematic literature review. *IEEE Transactions on Affective Computing*, *14*(3), 1876–1897. DOI: 10.1109/TAFFC.2022.3176135

Shatte, A. B., Hutchinson, D. M., & Teague, S. J. (2019). Machine learning in mental health: A scoping review of methods and applications. *Psychological Medicine*, *49*(9), 1426–1448. DOI: 10.1017/S0033291719000151 PMID: 30744717

Smith, K. A., Blease, C., Faurholt-Jepsen, M., Firth, J., Van Daele, T., Moreno, C., Carlbring, P., Ebner-Priemer, U. W., Koutsouleris, N., Riper, H., Mouchabac, S., Torous, J., & Cipriani, A. (2023). Digital mental health: Challenges and next steps. *BMJ Mental Health*, *26*(1), e300670. DOI: 10.1136/bmjment-2023-300670 PMID: 37197797

Subu, M. A., Holmes, D., Arumugam, A., Al-Yateem, N., Maria Dias, J., Rahman, S. A., Waluyo, I., Ahmed, F. R., & Abraham, M. S. (2022). Traditional, religious, and cultural perspectives on mental illness: A qualitative study on causal beliefs and treatment use. *International Journal of Qualitative Studies on Health and Well-being*, *17*(1), 2123090. DOI: 10.1080/17482631.2022.2123090 PMID: 36097886

Tsai, Y. Y., Chen, Y. J., Lin, Y. F., Hsiao, F. C., Hsu, C. H., & Liao, L. D. (2025). Photoplethysmography-based HRV analysis and machine learning for real-time stress quantification in mental health applications. *APL Bioengineering*, *9*(2), 026103. DOI: 10.1063/5.0256590 PMID: 40191605

Weiner, E. B., Dankwa-Mullan, I., Nelson, W. A., & Hassanpour, S. (2025). Ethical challenges and evolving strategies in the integration of artificial intelligence into clinical practice. *PLOS Digital Health*, *4*(4), e0000810. DOI: 10.1371/journal.pdig.0000810 PMID: 40198594

Section 5
Future Directions

Chapter 14
Scaling Digital Mental Health Solutions

ABSTRACT

Scaling digital mental health solutions requires more than technical readiness; it demands structured implementation frameworks. This chapter applies models like RE-AIM and CFIR to guide adoption, fidelity monitoring, and sustainability planning. Key strategies include stakeholder engagement, workflow integration, and iterative evaluation of usability and equity. Policy alignment and reimbursement models are addressed as prerequisites for scale. Practical tools scorecards, dashboards, and audit protocols support continuous improvement. The chapter emphasizes adaptive governance to manage emergent risks and performance drift. Scaling is reframed as a scientific process, ensuring that innovation translates into measurable, equitable impact at population level.

INTRODUCTION

This chapter reframes scaling as a clinical, organizational, and ethical challenge rather than a purely technical one. It introduces principle-based replication, emphasizing preservation of therapeutic mechanisms and ethical safeguards over uniformity of form. Implementation science frameworks are used to address workflow integration, governance, workforce readiness, and equity at scale. The chapter warns against silent failure modes such as alert fatigue and measurement drift. By positioning readiness, not enthusiasm, as the criterion for expansion, it offers a disciplined roadmap for sustainable scale.

DOI: 10.4018/979-8-3373-4997-8.ch014

MOVING TO SCALE

Scaling digital mental health interventions is often described as a technical challenge, framed in terms of platform capacity, interoperability, or algorithmic performance. While these elements matter, they represent only a narrow slice of what scale actually requires. In practice, scaling is a clinical, organizational, and moral undertaking. It demands that interventions preserve therapeutic integrity, contextual sensitivity, and ethical accountability as they move from controlled pilots into everyday care environments. Technologies that perform well in bespoke research settings frequently fail when introduced into complex health systems precisely because scale exposes tensions between personalization and standardization that are invisible at small scale.

This tension is particularly acute for digitally enabled mental health systems that rely on adaptation, real-time feedback, or continuous sensing. The very features that give these interventions their clinical promise, responsiveness, tailoring, and moment-to-moment adjustment, also complicate replication across settings. Scaling, therefore, cannot rely on simple duplication. Instead, it requires what might be called principle-based replication: preserving core therapeutic mechanisms and ethical guardrails while allowing surface features, workflows, and delivery modalities to adapt to local constraints. From an implementation science perspective, this distinction mirrors the difference between fidelity to form and fidelity to function. Effective scaling prioritizes the preservation of function, mechanisms of change, safety thresholds, and decision logic, rather than enforcing identical interfaces or identical workflows across disparate contexts.

As we stand at the intersection of neuroscience, artificial intelligence, extended reality, and wearable technology, the field of digital mental health is undergoing a profound transformation (Lindner et al., 2024). This transformation requires clear definitions of the technologies, their scope, and the problems they aim to solve in mental health care. Clarify that "digital mental health" here refers to interventions and platforms that use digital hardware, software, or data to assess, prevent, or treat mental health conditions (Poudel et al., 2025). Define "scaling" as expanding reach while maintaining effectiveness, safety, and equity across diverse settings. State that our focus is on practical strategies for sustainable adoption, not merely on technical possibility. What began as a series of experimental tools and pilot programs has evolved into a rapidly expanding ecosystem of interventions, platforms, and systems that are reshaping how mental health is understood, accessed, and supported. Yet, as this field matures, a new set of questions emerges, questions not only about what is possible, but about what is sustainable, equitable, and just. Part V of this volume, Future Directions, explores these questions with a dual focus: first, on the practical challenges of scaling digital mental health solutions across diverse populations and systems; and second, on the speculative horizon of neuroadaptive care, where emerging technologies may redefine the very nature of therapeutic engagement (Poudel et al., 2025).

The promise of digital mental health lies in its potential to transcend traditional barriers, geographic, economic, cultural, and clinical (Casson, 2019). Clarify that transcending barriers requires intentional design choices that address access, affordability, cultural fit, and clinical validity (Kargarandehkordi et al., 2025). Be explicit that improving access does not guarantee quality; both dimensions must be pursued in parallel. Stress that these technologies can augment rather than replace human-delivered care, enhancing reach while preserving therapeutic relationships. Mobile apps, virtual reality environments, AI-driven chatbots, and biosensor-integrated platforms offer unprecedented opportunities to deliver care that is personalized, scalable, and responsive (Kargarandehkordi et al., 2025). But realizing this promise at scale requires more than technological innovation. It demands a rigorous engagement with implementation science, the study of how evidence-based practices are adopted, adapted, and sustained in real-world settings (Kargarandehkordi et al., 2025). Implementation science provides the tools to navigate the complex terrain of health systems, policy environments, and community contexts. It helps us understand not only what works, but for whom, under what conditions, and why. Chapter 14, Scaling Digital Mental Health Solutions, delves into this terrain, examining the frameworks, strategies, and policy levers that can support the widespread and equitable adoption of digital therapeutics. It considers the role of public-private partnerships, regulatory pathways, reimbursement models, and global health initiatives in shaping the future of access and impact.

Figure 1. Clinician scale-up plan using the PLANE FRAMEWORK

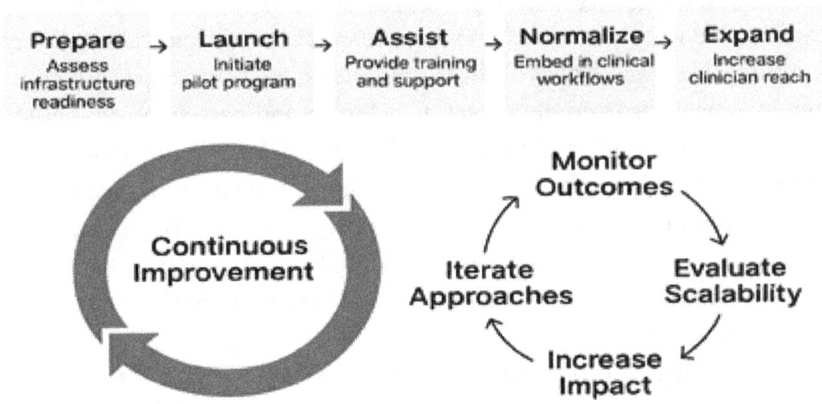

The top row illustrates five sequential phases: Prepare (assess infrastructure readiness), Launch (initiate pilot program), Assist (provide training and support), Normalize (embed in clinical workflows), and expand or increase clinician reach (Spytska, 2025). The bottom cycle emphasizes continuous improvement through monitoring outcomes, iterating approaches, evaluating scalability, and increasing impact. This visual highlight a structured roadmap for scaling digital mental health interventions across clinical settings (Engel, 1977).

The PLANE framework is most useful when understood not as a checklist, but as a lifecycle. Preparation extends beyond assessing technical readiness to include ethical, clinical, and organizational readiness. Systems must evaluate whether clinicians trust algorithmic supports, whether patients understand consent and data use, and whether escalation pathways are operational before deployment begins. Launch phases should prioritize learning rather than proof, using early pilots to surface misalignment, unintended effects, and workflow friction rather than to maximize performance metrics prematurely. Assistance phases formalize the human infrastructure required for scale. Training, supervision, and governance structures are not transitional scaffolds; they are enduring components of any scaled system. As tools move toward normalization, success is marked by cognitive invisibility, when clinicians experience digital supports as part of routine care rather than as add-ons competing for attention. Expansion, finally, must be conditional rather than assumed. Growth should occur only where systems demonstrate stability, equity, and accountability, with explicit clarity regarding which elements are fixed (such as safety thresholds and consent architecture) and which may adapt locally.

Implementation science also emphasizes the importance of stakeholder engagement. Stakeholders are broadly defined to include users, caregivers, clinicians, administrators, and policymakers. Involving stakeholders across planning, design, rollout, and evaluation phases reduces implementation risk and enhances cultural fit by ensuring that interventions align with real-world needs and values. Successful scaling requires the involvement of users, clinicians, administrators, policymakers, and community leaders from the outset. Co-design and participatory methods are not only valuable for product development but also for implementation planning. Stakeholders can help identify potential barriers, suggest culturally appropriate adaptations, and build local ownership. For example, in scaling a digital intervention for adolescent mental health in schools, involving teachers, parents, and students in the planning process can improve alignment with school routines, increase buy-in, and enhance relevance.

Scaling digital mental health systems introduces a problem that is often invisible in pilot studies: measurement drift. At scale, the data streams that drive adaptation, physiological signals, behavioral markers, self-report patterns, do not remain stable. Sensors degrade, users habituate, environments change, and symptom expression evolves in response to the very interventions designed to support it. Models trained on early adopters or controlled contexts can quietly lose validity as systems expand to more diverse populations and longer time horizons. This decay rarely presents as catastrophic failure; instead, it manifests as subtle misclassification, diminishing sensitivity, or biased responsiveness that erodes clinical value without triggering obvious alarms.

For neuroadaptive and closed-loop systems, drift is not a technical nuisance but a clinical risk. Scaled deployment therefore requires explicit revalidation strategies as part of routine operations. Thresholds, decision rules, and personalization logic must be periodically reassessed, not only against aggregate performance metrics, but against subgroup-level equity and safety indicators. Treating revalidation as an optional maintenance task undermines trust and exposes users to unintended harm. At scale, sustaining effectiveness means accepting that models are provisional and that clinical responsibility includes knowing when an algorithm's assumptions no longer hold.

Finally, implementation science is inherently iterative and data-driven (Lorke & Stefanou, 2025). Iterative approaches use cycles of testing, feedback, and refinement to improve contextual fit and clinical outcomes (Tsai et al., 2025). Implementers should plan short learning cycles, such as monthly reviews, with measurable indicators to enable rapid course correction. For example, a community rollout of a digital screening tool reduced attrition by 30% after monthly feedback sessions identified usability barriers and prompted interface adjustments. Data-driven iteration balances fidelity and adaptation by monitoring core outcomes (e.g., symptom reduction) alongside contextual metrics (e.g., engagement, cultural relevance; Tsai et al., 2025). It relies on continuous monitoring, stakeholder feedback, and adaptive decision-making to sustain effectiveness across diverse settings. Hybrid effectiveness-implementation trials, for example, evaluate both clinical outcomes and implementation processes simultaneously (Tsai et al., 2025). This allows researchers to understand not only whether an intervention works, but how and why it works, or doesn't, in specific settings. Implementation outcomes such as acceptability, feasibility, appropriateness, and cost are measured alongside clinical metrics, providing a more holistic view of success (Tsai et al., 2025).

These challenges intensify when scaling neuroadaptive and closed-loop systems. Interventions that continuously sense, interpret, and respond to user data introduce new layers of responsibility that traditional digital tools do not. Baseline personalization must operate reliably at population scale without flattening individual variability. Alert thresholds that function well in specialized settings may overwhelm primary care environments or community clinics. Without explicit governance, automation risks amplifying workload rather than reducing it.

Most critically, scaled adaptive systems must establish clear accountability chains. When a system adapts its behavior in response to sensor data or inferred states, responsibility for outcomes cannot remain implicit. Sustainable scale requires clarity about clinician override authority, organizational liability, and vendor responsibility before, not after, deployment. Without this clarity, trust erodes quickly, even when clinical outcomes appear favorable. Closed-loop and neuroadaptive interventions challenge static models of governance. When systems change their behavior in response to incoming data, oversight mechanisms must adapt as well. Traditional compliance models, built around one-time approval and periodic review, cannot adequately account for tools that learn, personalize, and evolve. Without adaptive governance, the pace of technological change outstrips the capacity to monitor ethical, clinical, and legal implications in real time.

Adaptive governance requires living protocols, clearly defined override authorities, and predefined ethical stopping points. It also requires routine audits that examine not only outcomes, but decision pathways, how and why systems responded under conditions of uncertainty. This approach treats governance as an active function rather than an external constraint. At scale, the credibility of digital mental health systems depends less on innovation and more on the visibility and rigor of the structures that hold them accountable. Implementation science provides the conceptual backbone for navigating this complexity. Rather than treating scale as a downstream phase that follows evidence generation, implementation frameworks emphasize that effectiveness and feasibility emerge together. Across digital mental health contexts, repeated patterns explain why promising interventions fail to move beyond pilots: misalignment with clinical workflows, excessive cognitive burden on clinicians, opaque algorithmic outputs that erode trust, and consent or governance processes that collapse under real-world constraints. Scaling fails not because interventions lack evidence, but because the systems designed to host them are not prepared to absorb the operational, ethical, and relational demands these tools introduce.

Technical readiness alone is a poor predictor of scalability in mental health systems. A platform may function flawlessly while remaining incompatible with clinical workflows, regulatory expectations, or reimbursement structures. To address this gap, the field would benefit from the articulation of implementation readiness levels that parallel, but do not conflate with, technology readiness. These levels would capture not just whether a system works, but whether it can be responsibly hosted by real-world care environments. Higher levels of readiness require evidence of governance alignment, workforce preparedness, liability clarity, and sustainable funding. A system is not fully ready for scale merely because it demonstrates effectiveness; it must also demonstrate that clinicians can use it without undue burden, that organizations can govern it without improvisation, and that patients understand how their data are collected and used. Framing scale in terms of readiness shifts the conversation from enthusiasm to preparedness, and from speed to responsibility.

When implementation is approached as an ongoing negotiation between technology, people, and organizations, scale becomes iterative rather than episodic. Feedback loops between clinicians, users, administrators, and developers are not optional enhancements; they are the mechanism by which a system remains clinically viable across environments. Implementation science reframes scale as adaptation with discipline, emphasizing learning velocity, stakeholder engagement, and continuous course correction over premature optimization.

Most digital mental health systems do not fail dramatically; they fail quietly. At scale, disengagement often becomes invisible, masked by nominal enrollment numbers and backend activity logs. Users may stop meaningfully interacting while remaining formally "active," and clinicians may develop informal workarounds to compensate for poorly integrated tools. Alert fatigue, particularly in adaptive systems, desensitizes staff to signals intended to support timely care. Over time, these patterns normalize dysfunction rather than correcting it, allowing systems to persist while delivering diminishing clinical benefit.

Another common failure mode is the redistribution of labor without recognition or support. Tasks such as data interpretation, ethical judgment, and exception handling quietly migrate to clinicians without corresponding time, training, or reimbursement. Governance processes may also erode, as consent procedures and escalation pathways that functioned in pilots buckle under operational pressure. These failures are rarely the result of bad intent; they are the predictable outcome of scaling systems without equal investment in human infrastructure, accountability, and oversight. Identifying failure modes early is therefore a prerequisite for responsible expansion.

Implementation science equips us with the frameworks, methods, and mindset needed to move digital mental health tools from innovation to impact. Achieving successful implementation requires both methodological rigor and operational pragmatism in equal measure. Teams must embed evaluation, stakeholder engagement, and policy alignment into development timelines to ensure feasibility and long-term impact. For example, a cross-functional team accelerated adoption of a digital therapeutic by coordinating clinical protocols, technical integration, and reimbursement policy updates in parallel (Pedram & Piatkowski, 2025). Sustainability planning should begin during initial development, not at scale-up, so that infrastructure, training, and funding models are in place before widespread deployment. It reminds us that scaling is not simply a matter of replication, but of thoughtful adaptation, stakeholder engagement, and systems integration. As we seek to expand access to mental health support through technology, implementation science ensures that our efforts are grounded in evidence, guided by context, and oriented toward equity and sustainability (De Kock et al., 2021).

A persistent myth in digital mental health is that technology scales itself. In reality, scale redistributes labor rather than eliminating it. Clinician time shifts from direct delivery toward interpretation, oversight, and ethical decision-making. As earlier chapters emphasize, future practitioners must be prepared to interpret physiological data, understand algorithmic uncertainty, manage XR-specific risks, and engage in nuanced consent conversations. Scaling without parallel investment in workforce development does not produce efficiency; it produces fragility. Digital mental health tools are often described as augmentative, yet the boundary between augmentation and substitution is rarely specified. At scale, ambiguity becomes dangerous. Tasks that involve pattern detection or routine monitoring may be well suited to automation, but activities requiring contextual judgment, ethical discernment, or relationship repair resist substitution. When systems quietly cross this boundary, they risk undermining care under the guise of efficiency.

Responsible scaling requires explicit articulation of which functions must remain human, and why. This includes complex risk assessment, consent negotiation, and response to ambiguous or conflicting data. Clear boundaries protect both clinicians and users by preventing the normalization of inappropriate reliance on automated inference. Scaling is not about replacing judgment; it is about reallocating it wisely.

Policy and reimbursement structures ultimately determine whether scaled systems endure. Programs dependent on pilot funding rarely transition into routine care unless payers recognize remote monitoring, data review, and digital intervention time as legitimate clinical labor. Sustainable scale is therefore an economic commitment as much as a technological one. Equity must function as a constraint rather than a goal: systems that presume broadband access, high digital literacy, or uninterrupted engagement will systematically exclude those with the greatest need. Equity in digital mental health is often articulated as a desired outcome rather than an operational constraint. At scale, this framing is not only insufficient, it is misleading. Systems implicitly assume access to broadband, stable housing, digital literacy, and normative physiological baselines, embedding structural bias into their core logic. The result is not simply exclusion, but systematic misclassification. When a model interprets signal loss as disengagement or atypical physiology as pathology, inequity becomes encoded as clinical inference rather than recognized as context. Operationalizing equity requires designing systems that anticipate variance rather than pathologize it. This includes stress-testing algorithms across populations that differ in culture, language, socioeconomic status, disability, and trauma exposure. It also demands transparency about where systems are likely to perform poorly and restraint in deploying tools beyond the environments for which they were designed. At scale, equity is not something that emerges through goodwill; it must function as a hard boundary that constrains design, deployment, and interpretation.

At its highest maturity, scaling represents a shift from projects to infrastructure, systems that are governed, maintained, audited, and trusted over time. The measure of success is not reach alone, but durability without erosion of care, trust, or dignity. At small scale, digital mental health systems can be protected by proximity, close supervision, motivated users, and bespoke support. At scale, those buffers disappear. What remains is the system itself: its assumptions, incentives, and priorities. Scale therefore functions as a moral test, revealing whose needs are centered, whose labor is invisible, and which harms are tolerated as acceptable trade-offs.

REFERENCES

Casson, A. J. (2019). Wearable EEG and beyond. *Biomedical Engineering Letters*, *9*(1), 53–71. DOI: 10.1007/s13534-018-00093-6 PMID: 30956880

De Kock, J. H., Latham, H. A., Leslie, S. J., Grindle, M., Munoz, S. A., Ellis, L., Polson, R., & O'Malley, C. M. (2021). A rapid review of the impact of COVID-19 on the mental health of healthcare workers: Implications for supporting psychological well-being. *BMC Public Health*, *21*(1), 104. DOI: 10.1186/s12889-020-10070-3 PMID: 33422039

Engel, G. L. (1977). The need for a new medical model: A challenge for biomedicine. *Science*, *196*(4286), 129–136. DOI: 10.1126/science.847460 PMID: 847460

Kargarandehkordi, A., Li, S., Lin, K., Phillips, K. T., Benzo, R. M., & Washington, P. (2025). Fusing wearable biosensors with artificial intelligence for mental health monitoring: A systematic review. *Biosensors (Basel)*, *15*(4), 202. DOI: 10.3390/bios15040202 PMID: 40277515

Lindner, P., Miloff, A., & Carlbring, P. (2024). The future of virtual reality therapy: Applications, challenges, and research directions. *Frontiers in Virtual Reality*, *5*, 112345.

Lorke, M., & Stefanou, T. (2025). Improving research and development of wearable assistive and rehabilitation technologies: A systematic review on diversity factors. *Journal of Neuroengineering and Rehabilitation*, *22*(1), 31. DOI: 10.1186/s12984-025-01562-7 PMID: 39985039

Pedram, S., & Piatkowski, T. (2025). Exploring the potential of virtual reality (Johnson et al., 2021) in mental healthcare: A systematic literature review. *Virtual Reality (Waltham Cross)*, *29*(3), 135. DOI: 10.1007/s10055-025-01181-6

Poudel, U., Jakhar, S., Mohan, P., & Nepal, A. (2025). AI in mental health: A review of technological advancements and ethical issues in psychiatry. *Issues in Mental Health Nursing*, *46*(7), 693–701. DOI: 10.1080/01612840.2025.2502943 PMID: 40378075

Spytska, L. (2025). The use of artificial intelligence in psychotherapy: Development of intelligent therapeutic systems. *BMC Psychology*, *13*(1), 175. DOI: 10.1186/s40359-025-02491-9 PMID: 40022267

Tsai, Y. Y., Chen, Y. J., Lin, Y. F., Hsiao, F. C., Hsu, C. H., & Liao, L. D. (2025). Photoplethysmography-based HRV analysis and machine learning for real-time stress quantification in mental health applications. *APL Bioengineering*, *9*(2), 026103. DOI: 10.1063/5.0256590 PMID: 40191605

Chapter 15
The Future of Neuroadaptive Mental Health Care

ABSTRACT

The closing chapter synthesizes technological, clinical, and ethical trajectories shaping the next decade of mental health care (Goktas & Grzybowski, 2025). It anticipates advances in multimodal neuroadaptive systems, federated learning for privacy-preserving AI, and immersive XR ecosystems (Engel, 1977). Ethical imperatives transparency, accountability, and justice are positioned as non-negotiable design constraints. Emerging risks such as behavioral surveillance, algorithmic bias, and digital dependency are analyzed alongside mitigation strategies. The chapter calls for global standards, participatory governance, and sustained research to ensure that innovation serves human dignity (Engel, 1977). The vision: a digital mental health ecosystem that is adaptive, inclusive, and anchored in care ethics.

INTRODUCTION

The final chapter synthesizes the book's core themes to envision the future of responsive, neuroadaptive mental health systems. It explores emerging technologies such as brain-computer interfaces alongside established tools, emphasizing cautious, ethically grounded evolution. The chapter reinforces clinician primacy, participatory governance, and continuous evaluation as conditions for legitimacy. By framing innovation as co-regulation rather than control, it articulates a future in which technology extends human capacity for care without eroding agency or dignity.

DOI: 10.4018/979-8-3373-4997-8.ch015

FROM THE PAST TO THE FUTURE

In the history of mental health care, the dominant model has long been reactive (Wibberly, 2024). This reactive model expects individuals to initiate contact and follow through with treatment when able (Ong et al., 2025). It assumes that people can recognize their own needs, navigate complex systems, and access care at the right moment. This dependence on user initiation systematically privileges those with health literacy, time, and social support. Even with the advent of digital tools, this reactive paradigm has largely persisted. Most mental health apps and platforms still rely on user-initiated engagement: log in, complete a module, track your mood. The system waits for you to act. In practical terms, clinicians should expect gaps in reach and engagement when care assumes self-starting behavior.

But what if the system could act first? This question reframes responsibility in care design, shifting some burden from the user to the system. It lies at the heart of neuroadaptive mental health care (Freeman et al., 2017). It signals a shift from static, one-size-fits-all interventions to dynamic, responsive systems that sense, interpret, and adapt to the user in real time. These systems are not passive repositories of content; they are active participants in the therapeutic process. They listen, learn, and respond. They are, in a very real sense, alive to the user's experience. Clinicians should therefore evaluate such systems not only for efficacy but also for how they redistribute agency and support.

To understand the promise of neuroadaptive systems, we must first understand their architecture (Bayor et al., 2025). This architecture is usefully conceptualized as three interdependent capabilities that together produce adaptive behavior. At their core, these systems are built on three interdependent capabilities: sensing, interpretation, and adaptation. Understanding these components clarifies design decisions and clinical trade-offs (Ienca et al., 2017). Each capability has distinct requirements for data quality, latency, and human oversight (Ienca et al., 2017). Together they form the technical backbone enabling timely, personalized interventions.

Sensing involves the continuous collection of data from the user (Freeman et al., 2017). This sensing covers multiple modalities that together create a richer signal than any single source could provide. This might include physiological signals (e.g., heart rate variability, galvanic skin response, EEG), behavioral data (e.g., typing speed, app usage patterns), and contextual information (e.g., time of day, location, ambient noise; Freeman et al., 2017). Continuous sensing requires calibration to individual baselines and safeguards for privacy (Freeman et al., 2017). These data streams provide a rich, multimodal picture of the user's internal and external state (Freeman et al., 2017). Clinicians should treat sensor outputs as probabilistic indicators requiring integration with clinical judgment (Freeman et al., 2017).

Interpretation is where artificial intelligence enters the equation. This interpretation layer translates signals into actionable insights using statistical models and domain knowledge. Machine learning algorithms analyze the incoming data to infer psychological states such as stress, anxiety, cognitive load, or emotional valence (Sheikh et al., 2021). These models must be validated against meaningful clinical outcomes to avoid misplaced confidence (Martinez-Martin et al., 2018). These inferences are not static diagnoses but dynamic assessments that evolve over time, shaped by both individual baselines and population-level patterns. Interpretations should be presented with uncertainty estimates and opportunities for clinician review

Figure 1. The future of neuroadaptive mental health care

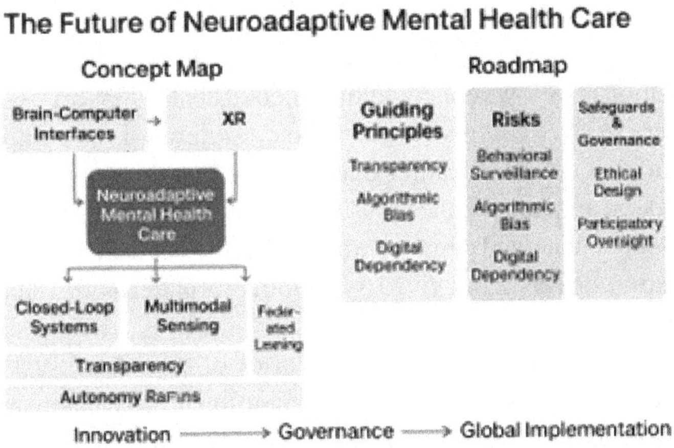

This integrated infographic combines a concept map and roadmap to illustrate emerging technologies (Brain-Computer Interfaces, XR, Wearables), core benefits (closed-loop systems, multimodal sensing, federated learning), and guiding principles (transparency, autonomy; Kargarandehkordi et al., 2025). Risks such as behavioral surveillance, algorithmic bias, and digital dependency are highlighted alongside safeguards and governance strategies. The roadmap shows progression from innovation through governance to global implementation, emphasizing ethical design and participatory oversight for scalable, inclusive mental health ecosystems.

Adaptation is the system's ability to respond to the interpreted data (Kargarandehkordi et al., 2025). In clinical design terms, adaptation must be proportional, contextualized, and discretely reversible to preserve user autonomy (Kargarandehkordi et al., 2025). This might mean adjusting the difficulty of a cognitive task, changing the tone of a chatbot, offering a grounding exercise, or prompting a check-in with a peer supporter. Designers should specify decision thresholds and allow clinician override to prevent inappropriate or unwanted interventions. The goal is not simply to react, but to respond in ways that are timely, personalized, and therapeutically meaningful. Implementation requires monitoring outcomes to confirm that adaptations produce the intended therapeutic effect.

This closed-loop architecture, sense, interpret, adapt, mirrors the feedback systems found in biological organisms. To make this comparison operational, map sensing to perception, interpretation to appraisal, and adaptation to behavior change. It is, in essence, a form of digital homeostasis: a system that seeks to maintain psychological equilibrium by continuously adjusting to the user's needs. Such systems must balance stability and flexibility to avoid oscillation or dependence. Clinicians should view homeostatic algorithms as partners that support, rather than replace, human clinical judgment (Kumar et al., 2024).

From a cognitive systems perspective, neuroadaptive technologies represent a profound evolution in how we conceptualize mental health support (Akhtar & Rawol, 2025). This perspective requires clinicians to consider tools as components within extended cognitive networks. Rather than treating cognition and emotion as static traits to be assessed and treated, these systems recognize them as dynamic processes, fluid, context-dependent, and deeply embedded in the environment. Practically, this shifts intervention targets from fixed symptoms to patterns of interaction across time and circumstance.

This view aligns with contemporary theories of cognition, such as embodied cognition, situated learning, and distributed cognition. Each framework foregrounds the role of action, context, and artifacts in shaping mental life. These frameworks emphasize that mental processes are not confined to the brain but are shaped by the body, the environment, and the tools we use. From a design perspective, then, technology becomes an environmental modifier that alters cognitive affordances. In this light, a neuroadaptive system is not just a tool, it is part of the cognitive system itself (Renuka et al., 2025). It extends the user's capacity for self-regulation, reflection, and resilience.

Consider, for example, a user navigating a high-stress workday. The example illustrates how timing and context determine intervention effectiveness. A traditional mental health app might offer a static library of coping strategies. A neuroadaptive system, by contrast, might detect rising stress through physiological signals, infer that the user is approaching cognitive overload, and intervene with a brief, personalized breathing exercise, delivered at the precise moment it is most needed (Saksena et al., 2021). After repeated interactions, the system updates its model, learning which exercises and prompts reliably reduce arousal for that individual (Martinez-Martin et al., 2018). Over time, the system learns which interventions are most effective for that individual, refining its responses through reinforcement learning or Bayesian optimization. This iterative learning fosters personalized co-regulation rather than one-size-fits-none solutions.

This is not just personalization, it is co-regulation. Co-regulation implies a mutual adjustment process where both parties influence outcomes in real time. In practice, co-regulation requires explicit mechanisms for feedback and user consent to the system's changing behaviors. Clinicians should view co-regulatory systems as collaborative tools that scaffold, rather than replace, self-regulation skills. The system and the user are engaged in a continuous dance of mutual adjustment, each shaping the other in real time. This mutual shaping creates opportunities for learning that are difficult to achieve in static interventions. Over time, measurable improvements in self-awareness and coping can emerge from this reciprocally adaptive process.

While the vision of fully neuroadaptive mental health systems may seem futuristic, the building blocks are already in place (Mohammad, 2021). Existing technologies provide modular components that designers can combine into adaptive architectures. Startups and research labs are integrating wearables, mobile apps, and cloud analytics to prototype responsive interventions (De Kock et al., 2021). A growing number of prototypes and early-stage products are demonstrating the feasibility, and the promise, of this approach. These prototypes offer proof-of-concept data that inform clinical trial design and implementation strategies (De Kock et al., 2021). Developers should prioritize interoperability and clinical validation when assembling these building blocks (De Kock et al., 2021).

Wearable-integrated apps such as BioBeats and Mindstrong use physiological and behavioral data to detect early signs of stress or mood shifts, prompting timely interventions (Kang & Exworthy, 2022). Such tools combine continuous sensing with simple, low-burden user interfaces to increase adherence. These applications typically require calibration periods and clear user education about what the sensors measure (Robinson et al., 2024). VR-based exposure therapies are being developed that adjust the intensity of stimuli based on real-time biometric feedback, helping users stay within their therapeutic window of tolerance (Robinson et al., 2024). Designers should document safety protocols and clinician oversight procedures for adaptive exposures. AI-powered chatbots like Woebot are beginning to incorporate sentiment analysis and natural language processing to tailor responses to the user's emotional tone (Robinson et al., 2024). These conversational systems should include escalation paths when risk indicators are detected.

These systems are still in their infancy, and rigorous evaluation is ongoing. Early pilots often demonstrate feasibility and acceptability but have limited statistical power for clinical efficacy (Zenker et al., 2022). Researchers should prioritize randomized, pragmatic trials that measure both clinical outcomes and implementation metrics such as engagement, equity, and cost-effectiveness (Fanarioti & Karpouzis, 2025). But the early evidence is promising (Fanarioti & Karpouzis, 2025). Preliminary findings suggest adaptive interventions can improve engagement, reduce dropout, and enhance clinical outcomes, particularly for users with complex or fluctuating needs (Fanarioti & Karpouzis, 2025). Such outcomes support further investment in scaled trials and real-world effectiveness studies. Careful attention to study design will clarify which user groups benefit most from adaptation (Fanarioti & Karpouzis, 2025).

Of course, the path forward is not without challenges. Technical complexity interacts with social, ethical, and clinical constraints in ways that can undermine implementation (Panarese et al., 2025). Neuroadaptive systems raise important questions about data privacy, algorithmic bias, user autonomy, and clinical oversight (Ong et al., 2025). Teams must implement privacy-preserving architectures and bias-auditing practices before deployment. These issues will be explored in depth in later sections of this chapter. For now, it is enough to acknowledge that the power of these systems must be matched by a commitment to ethical design, inclusive governance, and continuous evaluation. Robust governance structures should include stakeholder representation, transparent reporting, and mechanisms for redress.

Moreover, we must be cautious not to overpromise. Developers and clinicians should set realistic expectations about what adaptive systems can achieve. These technologies can augment care, but they rarely replace comprehensive assessment and human judgment. Early users should be informed about limitations, potential false positives, and the need for clinical backup when risk is detected (Morey et al., 2025). Clear framing reduces misconception and supports ethical adoption. Neuroadaptive tools should therefore be positioned as adjuncts to, not substitutes for, established therapeutic relationships (Mohr et al., 2017).

Neuroadaptive systems are not a panacea (Allgaier et al., 2023). Stakeholders must evaluate both benefits and harms before widescale implementation. Systems carry risks such as misclassification, overreliance, and potential erosion of patient autonomy. Risk mitigation should include iterative testing, stakeholder input, and monitoring for unintended consequences. Clinicians should establish protocols for oversight, escalation, and user education to manage these risks effectively. Responsible deployment requires continuous learning and governance aligned with ethical principles.

They are tools, powerful tools, to be sure, but tools nonetheless. Effective integration depends on training, workflow redesign, and clear role definitions for human and machine actors. Teams should co-develop practical guidelines that specify when automated responses are appropriate and when clinicians must intervene. Implementation plans must address data stewardship, clinician workload, and user consent processes to ensure safety (Correa et al., 2021). When used thoughtfully, these tools can extend therapeutic reach while preserving clinical integrity (Pedram & Piatkowski, 2025).

They must be integrated into broader systems of care, supported by human relationships, and grounded in the lived realities of users. Integration requires interoperable systems that communicate securely with electronic health records and clinician dashboards. Care models should embed human check-points where clinicians review algorithmic recommendations and contextualize them in therapy. Community resources and social supports must be linked to technological interventions to address social determinants of health. Ultimately, adaptive systems should strengthen, not fragment, existing care networks.

The rise of neuroadaptive systems signals a new paradigm in mental health care, one that is not only more technologically sophisticated but also more aligned with the complexity of human experience (Morgan et al., 2025). This paradigm invites multidisciplinary collaboration across engineering, clinical practice, ethics, and lived experience (De Kock et al., 2021). Translational pathways should include rigorous evaluation, implementation science, and equitable dissemination strategies. Clinical educators must prepare practitioners to interpret adaptive outputs and to engage clients in shared decision making around technology use (De Kock et al., 2021). The shift promises more responsive care while demanding vigilance to preserve human dignity and agency.

If neuroadaptive systems represent the shift from reactive to responsive care, then brain-computer interfaces (De Kock et al., 2021) represent the next frontier: the possibility of direct communication between the brain and digital systems. This next frontier reframes intervention possibilities by opening channels for earlier detection and more precise feedback. Once the domain of science fiction, BCIs are now emerging as a viable, if still nascent, technology with profound implications for mental health care. Early translational projects demonstrate how neural signals can complement behavioral and physiological markers to improve specificity. They offer a glimpse into a future where the boundary between mind and machine becomes increasingly porous, where thoughts, emotions, and neural signals can be sensed, interpreted, and even acted upon in real time. Developers and clinicians must therefore consider ethical safeguards alongside technical feasibility.

At their core, BCIs are systems that enable bidirectional communication between the brain and an external device. This bidirectionality distinguishes BCIs from passive monitoring systems and introduces distinct design considerations. This communication can be achieved through various means, ranging from invasive electrodes implanted in the brain to non-invasive technologies such as electroencephalography (EEG), functional near-infrared spectroscopy (fNIRS), and magnetoencephalography (MEG; Bibi, 2024). When selecting modalities, balance invasiveness, spatial and temporal resolution, and user acceptability. While invasive BCIs have shown remarkable results in clinical trials, such as enabling paralyzed individuals to control robotic limbs, their use in mental health is likely to be driven by non-invasive, wearable technologies that are safer, more scalable, and more acceptable to users (Ienca et al., 2017). Clinical deployment plans should therefore prioritize low-risk approaches with robust validation pathways (Ienca et al., 2017).

In the context of mental health, BCIs can serve three primary functions: Monitoring, Feedback, and Intervention. These functions form a continuum from observation to action and require separate validation and governance. Monitoring: Continuously tracking neural activity to detect patterns associated with mood, attention, or cognitive load. Establish clear clinical thresholds and uncertainty bounds for any monitoring output (Boda & Allam, 2022). Feedback: Providing users with real-time information about their brain states, enabling self-regulation through neurofeedback. Feedback protocols should incorporate learning principles and be paired with behavioral coaching. Intervention: Adjusting therapeutic content, environmental stimuli, or even neural stimulation based on brain activity. Any intervention must include clinician oversight and explicit consent procedures.

These functions are not mutually exclusive. Combining functions creates richer therapeutic possibilities but increases complexity and risk. In fact, the most promising applications of BCIs in mental health are those that integrate all three, creating closed-loop systems that monitor the brain, interpret its signals, and respond in ways that support psychological well-being. Pilot studies suggest that integrated systems can promote faster skill acquisition and more stable improvements in self-regulation. Creating such systems requires interdisciplinary teams that include clinicians, engineers, ethicists, and people with lived experience. This collaborative approach helps ensure that technical capabilities align with real-world clinical needs and values (Verma et al., 2023).

The potential applications of BCIs in mental health are vast and varied. Mapping applications to clear clinical targets will guide prioritization and evaluation (Engel, 1977). Some of the most promising areas include: Anxiety and Stress Regulation: BCIs can detect neural markers of stress and anxiety, such as increased beta wave activity or decreased alpha coherence, and prompt interventions such as guided breathing, mindfulness exercises, or environmental adjustments. Define measurable proximal outcomes for any regulation intervention. Depression Monitoring and Intervention: Changes in frontal alpha asymmetry have been associated with depressive states. Protocols should avoid deterministic claims and emphasize probabilistic risk indicators. BCIs could monitor these patterns and deliver personalized interventions, such as cognitive reframing prompts or mood-enhancing stimuli. Clinicians must integrate BCI outputs with clinical interviews and functional assessments (Engel, 1977).

ADHD and Cognitive Training: Neurofeedback using BCIs has shown promise in helping individuals with ADHD improve attention and executive function. Early protocols emphasize repeated, short training sessions with clear performance feedback to support neuroplastic changes. Trials often report modest effect sizes, so clinicians should interpret outcomes cautiously and monitor behavioral transfer. When designing programs, combine neurofeedback with behavioral strategies and environmental supports for sustained gains. Consider individualizing training targets and reinforcing skills that translate to daily functioning.

PTSD and Trauma Therapy: In exposure-based therapies, BCIs could help therapists monitor a client's neural arousal and adjust the intensity of stimuli to keep them within a therapeutic window, avoiding both under-engagement and re-traumatization. Implement threshold rules that prompt therapist review when neural markers exceed safe bounds. Use BCI feedback to pace exposure and to teach clients somatic regulatory skills during sessions. Ensure trauma-informed consent processes explain adaptive pacing and potential sensations during neurofeedback.

Sleep and Recovery: BCIs can track sleep architecture and detect disruptions in real time, enabling interventions that support rest and recovery, critical components of mental health. Integrate neural sleep markers with behavioral sleep interventions, such as stimulus control and cognitive strategies, for comprehensive care. Systems should provide clear, nonintrusive recommendations and avoid frequent nocturnal prompts that could worsen sleep fragmentation. Researchers should evaluate both subjective sleep quality and objective neural markers when assessing effectiveness.

These applications are not speculative; they are already being explored in research labs and early-stage startups (Lamb et al., 2025). Pilot projects often combine consumer-grade EEG with mobile platforms to test feasibility and acceptability in naturalistic settings (Radanliev, 2025). Early adopters report both opportunities and practical hurdles, including sensor placement variability and user burden (Radanliev, 2025). Scaling will require standardized protocols, clinician training, and robust evidence for clinical benefit (Radanliev, 2025). Developers should publish negative as well as positive findings to inform realistic expectations and iterative design.

For example, companies like Emotiv, Muse, and NeuroSky are developing consumer-grade EEG headsets that can be integrated into mental health apps and platforms (Omiyefa, 2025). These devices lower cost and improve access but vary widely in signal fidelity and software ecosystems. Clinicians and researchers should evaluate device validity in target populations before clinical use and document calibration procedures (Ienca et al., 2017). Integration into clinical workflows requires interoperability, data security, and clear documentation of limitations (Ienca et al., 2017).

A SYSTEMS VIEW: INTEGRATION AND INTEROPERABILITY

From a systems perspective, the true power of BCIs lies not in their standalone capabilities but in their integration with other technologies. Integration means designing interfaces and data pipelines that allow devices to share time-synchronized, semantically consistent signals (Chen et al., 2022). This requires explicit data schemas, standard timestamping, and agreed metadata fields so that multimodal streams can be meaningfully fused (Poudel et al., 2025). Clinicians should expect implementation teams to document integration points, error modes, and fallback procedures. When a BCI communicates with a wearable, a VR engine, and an AI agent, the therapeutic possibilities expand but so do coordination demands (Poudel et al., 2025).

For example, imagine a user engaging in a VR-based social anxiety intervention. The BCI detects rising neural arousal, the wearable confirms elevated heart rate, and the AI agent adjusts the scenario's intensity while offering calming prompts (Li et al., 2025). This coordinated response depends on low-latency messaging and clear decision hierarchies across components. Teams should specify which component has authority when signals conflict and how overrides are handled. Logging and audit trails ensure that clinicians can reconstruct decisions and explain interventions during clinical review (Fanarioti & Karpouzis, 2025). Such design practices support both safety and transparency.

Meanwhile, the system logs the data, updates the user's profile, and prepares a summary for their therapist (Freeman et al., 2017). These records should be interoperable with electronic health records and presented in clinically meaningful formats. Structured summaries that highlight trends, intervention timestamps, and confidence levels make clinician review efficient and clinically actionable. Consent processes must cover secondary uses of logged data, including research, quality improvement, and model retraining (Freeman et al., 2017). Users should have control over what summaries are shared and with whom.

Such integration requires interoperability standards, data governance frameworks, and user-centered design principles, all of which are essential for ethical and effective scaling (De Kock et al., 2021). Standards bodies, clinical leaders, and patient advocates should collaborate to define minimal viable interoperability requirements (Ienca et al., 2017). Governance frameworks must specify roles, responsibilities, and redress pathways when harms occur. User-centered design involves iterative testing with diverse populations to ensure the integrated system supports real-world workflows and cultural expectations. These practices reduce the risk of brittle systems that fail when scaled.

These issues will be addressed in later sections, but it is worth noting here that the success of BCIs in mental health will depend as much on systems thinking as on technological innovation. Investment in shared infrastructure, common protocols, and collaborative governance is as important as improvements in sensor fidelity (Radanliev, 2025). Funders and institutions should prioritize projects that demonstrate interoperable architectures and reproducible clinical workflows (Ricciardi &

Zomaya, 2025). Ultimately, a networked approach to development will accelerate safe, equitable, and scalable deployment.

Signal Quality and Noise: Non-invasive BCIs often struggle with low signal-to-noise ratios, making it difficult to extract reliable data in real-world settings (Kourtesis, 2024). Improving signal quality requires both hardware improvements and sophisticated preprocessing pipelines that remove artifacts while preserving meaningful neural features. Developers should report signal-to-noise metrics and common artifact sources so clinicians can interpret data confidence across contexts (Mohr et al., 2017). Field validation studies must assess performance during typical user activities, not only in laboratory conditions. Clinicians need clear guidance on when signals are too noisy to inform decisions and when to rely on complementary sensors. Wearable design should therefore prioritize stable contact, motion tolerance, and user comfort to minimize noise during daily use (Mohr et al., 2017). Documentation of failure modes assists teams in designing fallback procedures that maintain safety.

User Comfort and Accessibility: Wearing a headset for extended periods can be uncomfortable or stigmatizing. Design teams must prioritize ergonomics, lightweight materials, and discreet form factors to improve long-term acceptability. Accessibility also includes interface options for people with sensory sensitivities or movement limitations, which expand potential user populations. Training protocols should include gradual acclimatization periods and clear instructions to reduce frustration and increase adherence. Developers should collect qualitative feedback on comfort and perceived stigma to inform iterative design. Clinicians should screen for physical contraindications and offer alternative modalities when needed.

Data Privacy and Security: Neural data is among the most sensitive information a person can generate (Ma et al., 2025). Systems must implement end-to-end encryption, strict access controls, and transparent data retention policies to protect user privacy (Ricciardi & Zomaya, 2025). Consent procedures should explain potential secondary uses, anonymization limits, and mechanisms for data deletion upon request (Ricciardi & Zomaya, 2025). Governance frameworks must include independent oversight and audit capabilities to detect misuse or breaches. Clinicians should discuss data risks candidly with clients and document consent preferences in care plans (Ricciardi & Zomaya, 2025). Technical safeguards alone are insufficient; organizational policies and cultural practices must align to ensure responsible stewardship of neural data (Ricciardi & Zomaya, 2025).

Clinical Validation: Many BCI applications in mental health are still in the early stages of research (Boffet et al., 2025). Rigorous clinical trials are needed to establish efficacy, safety, and best practices for implementation (Kim & Backonja, 2025). Study designs should include diverse populations, ecologically valid settings, and both proximal neural and distal functional outcomes to demonstrate meaningful benefit (Kim & Backonja, 2025). Pre-registration of protocols and publication of null results will reduce publication bias and accelerate learning across the field. Clinicians should be cautious adopting devices without peer-reviewed evidence and prioritize use within research or supervised implementation frameworks (Kim & Backonja, 2025). Regulatory pathways must balance innovation with protection for vulnerable users.

Cost and Equity: As with all emerging technologies, there is a risk that BCIs will exacerbate existing disparities in access to care. Equitable deployment requires planning for affordability, distribution, and training in underserved communities. Public-private partnerships and tiered pricing models can support wider access while sustaining innovation. Implementation studies must report demographic characteristics and access barriers to reveal inequities early. Clinicians and policymakers should advocate for coverage models that include neuroadaptive interventions when evidence supports their effectiveness (Jain & Jain, 2025). Ensuring global accessibility aligns technological progress with ethical commitments to justice and inclusion.

Brain-computer interfaces represent a profound shift in how we understand and support mental health. This shift demands new frameworks for clinical assessment that include neural markers alongside behavioral measures (Ross et al., 2022). They offer the possibility of systems that are not only responsive but intimately attuned to the rhythms of the mind. Clinicians must therefore learn to interpret neural signals alongside subjective reports and functional outcomes. They challenge us to rethink the boundaries between thought and action, between self and system, between care and technology. Training programs should incorporate interpretive skills for neural data and ethical deliberation (Rajpal, 2025).

But with this power comes responsibility. Developers, clinicians, and institutions must collaborate to define ethical guardrails before widespread adoption. As we develop and deploy BCIs, we must do so with humility, foresight, and a deep commitment to ethical design. Oversight structures should include multidisciplinary review boards and processes for community input. We must ensure that these systems enhance, rather than diminish, human agency. Regular audits and transparent reporting will help maintain public trust and clinical accountability (Chaabene et al., 2025).

We must ensure that these systems enhance, rather than supplant, human connection. Design choices should prioritize augmenting therapeutic relationships and promoting meaningful human interactions. BCIs should support clinicians by providing additional data streams, not replace the relational competencies central to therapy (Kostadimas et al., 2025). Integrating technology into care must preserve opportunities for reflection, narrative, and mutual understanding with a human clinician. Patient preferences and cultural norms should guide when and how neural interfaces are used. Clear consent practices should explain how BCI data informs therapeutic decisions (Kim & Backonja, 2025).

That they are not only intelligent, but wise. Wisdom in design means prioritizing well-being, fairness, and long-term flourishing over narrow performance metrics. Systems must be evaluated for their broader impact on identity, autonomy, and social relationships, not just symptom reduction. Ethical frameworks should demand explainability, reversibility, and mechanisms for user control over adaptive behaviors. Interdisciplinary ethics committees can help translate abstract principles into operational standards for development teams. This commitment helps ensure technology aligns with values of care and dignity.

In the next section, we will explore another key component of neuroadaptive care: affective computing and empathic interfaces (Islam & Bae, 2024). This forthcoming discussion will detail how systems detect, interpret, and respond to emotional cues across modalities. These technologies are essential for creating digital environments that feel not only smart but emotionally intelligent. Readers should prepare to consider both technical mechanisms and ethical implications of emotion-sensitive systems. Together with BCIs, affective computing forms the emotional and cognitive scaffolding of future mental health care.

As neuroadaptive systems evolve, their ability to sense and respond to the user's cognitive state is only part of the equation (Adegoke et al., 2025). Designers must also account for affective dynamics that shape engagement and therapeutic progress. Equally important is their capacity to understand and engage with the user's emotional world, which requires multimodal sensing and context-aware interpretation. This is where affective computing, the interdisciplinary field focused on the recognition, interpretation, and simulation of human emotions, becomes central to clinical design (Martinez-Martin et al., 2018). In the context of digital mental health, affective computing enables systems to become not only intelligent but emotionally intelligent, enhancing therapeutic relevance. It allows for the creation of empathic interfaces: technologies that can perceive emotional cues, respond with sensitivity, and foster a sense of connection and care.

Affective computing draws on insights from psychology, neuroscience, computer science, and human-computer interaction. Practitioners should integrate theory and engineering early in design to ensure validity and utility. Its goal is to equip machines with the ability to detect and respond to affective states, such as joy, sadness, frustration, or anxiety, through a variety of input modalities. These modalities include facial expression analysis, voice tone and prosody, text sentiment analysis, and physiological signals, each requiring specific preprocessing and validation (Ong et al., 2025). Facial expression analysis: Using computer vision to detect micro-expressions and facial muscle movements (Robinson et al., 2024). Voice tone and prosody: Analyzing pitch, tempo, and rhythm to infer emotional tone. Text sentiment analysis: Using natural language processing (Robinson et al., 2024) to detect emotional valence in written or spoken language (Robinson et al., 2024).

These modalities can be used individually or in combination to create multimodal emotion recognition systems. Multimodal fusion increases robustness but requires careful alignment and weighting of inputs. When integrated into digital mental health platforms, they enable real-time emotional awareness, allowing systems to adjust their responses based not only on what the user says or does, but on how they feel. Clinicians should receive outputs with confidence intervals and contextual notes to guide interpretation. Multimodal systems should be validated in ecologically valid contexts reflecting typical user environments (Hiland, 2021).

The application of affective computing in mental health is already underway. Early deployments show promise across clinical and preventive settings, though generalizability remains under study (Bond et al., 2023). Consider the following examples: AI-powered chatbots like Woebot and Wysa are beginning to incorporate sentiment analysis to tailor their responses (De Kock et al., 2021). If a user expresses sadness or frustration, the chatbot can respond with increased empathy, offer validation, or suggest a coping strategy. Teletherapy platforms are exploring the use of emotion recognition to support clinicians with real-time analytics that highlight affective shifts, helping therapists attune more precisely to moments of distress or disengagement.

Empathic interfaces in practice extend beyond conversational agents to immersive and organizational tools. Implementation teams must define escalation protocols when affective signals indicate elevated risk. Immersive environments in virtual reality (Kargarandehkordi et al., 2025) can adapt based on the user's emotional state, altering sensory elements to promote regulation. A mindfulness app might adjust its visual and auditory elements to promote calm if it detects signs of anxiety. Educational and workplace wellness tools are using affective computing to monitor emotional well-being and prompt timely interventions such as breaks, motivational messages, or connections to support resources.

Empathy is not just a desirable feature in mental health care, it is a core mechanism of therapeutic change. Empathic attunement facilitates trust, supports alliance formation, and predicts better engagement and outcomes. Practitioners should therefore evaluate digital tools on their capacity to convey understanding, validate experience, and foster safety. In digital contexts, where the absence of human presence can lead to isolation, empathic interfaces can help bridge relational gaps. Designers must prioritize timing, phrasing, and cultural sensitivity to make machine responses feel authentic rather than hollow. Training datasets should include diverse expressions of distress to improve empathetic accuracy across populations. Clinicians need protocols to interpret machine empathy and to re-center human contact when needed.

From a cognitive systems perspective, empathy can be understood as a dynamic feedback loop: the system perceives the user's emotional state, adjusts its behavior accordingly, and receives feedback on the effectiveness of its response. Conceptualizing empathy this way highlights measurable mechanisms for design and evaluation. Systems should log responses and user reactions to refine empathic behaviors through iterative learning. Over time, this loop can foster a sense of being seen, heard, and understood, even in the absence of a human therapist. Designers must therefore include metrics for relational outcomes, such as perceived validation and trust, alongside symptom measures. Clinicians should review loop logs to verify therapeutic alignment and correct misattunements.

This is particularly important for populations that may be underserved or stigmatized in traditional care settings. Digital empathic tools can increase accessibility for adolescents, remote rural residents, and those hesitant to seek in-person care. However, accessibility gains are contingent on culturally appropriate design and language support. Systems should be localized and tested with representative users to avoid reinforcing disparities. For example, adolescents with social anxiety may prefer anonymous, empathic chat support as an initial engagement pathway. Clinicians should incorporate user preferences into deployment plans and maintain pathways for human referral when machine empathy is insufficient.

As with all powerful technologies, affective computing raises important ethical questions, particularly when deployed in sensitive domains like mental health. Accuracy and bias are primary concerns: models trained on narrow datasets may misinterpret emotions across cultures, ages, or neurotypes. Consent and transparency must be meaningful, explaining what is sensed and how responses are generated. Systems must avoid manipulative strategies that prioritize engagement over well-being. Design teams should adopt bias-auditing processes and publish performance metrics across demographic groups. Clinicians and organizations need governance structures to monitor for misuse and to respond to harm swiftly.

To build effective and ethical empathic interfaces, developers and designers must adopt a human-centered approach. Participatory design invites people with lived experience to shape system behaviors and priorities. Cultural sensitivity requires multiregional datasets and context-aware modeling techniques. Transparency and control give users agency to adjust or disable affective features. Context-aware adaptation ensures the same signal is interpreted differently across settings and relationships. Ethical oversight should be ongoing, with multidisciplinary review and community representation in decision-making.

CONCLUSION: TOWARD EMOTIONALLY INTELLIGENT SYSTEMS OF CARE

Affective computing and empathic interfaces represent a critical dimension of the future of neuroadaptive mental health care (Cristofaro & Giardino, 2025). This dimension requires evaluation metrics that capture both emotional attunement and clinical benefit (Ong et al., 2025). They enable systems to move beyond cognitive responsiveness to emotional attunement, to recognize not just what users are doing or thinking, but how they are feeling. Operational definitions of emotional attunement should guide model training and clinician interpretation (Ong et al., 2025). This capacity is essential for creating digital environments that are not only effective but humane. Implementations should therefore combine symptom monitoring with measures of perceived validation and trust.

As we integrate these technologies into mental health systems, we must do so with care. Implementation plans should include staged rollouts, usability testing, and continuous monitoring for harms. Emotional intelligence is not just a technical achievement, it is a relational and ethical commitment. It requires us to design systems that are sensitive, respectful, and grounded in the values of empathy, dignity, and trust. Design teams should include ethicists and lived-experience advisors to ensure these values are operationalized. It is also necessary to build clinician-facing tools that contextualize affective outputs and support shared decision making.

In the next section, we will explore how these emotionally intelligent systems can be embedded in immersive environments and embodied care, creating therapeutic experiences that engage the whole person, mind, body, and environment, in a unified, adaptive system of support. This integration will require coordination across hardware, software, and clinical workflows, with attention to safety and accessibility (Chithra & Bhambri, 2024). We will examine XR modalities, embodiment principles, and practical design constraints for neuroadaptive immersion (Martinez-Martin et al., 2018). Clinicians should prepare by assessing suitability, space, and contraindications for immersive work in their practices.

As digital mental health technologies evolve, they are increasingly moving beyond the screen, into spaces that are immersive, embodied, and multisensory. This shift is not merely aesthetic; it reflects a deeper understanding of how humans experience emotion, cognition, and healing. Immersive design must therefore be guided by therapeutic principles and empirical testing. Mental health is not just a matter of thoughts and feelings, it is lived through the body, shaped by the environment, and mediated by our interactions with the world. Therapeutic environments should therefore support interoception, safe movement, and paced engagement.

Immersive environments, particularly those enabled by extended reality (XR), offer a powerful medium for engaging the whole person in therapeutic processes (Subu et al., 2022). XR interventions should be designed with clear clinical goals, measurable outcomes, and safety checks (Kim & Backonja, 2025). When combined with biosensing and affective computing, these environments become neuroadaptive spaces of care, responsive, personalized, and deeply experiential (Kim & Backonja, 2025). Designers must ensure that adaptive behaviors remain transparent and reversible to users. Such systems can create novel pathways for embodiment-based interventions while requiring rigorous oversight and user-centered safeguards.

THE THERAPEUTIC POTENTIAL OF EXTENDED REALITY

Extended reality (Mahon, 2023) is an umbrella term that includes virtual reality (VR), augmented reality (AR), and mixed reality (MR; Ienca et al., 2017). In clinical planning, define XR modalities explicitly and match them to therapeutic goals and contraindications (Kargarandehkordi et al., 2025). These technologies allow users to enter or overlay digital environments that can simulate real-world scenarios, create entirely new worlds, or blend the physical and digital in seamless ways. Design teams should document sensory parameters, session durations, and escalation rules to safeguard users. In mental health, XR has already shown promise in a range of applications: exposure therapy for phobias and social anxiety, immersive mindfulness for stress reduction, and skills rehearsal for social interaction (Kargarandehkordi et al., 2025). Pilot studies should report both short-term engagement metrics and longer-term functional outcomes to guide clinical adoption (Kargarandehkordi et al., 2025).

In mental health, XR has already shown promise in a range of applications: exposure therapy, mindfulness and relaxation, psychoeducation and skills training, and trauma processing (Weiner et al., 2025). For each application, map XR affordances to specific therapeutic mechanisms, such as graded exposure, embodied practice, or narrative reconstruction (Ricciardi & Zomaya, 2025). Exposure therapy: VR environments can simulate anxiety-provoking situations, such as public speaking, flying, or social interactions, in a controlled and safe setting. Protocols must include criteria for progression and therapist-led debriefing to consolidate learning. Mindfulness and relaxation: Immersive nature scenes, guided meditations, and sensory-rich environments can support stress reduction and emotional regulation. Measures of physiological regulation and subjective calm should be collected to validate effects. Psychoeducation and skills training: XR can make abstract concepts tangible, allowing users to visualize cognitive distortions, practice coping strategies, or rehearse social skills (Ricciardi & Zomaya, 2025). Designers should integrate rehearsal with real-world transfer tasks to enhance generalization. Trauma processing: Carefully designed VR experiences can support narrative reconstruction, emotional processing, and integration in trauma therapy. Trauma-informed design requires slow titration, clinician oversight, and protocols for dissociation management.

These applications are not just novel, they are embodied. They engage the user's senses, movements, and spatial awareness. Embodiment amplifies experiential learning by linking cognitive processes to sensorimotor contingencies that support memory and regulation. They allow for presence, the feeling of "being there", which can enhance emotional engagement, memory consolidation, and therapeutic impact. To translate presence into clinical benefit, include pre- and post-session measures of distress, grounding techniques, and structured reflection to integrate experience (Kargarandehkordi et al., 2025). Immersive interventions require clinician training in both technical operation and embodied therapeutic facilitation to ensure safety and efficacy.

NEUROADAPTIVE IMMERSION: THE NEXT STEP (KARGARANDEHKORDI ET AL., 2025)

When XR is combined with biosensors and AI, it becomes more than immersive, it becomes adaptive (Akhtar & Rawol, 2024). Adaptive immersion requires engineering for low-latency feedback loops that can modulate sensory elements in meaningful ways. These neuroadaptive environments can sense the user's physiological and emotional state and adjust in real time to support therapeutic goals (Ong et al., 2025). Imagine a VR meditation app that monitors heart rate variability and adjusts the visual flow of a river scene to match the user's breathing. Or a social skills training simulation that detects signs of anxiety and pauses the interaction to offer coaching. Or a trauma therapy environment that modulates lighting, sound, and narrative pacing based on neural feedback. Each use case necessitates predefined safety thresholds, clinician oversight, and clear user controls.

These systems create a closed-loop between body, brain, and environment. They do not just deliver content, they co-create experience. Such co-creation enhances opportunities for just-in-time interventions, personalized pacing, and context-sensitive support that bridge in-session gains with daily life. They allow for just-in-time interventions, personalized pacing, and context-sensitive support. From a cognitive systems perspective, this is a profound development: it aligns with enactive cognition theories that treat cognition as emergent from embodied interaction. In neuroadaptive XR, the environment is not static, it is a partner in the therapeutic process that can scaffold learning and regulation in situ (Saganowski et al., 2022).

EMBODIMENT AND THE HEALING PROCESS

The importance of embodiment in mental health is increasingly recognized. This recognition invites clinicians to integrate somatic measures and movement-based assessments into treatment planning. Trauma, for example, is not only stored in memory, it is held in the body. Clinical protocols should therefore assess interoceptive awareness and somatic markers as routine components of intake (Agarwal et al., 2025). Practices such as somatic experiencing, yoga therapy, and sensorimotor psychotherapy emphasize the role of bodily awareness, movement, and interoception in healing. Implementation guides should specify pacing, contraindications, and integration strategies for combining somatic work with talk therapy. Immersive technologies can support these practices by creating environments that invite movement, enhance body awareness, and provide sensory feedback. Pilot programs should evaluate both subjective embodiment and objective physiological change to document therapeutic mechanisms.

For example: AR-guided breathing exercises can use visual overlays to guide inhalation and exhalation, helping users synchronize breath and attention. Developers must define visual pacing parameters, customize overlays for different lung capacities, and include fallback spoken guidance. VR movement therapies can support individuals with depression or PTSD in reconnecting with their bodies through gentle, guided motion. These interventions should include graded movement progressions and clinician-monitored safety checks to prevent exacerbation of symptoms. Biofeedback-enhanced environments can help users learn to regulate physiological responses by visualizing their own data in real time (APA, 2023). Research designs should test transfer of these skills to daily life and document adherence and acceptability metrics (Obermeyer et al., 2019).

These applications are not about replacing traditional therapies, they are about extending them into new modalities that are engaging, accessible, and embodied. Integration protocols should specify when to prefer embodied digital tools versus conventional in-person practices based on clinical presentation. They allow clinicians to tailor interventions to client preferences and somatic readiness, creating hybrid care pathways that combine human touch with adaptive technology. Such integration preserves the therapeutic relationship while leveraging novel affordances for regulation and learning. Training curricula must therefore include embodied facilitation skills alongside technical competencies to ensure clinicians can safely steward these combined approaches.

ACCESSIBILITY AND INCLUSION

While immersive technologies hold great promise, they also raise important questions about accessibility and inclusion. Ethical implementation requires assessment of who benefits and who may be excluded by design choices. Not everyone has access to high-end VR headsets or the physical space to move freely. Deployment strategies should include low-cost hardware options, community access points, and mobile adaptations to broaden reach. Some users may experience motion sickness, sensory overload, or discomfort in immersive environments. Screening tools and gradual acclimatization protocols reduce adverse reactions and support equitable participation. Designing BCIs and XR with universal design principles expands usability across sensory, motor, and cognitive differences (Watson, 2025). Offering alternative modalities and adjustable sensory settings allows clinicians to match interventions to diverse needs.

Designing for inclusion means offering multiple modes of interaction to accommodate different abilities and preferences. This multiplicity should be built into requirements from the outset rather than retrofitted post-hoc. Offer voice, gesture, gaze, and controller inputs so that users can select the mode that best matches their capacities and contexts. Provide adjustable sensory settings and simplified interaction modes for neurodiverse users who benefit from reduced stimulus complexity. Ensure low-bandwidth and mobile-compatible options for users in resource-limited settings, with offline capabilities where network access is unreliable. Create culturally relevant environments that reflect diverse identities, languages, and lived experiences, engaging community partners in content development to ensure authenticity and respect.

It also means involving users in the design process, especially those from marginalized communities. Participatory co-design reduces the risk of imposing assumptions and uncovers unanticipated barriers to uptake. Establish advisory panels, usability testing cohorts, and iterative feedback loops that center lived experience in decision-making at every stage. Collect demographic and accessibility outcome data to monitor who is reached and who remains underserved (Aiken et al., 2023). Commit to transparent reporting about limitations, modifications, and access initiatives so stakeholders can evaluate equity claims. Funders should require inclusion plans as part of implementation proposals to ensure resources match stated commitments.

ETHICAL CONSIDERATIONS

As with all neuroadaptive technologies, immersive environments raise ethical questions (Kim & Backonja, 2025). These questions must be addressed proactively with clear governance mechanisms and user protections. Informed consent: Users must understand what data is being collected, how it is used, and how the environment may adapt (Ong et al., 2025). Consent processes should be layered, allowing users to make granular choices about specific data streams and adaptive features (Ong et al., 2025). Psychological safety: Immersive experiences can be intense; systems must include safeguards to prevent overwhelm, dissociation, or re-traumatization. Safety features should include immediate exit options, clinician-triggered pauses, and automated de-escalation routines when physiological markers indicate distress.

Data privacy: XR systems often collect sensitive data, including gaze patterns, movement, and physiological signals (Ong et al., 2025). Maintain strict encryption, minimize retention, and transparently document secondary uses and sharing practices. Authentication and local data controls help users manage privacy preferences effectively (Ong et al., 2025).

Authenticity and trust: Users must feel that the environment is not only engaging but trustworthy. Build trust through transparent design, predictable adaptation rules, and accessible explanations of how the system responds. Provide clear avenues for users to question or contest system interpretations and to request human review. Implement audit trails and easy-to-understand logs that clinicians can review with clients during debriefing. Include mechanisms for reporting harms and for rapid remediation when adverse events occur. Ethical oversight should be continuous, involving ethicists, clinicians, technologists, and representatives of participant communities.

CONCLUSION: DESIGNING SPACES OF CARE

Immersive environments and embodied care represent a powerful frontier in digital mental health. Implementation roadmaps should link therapeutic rationale, safety protocols, and evaluation metrics to operational plans. They allow us to move beyond the limitations of text and screen into spaces that are sensory-rich, emotionally resonant, and deeply human. When combined with neuroadaptive technologies, these environments become not just tools but therapeutic ecosystems, spaces that listen, respond, and support healing in real time. Operationalizing this vision requires cross-sector partnerships, scalable training programs, and sustained investment in equitable access. As we design these spaces, we must do so with intention: centering user experience, honoring the body's wisdom, and creating environments that are safe, inclusive, and empowering.

As we've explored in the preceding sections, the future of neuroadaptive mental health care is being shaped by a constellation of emerging technologies: brain-computer interfaces, affective computing, immersive environments, and biosensing (Babu & Joseph, 2025). These technologies converge around the capacity to sense, interpret, and adapt at scale, creating new possibilities for timely support. Practitioners should therefore evaluate interventions not only for symptom reduction but for their capacity to integrate into existing care workflows and support continuity. Systems thinking helps identify where technologies add value and where human oversight remains essential. This section explores the architecture, applications, and implications of closed-loop systems in mental health. These systems represent the culmination of the neuroadaptive vision: care that is not only personalized and responsive, but self-adjusting, context-aware, and dynamically evolving (Engel, 1977).

In engineering and systems theory, a closed-loop system is one that uses feedback to regulate its behavior. In clinical work, the same logic supports iterative adjustments based on patient responses rather than one-off prescriptions (Hall et al., 2024). It continuously measures its output, compares it to a desired goal, and adjusts its inputs accordingly. Translating this into practice requires specifying measurable goals, acceptable error bounds, and clinician-defined fallback rules. This is in contrast to an open-loop system, which operates without feedback and cannot correct itself in response to changing conditions. Closed-loop designs therefore demand attention to latency, data quality, and human-in-the-loop checkpoints to ensure safety and relevance (Robinson et al., 2024).

In mental health, a closed-loop system might look like this: Sensing: The system collects real-time data from the user, physiological signals, behavioral patterns, emotional cues (Iwaya et al., 2023). Designers should document sensor calibration steps and baseline periods to improve interpretability (Pedram & Piatkowski, 2025). Interpretation: AI algorithms analyze the data to infer the user's current mental state (Pedram & Piatkowski, 2025). Interpretation layers must quantify uncertainty and provide rationale for alerts so clinicians can adjudicate responses. Adaptation: The system adjusts its behavior, delivering a calming prompt, modifying a VR scenario, or escalating to human support. Adaptation policies should include thresholds for clinician notification and options for user override. Evaluation: The system monitors the user's response to the intervention and uses that feedback to refine future actions. Incorporating evaluation metrics supports continuous learning and prevents maladaptive loops.

This loop can occur in milliseconds or over longer timeframes. Implementation teams must therefore choose sampling rates and decision windows that match clinical goals and user contexts (Inkster et al., 2023). It can be embedded in a single app or distributed across a network of devices and platforms. When distributed, teams must ensure synchronized timestamps and consistent semantics for shared signals. What defines it is the continuous, iterative nature of the interaction, a dynamic dance between user and system. This ongoing reciprocity creates opportunities for learning but also raises questions about long-term dependency, habituation, and shifting baselines that require monitoring and ethical oversight.

Closed-loop systems are already being explored in several areas of mental health care. Early translational projects demonstrate application in just-in-time support, adaptive exposure, and neurofeedback training. Just-in-Time Adaptive Interventions (JITAIs): These systems deliver support at the moment it is most needed, such as prompting a mindfulness exercise when stress is detected or suggesting a social connection when loneliness is inferred. Implementation should include user-configurable sensitivity settings and documented escalation pathways. Neurofeedback and Cognitive Training: Closed-loop neurofeedback systems allow users to learn self-regulation by providing real-time feedback on brain activity. These programs should combine practice schedules with behavioral coaching for transfer to daily life. Therapeutic XR Environments: In VR-based therapy, closed-loop systems can adjust the intensity of exposure, the pacing of narrative, or the sensory environment based on physiological and emotional feedback, keeping the user within their therapeutic window (Khoo et al., 2024). Crisis Detection and Escalation: Systems can monitor for signs of acute distress and trigger alerts, connect users to crisis lines, or notify caregivers. Protocols must balance timely support with respect for privacy and user consent.

These applications are not speculative, they are being piloted in research labs, startups, and clinical settings around the world (Freeman et al., 2017). Early translational work demonstrates feasibility but also highlights the importance of rigorous implementation protocols and clinician involvement. Pilot projects often focus on feasibility, acceptability, and safety before moving to efficacy trials, which helps identify practical barriers early. Researchers should publish detailed methods, including calibration procedures and failure modes, to support reproducibility and clinician interpretation (Freeman et al., 2017). Implementation teams must plan for training, maintenance, and integration with clinical workflows to avoid fragmented care (Freeman et al., 2017). Funders should support replication studies and transparent reporting to accelerate reliable evidence synthesis (Freeman et al., 2017).

What they share is a commitment to timeliness, personalization, and responsiveness, hallmarks of effective mental health care. These shared goals guide both technology design and clinical evaluation frameworks. Design specifications should map intervention components to measurable proximal outcomes and user experience metrics. Clinical teams need decision rules that define when automated actions are appropriate and when human clinicians must intervene (Ricciardi & Zomaya, 2025). Evaluation frameworks should therefore include mixed-methods approaches that capture quantitative outcomes and qualitative user experiences. Over time, comparative effectiveness studies will clarify which adaptive features drive meaningful benefits.

Despite promising early work, scaling neuroadaptive interventions requires addressing governance, training, and infrastructure barriers (Lay et al., 2025). Scaling plans must anticipate needs for clinician education, data interoperability, and equitable device distribution (Martinez-Martin et al., 2018). Institutions should develop credentialing pathways that certify clinicians in neuroadaptive competencies and ethical oversight (Martinez-Martin et al., 2018). Technical infrastructure must support secure data exchange, standardized schemas, and audit trails to maintain safety across distributed deployments (Martinez-Martin et al., 2018). Policies should encourage open standards and shared libraries to reduce duplication and accelerate best-practice diffusion. Community partnerships are essential to ensure local relevance and sustainable adoption.

Technical complexity interacts with social, ethical, and clinical constraints in ways that can undermine implementation if not proactively managed (Baka et al., 2025). Multidisciplinary teams should include ethicists, legal experts, and community representatives from the start to anticipate unintended consequences. Conducting staged rollouts with iterative user feedback helps identify equity gaps and cultural mismatches before full deployment. Continuous monitoring for bias, differential performance, and adverse events must be built into post-deployment surveillance. Organizations should create clear channels for user complaints, redress, and system updates to maintain trust and accountability. These governance practices support responsible innovation and user safety.

Ultimately, the future of neuroadaptive mental health care depends on aligning technological possibility with human values, clinical judgment, and equitable access (Livieri et al., 2025). This alignment requires deliberate design choices, robust evaluation, and ongoing dialogue among stakeholders. Clinicians must be prepared to interpret adaptive outputs, communicate limitations, and preserve the therapeutic relationship amid technological augmentation. Policymakers should establish frameworks that protect privacy, ensure fairness, and incentivize inclusive distribution. When these elements converge, neuroadaptive systems can extend reach and responsiveness without sacrificing dignity or autonomy (Poudel et al., 2025).

As we stand at the threshold of a new era in mental health care, one shaped by neuroadaptive systems, brain-computer interfaces, affective computing, and immersive environments, we are called not only to innovate, but to reflect (Liu & Schueller, 2023). This moment requires deliberate attention to ethical design, governance, and the lived realities of users to avoid harm. The technologies we have explored in this chapter are powerful. They promise to transform how care is delivered, how suffering is understood, and how healing unfolds. But with this power comes profound responsibility. Ethical frameworks should guide design choices from prototype to deployment and include mechanisms for user feedback and remediation.

This final section invites us to consider the ethical, philosophical, and societal dimensions of neuroadaptive care (Smith et al., 2023). It asks: What kind of future are we building? Who is it for? And how can we ensure that it is inclusive, participatory, and grounded in care? These questions require multidisciplinary deliberation that centers both empirical evidence and moral reasoning (Robinson et al., 2024). Reflective processes should be iterative, documented, and open to critique from diverse stakeholders. They should also translate theoretical principles into operational checklists that guide teams in practice.

At its core, mental health care is a relational practice. It is built on trust, empathy, and the shared work of meaning-making. As we introduce increasingly intelligent and responsive technologies into this space, we must ask: What does it mean to receive care from a system? Can a machine be empathic? Can an algorithm understand suffering (Robinson et al., 2024)? Teams should test how digital interactions alter relational dynamics and report findings transparently. Researchers and clinicians must jointly evaluate whether technological affordances enhance or diminish the therapeutic relationship in measurable ways.

These are not merely abstract questions. They shape how we design, deploy, and relate to neuroadaptive systems (Robinson et al., 2024). If we treat care as a transaction, an input-output process to be optimized, we risk reducing the richness of human experience to a set of data points (Robinson et al., 2024). But if we treat care as a relationship, dynamic, contextual, and co-created, we open the door to technologies that support, rather than supplant, the human spirit. Design processes should therefore preserve spaces for narrative, reflection, and human judgment within digitally mediated care pathways.

This requires a shift in mindset. We must move from designing systems that are merely efficient to designing systems that are wise, systems that are attuned to context, sensitive to complexity, and guided by ethical principles. Operationally, this means embedding multidisciplinary ethics review, participatory design, and long-term impact evaluation into development lifecycles. Teams should define metrics for wisdom that include dignity, autonomy, and social connectedness alongside clinical symptom measures (Shatte et al., 2019).

DESIGNING FOR EQUITY AND INCLUSION

One of the greatest risks of neuroadaptive technologies is that they will deepen existing inequities (Obermeyer et al., 2019). Design teams must therefore embed equity objectives from project inception, setting measurable access and inclusion targets. Co-design with underserved communities ensures that interventions reflect diverse priorities, languages, and care norms. Funding proposals should require concrete plans for distribution, training, and evaluation in low-resource settings. Audit processes must evaluate algorithmic performance across demographic groups to detect and mitigate disparate impacts. Policymakers and institutions should prioritize subsidized deployment models that reduce cost barriers for marginalized populations. Clinicians and researchers must report demographic reach and access metrics in publications and implementation reports to promote transparency.

PARTICIPATORY FUTURES AND COLLECTIVE IMAGINATION

The future of mental health should not be dictated by technologists, clinicians, or policymakers alone. Convene community panels and lived-experience advisory boards early to surface values, fears, and preferences that shape acceptable interventions. It should be co-created with the people it is meant to serve. Use scenario planning exercises to explore diverse futures and identify social trade-offs before scaling technologies. What do users want from neuroadaptive care (Ball et al., 2025)? Ask structured, iterative questions and record responses as part of design documentation. What fears, hopes, and values do they bring? Translate these insights into design constraints and governance principles. How can we create spaces for dialogue, deliberation, and shared imagination? Allocate budget and time for ongoing public engagement rather than one-off consultations.

THE ETHICS OF KNOWING AND NOT KNOWING

The future of mental health care involves systems that may predict states before users are consciously aware of them (Fanarioti & Karpouzis, 2025). This predictive capacity raises questions about autonomy, surveillance, and informed consent that require procedural safeguards. What does it mean to be known in this way? Establish consent processes that are layered, ongoing, and revocable, enabling users to opt into specific sensing streams. What are the risks of being misread, misdiagnosed, or manipulated? Implement audit logs and human-review checkpoints to catch and correct misclassifications. How do we ensure that users retain control over their data, their choices, and their narratives (Obermeyer et al., 2019)? Provide simple interfaces for data export, deletion, and granular sharing preferences aligned with clinical workflows (Obermeyer et al., 2019).

A VISION FOR THE FUTURE

We envision a future where mental health care is responsive, relational, inclusive, empowering, and ethical. Translate this vision into operational principles by specifying measurable criteria for each value, such as responsiveness metrics, equity indices, and user-reported empowerment scales. In this future, neuroadaptive systems are partners in care rather than replacements for human clinicians (Gkintoni et al., 2025). Define roles and handoff rules that clarify when systems prompt human involvement and how responsibility is shared. They extend our capacity to listen, to understand, and to support one another. Build evaluation frameworks that assess both technical performance and relational outcomes, including trust, perceived dignity, and social connectedness.

BUILDING FUTURES WORTH LIVING

So, what kind of future do we want to build? Use participatory impact assessments to decide which trajectories align with community priorities. We envision systems that are not only innovative, but just; not only intelligent, but wise; not only scalable, but human. Operationalize justice through equitable procurement practices, inclusive hiring, and community benefit agreements tied to deployment. In this future, neuroadaptive systems augment human care and strengthen social supports rather than displace them (Ricciardi & Zomaya, 2025). Let us build technologies that advance well-being while preserving agency, dignity, and meaningful connection.

REFERENCES

Adegoke, K., Adegoke, A., Dawodu, D., Adekoya, A., Bayowa, A., Kayode, T., & Singh, M. (2025). Interoperability as a catalyst for digital health and therapeutics: A scoping review of emerging technologies and standards (2015–2025). *International Journal of Environmental Research and Public Health, 22*(10), 1535. DOI: 10.3390/ijerph22101535 PMID: 41154939

Agarwal, S., Jalan, M., Hill, R., Pantalone, E., Thrul, J., Sharma, R., Wilcox, H. C., & Robinson, K. A. (2025). Framework to Assist Stakeholders in Technology Evaluation for Recovery (Freeman et al., 2017) to Mental Health and Wellness. *BMC Health Services Research, 25*, 623. Advance online publication. DOI: 10.1186/s12913-025-12418-0 PMID: 40307807

Aiken, L. H., Lasater, K. B., Sloane, D. M., Pogue, C. A., Rosenbaum, K. E. F., & Muir, K. J.US Clinician Wellbeing Study Consortium. (2023, July). Physician and nurse well-being and preferred interventions to address burnout in hospital practice: Factors associated with turnover, outcomes, and patient safety. [). American Medical Association.]. *JAMA Health Forum, 4*(7), e231809–e231809. DOI: 10.1001/jamahealthforum.2023.1809 PMID: 37418269

Akhtar, Z. B., & Rawol, A. T. (2025). Artificial Intelligence (Leivaditis & Sepetis, 2025) & Extended Reality (Reddy, 2025) within Healthcare: A Multidimensional Biomedical Engineering (Rajpal, 2025) Investigative Exploration. *Biomed. Clin. Res. J, 1*, 1–22.

Allgaier, J., Mulansky, L., Draelos, R. L., & Pryss, R. (2023). How does the model make predictions? A systematic literature review on the explainability power of machine learning in healthcare. *Artificial Intelligence in Medicine, 143*, 102616. DOI: 10.1016/j.artmed.2023.102616 PMID: 37673561

American Psychiatric Association. (2023). Digital [Resource Document. APA.]. *Mental Health (Detroit, Mich.)*, •••, 101.

Babu, A., & Joseph, A. P. (2025). Digital wellness or digital dependency? A critical examination of mental health apps and their implications. *Frontiers in Psychiatry, 16*, 1581779. DOI: 10.3389/fpsyt.2025.1581779 PMID: 40248604

Baka, E., Tan, Y.-R., Wong, B. L. H., Xing, Z., & Yap, P. (2025). A scoping review of digital interventions for the promotion of mental health and prevention of mental health conditions for young people. *Oxford Open Digital Health, 3*, oqaf005. DOI: 10.1093/oodh/oqaf005 PMID: 40230873

Ball, H., Eisner, E., Nicholas, J., Wilson, P., & Bucci, S. (2025). How theories, models, and frameworks have been used to implement digital health interventions in services for people with severe mental health problems: A scoping review. *BMC Public Health*, *25*(1), 1023. DOI: 10.1186/s12889-025-22189-2 PMID: 40098003

Bayor, A. A., Li, J., Yang, I. A., & Varnfield, M. (2025). Designing Clinical Decision Support Systems (CDSS)—A User-Centered Lens of the Design Characteristics, Challenges, and Implications: Systematic Review. *Journal of Medical Internet Research*, *27*, e63733. DOI: 10.2196/63733 PMID: 40540451

Bibi, P (2024). Establishing Transparency and Accountability in AI: Ethical Standards for Data Governance and Automated Systems. In.

Boda, V. V. R., & Allam, H. (2022). Ready for Anything: Disaster Recovery Strategies Every Healthcare IT Team Should Know. *International Journal of Emerging Trends in Computer Science and Information Technology*, *3*(1), 38–46. DOI: 10.63282/3050-9246.IJETCSIT-V3I1P105

Boffet, A., Arsac, L. M., Ibanez, V., Sauvet, F., & Deschodt-Arsac, V. (2025). Detection of Cognitive Load Modulation by EDA and HRV. *Sensors (Basel)*, *25*(8), 2343. DOI: 10.3390/s25082343 PMID: 40285033

Bond, R. R., Mulvenna, M. D., Potts, C., O'Neill, S., Ennis, E., & Torous, J. (2023). Digital transformation of mental health services. *Npj Mental Health Research*, *2*(1), 13. DOI: 10.1038/s44184-023-00033-y PMID: 38609479

Chaabene, S., Boudaya, A., Bouaziz, B., & Chaari, L. (2025). An overview of methods and techniques in multimodal data fusion with application to healthcare. *International Journal of Data Science and Analytics*, *20*(4), 1–25. DOI: 10.1007/s41060-025-00715-0

Chen, Z. S., Galatzer-Levy, I. R., Bigio, B., Nasca, C., & Zhang, Y. (2022). Modern views of machine learning for precision psychiatry. *Patterns (New York, N.Y.)*, *3*(11), 100602. DOI: 10.1016/j.patter.2022.100602 PMID: 36419447

Chithra, N., & Bhambri, P. (2024). Ethics in sustainable technology. In *Handbook of Technological Sustainability* (pp. 245–256). CRC Press. DOI: 10.1201/9781003475989-21

Correa, T., Pavez, I., & Contreras, J. (2021). Digital inequality and mobiles: opportunities and challenges of relying on smartphones for digital inclusion in disadvantaged contexts. Handbook of digital inequality, 62-74.

Cristofaro, M., & Giardino, P. L. (2025). Surfing the AI waves: The historical evolution of artificial intelligence in management and organizational studies and practices. *Journal of Management History*. Advance online publication. DOI: 10.1108/JMH-01-2025-0002

De Kock, J. H., Latham, H. A., Leslie, S. J., Grindle, M., Munoz, S. A., Ellis, L., Polson, R., & O'Malley, C. M. (2021). A rapid review of the impact of COVID-19 on the mental health of healthcare workers: Implications for supporting psychological well-being. *BMC Public Health*, *21*(1), 104. DOI: 10.1186/s12889-020-10070-3 PMID: 33422039

Engel, G. L. (1977). The need for a new medical model: A challenge for biomedicine. *Science*, *196*(4286), 129–136. DOI: 10.1126/science.847460 PMID: 847460

Fanarioti, A. K., & Karpouzis, K. (2025). Artificial Intelligence and the Future of Mental Health in a Digitally Transformed World. *Computers*, *14*(7), 259. DOI: 10.3390/computers14070259

Freeman, D., Reeve, S., Robinson, A., Ehlers, A., Clark, D., Spanlang, B., & Slater, M. (2017). Virtual reality in the assessment, understanding, and treatment of mental health disorders. *Psychological Medicine*, *47*(14), 2393–2400. DOI: 10.1017/S003329171700040X PMID: 28325167

Gkintoni, E., Vassilopoulos, S. P., & Nikolaou, G. (2025). Next-generation cognitive-behavioral therapy for depression: Integrating digital tools, teletherapy, and personalization for enhanced mental health outcomes. *Medicina (Kaunas, Lithuania)*, *61*(3), 431. DOI: 10.3390/medicina61030431 PMID: 40142242

Hall, C. L., Gómez Bergin, A. D., & Rennick-Egglestone, S. (2024). Research into digital health intervention for mental health: 25-year retrospective on the ethical and legal challenges. *Journal of Medical Internet Research*, *26*, e58939. DOI: 10.2196/58939 PMID: 39250796

Hiland, E. B. (2021). *Therapy tech: The digital transformation of mental healthcare*. U of Minnesota Press. DOI: 10.5749/j.ctv1xp9q3t

Ienca, M., Fabrice, J., Elger, B., Caon, M., Scoccia Pappagallo, A., Kressig, R. W., & Wangmo, T. (2017). Intelligent assistive technology for Alzheimer's disease and other dementias: A systematic review. *Journal of Alzheimer's Disease*, *56*(4), 1301–1340. DOI: 10.3233/JAD-161037 PMID: 28222516

Inkster, B., Knibbs, C., & Bada, M. (2023). Cybersecurity: A critical priority for digital mental health. *Frontiers in Digital Health*, *5*, 1242264. DOI: 10.3389/fdgth.2023.1242264 PMID: 37781452

Iwaya, L. H., Babar, M. A., Rashid, A., & Wijayarathna, C. (2023). On the privacy of mental health apps: An empirical investigation and its implications for app development. *Empirical Software Engineering*, *28*(1), 2. DOI: 10.1007/s10664-022-10236-0 PMID: 36407814

Kang, H. S., & Exworthy, M. (2022). Wearing the future—wearables to empower users to take greater responsibility for their health and care: Scoping review. *JMIR mHealth and uHealth*, *10*(7), e35684. DOI: 10.2196/35684 PMID: 35830222

Kargarandehkordi, A., Li, S., Lin, K., Phillips, K. T., Benzo, R. M., & Washington, P. (2025). Fusing wearable biosensors with artificial intelligence for mental health monitoring: A systematic review. *Biosensors (Basel)*, *15*(4), 202. DOI: 10.3390/bios15040202 PMID: 40277515

Khoo, Y. X., Kang, R. M., Reynolds, T. L., & Mentis, H. M. (2024). The comprehensiveness of mental health application users' privacy and security concerns. *CHI Conference on Human Factors in Computing Systems*, 16 pages.

Kim, J., & Backonja, U. (2025). Digital health equity frameworks and key concepts: A scoping review. *Journal of the American Medical Informatics Association : JAMIA*, *32*(1), 45–59. DOI: 10.1093/jamia/ocaf017 PMID: 39936843

Kostadimas, D., Kasapakis, V., & Kotis, K. (2025). A systematic review on the combination of VR, IoT and AI technologies, and their integration in applications. *Future Internet*, *17*(4), 163. DOI: 10.3390/fi17040163

Kumar, T., Arora, M., Verma, V., Bhushan, S., & Lalar, S. (2024). Biometric System Integration in Public Health: Challenges and Solutions. In Computational Intelligence and Mathematical Applications (pp. 168-173). CRC Press.

Lamb, R., Choi, I., & Owens, T (2025). Convergence of Extended Reality, Artificial Intelligence, Machine Leaning, and Wearable Sensors in the Field of Education. Mental Health Virtual Reality: The Power of Immersive Worlds, 113-128.

Lay, W., Gasparini, L., Siero, W., & Hughes, E. K. (2025). A rapid review of the benefits and challenges of dynamic consent. *Research Ethics*, *21*(1), 180–202. DOI: 10.1177/17470161241278064

Li, M., Patel, J., & Katapally, T. R. (2025). The impact of extended reality cognitive behavioral therapy on mental disorders among children and youth: A systematic review and meta-analysis protocol. *PLoS One*, *20*(3), e0315313. DOI: 10.1371/journal.pone.0315313 PMID: 40048453

Liu, M., & Schueller, S. M. (2023). Moving evidence-based mental health interventions into practice: Implementation of digital mental health interventions. *Current Treatment Options in Psychiatry, 10*(4), 333–345. DOI: 10.1007/s40501-023-00298-2

Livieri, G., Mangina, E., Protopapadakis, E. D., & Panayiotou, A. G. (2025). The gaps and challenges in digital health technology use as perceived by patients: A scoping review and narrative meta-synthesis. *Frontiers in Digital Health, 7*, 1474956. DOI: 10.3389/fdgth.2025.1474956 PMID: 40212901

Ma, C.-B., Shang, X., Sun, M., Bo, X., Bai, J., Du, Y., & Zhou, M. (2025). Emerging Multifunctional Wearable Sensors: Integrating Multimodal Sweat Analysis and Advanced Material Technologies for Next-Generation Health Monitoring. *ACS Sensors, 10*(4), 2388–2408. DOI: 10.1021/acssensors.4c03396 PMID: 40162570

Martinez-Martin, N., Marcandalli, J., Huang, C. S., Arthur, C. P., Perotti, M., Foglierini, M., Ho, H., Dosey, A. M., Shriver, S., Payandeh, J., Leitner, A., Lanzavecchia, A., Perez, L., & Ciferri, C. (2018). An unbiased screen for human cytomegalovirus identifies neuropilin-2 as a central viral receptor. *Cell, 174*(5), 1158–1171. DOI: 10.1016/j.cell.2018.06.028 PMID: 30057110

Mohammad, N. (2021). Enhancing security and privacy in multi-cloud environments: A comprehensive study on encryption techniques and access control mechanisms. [IJCET]. *International Journal of Computer Engineering and Technology, 12*(2), 51–63.

Mohr, D. C., Zhang, M., & Schueller, S. M. (2017). Personal sensing: Understanding mental health using ubiquitous sensors and machine learning. *Annual Review of Clinical Psychology, 13*(1), 23–47. DOI: 10.1146/annurev-clinpsy-032816-044949 PMID: 28375728

Morey, D. A., Rayo, M. F., & Woods, D. D. (2025). Empirically derived evaluation requirements for responsible deployments of AI in safety-critical settings. *NPJ Digital Medicine, 8*(1), 374. DOI: 10.1038/s41746-025-01784-y PMID: 40533485

Morgan, J. W., Patel, R. A., & Campbell, S. (2025). Practical considerations of clinical XR (Singh & Chandra, 2025) deployments. *Frontiers in Virtual Reality, 6*, 1517402. DOI: 10.3389/frvir.2025.1517402

Obermeyer, Z., Powers, B., Vogeli, C., & Mullainathan, S. (2019). Dissecting racial bias in an algorithm used to manage the health of populations. *Science, 366*(6464), 447–453. DOI: 10.1126/science.aax2342 PMID: 31649194

Omiyefa, S. (2025). Artificial intelligence and machine learning in precision mental health diagnostics and predictive treatment models. *Int J Res Publ Rev*, *6*(3), 85–99. DOI: 10.55248/gengpi.6.0325.1107

Ong, T., Ivanova, J., Soni, H., Barrera, J., Cummins, M., Welch, B. M., & Bunnell, B. E. (2025). Mental health clients' perspectives on telehealth-based virtual reality therapy. *Frontiers in Virtual Reality*, *6*, 1595326. DOI: 10.3389/frvir.2025.1595326

Panarese, P., Grasso, M. M., & Solinas, C. (2025). Algorithmic bias, fairness, and inclusivity: A multilevel framework for justice-oriented AI. *AI & Society*, ●●●, 1–23. DOI: 10.1007/s00146-025-02451-2

Pedram, S., & Piatkowski, T. (2025). Exploring the potential of virtual reality (Johnson et al., 2021) in mental healthcare: A systematic literature review. *Virtual Reality (Waltham Cross)*, *29*(3), 135. DOI: 10.1007/s10055-025-01181-6

Poudel, U., Jakhar, S., Mohan, P., & Nepal, A. (2025). AI in mental health: A review of technological advancements and ethical issues in psychiatry. *Issues in Mental Health Nursing*, *46*(7), 693–701. DOI: 10.1080/01612840.2025.2502943 PMID: 40378075

Radanliev, P. (2025). Privacy, ethics, transparency, and accountability in AI systems for wearable devices. *Frontiers in Digital Health*, *7*, 1431246. DOI: 10.3389/fdgth.2025.1431246 PMID: 40599875

Rajpal, S. (2025). Exploring the Role of Virtual Reality and Metaverse in Treating Mental Health: Operating Models and Challenges in Adoption. *Journal of Computer and Communications*, *13*(10), 1–22. DOI: 10.4236/jcc.2025.1310001

Ricciardi, F., & Zomaya, A. (2025). Perspectives on Managing AI Ethics in the Digital Age. *Information (Basel)*, *16*(2), 89. DOI: 10.3390/info16040318

Robinson, A., Flom, M., Forman-Hoffman, V. L., Histon, T., Levy, M., Darcy, A., Ajayi, T., Mohr, D. C., Wicks, P., Greene, C., & Montgomery, R. M. (2024). Equity in digital mental health interventions in the United States: Where to next? *Journal of Medical Internet Research*, *26*, e59939. DOI: 10.2196/59939 PMID: 39316436

Ross, G., Zhao, Y., Bosman, A., Geballa-Koukoula, A., Zhou, H., Elliott, C., Nielen, M., Rafferty, K., & Salentijn, G (2022). Data handling and ethics of emerging smartphone-based (Glass et al., 2022) sensors–Part 1: best practices and current implementation.

Saganowski, S., Perz, B., Polak, A. G., & Kazienko, P. (2022). Emotion recognition for everyday life using physiological signals from wearables: A systematic literature review. *IEEE Transactions on Affective Computing, 14*(3), 1876–1897. DOI: 10.1109/TAFFC.2022.3176135

Saksena, N., Matthan, R., Bhan, A., & Balsari, S. (2021). Rebooting consent in the digital age: A governance framework for health data exchange. *BMJ Global Health, 6*(Suppl 5), e005057. DOI: 10.1136/bmjgh-2021-005057 PMID: 34301754

Shatte, A. B., Hutchinson, D. M., & Teague, S. J. (2019). Machine learning in mental health: A scoping review of methods and applications. *Psychological Medicine, 49*(9), 1426–1448. DOI: 10.1017/S0033291719000151 PMID: 30744717

Sheikh, M., Qassem, M., & Kyriacou, P. A. (2021). Wearable, environmental, and smartphone-based passive sensing for mental health monitoring. *Frontiers in Digital Health, 3*, 662811. DOI: 10.3389/fdgth.2021.662811 PMID: 34713137

Smith, K. A., Blease, C., Faurholt-Jepsen, M., Firth, J., Van Daele, T., Moreno, C., Carlbring, P., Ebner-Priemer, U. W., Koutsouleris, N., Riper, H., Mouchabac, S., Torous, J., & Cipriani, A. (2023). Digital mental health: Challenges and next steps. *BMJ Mental Health, 26*(1), e300670. DOI: 10.1136/bmjment-2023-300670 PMID: 37197797

Subu, M. A., Holmes, D., Arumugam, A., Al-Yateem, N., Maria Dias, J., Rahman, S. A., Waluyo, I., Ahmed, F. R., & Abraham, M. S. (2022). Traditional, religious, and cultural perspectives on mental illness: A qualitative study on causal beliefs and treatment use. *International Journal of Qualitative Studies on Health and Well-being, 17*(1), 2123090. DOI: 10.1080/17482631.2022.2123090 PMID: 36097886

Verma, H., Mlynar, J., Schaer, R., Reichenbach, J., Jreige, M., Prior, J., Evéquoz, F., & Depeursinge, A. (2023). Rethinking the role of AI with physicians in oncology: revealing perspectives from clinical and research workflows. *Proceedings of the 2023 CHI conference on human factors in computing systems*. DOI: 10.1145/3544548.3581506

Watson, D (2025). The dark side of mental health apps: Privacy concerns and therapeutic limitations. MentalHealthSigns.com.

Weiner, E. B., Dankwa-Mullan, I., Nelson, W. A., & Hassanpour, S. (2025). Ethical challenges and evolving strategies in the integration of artificial intelligence into clinical practice. *PLOS Digital Health, 4*(4), e0000810. DOI: 10.1371/journal.pdig.0000810 PMID: 40198594

Wibberly, K. H. (2024). Preparing mental health providers for the future: The case for moving beyond the elective telehealth course to integrating telehealth training throughout the curriculum. *Frontiers in Psychology*, *14*, 1301569. DOI: 10.3389/fpsyg.2023.1301569 PMID: 38235285

Zenker, S., Strech, D., Ihrig, K., Jahns, R., Müller, G., Schickhardt, C., Schmidt, G., Speer, R., Winkler, E., von Kielmansegg, S. G., & Drepper, J. (2022). Data protection-compliant broad consent for secondary use of health care data and human biosamples for (Mulukuntla, 2025) medical research: Towards a new German national standard. *Journal of Biomedical Informatics*, *131*, 104096. DOI: 10.1016/j.jbi.2022.104096 PMID: 35643273

Compilation of References

Abdul Rahman, N. F., Davies, N., Suhaimi, J., Idris, F., Syed Mohamad, S. N., & Park, S. (2023). Transformative learning in clinical reasoning: A meta-synthesis in undergraduate primary care medical education. *Education for Primary Care : An Official Publication of the Association of Course Organisers, National Association of GP Tutors, World Organisation of Family Doctors*, *34*(4), 211–219. DOI: 10.1080/14739879.2023.2248070 PMID: 37742228

Adegoke, K., Adegoke, A., Dawodu, D., Bayowa, A., & Adekoya, A (2025). Interoperability in digital healthcare: Enhancing consumer health and transforming care systems.

Adegoke, K., Adegoke, A., Dawodu, D., Adekoya, A., Bayowa, A., Kayode, T., & Singh, M. (2025). Interoperability as a catalyst for digital health and therapeutics: A scoping review of emerging technologies and standards (2015–2025). *International Journal of Environmental Research and Public Health*, *22*(10), 1535. DOI: 10.3390/ijerph22101535 PMID: 41154939

Adepoju, D. A., & Adepoju, A. G. (2025). Establishing ethical frameworks for scalable data engineering and governance in AI-driven healthcare systems. *Int. J. Res. Publ. Rev*, *6*(4), 8710–8726. DOI: 10.55248/gengpi.6.0425.1547

Agarwal, S., Jalan, M., Hill, R., Pantalone, E., Thrul, J., Sharma, R., Wilcox, H. C., & Robinson, K. A. (2025). Framework to Assist Stakeholders in Technology Evaluation for Recovery (Freeman et al., 2017) to Mental Health and Wellness. *BMC Health Services Research*, *25*, 623. Advance online publication. DOI: 10.1186/s12913-025-12418-0 PMID: 40307807

Aiken, L. H., Lasater, K. B., Sloane, D. M., Pogue, C. A., Rosenbaum, K. E. F., & Muir, K. J.US Clinician Wellbeing Study Consortium. (2023, July). Physician and nurse well-being and preferred interventions to address burnout in hospital practice: Factors associated with turnover, outcomes, and patient safety. [). American Medical Association.]. *JAMA Health Forum*, *4*(7), e231809–e231809. DOI: 10.1001/jamahealthforum.2023.1809 PMID: 37418269

Akhtar, Z. B., & Rawol, A. T. (2024). Artificial intelligence (Tizzard, 2025) and extended reality (XR): A biomedical engineering perspective investigation analysis. *Indonesian Journal of Electronics, Electromedical Engineering, and Medical Informatics*, *6*(3). Advance online publication. DOI: 10.35882/ijeeemi.v6i3.5

Akhtar, Z. B., & Rawol, A. T. (2025). Artificial Intelligence (Leivaditis & Sepetis, 2025) & Extended Reality (Reddy, 2025) within Healthcare: A Multidimensional Biomedical Engineering (Rajpal, 2025) Investigative Exploration. *Biomed. Clin. Res. J*, *1*, 1–22.

Akinode, A. O., Ayadi, O. E., Ezerioha, C. C., & Chika, P (2025). Machine Learning Approaches for Early Detection of Mental Health Disorders Using Wearable Devices and Big Data Analytics. environments, 4, 5.

Alhammad, N., Alajlani, M., Abd-alrazaq, A., Epiphaniou, G., & Arvanitis, T. (2024). Patients' perspectives on the data confidentiality, privacy, and security of mHealth apps: Systematic review. *Journal of Medical Internet Research*, *26*, e50715. DOI: 10.2196/50715 PMID: 38820572

Alifia, R. R., Sadeghi, M., Eluru, M., Jafari, M., & Grando, M. A. (2025). Bridging ethical gaps in digital health research: A framework for informed consent aligned with NIH guidance. *BMC Medical Ethics*, *26*(1), 132. DOI: 10.1186/s12910-025-01291-5 PMID: 41063017

Allgaier, J., Mulansky, L., Draelos, R. L., & Pryss, R. (2023). How does the model make predictions? A systematic literature review on the explainability power of machine learning in healthcare. *Artificial Intelligence in Medicine*, *143*, 102616. DOI: 10.1016/j.artmed.2023.102616 PMID: 37673561

Almadani, B., Kaisar, H., Thoker, I. R., & Aliyu, F. (2025). A systematic survey of distributed decision support systems in healthcare. *Systems*, *13*(3), 157. DOI: 10.3390/systems13030157

Alzghaibi, H. (2025). Nurses' perspectives on AI-enabled wearable health technologies: Opportunities and challenges in clinical practice. *BMC Nursing*, *24*(1), 799. DOI: 10.1186/s12912-025-03343-y PMID: 40598216

American Psychiatric Association. (2023). Digital [Resource Document. APA.]. *Mental Health (Detroit, Mich.)*, •••, 101.

Anklam, E., Bahl, M. I., Ball, R., Beger, R. D., Cohen, J., Fitzpatrick, S., Girard, P., Halamoda-Kenzaoui, B., Hinton, D., Hirose, A., Hoeveler, A., Honma, M., Hugas, M., Ishida, S., Kass, G. E. N., Kojima, H., Krefting, I., Liachenko, S., Liu, Y., & Slikker, W.Jr. (2022). Emerging technologies and their impact on regulatory science. *Experimental Biology and Medicine (Maywood, N.J.)*, *247*(1), 1–75. DOI: 10.1177/15353702211052280 PMID: 34783606

Armontrout, J. A., Torous, J., Cohen, M., McNiel, D. E., & Binder, R. (2018). Current Regulation of Mobile Mental Health Applications. *The Journal of the American Academy of Psychiatry and the Law*, *46*(2), 204–211. DOI: 10.29158/JAAPL.003748-18 PMID: 30026399

ASPE (2024). How health information exchanges support integration for behavioral health settings.

Auf, H., Svedberg, P., Nygren, J., Nair, M., & Lundgren, L. E. (2025). The use of AI in mental health services to support decision-making: Scoping review. *Journal of Medical Internet Research*, *27*, e63548. DOI: 10.2196/63548 PMID: 39854710

Babu, A., & Joseph, A. P. (2025). Digital wellness or digital dependency? A critical examination of mental health apps and their implications. *Frontiers in Psychiatry*, *16*, 1581779. DOI: 10.3389/fpsyt.2025.1581779 PMID: 40248604

Back, S. E., Acierno, R., Saraiya, T. C., Harley, B., Wangelin, B., Jarnecke, A. M., McTeague, L. M., Brown, D. G., Santa Ana, E., & Rothbaum, A. O. (2022). Enhancing Prolonged Exposure therapy for PTSD using physiological biomarker-driven technology. *Contemporary Clinical Trials Communications*, *28*, 100940. DOI: 10.1016/j.conctc.2022.100940 PMID: 35664505

Baka, E., Tan, Y.-R., Wong, B. L. H., Xing, Z., & Yap, P. (2025). A scoping review of digital interventions for the promotion of mental health and prevention of mental health conditions for young people. *Oxford Open Digital Health*, *3*, oqaf005. DOI: 10.1093/oodh/oqaf005 PMID: 40230873

Balcombe, L. (2023). AI chatbots in digital mental health. *Informatics (MDPI)*, *10*(4), 82. DOI: 10.3390/informatics10040082

Ball, H., Eisner, E., Nicholas, J., Wilson, P., & Bucci, S. (2025). How theories, models, and frameworks have been used to implement digital health interventions in services for people with severe mental health problems: A scoping review. *BMC Public Health*, *25*(1), 1023. DOI: 10.1186/s12889-025-22189-2 PMID: 40098003

Bapat, C., & Jog, S (2025). Data-driven ethical guidelines for digitized mental health services: Principal components analysis. Frontiers in Human Dynamics, 7, Article 1549325.

Basystiuk, O., Rybchak, Z., Zavushchak, I., & Marikutsa, U. (2024). Evaluation of multimodal data synchronization tools. *Comput. Des. Syst. Theory Pract*, *6*(3), 104–111. DOI: 10.23939/cds2024.03.104

Baumann, S., Stone, R. T., & Abdelall, E. (2024). Introducing a remote patient monitoring usability impact model to overcome challenges. *Sensors (Basel)*, *24*(12), 3977. DOI: 10.3390/s24123977 PMID: 38931760

Baydili, İ., Tasci, B., & Tasci, G. (2025). Artificial intelligence in psychiatry: A review of biological and behavioral data analyses. *Diagnostics (Basel)*, *15*(4), 434. DOI: 10.3390/diagnostics15040434 PMID: 40002587

Bayor, A. A., Li, J., Yang, I. A., & Varnfield, M. (2025). Designing Clinical Decision Support Systems (CDSS)—A User-Centered Lens of the Design Characteristics, Challenges, and Implications: Systematic Review. *Journal of Medical Internet Research*, *27*, e63733. DOI: 10.2196/63733 PMID: 40540451

Berardi, C., Antonini, M., Jordan, Z., Wechtler, H., Paolucci, F., & Hinwood, M. (2024). Barriers and facilitators to the implementation of digital technologies in mental health systems: A qualitative systematic review to inform a policy framework. *BMC Health Services Research*, *24*(1), 243. DOI: 10.1186/s12913-023-10536-1 PMID: 38408938

Bezyl, E. H. (2024). Mental health apps: Regulation and validation are needed. Global Forum DIA.

BHM Healthcare Solutions. (2025). Technology and the behavioral health shortage. Retrieved from https://bhmpc.com/2025/05/technology-and-the-behavioral-health-shortage/

Bibi, P (2024). Establishing Transparency and Accountability in AI: Ethical Standards for Data Governance and Automated Systems. In.

Boda, V. V. R., & Allam, H. (2022). Ready for Anything: Disaster Recovery Strategies Every Healthcare IT Team Should Know. *International Journal of Emerging Trends in Computer Science and Information Technology*, *3*(1), 38–46. DOI: 10.63282/3050-9246.IJETCSIT-V3I1P105

Boffet, A., Arsac, L. M., Ibanez, V., Sauvet, F., & Deschodt-Arsac, V. (2025). Detection of Cognitive Load Modulation by EDA and HRV. *Sensors (Basel)*, *25*(8), 2343. DOI: 10.3390/s25082343 PMID: 40285033

Bond, R. R., Mulvenna, M. D., Potts, C., O'Neill, S., Ennis, E., & Torous, J. (2023). Digital transformation of mental health services. *Npj Mental Health Research*, *2*(1), 13. DOI: 10.1038/s44184-023-00033-y PMID: 38609479

Bouderhem, R. (2023). Privacy and regulatory issues in wearable health technology. *Engineering Proceedings*, *58*(1), 87.

Brasier, N. K., Mahato, K., Princip, M., Matos Gonçalves, V., Mutuyimana, C., Bourke, S., Schaffarczyk, D., Goldhahn, J., Barata, F., von Känel, R., Kowatsch, T., & Wang, J. (2025). Next-generation wearable sensors for biopsychosocial care in mental health: A narrative review. *BMJ Digital Health & AI*, *1*(1), e000018. DOI: 10.1136/bmjdhai-2025-000018

Brotherdale, R., Berry, K., Branitsky, A., & Bucci, S. (2024). Co-producing digital mental health interventions: A systematic review. *Digital Health*, *10*, 128–145. DOI: 10.1177/20552076241239172 PMID: 38665886

Bunyi, J., Ringland, K. E., & Schueller, S. M. (2021). Accessibility and digital mental health: Considerations for more accessible and equitable mental health apps. *Frontiers in Digital Health*, *3*, 742196. DOI: 10.3389/fdgth.2021.742196 PMID: 34713206

Camacho, E., Cohen, A., & Torous, J. (2022). Assessment of mental health services available through smartphone apps. *JAMA Network Open*, *5*(12), e2248784. DOI: 10.1001/jamanetworkopen.2022.48784 PMID: 36576737

Canali, S., Schiaffonati, V., & Aliverti, A. (2022). Challenges and recommendations for wearable devices in digital health: Data quality, interoperability, health equity, fairness. *PLOS Digital Health*, *1*(10), e0000104. DOI: 10.1371/journal.pdig.0000104 PMID: 36812619

Carl, E., Stein, A. T., Levihn-Coon, A., Pogue, J. R., Rothbaum, B., Emmelkamp, P., Asmundson, G. J. G., Carlbring, P., & Powers, M. B. (2019). Virtual reality exposure therapy for anxiety and related disorders: A meta-analysis of randomized controlled trials. *Journal of Anxiety Disorders*, *61*, 27–36. DOI: 10.1016/j.janxdis.2018.08.003 PMID: 30287083

Casson, A. J. (2019). Wearable EEG and beyond. *Biomedical Engineering Letters*, *9*(1), 53–71. DOI: 10.1007/s13534-018-00093-6 PMID: 30956880

CDC. (2023). Health workers face a mental health crisis. *VitalSigns*.

Chaabene, S., Boudaya, A., Bouaziz, B., & Chaari, L. (2025). An overview of methods and techniques in multimodal data fusion with application to healthcare. *International Journal of Data Science and Analytics*, *20*(4), 1–25. DOI: 10.1007/s41060-025-00715-0

Chennupati, N. (2025). Securing the Automated Enterprise: A Framework for Mitigating Security and Privacy Risks in AI-Driven Workflow Automation. *Journal of Computer Science and Technology Studies*, *7*(3), 624–632. DOI: 10.32996/jcsts.2025.7.3.71

Chen, Z. S., Galatzer-Levy, I. R., Bigio, B., Nasća, C., & Zhang, Y. (2022). Modern views of machine learning for precision psychiatry. *Patterns (New York, N.Y.)*, *3*(11), 100602. DOI: 10.1016/j.patter.2022.100602 PMID: 36419447

Chithra, N., & Bhambri, P. (2024). Ethics in sustainable technology. In *Handbook of Technological Sustainability* (pp. 245–256). CRC Press. DOI: 10.1201/9781003475989-21

Clemens-Meyer, F. H., Lepot, M., Blumensaat, F., Leutnant, D., & Gruber, G. (2021). In Bertrand-Krajewski, J.-L., Clemens-Meyer, F., Lepot, M., & Publishing, I. W. A. (Eds.), *Data validation and data quality assessment. Metrology in Urban Drainage and Stormwater Management: Plug and Pray* (pp. 327–390).

CMS (2024). Interoperability Framework.

Correa, T., Pavez, I., & Contreras, J. (2021). Digital inequality and mobiles: opportunities and challenges of relying on smartphones for digital inclusion in disadvantaged contexts. Handbook of digital inequality, 62-74.

County Health Rankings & Roadmaps. (2025). Mental health providers: Ratio of population to providers. Retrieved from https://www.countyhealthrankings.org

Crameri, L., Hettiarachchi, I. T., & Hanoun, S. (2021). Effects of dynamic resilience on the reactivity of vagally mediated heart rate variability. *Frontiers in Psychology*, *11*, 579210. DOI: 10.3389/fpsyg.2020.579210 PMID: 33551903

Cristofaro, M., & Giardino, P. L. (2025). Surfing the AI waves: The historical evolution of artificial intelligence in management and organizational studies and practices. *Journal of Management History*. Advance online publication. DOI: 10.1108/JMH-01-2025-0002

Crocker, K. M., Gnatt, I., Haywood, D., Butterfield, I., Bhat, R., Lalitha, A. R. N., Jenkins, Z. M., & Castle, D. J. (2023). The impact of COVID-19 on the mental health workforce: A rapid review. *International Journal of Mental Health Nursing*, *32*(2), 420–445. DOI: 10.1111/inm.13097 PMID: 36461629

Cruz-Gonzalez, P., He, A. W. J., Lam, E. P., Ng, I. M. C., Li, M. W., Hou, R., & Vidaña, D. I. S. (2025). Artificial intelligence in mental health care: A systematic review of diagnosis, monitoring, and intervention applications. *Psychological Medicine*, *55*, e18. DOI: 10.1017/S0033291724003295 PMID: 39911020

Cruz, S., Redding, A., Chau, C. W., Lu, C., Persche, J., Hester, J., & Jacobs, M. (2023, April). EquityWare: Co-designing wearables with and for low income communities in the US. In *Proceedings of the 2023 CHI Conference on Human Factors in Computing Systems* (pp. 1-18). DOI: 10.1145/3544548.3580980

Cushnan, J., McCafferty, P., & Best, P. (2024). Clinicians' perspectives of immersive tools in clinical mental health settings: A systematic scoping review. *BMC Health Services Research*, *24*(1), 1091. DOI: 10.1186/s12913-024-11481-3 PMID: 39294727

De Kock, J. H., Latham, H. A., Leslie, S. J., Grindle, M., Munoz, S. A., Ellis, L., Polson, R., & O'Malley, C. M. (2021). A rapid review of the impact of COVID-19 on the mental health of healthcare workers: Implications for supporting psychological well-being. *BMC Public Health*, *21*(1), 104. DOI: 10.1186/s12889-020-10070-3 PMID: 33422039

Dehbozorgi, R., Zangeneh, S., Khooshab, E., Nia, D. H., Hanif, H. R., Samian, P., Yousefi, M., Hashemi, F. H., Vakili, M., Jamalimoghadam, N., & Lohrasebi, F. (2025). The application of artificial intelligence in the field of mental health: A systematic review. *BMC Psychiatry*, *25*(1), 132. DOI: 10.1186/s12888-025-06483-2 PMID: 39953464

Dewa, Z. (2025). The relationship between biometric technology and privacy: A systematic review. *SAI Conference Proceedings.*

Dima, E. (2025). The impact of burnout in healthcare professionals on patient care quality: A review. *World Journal of Advanced Research and Reviews*, *25*(02), 2706–2710. DOI: 10.30574/wjarr.2025.25.2.0633

El Khoury-Malhame, M., Sawma, T., Hallit, S., Younis, C. J., Jaber, J., & Doumit, R. (2025). Cultural stigma, psychological distress and help-seeking: Moderating role of self-esteem and self-stigma in Lebanon. *PLoS One*, *20*(9), e0315063. DOI: 10.1371/journal.pone.0315063 PMID: 40997115

Elfouly, T., & Alouani, A. (2025). A comprehensive survey on wearable computing for mental and physical health monitoring. *Electronics (Basel)*, *14*(17), 3443. DOI: 10.3390/electronics14173443

Ellis, D. M., Draheim, A. A., & Anderson, P. L. (2022). Culturally adapted digital mental health interventions for ethnic/racial minorities: A systematic review and meta-analysis. *Journal of Consulting and Clinical Psychology*, *90*(10), 717–733. DOI: 10.1037/ccp0000759 PMID: 36227330

Engel, G. L. (1977). The need for a new medical model: A challenge for biomedicine. *Science*, *196*(4286), 129–136. DOI: 10.1126/science.847460 PMID: 847460

Fanarioti, A. K., & Karpouzis, K. (2025). Artificial Intelligence and the Future of Mental Health in a Digitally Transformed World. *Computers*, *14*(7), 259. DOI: 10.3390/computers14070259

Ferrara, E. (2024). Large language models for wearable sensor-based human activity recognition, health monitoring, and behavioral modeling: A survey of early trends, datasets, and challenges. *Sensors (Basel)*, *24*(15), 5045. DOI: 10.3390/s24155045 PMID: 39124092

Ferrar, J., Griffith, G. J., Skirrow, C., Cashdollar, N., Taptiklis, N., Dobson, J., Cree, F., Cormack, F. K., Barnett, J. H., & Munafò, M. R. (2021). Developing digital tools for remote clinical research: How to evaluate the validity and practicality of active assessments in field settings. *Journal of Medical Internet Research*, *23*(6), e26004. DOI: 10.2196/26004 PMID: 34142972

Fischer, L., Mann, P. A., Nguyen, M. H. H., Becker, S., Khodadadi, S., Schulz, A., Edwin Thanarajah, S., Repple, J., Hahn, T., Reif, A., Salamikhanshan, A., Kittel-Schneider, S., Rief, W., Mulert, C., Hofmann, S. G., Dannlowski, U., Kircher, T., Bernhard, F. P., & Jamalabadi, H. (2025). AI for mental health: Clinician expectations and priorities in computational psychiatry. *BMC Psychiatry*, *25*(1), 584. DOI: 10.1186/s12888-025-06957-3 PMID: 40481455

Fleming, L. E., Maycock, B., White, M. P., & Depledge, M. H. (2019). Fostering human health through ocean sustainability in the 21st century. *People and Nature*, *1*(3), 276–283. DOI: 10.1002/pan3.10038

Flores-Castañeda, R. O., Olaya-Cotera, S., & Iparraguirre-Villanueva, O. (2025). Exploring wearable technologies for health monitoring: A systematic review of applications, advantages and disadvantages. *Neural Computing & Applications*, *37*(33), 27957–27983. DOI: 10.1007/s00521-025-11605-8

Freeman, D., Reeve, S., Robinson, A., Ehlers, A., Clark, D., Spanlang, B., & Slater, M. (2017). Virtual reality in the assessment, understanding, and treatment of mental health disorders. *Psychological Medicine*, *47*(14), 2393–2400. DOI: 10.1017/S003329171700040X PMID: 28325167

Freyer, N., Groß, D., & Lipprandt, M. (2024). The ethical requirement of explainability for AI-DSS in healthcare: A systematic review of reasons. *BMC Medical Ethics*, *25*(1), 104. DOI: 10.1186/s12910-024-01103-2 PMID: 39354512

Friend, S. H., Ginsburg, G. S., Picard, R. W., & Drazen, J. M. (2024). Key issues as wearable digital health technologies enter clinical care. *The New England Journal of Medicine*, *390*(12), 1118–1127. DOI: 10.1056/NEJMra2307160 PMID: 38507754

Funda, V. (2025). A systematic review of algorithm auditing processes to assess bias and risks in AI systems. Journal of Infrastructure. *Policy and Development*, *9*(2), 11489.

GAO (2022). Mental health care: Access challenges for covered consumers and relevant federal efforts.

GDPR Advisor (2025). GDPR compliance for mental health apps: Safeguarding sensitive data.

Ghadi, Y. Y., Shah, S. F. A., Waheed, W., Mazhar, T., Ahmad, W., Saeed, M. M., & Hamam, H. (2025). Integration of wearable technology and artificial intelligence in digital health for remote patient care. *Journal of Cloud Computing (Heidelberg, Germany)*, *14*(1), 39. DOI: 10.1186/s13677-025-00759-4

Ghanim, R., Kaushik, A., Park, J., & Abramson, A. (2023). Communication protocols integrating wearables, ingestibles, and implantables for closed-loop therapies. *Device*, *1*(3), 100092. DOI: 10.1016/j.device.2023.100092

Gilbert, P., & Van Gordon, W. (2023). Compassion as a skill: A comparison of contemplative and evolution-based approaches. *Mindfulness*, *14*(10), 2395–2416. DOI: 10.1007/s12671-023-02173-w

Gkintoni, E., Vassilopoulos, S. P., & Nikolaou, G. (2025). Next-generation cognitive-behavioral therapy for depression: Integrating digital tools, teletherapy, and personalization for enhanced mental health outcomes. *Medicina (Kaunas, Lithuania)*, *61*(3), 431. DOI: 10.3390/medicina61030431 PMID: 40142242

Glass, J. E., Tiffany, B., Matson, T. E., Lim, C., Gundersen, G., Kimbel, K., Hartzler, A. L., Curran, G. M., McWethy, A. G., Caldeiro, R. M., & Bradley, K. A. (2022). Approaches for implementing digital interventions for alcohol use disorders in primary care: A qualitative, user-centered design study. *Implementation Research and Practice*, *3*, 26334895221135264. DOI: 10.1177/26334895221135264 PMID: 37091101

Godfrey, A., Vandendriessche, B., Bakker, J. P., Fitzer-Attas, C., Gujar, N., Hobbs, M., Liu, Q., Northcott, C. A., Parks, V., Wood, W. A., Zipunnikov, V., Wagner, J. A., & Izmailova, E. S. (2021). Fit-for-purpose biometric monitoring technologies: Leveraging the laboratory biomarker experience. *Clinical and Translational Science*, *14*(1), 62–74. DOI: 10.1111/cts.12865 PMID: 32770726

Goktas, P., & Grzybowski, A. (2025). Shaping the future of healthcare: Ethical clinical challenges and pathways to trustworthy AI. *Journal of Clinical Medicine*, *14*(5), 1605. DOI: 10.3390/jcm14051605 PMID: 40095575

Hall, C. L., Gómez Bergin, A. D., & Rennick-Egglestone, S. (2024). Research into digital health intervention for mental health: 25-year retrospective on the ethical and legal challenges. *Journal of Medical Internet Research*, *26*, e58939. DOI: 10.2196/58939 PMID: 39250796

Hassan Almansour, H. A., Almanajam, F. A., Alyami, M. A., Shawil Al-Mahamad, A. H., Saleh Al Zabid, N. H., Hamad Al-Mahamad, M. S., Yahya Al Hammam, H. N., Al Matif, M. Y., Almansour, M. A., & Mohammed Almansour, A. H (2024). Evaluating the Impact of Wearable Health Devices on Mental Health Outcomes: A Collaborative Study between Psychologists, Social Workers, and Nursing Staff. Journal of International Crisis & Risk Communication Research (JICRCR), 7.

Henderson, J. T., & Bekhuis, T. (2023). *Historical concepts of mental illness*. EBSCO Research Starters.

Hickey, B. A., Chalmers, T., Newton, P., Lin, C.-T., Sibbritt, D., McLachlan, C. S., Clifton-Bligh, R., Morley, J., & Lal, S. (2021). Smart devices and wearable technologies to detect and monitor mental health conditions and stress: A systematic review. *Sensors (Basel)*, *21*(10), 3461. DOI: 10.3390/s21103461 PMID: 34065620

Hiland, E. B. (2021). *Therapy tech: The digital transformation of mental healthcare*. U of Minnesota Press. DOI: 10.5749/j.ctv1xp9q3t

Hilty, D. M., Armstrong, C. M., Luxton, D. D., Gentry, M. T., & Krupinski, E. A. (2021). A scoping review of sensors, wearables, and remote monitoring for behavioral health: Uses, outcomes, clinical competencies, and research directions. *Journal of Technology in Behavioral Science*, *6*(2), 278–313. DOI: 10.1007/s41347-021-00199-2 PMID: 33501372

Holly, L., Thom, S., Elzemety, M., Murage, B., Mathieson, K., & Iñigo Petralanda, M. I. (2023). Strengthening health data governance: New equity and rights-based principles. *International Journal of Health Governance*, *28*(3), 225–237. DOI: 10.1108/IJHG-11-2022-0104

Huang, J., Wang, H., Wu, Q., Yin, J., Zhou, H., & He, Y. (2024). Clinical research on neurological and psychiatric diagnosis and monitoring using wearable devices: A literature review. *Interdisciplinary Medicine*, *2*(4), e20230037. DOI: 10.1002/INMD.20230037

Hughes, N., & Kalra, D. (2023). Data standards and platform interoperability. In *Real-World Evidence in Medical Product Development* (pp. 79–107). Springer. DOI: 10.1007/978-3-031-26328-6_6

Humayun, A., Madawana, A. M., Hassan, A., Mahmud, A., Kamaruddin, N., Noor, S. H., Noor, S. H., & Awang Nawi, M. A. (2025). Artificial intelligence as a predictive tool for mental health status: Insights from a systematic review and meta-analysis. *PLoS One*, *20*(9), e0332207. DOI: 10.1371/journal.pone.0332207 PMID: 41004515

Ienca, M., Fabrice, J., Elger, B., Caon, M., Scoccia Pappagallo, A., Kressig, R. W., & Wangmo, T. (2017). Intelligent assistive technology for Alzheimer's disease and other dementias: A systematic review. *Journal of Alzheimer's Disease*, *56*(4), 1301–1340. DOI: 10.3233/JAD-161037 PMID: 28222516

Ikwuanusi, U. F., Adepoju, P. A., & Odionu, C. S (2023). Advancing ethical AI practices to solve data privacy issues in library systems. International journal of multidisciplinary research updates, 6(1), 033-044.

Immanuel, S., Teferra, M. N., Baumert, M., & Bidargaddi, N. (2023). Heart rate variability for evaluating psychological stress changes in healthy adults: A scoping review. *Neuropsychobiology*, *82*(4), 187–202. DOI: 10.1159/000530376 PMID: 37290411

Inkster, B., Knibbs, C., & Bada, M. (2023). Cybersecurity: A critical priority for digital mental health. *Frontiers in Digital Health*, *5*, 1242264. DOI: 10.3389/fdgth.2023.1242264 PMID: 37781452

Islam, R., & Bae, S. W. (2024). Revolutionizing mental health support: An innovative affective mobile framework for dynamic, proactive, and context-adaptive conversational agents. arXiv preprint arXiv:2406.15942.

Iwaya, L. H., Babar, M. A., Rashid, A., & Wijayarathna, C. (2023). On the privacy of mental health apps: An empirical investigation and its implications for app development. *Empirical Software Engineering*, *28*(1), 2. DOI: 10.1007/s10664-022-10236-0 PMID: 36407814

Jain, A., & Jain, A (2025). AI-Based Emotion Detection System in Healthcare for Patient. Generative Artificial Intelligence for Biomedical and Smart Health Informatics, 455-470.

Jena, N. (2024). Promoting Health Equity in Digital Mental Health: Insights from Medical Anthropology for Global Mental Health. *Journal of Social Research*, *17*(4), 155258.

Jiao, C. (2024). A mental health monitoring system based on intelligent algorithms and biosensors: Algorithm behaviour analysis and intervention strategies. *Molecular & Cellular Biomechanics*, *21*(1), 357–357. DOI: 10.62617/mcb.v21i1.357

Johnson, K. B., Wei, W. Q., Weeraratne, D., Frisse, M. E., Misulis, K., Rhee, K., Zhao, J., & Snowdon, J. L. (2021). Precision medicine, AI, and the future of personalized health care. *Clinical and Translational Science*, *14*(1), 86–93. DOI: 10.1111/cts.12884 PMID: 32961010

Jones, A. (2024). *Ensuring that digital mental health benefits everyone*. APA Services.

Kang, H. S., & Exworthy, M. (2022). Wearing the future—wearables to empower users to take greater responsibility for their health and care: Scoping review. *JMIR mHealth and uHealth*, *10*(7), e35684. DOI: 10.2196/35684 PMID: 35830222

Kargarandehkordi, A., Li, S., Lin, K., Phillips, K. T., Benzo, R. M., & Washington, P. (2025). Fusing wearable biosensors with artificial intelligence for mental health monitoring: A systematic review. *Biosensors (Basel)*, *15*(4), 202. DOI: 10.3390/bios15040202 PMID: 40277515

Kelshiker, A., Cheng, S., Achar, J., Celi, L. A., Jain, D., Nguyen, T., . . . Evans, B. (2025). Bridging the Regulatory Divide: Ensuring Safety and Equity in Wearable Health Technologies. *arXiv preprint arXiv:2508.20031*.

Khoo, Y. X., Kang, R. M., Reynolds, T. L., & Mentis, H. M. (2024). The comprehensiveness of mental health application users' privacy and security concerns. *CHI Conference on Human Factors in Computing Systems*, 16 pages.

Kim, J., & Backonja, U. (2025). Digital health equity frameworks and key concepts: A scoping review. *Journal of the American Medical Informatics Association : JAMIA*, *32*(1), 45–59. DOI: 10.1093/jamia/ocaf017 PMID: 39936843

Kostadimas, D., Kasapakis, V., & Kotis, K. (2025). A systematic review on the combination of VR, IoT and AI technologies, and their integration in applications. *Future Internet*, *17*(4), 163. DOI: 10.3390/fi17040163

Kourtesis, P. (2024). A comprehensive review of multimodal XR applications, risks, and ethical challenges in the metaverse. *Multimodal Technologies and Interaction*, *8*(11), 98. DOI: 10.3390/mti8110098

Kumar, T., Arora, M., Verma, V., Bhushan, S., & Lalar, S. (2024). Biometric System Integration in Public Health: Challenges and Solutions. In Computational Intelligence and Mathematical Applications (pp. 168-173). CRC Press.

Kumar, P. (2025). Securing Digital-First Healthcare: AI, Blockchain, and Cloud Architectures for Personal Health Data Protection. *International Journal of Applied Mathematics*, *38*(7s).

Lacmanovic, S., & Skare, M. (2025). Artificial intelligence bias auditing – current approaches, challenges and lessons from practice. *Review of Accounting and Finance*, *24*(3), 375–400. DOI: 10.1108/RAF-01-2025-0006

Lamb, R., Choi, I., & Owens, T (2025). Convergence of Extended Reality, Artificial Intelligence, Machine Leaning, and Wearable Sensors in the Field of Education. Mental Health Virtual Reality: The Power of Immersive Worlds, 113-128.

Langat, C. A. (2025). Critical analysis of current global trends in mental health: Challenges, innovations, and future directions. *International Journal of Innovative Science and Research Technology*, *10*(1), 2493–2515.

Layode, O., Naiho, H. N. N., Adeleke, G. S., Udeh, E. O., & Labake, T. T. (2024). Data privacy and security challenges in environmental research: Approaches to safeguarding sensitive information. *International Journal of Applied Research in Social Sciences*, *6*(6), 1193–1214. DOI: 10.51594/ijarss.v6i6.1210

Lay, W., Gasparini, L., Siero, W., & Hughes, E. K. (2025). A rapid review of the benefits and challenges of dynamic consent. *Research Ethics*, *21*(1), 180–202. DOI: 10.1177/17470161241278064

Lazarou, E., & Exarchos, T. P. (2024). Predicting stress levels using physiological data: Real-time stress prediction models utilizing wearable devices. *AIMS Neuroscience*, *11*(2), 76–102. DOI: 10.3934/Neuroscience.2024006 PMID: 38988886

Leivaditis, V., & Sepetis, A (2025). Digital Transformation As A Catalyst For Sustainable Health Care Systems: A Narrative Review Of Current Evidence. International Journal of Innovation Management, 29(05n06), 2540009.

Li, M., Patel, J., & Katapally, T. R. (2025). The impact of extended reality cognitive behavioral therapy on mental disorders among children and youth: A systematic review and meta-analysis protocol. *PLoS One*, *20*(3), e0315313. DOI: 10.1371/journal.pone.0315313 PMID: 40048453

Lindner, P., Miloff, A., & Carlbring, P. (2024). The future of virtual reality therapy: Applications, challenges, and research directions. *Frontiers in Virtual Reality*, *5*, 112345.

Liu, M., & Schueller, S. M. (2023). Moving evidence-based mental health interventions into practice: Implementation of digital mental health interventions. *Current Treatment Options in Psychiatry*, *10*(4), 333–345. DOI: 10.1007/s40501-023-00298-2

Livieri, G., Mangina, E., Protopapadakis, E. D., & Panayiotou, A. G. (2025). The gaps and challenges in digital health technology use as perceived by patients: A scoping review and narrative meta-synthesis. *Frontiers in Digital Health, 7*, 1474956. DOI: 10.3389/fdgth.2025.1474956 PMID: 40212901

Löchner, J., Carlbring, P., Schuller, B., Torous, J., & Sander, L. B. (2025). Digital interventions in mental health: An overview and future perspectives. *Internet Interventions : The Application of Information Technology in Mental and Behavioural Health, 40*, 100824. DOI: 10.1016/j.invent.2025.100824 PMID: 40330743

Lorke, M., & Stefanou, T. (2025). Improving research and development of wearable assistive and rehabilitation technologies: A systematic review on diversity factors. *Journal of Neuroengineering and Rehabilitation, 22*(1), 31. DOI: 10.1186/s12984-025-01562-7 PMID: 39985039

Loud, G. (2025). *The promise and policy challenges of digital mental health solutions*. Bipartisan Policy Center.

Lyndon, A (2015). Burnout among health professionals and its effect on patient safety. PSNet Perspectives.

Ma, C.-B., Shang, X., Sun, M., Bo, X., Bai, J., Du, Y., & Zhou, M. (2025). Emerging Multifunctional Wearable Sensors: Integrating Multimodal Sweat Analysis and Advanced Material Technologies for Next-Generation Health Monitoring. *ACS Sensors, 10*(4), 2388–2408. DOI: 10.1021/acssensors.4c03396 PMID: 40162570

Mackey, S., Aghaeepour, N., Gaudilliere, B., Kao, M.-C., Kaptan, M., Lannon, E., Pfyffer, D., & Weber, K. (2025). Innovations in acute and chronic pain biomarkers: Enhancing diagnosis and personalized therapy. *Regional Anesthesia and Pain Medicine, 50*(2), 110–120. DOI: 10.1136/rapm-2024-106030 PMID: 39909549

Mahon, D. (2023). Empirically Supported Treatments: A Brief History. In Evidence Based Counselling & Psychotherapy for the 21st Century Practitioner (pp. 3-14). Emerald Publishing Limited. DOI: 10.1108/978-1-80455-732-720231001

Malgaroli, M., Hull, T. D., Zech, J. M., & Althoff, T. (2023). Natural language processing for mental health interventions: A systematic review and research framework. *Translational Psychiatry, 13*(1), 309. DOI: 10.1038/s41398-023-02592-2 PMID: 37798296

Marriott, B. R., Meyer, A. E., Feagans, A., Batch, B. L., & Adams, Z. W. (2025). Characterizing fidelity monitoring practices in community behavioral health care. *The Journal of Behavioral Health Services & Research*. PMID: 40931317

Martinez-Martin, N., Marcandalli, J., Huang, C. S., Arthur, C. P., Perotti, M., Foglierini, M., Ho, H., Dosey, A. M., Shriver, S., Payandeh, J., Leitner, A., Lanzavecchia, A., Perez, L., & Ciferri, C. (2018). An unbiased screen for human cytomegalovirus identifies neuropilin-2 as a central viral receptor. *Cell, 174*(5), 1158–1171. DOI: 10.1016/j.cell.2018.06.028 PMID: 30057110

Martí-Noguera, J. J. (2025). *Governing Digital Mental Health: Introducing the.* Model and the Digital Behavioral Health Expert. SpringerBriefs in Public Health. DOI: 10.1007/978-3-031-94763-6

Megahed Ibrahim, A., Ramadan Abdel-Aziz, H., Mohamed, H. A. H., Zaghamir, D. E. F., Wahba, N. M. I., Hassan, G. A., & Shaban, M. (2024). Balancing confidentiality and care coordination: Challenges in patient privacy. *BMC Nursing*, *23*(1), 564. Advance online publication. DOI: 10.1186/s12912-024-02231-1 PMID: 39148055

Mescher, T., Hacker, R. L., Martinez, L. A., Morris, C. D., Mishkind, M. C., & Garver-Apgar, C. E. (2025). Mobile health apps: Guidance for evaluation and implementation by healthcare workers. *Journal of Technology in Behavioral Science*, *10*(2), 224–235. DOI: 10.1007/s41347-024-00441-7

Mitsea, E., Drigas, A., & Skianis, C. (2024). Artificial intelligence, immersive technologies, and neurotechnologies in breathing interventions for mental and emotional health: A systematic review. *Electronics (Basel)*, *13*(12), 2253. DOI: 10.3390/electronics13122253

Mohammad, N. (2021). Enhancing security and privacy in multi-cloud environments: A comprehensive study on encryption techniques and access control mechanisms. [IJCET]. *International Journal of Computer Engineering and Technology*, *12*(2), 51–63.

Mohr, D. C., Zhang, M., & Schueller, S. M. (2017). Personal sensing: Understanding mental health using ubiquitous sensors and machine learning. *Annual Review of Clinical Psychology*, *13*(1), 23–47. DOI: 10.1146/annurev-clinpsy-032816-044949 PMID: 28375728

Mone, V., & Fayazullaeva, S. (2023). Health data on the go: Navigating privacy concerns with wearable technologies. *Legal Information Management*, *23*(3), 179–188. DOI: 10.1017/S1472669623000427

Morey, D. A., Rayo, M. F., & Woods, D. D. (2025). Empirically derived evaluation requirements for responsible deployments of AI in safety-critical settings. *NPJ Digital Medicine*, *8*(1), 374. DOI: 10.1038/s41746-025-01784-y PMID: 40533485

Morgan, J. W., Patel, R. A., & Campbell, S. (2025). Practical considerations of clinical XR (Singh & Chandra, 2025) deployments. *Frontiers in Virtual Reality*, *6*, 1517402. DOI: 10.3389/frvir.2025.1517402

Moriarty, A. S., Meader, N., Snell, K. I., Riley, R. D., Paton, L. W., Dawson, S., Hendon, J., Chew-Graham, C. A., Gilbody, S., Churchill, R., Phillips, R. S., Ali, S., & McMillan, D. (2022). Predicting relapse or recurrence of depression: Systematic review of prognostic models. *The British Journal of Psychiatry : The Journal of Mental Science*, *221*(2), 448–458. DOI: 10.1192/bjp.2021.218 PMID: 35048843

Mulukuntla, S. (2025). Monitoring and Remote Patient Management with Immersive Technologies. In Augmented Wellness: Exploring the Power of VR and AR in Healthcare (pp. 197-218). Springer. DOI: 10.1007/978-981-96-2952-7_9

Naderbagi, A., Loblay, V., Zahed, I. U. M., Ekambareshwar, M., Poulsen, A., Song, Y. J., Ospina-Pinillos, L., Krausz, M., Mamdouh Kamel, M., Hickie, I. B., & LaMonica, H. M. (2024). Cultural and contextual adaptation of digital health interventions: Narrative review. *Journal of Medical Internet Research*, *26*, e55130. DOI: 10.2196/55130 PMID: 38980719

NASHP (2025). Key strategies for strengthening the behavioral health workforce.

National Academy of Medicine. (2020). Taking action against clinician burnout: A systems approach to professional well-being.

Nittas, V., Daniore, P., Chavez, S. J., & Wray, T. B. (2023). *Challenges in implementing cultural adaptations of digital health interventions*. Nature Human Behaviour Perspectives.

Ni, Y., & Jia, F. (2025). A scoping review of AI-driven digital interventions in mental health care: Mapping applications across screening, support, monitoring, prevention, and clinical education. *Health Care*, *13*(10), 1205. PMID: 40428041

Obermeyer, Z., Powers, B., Vogeli, C., & Mullainathan, S. (2019). Dissecting racial bias in an algorithm used to manage the health of populations. *Science*, *366*(6464), 447–453. DOI: 10.1126/science.aax2342 PMID: 31649194

Okposio, B. O., Richard, G. A., Olatokun, T. P., Akadiri, O. O., Akpevba, E. A., John, J. O., & Okonkwo, B. A. (2025). Enhancing Mental health Outcomes through AI-Driven Predictive Analytics: A review of applications in neuroscience and substance abuse prevention. *International Journal of Biological and Pharmaceutical Sciences Archive, 10*(2), 024-048.

Omiyefa, S. (2025). Artificial intelligence and machine learning in precision mental health diagnostics and predictive treatment models. *Int J Res Publ Rev*, *6*(3), 85–99. DOI: 10.55248/gengpi.6.0325.1107

Ong, T., Ivanova, J., Soni, H., Barrera, J., Cummins, M., Welch, B. M., & Bunnell, B. E. (2025). Mental health clients' perspectives on telehealth-based virtual reality therapy. *Frontiers in Virtual Reality*, *6*, 1595326. DOI: 10.3389/frvir.2025.1595326

Ostrowski, K., & Goldberg, R. (2022). Designing an effective statewide data sharing agreement. California Health Care Foundation. https://www.chcf.org/wp-content/uploads/2022/03/DataExchangeExplainerDesigningStatewideAgreement.pdf

Pal, D. K. D., Saini, V., & Aakula, A. (2020). API-led integration for improved healthcare interoperability. *vol, 6*, 488-523.

Panarese, P., Grasso, M. M., & Solinas, C. (2025). Algorithmic bias, fairness, and inclusivity: A multilevel framework for justice-oriented AI. *AI & Society*, •••, 1–23. DOI: 10.1007/s00146-025-02451-2

Pedram, S., & Piatkowski, T. (2025). Exploring the potential of virtual reality (Johnson et al., 2021) in mental healthcare: A systematic literature review. *Virtual Reality (Waltham Cross)*, *29*(3), 135. DOI: 10.1007/s10055-025-01181-6

Poudel, U., Jakhar, S., Mohan, P., & Nepal, A. (2025). AI in mental health: A review of technological advancements and ethical issues in psychiatry. *Issues in Mental Health Nursing*, *46*(7), 693–701. DOI: 10.1080/01612840.2025.2502943 PMID: 40378075

Price, A., & Van Heerden, A. (2025). Editorial perspective: Digital technology and the future of mental health treatment. *BMC Digital Health*, *3*(5), 5. DOI: 10.1186/s44247-024-00146-0

Pruden, S (2025). Implementing Depression Screening and Treatment Algorithms to Reduce Post-Operative Complications for Patients Undergoing Cardiac Surgery The University of North Carolina at Chapel Hill].

Radanliev, P. (2025). Privacy, ethics, transparency, and accountability in AI systems for wearable devices. *Frontiers in Digital Health*, *7*, 1431246. DOI: 10.3389/fdgth.2025.1431246 PMID: 40599875

Rajpal, S. (2025). Exploring the Role of Virtual Reality and Metaverse in Treating Mental Health: Operating Models and Challenges in Adoption. *Journal of Computer and Communications*, *13*(10), 1–22. DOI: 10.4236/jcc.2025.1310001

Reddy, K. J. (2025). Integrating Technology into Clinical Practice. In Innovations in Neurocognitive Rehabilitation: Harnessing Technology for Effective Therapy (pp. 329-350). Springer. DOI: 10.1007/978-3-031-88117-6_15

Renuka, O., RadhaKrishnan, N., Priya, B. S., Jhansy, A., & Ezekiel, S (2025). Data privacy and protection: Legal and ethical challenges. Emerging Threats and Countermeasures in Cybersecurity, 433-465.

Ricciardi, F., & Zomaya, A. (2025). Perspectives on Managing AI Ethics in the Digital Age. *Information (Basel), 16*(2), 89. DOI: 10.3390/info16040318

Robinson, A., Flom, M., Forman-Hoffman, V. L., Histon, T., Levy, M., Darcy, A., ... & Montgomery, R. M. (2024). Equity in digital mental health interventions in the United States: Where to next?. *Journal of Medical Internet Research, 26*, e59939. Lamb, R., Choi, I., & Owens, T (2025). Convergence of Extended Reality, Artificial Intelligence, Machine Leaning, and Wearable Sensors in the Field of Education. Mental Health Virtual Reality: The Power of Immersive Worlds, 113-128.

Robinson, A., Flom, M., Forman-Hoffman, V. L., Histon, T., Levy, M., Darcy, A., Ajayi, T., Mohr, D. C., Wicks, P., Greene, C., & Montgomery, R. M. (2024). Equity in digital mental health interventions in the United States: Where to next? *Journal of Medical Internet Research, 26*, e59939. DOI: 10.2196/59939 PMID: 39316436

Ross, G., Zhao, Y., Bosman, A., Geballa-Koukoula, A., Zhou, H., Elliott, C., Nielen, M., Rafferty, K., & Salentijn, G (2022). Data handling and ethics of emerging smartphone-based (Glass et al., 2022) sensors–Part 1: best practices and current implementation.

Sadeh, Y., Denejkina, A., Karyotaki, E., Lenferink, L. I., & Kassam-Adams, N. (2023). Opportunities for improving data sharing and FAIR data practices to advance global mental health. *Cambridge Prisms: Global Mental Health, 10*, e14. PMID: 37860102

Saeidnia, H. R., Fotami, S. G. H., Lund, B., & Ghiasi, N. (2024). Ethical considerations in artificial intelligence interventions for mental health and well-being: Ensuring responsible implementation and impact. *Social Sciences (Basel, Switzerland), 13*(7), 381. DOI: 10.3390/socsci13070381

Saganowski, S., Perz, B., Polak, A. G., & Kazienko, P (2022). Emotion recognition for everyday life using physiological signals from wearables: A systematic literature review. IEEE Transactions on Affective Computing, 14(3), 1876-1897. Pinel, P (1793). Traité médico-philosophique sur l'aliénation mentale.

Saganowski, S., Perz, B., Polak, A. G., & Kazienko, P. (2022). Emotion recognition for everyday life using physiological signals from wearables: A systematic literature review. *IEEE Transactions on Affective Computing*, *14*(3), 1876–1897. DOI: 10.1109/TAFFC.2022.3176135

Saksena, N., Matthan, R., Bhan, A., & Balsari, S. (2021). Rebooting consent in the digital age: A governance framework for health data exchange. *BMJ Global Health*, *6*(Suppl 5), e005057. DOI: 10.1136/bmjgh-2021-005057 PMID: 34301754

Sangraula, M., Chauhan, J., Best, C., McEneaney, C., Shah, C., Brown, A. D., & Kohrt, B. A. (2024). The impact of task-sharing scalable mental health interventions on non-specialist providers: A scoping review. *Global Mental Health (Cambridge, England)*, *11*, e134. DOI: 10.1017/gmh.2024.129 PMID: 39811624

Saxena, S. (2016). Challenges and opportunities in global mental health: A perspective from WHO. *Epidemiology and Psychiatric Sciences*, *25*(6), 495–498. DOI: 10.1017/S2045796016000536 PMID: 27666668

Scholle, S. H (2024). Digital mental health technologies: Gaps and opportunities in current U. S. regulatory authorities. Leavitt Partners Report.

Shah, B., Allen, J. L. Y., Chaudhury, H., O'Shaughnessy, J., & Tyrrell, C. S. (2022). The role of digital health in the future of integrated care. *Clinics in Integrated Care*, *15*, 100131. DOI: 10.1016/j.intcar.2022.100131

Shah, R. V., Grennan, G., Zafar-Khan, M., Alim, F., Dey, S., Ramanathan, D., & Mishra, J. (2021). Personalized machine learning of depressed mood using wearables. *Translational Psychiatry*, *11*(1), 338. DOI: 10.1038/s41398-021-01445-0 PMID: 34103481

Shahsavar, Y., & Choudhury, A. (2025). Effectiveness of evidence-based mental health apps on user health outcomes: A systematic literature review. *PLoS One*, *20*(3), e0319983. DOI: 10.1371/journal.pone.0319983 PMID: 40131942

Sharma, R., & Meena, H. K. (2024). Emerging trends in EEG signal processing: A systematic review. *SN Computer Science*, *5*(4), 415. DOI: 10.1007/s42979-024-02773-w

Shatte, A. B., Hutchinson, D. M., & Teague, S. J. (2019). Machine learning in mental health: A scoping review of methods and applications. *Psychological Medicine*, *49*(9), 1426–1448. DOI: 10.1017/S0033291719000151 PMID: 30744717

Sheikh, M., Qassem, M., & Kyriacou, P. A. (2021). Wearable, environmental, and smartphone-based passive sensing for mental health monitoring. *Frontiers in Digital Health*, *3*, 662811. DOI: 10.3389/fdgth.2021.662811 PMID: 34713137

Shen, S., Qi, W., Zeng, J., Li, S., Liu, X., Zhu, X., Dong, C., Wang, B., Shi, Y., Yao, J., Wang, B., Lou, X., Gu, S., Li, P., Wang, J., Jiang, G., & Cao, S. (2025). Passive Sensing for Mental Health Monitoring Using Machine Learning With Wearables and Smartphones: Scoping Review. *Journal of Medical Internet Research*, *27*, e77066. DOI: 10.2196/77066 PMID: 40811794

Simbo AI (2025). Exploring the impact of clinician burnout on patient safety and satisfaction.

Singh, B., & Chandra, S. (2025). Strengthening Sensors and Wearable Technologies in Gauging Healthcare Transmuting Digital Health Technologies: Human Augmentation via Innovation and Implementations of AI. In Cases on AI Innovations in Occupational Health and Safety (pp. 289-308). IGI Global Scientific Publishing.

Sit, H. F., Ling, R., Lam, A. I. F., Chen, W., Latkin, C. A., & Hall, B. J. (2020). The cultural adaptation of step-by-step: An intervention to address depression among Chinese young adults. *Frontiers in Psychiatry*, *11*, 650. DOI: 10.3389/fpsyt.2020.00650 PMID: 32733296

Smith, K. A., Blease, C., Faurholt-Jepsen, M., Firth, J., Van Daele, T., Moreno, C., Carlbring, P., Ebner-Priemer, U. W., Koutsouleris, N., Riper, H., Mouchabac, S., Torous, J., & Cipriani, A. (2023). Digital mental health: Challenges and next steps. *BMJ Mental Health*, *26*(1), e300670. DOI: 10.1136/bmjment-2023-300670 PMID: 37197797

Smuck, M., Odonkor, C. A., Wilt, J. K., Schmidt, N., & Swiernik, M. A. (2021). The emerging clinical role of wearables: Factors for successful implementation in healthcare. *NPJ Digital Medicine*, *4*(1), 45. DOI: 10.1038/s41746-021-00418-3 PMID: 33692479

Souther, R., & Boughton, J. (2025). *The evolution of mental health services and modern therapies*. Mental Health Center of San Diego.

Spahl, W., & Rubeis, G. (2025). Integrating ethics in digital mental healthcare technologies: A principle-based empirically grounded roadmap approach. *Medicine, Health Care, and Philosophy*, *28*(3), 411–424. DOI: 10.1007/s11019-025-10283-6 PMID: 40736629

Spuskanyuk, A. (2024). Ethical implications of wearable digital health technology: Balancing innovation and patient autonomy. *American Journal of Health Care Studies*, *1*(2), 46–57. DOI: 10.61449/ajhcs.2024.7

Spytska, L. (2025). The use of artificial intelligence in psychotherapy: Development of intelligent therapeutic systems. *BMC Psychology*, *13*(1), 175. DOI: 10.1186/s40359-025-02491-9 PMID: 40022267

Stanford Law School. (2025). Digital diagnosis: Health data privacy in the U. S.

Stirman, S. W. (2022). Implementing evidence-based mental-health treatments: Attending to training, fidelity, adaptation, and context. *Current Directions in Psychological Science*, *31*(5), 436–442. DOI: 10.1177/09637214221109601

Subu, M. A., Holmes, D., Arumugam, A., Al-Yateem, N., Maria Dias, J., Rahman, S. A., Waluyo, I., Ahmed, F. R., & Abraham, M. S. (2022). Traditional, religious, and cultural perspectives on mental illness: A qualitative study on causal beliefs and treatment use. *International Journal of Qualitative Studies on Health and Well-being*, *17*(1), 2123090. DOI: 10.1080/17482631.2022.2123090 PMID: 36097886

Sun, J., Lu, T., Shao, X., Han, Y., Xia, Y., Zheng, Y., Wang, Y., Li, X., Ravindran, A., Fan, L., Fang, Y., Zhang, X., Ravindran, N., Wang, Y., Liu, X., & Lu, L. (2025). Practical AI application in psychiatry: Historical review and future directions. *Molecular Psychiatry*, *30*(9), 4399–4408. DOI: 10.1038/s41380-025-03072-3 PMID: 40456953

Surani, A., Bawaked, A., Wheeler, M., Kelsey, B., Roberts, N., Vincent, D., & Das, S. (2023, July). Security and privacy of digital mental health: An analysis of web services and mobile applications. In *IFIP annual conference on data and applications security and privacy* (pp. 319-338). Cham: Springer Nature Switzerland.

Tabassum, A., Ghaznavi, I., Abd-Alrazaq, A., & Qadir, J. (2025). Exploring the application of AI and extended reality technologies in metaverse-driven mental health solutions: Scoping review. *Journal of Medical Internet Research*, *27*, e72400. DOI: 10.2196/72400 PMID: 40829151

Tavory, T. (2024). Regulating AI in mental health: Ethics of care perspective. *JMIR Mental Health*, *11*, e58493. DOI: 10.2196/58493 PMID: 39298759

Tizzard, C. L. (2025). Re-imagining Care for Aging Disabled Adults.

Tsai, Y. Y., Chen, Y. J., Lin, Y. F., Hsiao, F. C., Hsu, C. H., & Liao, L. D. (2025). Photoplethysmography-based HRV analysis and machine learning for real-time stress quantification in mental health applications. *APL Bioengineering*, *9*(2), 026103. DOI: 10.1063/5.0256590 PMID: 40191605

Vaidyam, A. N., Wisniewski, H., Halamka, J. D., Kashavan, M. S., & Torous, J. B. (2019). Chatbots and conversational agents in mental health: A review of the psychiatric landscape. *Canadian Journal of Psychiatry. Revue Canadienne de Psychiatrie*, *64*(7), 456–464. DOI: 10.1177/0706743719828977 PMID: 30897957

van Genugten, C. R., Thong, M. S., Van Ballegooijen, W., Kleiboer, A. M., Spruijt-Metz, D., Smit, A. C., Sprangers, M. A. G., Terhorst, Y., & Riper, H. (2025). Beyond the current state of just-in-time adaptive interventions in mental health: A qualitative systematic review. *Frontiers in Digital Health*, *7*, 1460167. DOI: 10.3389/fdgth.2025.1460167 PMID: 39935463

Verma, H., Mlynar, J., Schaer, R., Reichenbach, J., Jreige, M., Prior, J., Evéquoz, F., & Depeursinge, A. (2023). Rethinking the role of AI with physicians in oncology: revealing perspectives from clinical and research workflows. *Proceedings of the 2023 CHI conference on human factors in computing systems* DOI: 10.1145/3544548.3581506

Volckens, J., Haynes, E. N., Croisant, S. P., Cui, Y., Errett, N. A., Henry, H. F., Horney, J. A., Kwok, R. K., Magzamen, S., Rappold, A. G., Ravichandran, L., Reinlib, L., Ryan, P. H., & Shaughnessy, D. T. (2023). Health research in the wake of disasters: Challenges and opportunities for sensor science. *Environmental Health Perspectives*, *131*(6), 065002. DOI: 10.1289/EHP12270 PMID: 37389972

Walter, J. R., Xu, S., & Rogers, J. A. (2023). From lab to life: How wearable devices can improve health equity. *Nature Communications*, *14*, 44634. PMID: 38167483

Wang, Z., Xiong, H., Zhang, J., Yang, S., Boukhechba, M., Zhang, D., Barnes, L. E., & Dou, D. (2022). From personalized medicine to population health: A survey of mHealth sensing techniques. *IEEE Internet of Things Journal*, *9*(17), 15413–15434. DOI: 10.1109/JIOT.2022.3161046

Watson, D (2025). The dark side of mental health apps: Privacy concerns and therapeutic limitations. MentalHealthSigns.com.

Weiner, E. B., Dankwa-Mullan, I., Nelson, W. A., & Hassanpour, S. (2025). Ethical challenges and evolving strategies in the integration of artificial intelligence into clinical practice. *PLOS Digital Health*, *4*(4), e0000810. DOI: 10.1371/journal.pdig.0000810 PMID: 40198594

Wibberly, K. H. (2024). Preparing mental health providers for the future: The case for moving beyond the elective telehealth course to integrating telehealth training throughout the curriculum. *Frontiers in Psychology*, *14*, 1301569. DOI: 10.3389/fpsyg.2023.1301569 PMID: 38235285

World Economic Forum. (2022). Global Governance Toolkit for Digital Mental Health. WEF.

Wykes, T., Lipshitz, J., & Schueller, S. M. (2019). Towards the design of ethical standards related to digital mental health and all its applications. *Current Treatment Options in Psychiatry*, *6*(3), 232–242. DOI: 10.1007/s40501-019-00180-0

Xing, Y., Yang, Y., Yang, K., Lu, A., Xing, L., Mackie, K., & Guo, F. (2025). Intelligent sensing devices and systems for personalized mental health. *Med-X*, *3*(1), 10. DOI: 10.1007/s44258-025-00057-3 PMID: 40837134

Yhang, F. (2023). Safeguarding biometric data: Privacy, security and ethical considerations. *Journal of Biometrics & Biostatistics*, *14*(2).

Zenker, S., Strech, D., Ihrig, K., Jahns, R., Müller, G., Schickhardt, C., Schmidt, G., Speer, R., Winkler, E., von Kielmansegg, S. G., & Drepper, J. (2022). Data protection-compliant broad consent for secondary use of health care data and human biosamples for (Mulukuntla, 2025) medical research: Towards a new German national standard. *Journal of Biomedical Informatics*, *131*, 104096. DOI: 10.1016/j.jbi.2022.104096 PMID: 35643273

About the Author

Richard Lamb, Ph.D. is a faculty member in both the Department of Physiology and Pharmacology and the Department of Clinical and Administrative Pharmacy at the University of Georgia, where he holds appointments in the College of Pharmacy and the College of Veterinary Medicine. He currently serves as the Director of the Neurocognition Science Laboratory. Dr. Lamb earned his Ph.D. in Science Education and Measurement from the College of Education and Human Development at George Mason University in 2013. His interdisciplinary research integrates psychophysiological measurement, artificial intelligence, and emerging technologies—including virtual and synthetic environments—to support clinical mental health treatment, assess mental status, and explore socioemotional health across pediatric, adult, and geriatric populations. A second focus of his work involves identifying cognitive and physiological markers for mental health treatment to enhance the efficacy and efficiency related to information processing, decision-making, and cognition in high-stress environments. His work also seeks to leverage advanced technologies such as machine learning and artificial intelligence, aiming to shape the biopsychosocial dimensions of learning and mental health, promoting wellbeing across the lifespan. He has received recognition for his research from organizations such as the Association for Child and Adolescent Mental Health and the Foundation for Health Leadership & Innovation and has been featured in various media outlets.

Index

A

B

C

D

E

F

G

H

I

M

N

O

P

R

S

T

W

www.ingramcontent.com/pod-product-compliance
Lightning Source LLC
LaVergne TN
LVHW081316300926
849161LV00008B/1781